Handbuch der experimentellen Pharmakologie

Vol. 46 Heffter-Heubner New Series

Handbook of Experimental Pharmacology

Fibrinolytics and Antifibrinolytics

Contributors

B. Blombäck · P. C. Comp · P. D. Desnoyers · F. Duckert
U. Hedner · K. N. Kaulla von · H. P. Klöcking · M. Kopeć
H. Landmann · Z. B. Latallo · F. Markwardt · I. M. Nilsson
M. Pandolfi · K. C. Robbins · W. H. E. Roschlau
K. Stocker · F. B. Taylor · G. Vogel

Editor
Fritz Markwardt

With 164 Figures

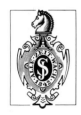

Springer-Verlag Berlin Heidelberg New York 1978

Prof. Dr. Dr. F. MARKWARDT,
Institut für Pharmakologie und Toxikologie, Medizinische Akademie Erfurt
Nordhäuser Straße 74, Erfurt, German Democratic Republic

ISBN 3-540-08608-0 Springer-Verlag Berlin Heidelberg New York
ISBN 0-387-08608-0 Springer-Verlag New York Heidelberg Berlin

Library of Congress Cataloging in Publication Data. Main entry under title: Fibrinolytics and antifibrinolytics. (Handbook of experimental pharmacology: New series; v. 46). Includes bibliographies and index. 1. Fibrinolytic agents. 2. Antifibrinolytic agents. I. Blombäck, Birger. II. Markwardt, Fritz. III. Series: Handbuch der experimentellen Pharmakologie: New series; v. 46. QP905.H3 vol. 46 [RM340] 615'.1'08s [615'.718] 78-9492.

Typesetting, printing, and binding: Brühlsche Universitätsdruckerei, Lahn-Gießen
2122/3130-543210

Preface

Disturbances of haemostasis and thromboembolic disorders still constitute a great problem in clinical practice. Increasing insight into the mechanism of blood coagulation has led to more effective therapy and prophylaxis. Particularly, the understanding of the biochemistry of fibrinolysis has provided possibilities for the pharmacological interference of these processes, which has resulted in effective haemostatic agents and useful antithrombotic ones.

The development of antifibrinolytics for interfering with pathological fibrinolytic processes is nearly complete and has led to the development of drugs essential to the therapy of hyperfibrinolytic bleeding. The search for fibrinolytics for dissolving intravascular thrombi has led to highly effective compounds. This development is still under way and promising results are hoped.

Spontaneous dissolution of blood clots is a phenomenon which was described a century ago. First investigations of this process assured that there is in the organism a system capable of removing the fibrin which is formed during blood coagulation after it has fulfilled its physiological function. This fibrinolytic system is specifically adapted to the degradation of insoluble fibrin into soluble degradation products. In the past 30 years, thorough investigation of this system has clarified the fibrinolytic process, its physiological role and its meaning as a pathogenetic principle. A good knowledge of these processes is required for an understanding of the effects and side effects of fibrinolytics and antifibrinolytics, which comprise the basis of methods for the detection of fibrinolytic processes in the organism and of the control of therapy with these drugs.

In the section "Activators of Fibrinolysis", therapeutically used preparations such as streptokinase and urokinase, are described. Synthetic, indirectly acting fibrinolytic agents, providing new approaches to antithrombotic therapy are also discussed. The section "Fibrinolytically Active Enzymes" covers fungal proteases, though these are not specifically adapted to the hydrolysis of fibrin, and the special enzymes from snake venoms that lead to therapeutic defibrination.

Although antifibrinolytic therapy uses predominantly synthetic antifibrinolytics, the section "Antifibrinolytics" discusses also the naturally occurring, mainly polyvalent inhibitors of the fibrinolytic system. In spite of their limited use as antifibrinolytics, these inhibitors are an interesting object of research.

The aim of this book is to provide more information about fibrinolytics and antifibrinolytics and to make not only specialist research workers but also clinicians involved in the study and medicamentous therapy of thrombosis and bleeding disorders more familiar with these classes of drugs.

Erfurt, May 1978   F. MARKWARDT

Table of Contents

The Fibrinolytic Process

Biochemistry of the Factors of the Fibrinolytic System. H. LANDMANN.
With 3 Figures

Fibrinogen and Fibrin Degradation Products. Maria Kopeć and Z. S. Latallo.
With 2 Figures

The Measurement of Fibrinolytic Activities. INGA MARIE NILSSON, ULLA HEDNER and M. PANDOLFI. With 7 Figures

Activators of Fibrinolysis

Biochemistry of Streptokinase. F. B. TAYLOR and P. C. COMP. With 2 Figures

* Erratum: For citrate buffer pH 3.0 on line 7, page 145; read: bicarbonate buffer pH 10.7.

Urokinase. F. DUCKERT

Synthetic Fibrinolytic Agents. Induction of Fibrinolytic Activity In Vitro.
K. N. von Kaulla. With 16 Figures

Indirect Fibrinolytic Agents. P. C. Desnoyers

Fibrinolytically Active Enzymes

Plasmin. K. C. ROBBINS

Fungal Proteases. W. H. E. ROSCHLAU. With 84 Figures

Defibrinogenation with Thrombin-like Snake Venom Enzymes. K. STOCKER

Antifibrinolytics

Naturally Occurring Inhibitors of Fibrinolysis. F. MARKWARDT. With 6 Figures

Synthetic Inhibitors of Fibrinolysis. F. MARKWARDT. With 18 Figures

List of Contributors

B. BLOMBÄCK, Professor Dr., Karolinska Institutet, Department of Blood Coagulation Research, S-10401 Stockholm, Sweden

P.C.COMP, Ph. D., Assistant Professor of Medicine, University of Oklahoma Health Sciences Center, Department of Medicine, P.O.Box 26901, Oklahoma City, Oklahoma 73190

P.C.DESNOYERS, Dr., Institut de Recherches Servier, 14, Rue du Val d'Or, F-92150 Suresnes

F.DUCKERT, Professor Dr., Gerinnungs- und Fibrinolyse-Laboratorium, Kantonspital, CH-4031 Basel

U.HEDNER, Dr., Associate Professor, Koagulationslaboratoriet, Allmänna Sjukhuset, S-21401 Malmö

K.N.v.KAULLA, Professor Dr., Stechertweg 2, D-7800 Freiburg

H.-P. KLÖCKING, Dr. Dr., Medizinische Akademie Erfurt, Institut für Pharmakologie und Toxikologie, Nordhäuser Str. 74, GDR-506 Erfurt

MARIA KOPEĆ, Professor Dr., Department of Radiobiology and Health Protection, Institute of Nuclear Research, Ulica Dorodna 16, PL-03-195 Warszawa 91

H.LANDMANN, Dr., VEB Arzneimittelwerk Dresden, Wilhelm-Pieck-Straße 35, GDR-8122 Radebeul

Z.S.LATALLO, Dozent Dr., Department of Radiobiology and Health Protection, Institute of Nuclear Research, Ulica Dorodna 16, PL-03-195 Warszawa 91

F. MARKWARDT, Professor Dr. Dr., Institut für Pharmakologie und Toxikologie, Medizinische Akademie Erfurt, Nordhäuser Str. 74, GDR-506 Erfurt

INGA M. NILSSON, Professor Dr., Koagulationslaboratoriet, Allmänna Sjukhuset, S-214 01 Malmö

M.PANDOLFI, Dr., Associate Professor, Koagulationslaboratoriet, Allmänna Sjukhuset, S-21401 Malmö

K.C.ROBBINS, Professor, Michael Reese Research Foundation, 530 East, 31st Street, Chicago, Ill 60616, USA

W.H.E.ROSCHLAU, Professor Dr., University of Toronto, Department of Pharmacology, Medical Sciences Building, Toronto 5, Ontario, Canada M5S 1A8

K.STOCKER, Dr., Pentapharm A.G., Engelgasse 109, CH-4002 Basel

F.B.TAYLOR, Jr., Dr., Professor of Pathology, Department of Pathology, University of Oklahoma, Health Sciences Center, P.O. Box 26901, Oklahoma City, OK 73190, USA

G.VOGEL, Dr. sc. med., Leiter der Hämostaselogischen Abteilung der medizinischen Klinik der Med. Akademie Erfurt, Nordhäuser Str. 74, GDR-506 Erfurt

The Fibrinolytic Process

Biochemistry of the Factors of the Fibrinolytic System

H. LANDMANN

Introduction

The ability of the organism to liquefy deposited fibrin is a phenomenon that has been known for more than a century (DENIS, 1838; DASTRE, 1893). Early investigations on this process led to the conclusion that the organism possesses a special system, the function of which is the removal of the end product of blood coagulation, fibrin, after having fulfilled its physiologic function (DENYS and DE MARBAIX, 1889; DELEZENNE and POZERSKI, 1903; NOLF, 1908; SCHMITZ, 1937). This fibrinolytic system which is specifically adapted to the fragmentation of the insoluble fibrin into soluble split products has been investigated very intensively in the past 30 years. In these studies, its underlying biochemic mechanism, physiologic role, and significance as a pathogenetic principle in certain hemorrhagic disorders became much clearer. This review summarizes some important data of the biochemistry of the factors of the fibrinolytic system and of the mechanisms of their interaction and cooperative action, in order to provide a basis for the understanding of the effects of fibrinolytic and antifibrinolytic therapeutic agents. Detailed descriptions of the fibrinolytic process and its biochemistry were also given by other authors (ASTRUP, 1956, 1959, 1967; SHERRY et al., 1959; ABLONDI and HAGAN, 1960; MACFARLANE, 1964; FEARNLEY, 1965; SHERRY, 1965, 1968; SCHWICK, 1967; KONTTINEN, 1968; ROBBINS and SUMMARIA, 1970, 1971; BANG, 1971; MARDER and SHERRY, 1972; ASTRUP and THORSEN, 1972). Very recently the biochemistry of plasminogen and of its activation process was extensively reviewed by RICKLI (1975), COLLEN and DE MAYER (1975) and COLLEN and VERSTRAETE (1975).

The coagulation of blood and the redissolution of the clots are mediated by sequences of specific proteolytic reactions. Both processes are not only connected with each other causally, since fibrin is the substrate of fibrinolysis, but also show a number of remarkable similarities (Fig. 1). They become activated only under certain circumstances and are maintained by specific enzyme systems. These enzymes are not normally present in blood in an active form, but they can be formed rapidly by specific activators and abolished by inhibitors after accomplishing their physiologic effects. The complex cooperative action of activators and inhibitors is the basis of the physiologic functioning of the coagulation and fibrinolytic system.

The coagulation of blood is the result of the conversion of the soluble blood plasma protein, fibrinogen, into the insoluble protein aggregate, fibrin. This conversion is triggered by the clotting enzyme, thrombin, which is formed from its inactive precursor prothrombin by the action of specific activator enzymes. Thrombin splits off four small peptides from the fibrinogen molecule. By this process reactive groups

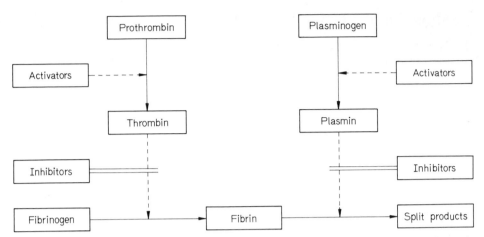

Figure 1. Scheme of blood coagulation and fibrinolysis. - - -→: action on; ——→: transformation into

become unmasked in the molecules of the formed fibrin monomers which enable them to aggregate and to form in this way an insoluble precipitate, fibrin. In this type of fibrin the monomer units are held together predominantly by hydrogen bonds. It can be desaggregated and resolubilized by hydrogen bond-breaking agents. Under physiologic conditions a blood plasma transpeptidase (clotting factor XIII) stabilizes the aggregate by the insertion of covalent peptide bonds. Therefore, fibrin formed from blood plasma is insoluble in hydrogen bond-breaking media.

The process of fibrinolysis represents the counterpart of the blood-clotting mechanism. Blood coagulation produces, and fibrinolysis destroys fibrin. Generally no fibrinolytic activity is present in the circulating blood. The proteolytic enzyme plasmin, catalyzing the degradation of fibrin, is found in blood plasma in the form of its inactive precursor, plasminogen. It is activated by specific activators under certain physiologic or pathologic circumstances.

A. Factors of the Fibrinolytic System

I. Plasminogen — Plasmin

1. Plasminogen

Plasminogen (profibrinolysin) is a plasma protein with the properties of a globulin (MILSTONE, 1941). It is an essential component of Cohn-plasma fraction III-3. It is precipitated from diluted plasma at pH 5.3 together with fibrinogen and other "euglobulins." Utilizing its high acid stability (CHRISTENSEN and SMITH, 1950) the proenzyme was prepared in a crystalline state by KLINE (1953). Highly purified plasminogen preparations were obtained from Cohn-fraction III by similar procedures (HAGAN et al., 1960; KLINE and FISHMAN, 1961a; ROBBINS and SUMMARIA, 1963). Acid treatment causes a slight denaturation of the protein, so that these plasminogen preparations are only poorly soluble at neutral pH (SLOTTA et al., 1962; SLOTTA and GONZALES, 1964).

Soluble preparations were obtained by extraction of plasminogen-containing plasma fractions with solutions of the amino acids lysine or ε-aminocaproic acid (WALLÉN and BERGSTRÖM, 1960; DERECHIN, 1962; DERECHIN et al., 1962; WALLÉN, 1962a, 1962b; ROBBINS and SUMMARIA, 1963). These amino acids specifically promote the solubility of plasminogen, so that it can be easily extracted relatively free of impurities (WALLÉN and BERGSTRÖM, 1959). Highly purified human plasminogen was obtained from those extracts by the use of chromatographic procedures mainly by two groups of workers: that of ROBBINS and SUMMARIA in the United States, and that of WALLÉN and WIMAN in Sweden. The former group prepared plasminogen from Cohn-fraction III-2,3 through extraction by means of lysine solutions, isoelectric precipitation of the extract at pH 6.2, repeated lysine extraction, chromatography on DEAE-Sephadex and final gel filtration on Sephadex G-100 (ROBBINS et al., 1965; ROBBINS and SUMMARIA, 1970). The WALLÉN group started from Cohn-fraction III; plasminogen was isolated through extraction by means of ε-aminocaproic acid, ethanol and salt fractionation, and finally DEAE-Sephadex chromatography (WALLÉN and WIMAN, 1970, 1972). The latter authors also used affinity chromatography methods for the isolation of the proenzyme (WIMAN and WALLÉN, 1973). A great number of modifications of these plasminogen isolation procedures have been described.

Preparations of human plasminogen obtained in this manner proved to be homogenous, when investigated immunologically or by ultracentrifugation (ROBBINS et al., 1965; BARLOW et al., 1969; WALLÉN and WIMAN, 1972). Some molecular data are summarized in Table 1. However, in electrophoretic studies, the highly purified plasminogen of human and animal sources exhibited remarkable heterogeneity (WALLÉN, 1962b; RYBAK and PETAKOVA, 1963; SLOTTA and GONZALES, 1964; BARG et al., 1965; CHAN and MERTZ, 1966a, 1966b; HEBERLEIN and BARNHART, 1968; DEUTSCH and MERTZ, 1970; BROCKWAY and CASTELLINO, 1972; WALLÉN and WIMAN, 1972; SODETZ et al., 1972; McCLINTOCK et al., 1974). The reason is the heterogeneity of the plasminogen molecule, which was shown to exist in a number of modifications in the plasma of each species. In human plasma eight different plasminogens were demon-

Table 1. Physicochemical data on human plasminogen and plasmin

	Plasminogen	Plasmin	References
Molecular weight	81000 ± 2900	75000 ± 2800	BARLOW et al. (1969)
Specific activity (caseinolytic units/mg protein)		25–28	SJÖHOLM et al. (1973) ROBBINS et al. (1965)
Sedimentation constant, $S_{20,w}^{0}(S)$	4.2	3.9	BARLOW et al. (1969)
Partial specific volume $\overline{V}$ (ml/g)	0.714–0.720	0.709–0.717	ROBBINS et al. (1965) BARLOW et al. (1969)
Frictional ratio, f/f_0	1.8	1.5	ROBBINS et al. (1965)
Electrophoretic mobility (cm²/V/s; pH 2.9)	$+9.4 \times 10^{-5}$	$+7.63 \times 10^{-5}$	ROBBINS et al. (1965)
Isoelectric point, pH	6.4–8.5		SUMMARIA et al. (1972)
Extinction coefficient: $E_{1\,cm}^{1\%}$, 280 nm	17.0 ± 0.3	17.0 ± 0.3	ROBBINS and SUMMARIA (1970)

Table 2. Amino-acid sequences in human plasminogen

Localization	Sequence	References
I. N-terminal sequence of native plasminogen (plasminogen A)	Glu-Pro-Leu-Asp-Asp-Tyr-Val-Asn-Thr-Gln- 11 Gly-Ala-Ser-Leu-Phe-Ser-Val-Thr-Lys-Lys- 21 Gln-Leu-Gly-Ala-Gly-Ser-Ile-Glu-Glu-Cys[1]- 31 Ala-Gln-Ala-Lys-Cys[2])-Glu-Glu-Asp-Glu-Glu- 41 Phe-Thr-Cys[3])-Arg-Ala-Phe-Gln-Tyr-His-Ser- 51 Lys-Glu-Gln-Glu-Cys[4]-Val-Ile-Met-Ala-Glu- 61 Asn-Arg-Lys[5]-Ser-Ser-Ile-Ile-Arg-Arg[5])-Met[6])-Arg[7])- 71 Asp-Val-Val-Leu-Phe-Glu-Lys[8])-	WIMAN (1973) WIMAN and WALLÉN (1975c)
II. N-terminal sequence of altered plasminogen (plasminogen B) (= N-terminal sequence of the heavy chain of plasmin)	Lys[9])-Val[10])-Tyr- 81 Leu-Ser[11])-Glu-Cys[12])-Lys-Thr-Gly	ROBBINS et al. (1972) (78–82) WALTHER et al. (1974) (78–85) WIMAN and WALLÉN (1975d) (78–81)
III. Sequence preceding the "activation bond" (= C-terminus of the heavy chain of plasmin)	Phe-Gly-Asn-Gly-Lys-Gly-Tyr-Arg-Gly-Lys- 11 Arg-Ala-Thr-Thr-Val-Thr-Gly-Thr-Pro-Cys- 21 Gln-Asp-Trp-Ala-Ala-Glu-Glu-Pro-His-Arg- 31 His-Ser-Ile-Phe-Thr-Pro-Glu-Thr-Asn-Pro- 41 Arg-Ala-Gly-Leu-Glu-Lys-Asn-Tyr-Cys-Arg- 51 Asn-Pro-Asp-Gly-Asp-Val-Gly-Gly-Pro-Trp- 61 Cys-Tyr-Thr-Thr-Asn-Pro-Arg-Lys-Leu-Tyr- 71 Asp-Tyr-Cys-Asp[13])-Val-Pro-Gln[14])-Cys-Ala-Ala- 81 Pro-Ser-Phe-Asp-Cys-Gly-Lys-Pro-Gln[14])-Val- 91 Glu[15])-Pro-Lys-Lys-Cys-Pro-Gly-Arg[16])-	WIMAN and WALLÉN (1975b, 1975e) SOTTRUP-JENSEN et al. (1975) (71–98)
IV. Sequence following the "activation bond"[17] (N-terminal sequence of the light chain of plasmin)	Val[18]-Val- 101 Gly-Gly-Cys[19])-Val-Ala-His-Pro-His-Ser-Trp- 111 Pro-Trp-Gln-Val-Ser[20])-Leu-Arg[21])-Thr[22])-Arg-Phe- 121 Gly-Met	ROBBINS et al. (1972, 1973b) (98–117) WALTHER et al. (1974) (98–105) WIMAN and WALLÉN (1975e) (98–122) SOTTRUP-JENSEN et al. (99–108)
V. Histidine-loop[17]	His-Phe-Cys-Gly-Gly-Thr-Ile-Ser-Pro- 11 Glu-Trp-Val-Leu-Ser-Ala-Ala-His[23])-Cys-Leu	ROBBINS et al. (1973a)
VI. Vicinity of the active serine residue[17]	Val-Glx-(Ser-Thr, Glx)-Leu-(Gly, Ala)-His-Leu- 11 Ala-Cys-Asn-(Thr, Gly, Gly)-Ser-Cys-Gln-Gly- 21 Asp-Ser[24])-Gly-Gly-Pro-Leu-Val-Cys-Phe-Glu- 31 Lys-Asp-Lys-Tyr	GROSKOPF et al. (1969b)
VII. C-terminal sequence	Leu-Asn	ROBBINS et al. (1967)

Table 2 (continued)

[1] Disulfide bridge to Cys-55.
[2] Disulfide bridge to Cys-43.
[3] Disulfide bridge to Cys-35.
[4] Disulfide bridge to Cys-30.
[5] Points of attack of activators; C-terminal residues of "pre-activation peptides".
[6] N-terminus of Met-plasmin or of the enzymatically inactive intermediate produced during the activation of native plasminogen.
[7] Not Ser as noted in the text of WIMAN and WALLÉN (1975c); see footnote of that paper.
[8] Bond predominantly split in proteolytically altered plasminogen.
[9] N-terminus of proteolytically altered plasminogen.
[10] N-terminus of Val-plasmin(ogen) = des-lysyl-plasmin(ogen).
[11] Leu was found by ROBBINS et al. (1972).
[12] Phe was found by WALTHER et al. (1974).
[13] Asn was found by SOTTRUP-JENSEN et al. (1975).
[14] Originally described as Glu (WIMAN and WALLÉN, 1975b); Glu was also found by SOTTRUP-JENSEN et al. (1975).
[15] Gln was found by SOTTRUP-JENSEN et al. (1975).
[16] "Activation bond" (ROBBINS et al., 1967); C-terminal residue of the heavy chain of plasmin.
[17] These parts show extensive homologies to the corresponding segments of pancreatic and blood serine proteinases (trypsin, thrombin etc.).
[18] N-terminus of the light chain of plasminogen.
[19] In the first study (ROBBINS et al., 1972) reported as Gln. The Cys residue, now determined, is presumably part of the "hinge" disulfide bond connecting the heavy and light chains of plasmin (ROBBINS et al., 1973b).
[20] Val was found by ROBBINS et al. (1972, 1973b).
[21] Leu was found by ROBBINS et al. (1972, 1973b).
[22] Arg was found by ROBBINS et al. (1972, 1973b).
[23] "Active" histidine residue.
[24] "Active" serine residue.

strated by isoelectric focusing. All these forms could be activated to plasmin isoenzymes with similar proteolytic activity, showing isoelectric points between pH 6.4 and 8.5 (SUMMARIA et al., 1972).

Estimations of the molecular weight of highly purified human plasminogen resulted in values varying between 81000 and 93000 (DAVIES and ENGLERT, 1960; DAVIES et al., 1964; SLOTTA and GONZALES, 1964; ROBBINS et al., 1965; BARLOW et al., 1969; WALLÉN and WIMAN, 1972; SJÖHOLM et al., 1973). Lysine was found to be the N-terminal amino acid of human plasminogen prepared according to the ROBBIN, group's isolation method (ROBBINS et al., 1967; SUMMARIA et al., 1967a, 1967b, 1971b, 1972). Later it was demonstrated that this plasminogen does not correspond to the native protein, but is a plasminogen derivative (plasminogen B) which has become altered proteolytically in its N-terminal portion by traces of plasmin during the isolation procedure (CHAN and MERTZ, 1966c; WALLÉN and WIMAN, 1970, 1972; CLAEYS et al., 1973). If plasmin is excluded carefully during the process of preparation or isolated in the presence of plasmin inhibitors, native plasminogen (plasminogen A) with N-terminal glutamic acid is obtained (RICKLI and CUENDET, 1971; WALLÉN and WIMAN, 1972; WIMAN and WALLÉN, 1973; ROBBINS et al., 1973b; SUMMARIA et al., 1974; McCLINTOCK et al., 1974). The proteolytic alteration results in a removal from the N-terminal part of a polypeptide amounting to 10% of the total plasminogen molecule. By this modification the tertiary structure of the plasminogen is changed drastically. According to these facts, the big differences in the molecular weight determined by different authors can be explained. During the activation of the proenzyme, peptide material which in most cases is identical with that removed during the formation of plasminogen B is also split off from the N-terminus of the plasminogen molecule (Table 2; see p. 23f) (WALLÉN and WIMAN, 1972; WIMAN, 1972, 1973; WIMAN and WALLÉN, 1973, 1975c; SJÖHOLM et al., 1973; RICKLI and OTAVSKI, 1973).

The plasminogen molecule consists of a single polypeptide chain, the quantitative amino-acid composition of which (see Table 4) has been known for a long time (SLOTTA and GONZALES, 1964; ROBBINS et al., 1965; WALLÉN and WIMAN, 1972). A number of groups are presently studying the primary structure. The amino-acid sequences of the following parts of human plasminogen are known (Table 2): The N-terminal sequence of native plasminogen, i.e., the primary structure of the peptides released during proteolytic alteration or during activation (WIMAN, 1972, 1973; WIMAN and WALLÉN, 1973, 1975c); the N-terminal sequence of plasminogen B (ROBBINS et al., 1972; WALTHER et al., 1974; WIMAN and WALLÉN, 1975c, 1975d); and some sequences in the middle of the chain (GROSKOPF et al., 1969b; ROBBINS et al., 1972a, 1973a, 1973b; WALTHER et al., 1974; WIMAN and WALLÉN, 1975b, 1975e). The C-terminal amino acid is asparagin (ROBBINS et al., 1967). Clarification of the primary structure of the whole molecule, which consists of approximately 750 amino-acid residues, is expected in the near future (WIMAN and WALLÉN, 1975a, MAGNUSSON et al., 1975a, 1975b).

Plasminogen contains 21 or 22 disulfide bridges and 1.45% carbohydrate (ROBBINS et al., 1965). Heterogeneities of the latter are thought to be partially responsible for the existence of multiple molecular forms of plasminogen (CASTELLINO et al., 1973b; SIEFRING and CASTELLINO, 1974; HAYES et al., 1975). Some sequences of animal plasminogens are also known (NAGASAWA and SUZUKI, 1970; SUMMARIA et al., 1973; ROBBINS et al., 1973b). In sheep plasminogen a peptide which represents 30% of the whole molecule can be removed N-terminally without disturbing the ability of the remainder to be activated to plasmin (PAONI and CASTELLINO, 1975).

Antifibrinolytic amino acids, such as ε-aminocaproic acid, p-aminomethyl benzoic acid, and trans-4-aminomethyl cyclohexane carboxylic acid (see also MARKWARDT: "Synthetic Inhibitors of Fibrinolysis" in this volume), are able to form stoichiometric complexes with plasminogen in a molecular ratio of 1:1 (ABIKO et al., 1969; BROCKWAY and CASTELLINO, 1971). In these complexes plasminogen undergoes conformational changes (ALKJAERSIG, 1964; IWAMOTO et al., 1968; BROCKWAY and CASTELLINO, 1972; CASTELLINO et al., 1973a; SJÖHOLM et al., 1973) which seem to be related to the improved solubility of plasminogen in the presence of ε-aminocaproic acid and to the mechanism of the antifibrinolytic action of these compounds. Plasminogen possesses a high affinity for fibrinogen. Therefore, the preparation of fibrinogen free of plasminogen is difficult (BLOMBÄCK and BLOMBÄCK, 1957; MOSESSON, 1962; BALL et al., 1971). For that reason, the proenzyme is enriched specifically within the fibrin deposits of the organism.

Plasminogen is present in all body fluids. Its concentration in human plasma amounts to 0.1–0.2 mg/ml (NANNINGA, 1967; SCHWICK, 1968; RABINER et al., 1969). Furthermore, the proenzyme was demonstrated to occur in human tissues and granulocytes (KOWALSKI et al., 1958; BARNHART and RIDDLE, 1963; PROKOPOWICZ, 1968).

2. Plasmin

The fibrinolytic enzyme, plasmin, the activation product of plasminogen, is a proteolytic enzyme with the physiologic function of degrading the insoluble fibrin into soluble split products. This mechanism is described subsequently (see p. 30f; for further details see ROBBINS: "Plasmin" in this volume).

The action of plasmin is not restricted to fibrin, but the enzyme splits peptide bonds in practically all protein substrates. In these reactions plasmin proved to be a proteolytic enzyme with trypsin-like substrate specificity, i.e., it hydrolyzes like trypsin peptide bonds of the basic amino acids arginine and lysine (BLOMBÄCK et al., 1967; IWANAGA et al., 1967; GROSKOPF et al., 1968). Plasmin cleaves only a limited number of the peptide bonds of basic amino acids present in protein substrates, whereas they are split by trypsin to a much higher extent (CHRISTENSEN and MCLEOD, 1945; WALLÉN and BERGSTRÖM, 1958; IWANAGA et al., 1967, WALLÉN and IWANAGA, 1968). Presumably, the large plasmin molecule does not possess the same flexibility as that of trypsin, and thus, the active center of the enzyme reaches only part of the total number of bonds being potentially split. Especially well investigated is the degradation of fibrinogen by plasmin. This process showing a Michaelis-constant of $K_m = 3 \times 10^{-5}\,M$ (BICKFORD et al., 1964; NANNINGA and GUEST, 1968) leads to defined products with biologic activity (see chapter by KOPEC and LATALLO, in this volume). Furthermore, plasmin was used in structure analysis of the fibrinogen molecule (see chapter by BLOMBÄCK, in this volume).

Like trypsin and other related proteolytic enzymes (thrombin, kallikrein, acrosin), plasmin hydrolyzes, in addition to protein substrates, esters of arginine and lysine (TROLL et al., 1954; ROBERTS, 1958; SCHERAGA et al., 1958; SHERRY et al., 1965, 1966; ROBBINS et al., 1965; SILVERSTEIN, 1973, 1975), as well as the 4-nitroanilides and β-naphthylamides of those amino acids (MARKWARDT et al., 1968; SZCZEKLIK et al., 1968; LATALLO and THEISSEYRE, 1974). Histidine esters are also cleaved (COLE and OLWIN, 1967; COLE, 1968). Kinetic constants of the reactions of plasmin with a number of these substrates were determined. In proteolytic and esterolytic reactions plasmin showed a preference for lysine residues (WALLÉN and IWANAGA, 1968; WEINSTEIN and DOOLITTLE, 1972; NAGAMATSU and HAYASHIDA, 1974).

Plasmin is inhibited by diisopropylfluorophosphate (DFP) and other organo-phosphorus compounds (MOUNTER and SHIPLEY, 1958; MOUNTER and MOUNTER, 1963). Accordingly, the enzyme can be characterized as a serine proteinase. The molecular mechanism of the catalytic action of this group of proteolytic enzymes is well-known from extensive studies on the structure and activity of chymotrypsin (SMILLIE et al., 1968; BIRKTOFT et al., 1970; HENDERSON, 1970; HENDERSON et al., 1971). Though detailed investigations on the catalytic mechanism of plasmin have not yet been undertaken, all experimental data are in accordance with the assumption that it functions in an analogous manner. The catalytic mechanism of these enzymes is brought about by the transfer of a negative charge of the side chain of an aspartic acid residue via a histidine residue to the β-hydroxyl group of a serine residue ("charge relay system"). In this way, this group becomes highly electronegative, so that it reacts by nucleophilic attack with amide or ester bonds.

These bonds are split under formation of an intermediate ester bond between the carboxyl group of the amino acid in the substrate molecule and the serine hydroxyl group of the enzyme (acyl enzyme). The reaction proceeds according to the following general scheme (CHASE and SHAW, 1969):

$$
\begin{array}{ccc}
\text{Formation of an} & \text{acylation} & \text{deacylation} \\
\text{adsorption complex} & &
\end{array}
$$

$$
E + S \rightleftharpoons ES \quad \rightarrow \quad ES' \quad \rightarrow \quad E + P_2 \\
\qquad\qquad\qquad\qquad + P_1
$$

(E = enzyme; S = substrate; ES = noncovalent adsorption complex — "Michaelis-complex"; ES′ = acyl enzyme; P_1 = split product liberated during the formation of acyl enzyme: i.e., H_2N-peptide, amine, alcohol; P_2 = split product liberated during the deacylation process: i.e., peptide-COOH, amino acid).

Plasmin is inhibited by a great number of naturally occurring protein-like proteinase inhibitors (reviews: VOGEL et al., 1966; MARKWARDT et al., 1972a). The physiologic plasmin inactivators of blood plasma (see p. 22) are inhibitors of the same type. Like other trypsin-like proteolytic enzymes, plasmin is inhibited by a number of small molecular synthetic substances structurally related to lysine or arginine (ABLONDI et al., 1959; NAGAMATSU et al., 1963, 1968; BICKFORD et al., 1964; MURA-MATU et al., 1965a, 1965b, 1967; LANDMANN, 1967, 1973; IWAMOTO et al., 1968; MURAMATU and FUJII, 1968, 1969, 1971, 1972; GROSKOPF et al., 1969a; AOYAGI et al., 1969a, b; OKANO et al., 1972; UMEZAWA, 1972; OKAMOTO et al., 1975). Other groups of synthetic plasmin inhibitors are derivatives of benzylamine, phenylguanidine, and benzamidine. They also can be regarded as substrate analogs (MARKWARDT et al., 1968, 1970a, 1970b, 1971, 1972b, 1973; CHASE and SHAW, 1969; LANDMANN, 1970,

1973; GERATZ, 1970, 1971, 1972, 1973; SODETZ and CASTELLINO, 1972; WALSMANN et al., 1974a, 1974b, 1975; STÜRZEBECHER et al., 1974).

Most of the synthetic inhibitors act in a competitive manner. However, some of them possess, in addition to substrate analogous structures, reactive groups which enable these substances to form covalent bonds with the enzyme after being fixed at the substrate binding center ("affinity labeling"). Those inhibitors react irreversibly with the enzyme. The best known member of this type of inhibitors is L-1-chloro-3-toluenesulfonylamido-7-amino-2-heptanone (tosyl-L-lysyl-chloromethylketone—TLCK) (GROSKOPF et al., 1969b; ROBBINS et al., 1973a). Other inhibitors react with the enzyme like substrates, but form very stable acyl enzymes, so that the reaction stops at this stage. Depending on the velocity of the deacylation process, temporary or irreversible inhibitory effects can occur. 4'-Nitrophenyl-4-guanidinobenzoate (CHASE and SHAW, 1969; SODETZ and CASTELLINO, 1972) and related guanidino compounds (MARKWARDT et al., 1970a, 1973) are representatives of this type. Because of their substrate-analogous structures, the synthetic inhibitors mentioned react primarily with the substrate binding center of plasmin. The antiplasmin activity of the inhibitors runs parallel with an analogous inhibitory effect against trypsin. Therefore, the substrate binding area of both enzymes is assumed to have similar structures in plasmin and trypsin (MARKWARDT et al., 1968; CHASE and SHAW, 1969; COATS, 1972). Its geometry is very well-known in the case of trypsin (KRIEGER et al., 1974).

As a result of the molecular changes of the plasminogen molecule during the process of activation (see p. 23ff) the plasmin molecule consists of two amino-acid chains of different size. Both chains are connected with each other by a single disulfide bond (ROBBINS et al., 1967). In this way, plasmin possesses two N-terminal amino acids, lysine and valine. Lysine is the N-terminus of the "heavy" chain (A-chain) with a molecular weight of approximately 60000 comprising the major part of the parent plasminogen molecule (N-terminal portion). This lysine residue corresponds to N-terminal lysine of plasminogen B (WIMAN and WALLÉN, 1975c). Valine is the N-terminus of the "light" chain (B-chain) with a molecular weight of approximately 26000; it represents the C-terminal portion of the parent plasminogen molecule. In solution plasmin undergoes autolytic alterations. The removal of the N-terminal lysine residue (formation of des-lysyl-plasmin = Val-plasmin, see, p. 24) is common. Furthermore, bond splitting in the C-terminal part of the A-chain was seen (ROBBINS et al., 1973b). An autolytic cleavage in the B-chain was found to be responsible for the rapid inactivation of plasmin in solution. This reaction is accompanied by the removal of a peptide with a molecular weight of 6500 remaining bound to the main portion of the molecule by a disulfide bond (WALTHER et al., 1974).

The catalytic activity of the enzyme is brought about by the cooperative effect of a number of amino-acid side chains which are localized completely in the B-chain. With regard to size, amino-acid composition and sequences, this chain shows a number of remarkable similarities to the molecules of the serine proteinases trypsin and chymotrypsin (SUMMARIA et al., 1967b; GROSKOPF et al., 1969a, 1969b; ROBBINS et al., 1972, 1973a). This led to the well-founded hypothesis that this part of the plasmin molecule can be considered an evolutionary derivative of an ancestral protein common to all serine proteinases in pancreas and blood plasma. So far studied, all these enzyme molecules possess obvious homologies in their primary structure

(HARTLEY, 1964, 1970). Recently, sequence homologies were also demonstrated in parts of the A-chain of plasmin and that portion of the prothrombin molecule not entering the thrombin entity. In that part of the prothrombin molecule two structurally related segments were demonstrated ("kringles") which also occur in four positions of the A-chain of plasmin (MAGNUSSON et al., 1975a, 1975b). Thus, this part of the molecules of blood proteinases lacking the molecules of pancreas proteinases seems to be derived from a common ancestral protein, too.

Plasmin is unstable at neutral pH (SHERRY, 1954; KOWALSKI et al., 1957; WALTHER et al., 1974). At pH values below 4 (ROBBINS and SUMMARIA, 1970) as well as in the presence of casein (REMMERT and COHEN, 1949; ABIKO et al., 1968), glycerol (ALKJAERSIG et al., 1958a; GROSKOPF et al., 1968; ROBBINS and SUMMARIA, 1970) or neutral salts (ROBERTS and BURKAT, 1966) its stability increases. At pH2 plasmin can be precipitated by 1 M NaCl solution without significant loss of activity. In this way it is possible to remove activators which do not endure this procedure (TROLL and SHERRY, 1955). The pH optimum of plasmin activity depends on the type of substrate. Protein substrates are hydrolyzed optimally at pH 7–8, arginine esters at pH 8–9 and lysine esters at pH 6.5 (TROLL et al., 1954; RONWIN, 1956; SCHERAGA et al., 1958).

The activity of plasmin is measured in caseinolytic units. One unit is defined as that quantity of plasmin which liberates 450 μg of trichloroacetic acid soluble tyrosine from a 4% casein solution at pH 7.4 and 35° C within 1 h (REMMERT and COHEN, 1949; ROBBINS and SUMMARIA, 1970; KLINE, 1971). Plasmin preparations of highest purity possess a specific activity of 26–28 caseinolytic units per mg of protein. In addition to the caseinolytic assay there are a number of other standardization procedures and calibration units. They are partially based upon comparing plasmin activities with international standards (WALLÉN and WIMAN, 1972). From 1 ml of plasma from healthy subjects a plasmin quantity is produced, corresponding to 3–4 caseinolytic units (FLETCHER et al., 1959, 1962). This quantity amounts to a concentration of 20.3 ± 2.6 mg/100 ml of plasma (COLLEN and VERSTRAETE, 1975) or to a molar concentration of 8×10^{-7} M (NANNINGA, 1975).

II. Plasminogen Activators

The activation of plasminogen is a proteolytic mechanism mediated by plasminogen activators which are proteolytic enzymes catalyzing the activation process with high specificity. Activators are found in body fluids, tissues, and certain bacteria.

1. Activators in Body Fluids

a) Blood Activator

In early investigations on the activation of the fibrinolytic process by FEARNLEY and TWEED (1953), MÜLLERTZ (1956, 1957), and FEARNLEY and FERGUSON (1957) a plasminogen activator in human blood was demonstrated and characterized. The factor precipitates with the euglobulines from diluted plasma at pH 5.3 and causes a spontaneous lysis of euglobulin clots with low inhibitor content. The circulating activator was characterized as an enzyme catalyzing the hydrolysis of N-acetyl-L-lysine methyl ester (COUGHLIN, 1966). Later it was demonstrated that the endothelium of venous vessels contains high amounts of plasminogen activators (see p. 17ff). This led to the assumption that the blood activator is a product of the venous vessel wall (TODD, 1964; WARREN, 1964; FEARNLEY, 1965). If this is proved to be exact, the relative inactivity of the fibrinolytic system in blood under normal conditions would be realized in contrast to blood coagulation by means of a compartment effect. However, up to now it cannot be excluded completely that an activation mode of the fibrinolytic system comparable to that of the intrinsic blood clotting mechanism does exist. Recent experimental data show that the surface-activated blood clotting factor XII (Hageman factor) is able to activate plasminogen indirectly by converting additional factors into directly acting plasminogen activators (OGSTON et al., 1969; MOVAT et al., 1972; LAAKE and VENNERÖD, 1974; ASTRUP and ROSA, 1974). The knowledge of these "proactivators", i.e., precursors of a blood plasma plasminogen activator, is extremely limited.

b) Urine Activator (Urokinase)

The fibrinolytic activity of urine has been known for almost a century (SAHLI, 1885). This activity was shown to result from a plasminogen activator (MACFARLANE and PILLING, 1947; WILLIAMS, 1951; CELANDER et al., 1955) which was named "urokinase" (SOBEL et al., 1952).

Crude preparations of urokinase were obtained by treatment of the urine with organic solvents (SOBEL et al., 1952; CELANDER et al., 1955) or by means of a special foam technique (CELANDER and GUEST, 1960; GUEST and CELANDER, 1961). Further purification was attained by adsorption methods and chromatographic procedures (VON KAULLA, 1954, 1956a, 1956b; PLOUG and KJELDGAARD, 1956, 1957; SGOURIS et al., 1960, 1962). In this manner, urokinase was separated from a thromboplastic activity uroplastin, which is still present in the crude preparations. Highly purified human urokinase was prepared by WHITE et al. (1966) by salt precipitation of urine foam, chromatography on Amberlite IRC-50 and final gel filtration on Sephadex G-100 (WHITE and BARLOW, 1970). Another method for the preparation of highly purified human urokinase yielding a crystalline product was described by LESUK et al. (1965).

Urokinase preparations obtained by these isolation procedures differ in some molecular parameters (Table 3). The enzyme prepared according to WHITE et al. (1966) is homogeneous in Sephadex gel filtration, but proves to consist of two components with a molecular weight of 31700 and 54700 in ultracentrifugal and immunologic studies. Both components can be prepared separately by chromatography on hydroxyl apatite at pH 6.8. The low molecular and the high molecular forms of urokinase possess specific activities of 218000 and 93500 CTA units (see p. 15) per mg of protein, respectively. They are partially identical, as was concluded from their cross-reactivity with specific antisera against urokinase. The heavy molecular form is supposed to be the native protein. It corresponds to the crystalline product of LESUK et al. (1965) in molecular size and specific activity. The smaller form is considered an enzymatically active fragment formed proteolytically by the action of uropepsin. This view is supported by the finding that degradation of the heavy molecular form of urokinase with trypsin yields a light fragment with high activator activity (175000 CTA units per mg of protein). Thus, during the proteolytic process those parts of the urokinase molecule seem to be removed which are not necessary for catalytic action,

Table 3. Physicochemical data on urokinase

	"Light" form	"Heavy" form	References
Molecular weight	31,700	54,700	WHITE et al. (1966)
	34,500		BURGES et al. (1965)
	(27,000)[a]	54,000	DOLESCHEL and
		(104,000, 200,000)[b]	AUERSWALD (1967)
	22,000 32,000	54,000	DOLESCHEL (1975)
		54,000	LESUK et al. (1965, 1967b)
Specific activity (CTA-units/mg protein)	218,000	93,500	WHITE et al. (1966)
		104,000	LESUK et al. (1967)
Sedimentation constant, $S^0_{20,w}(S)$	2.66–2.75	3.18–3.33	WHITE et al. (1966)
Diffusion coefficient, $D^0_{20,w}(cm^2/s)$	$7.41 \cdot 10^{-7}$		WHITE et al. (1966)
Partial specific volume, $\bar{V}$ (ml/g)	0.724	0.728	WHITE et al. (1966)
Frictional ratio, f/f_0	1.35		WHITE et al. (1966)
Electrophoretic mobility, (cm^2/V/s; pH 4.8)	+ 3.5	+ 2.2	WHITE et al. (1966)
Extinction coefficient, $E^{1\%}_{1cm}$ (280 nm, pH 6.5)	13.2	13.6	WHITE et al. (1966)

[a] Mixture of the 22,000 and 32,000 components (DOLESCHEL, 1975).
[b] Aggregation products (DOLESCHEL, 1975).

while the active center remains unaffected (LESUK et al., 1967a, 1967b). Further types of urokinase with either smaller or larger molecules have been described by other authors (BURGES et al., 1965; DOLESCHEL and AUERSWALD, 1967; DOLESCHEL, 1975). Those forms with a molecular weight higher than 55000 (DOLESCHEL and AUERSWALD, 1967) are thought to be aggregation products (DOLESCHEL, 1975).

Amino acid analyses have been performed with both the high molecular and low molecular weight urokinase forms (WHITE et al., 1966). The amino-acid compositions were found to be very similar (Table 4). The molecules consist of single polypeptide chains with isoleucine as the N-terminal residue (LESUK et al., 1967a).

Urokinase solutions are relatively stable against pH changes in the range 1–10 and against temperature up to 50° C. Stability decreases, if salt concentration falls below 0.03 M. In the slightly acidic urine medium, urokinase undergoes proteolytic inactivation through uropepsin (KICKHÖFEN et al., 1958; CELANDER and GUEST, 1960; WHITE and BARLOW, 1970). The biologic function of urokinase consists in the formation of active plasmin from the inactive precursor, plasminogen (SHERRY and ALKJAERSIG, 1956; KJELDGAARD and PLOUG, 1957). According to ROBBINS et al. (1967) and SUMMARIA et al. (1967b) this process is brought about by the cleavage of a single arginyl-valine peptide bond in the C-terminal part of the proenzyme polypeptide chain (see p. 23). The Michaelis constant of that process was shown to be 1.5×10^{-4} M at pH 7.4, assuming a molecular weight of 90000 for plasminogen (NANNINGA and GUEST, 1968). Urokinase can activate plasminogen at pH values between 5.5 and 9; the process functions more rapidly at basic pH values (KJELD-

GAARD and PLOUG, 1957; ALKJAERSIG et al., 1958b). With low urokinase concentrations the amount of plasmin produced does not completely reach the value expected from the quantity of plasminogen present, presumably due to the autolytic destruction of part of the plasmin formed (BERG, 1968). Recently urokinase was successfully fixed on carriers. Insoluble preparations of high enzymatic activity were obtained and used in plasminogen activation studies (AMBRUS et al., 1972; DEUTSCH and MERTZ, 1972; CAPET-ANTONINI et al., 1973; WIMAN and WALLÉN, 1973). These insoluble urokinase preparations can be easily and completely removed from plasminogen activation mixtures.

Besides plasminogen, urokinase hydrolyzes esters of the amino acids lysine, arginine, and histidine. Among these synthetic substrates the following especially are used for the measurement of urokinase activity: N^α-acetyl-L-lysine methyl ester and N^α-acetylglycyl-L-lysine methyl ester (KJELDGAARD and PLOUG, 1957; SHERRY et al., 1964; WALTON, 1967; COLE and OLWIN, 1967; COLE, 1968; GERATZ and CHENG, 1975). Furthermore, N^α-benzyloxycarbonyl-L-tyrosine-4-nitrophenyl ester was shown to be split by urokinase (LORAND and MOZEN, 1964; LORAND and CONDIT, 1965). The cleavage of a series of N^α-acetyl-L-lysine-anilides by urokinase was recently described (PETKOV et al., 1975). Plasminogen activation and hydrolysis of synthetic substrates catalyzed by urokinase are inhibited competitively, temporarily, or irreversibly by substances structurally similar to the amino acids arginine and lysine as well as by derivatives of benzamidine or phenylguanidine. This takes place in a manner analogous to that described for plasmin (KJELDGAARD and PLOUG, 1957; SHERRY et al., 1964; LANDMANN and MARKWARDT, 1970; LANDMANN, 1973; GERATZ and CHENG, 1975). In contrast to plasmin, urokinase is not inhibited by TLCK (LANDMANN and MARKWARDT, 1970; HIJIKATA et al., 1974). Also in discordance with plasmin, an inhibition of urokinase is not produced by protein-like proteinase inhibitors from bovine organs, from urine, and from soy beans (LORAND and CONDIT, 1965; WALTON, 1967; DUCKERT, 1968). A special protein-like urokinase inhibitor seems to be present only in blood plasma (LAURITSEN, 1968; KAWANO et al., 1968, 1970, 1971). In accordance with plasmin, trypsin, and related enzymes, urokinase is inhibited by DFP and can be thus considered a serine proteinase with trypsin-like specificity (LANDMANN and MARKWARDT, 1970). Evolutionary relations between urokinase and other serine proteinases and, consequently, homologies in primary structure are hypothesized.

Urokinase attacks proteins other than plasminogen either mildly or not at all (KJELDGAARD and PLOUG, 1957). The enzyme seems to possess a special affinity for fibrinogen and fibrin. Thus it might be enabled to activate easily intrinsic clot plasminogen and to produce a fibrinolytic reaction (BALL et al., 1971; CHESTERMAN et al., 1972).

Quite a number of different units for the measurement of urokinase activity have been described (PLOUG and KJELDGAARD, 1957; GUEST and CELANDER, 1961; SHERRY et al., 1964; for review see MARKWARDT et al., 1972). The most frequently used reference is now the CTA unit proposed by the Committee on Thrombolytic Agents (JOHNSON et al., 1969; WHITE and BARLOW, 1970). One ml of human urine contains 10 CTA units of urokinase.

Earlier investigations demonstrated that the plasminogen activator content of urine was increased after the occurrence of fibrinolytic activity in blood. According

Table 4. Amino-acid composition of purified fibrinolytic factors (number of residues per molecule)

| | Plasminogen | | Plasmin | Urokinase | | Streptokinase | | | | | |
	ROBBINS et al. (1965)	WALLÉN and WIMAN (1972)	ROBBINS et al. (1965)	WHITE et al. (1966) "light"	"heavy"	SCHWICK (1964)	DE RENZO et al. (1967b)	TAYLOR and BOTTS (1968)	MORGAN and HENSCHEN (1969)	BILINSKI et al. (1968)	BROCKWAY and CASTELLINO (1974)
Ala	32	38–39	31–32	10	20	18	23	24	22	27	21
Arg	37	39–42	38	14	22	4	21	18	19	20	18
Asx	71[a]	76–78[b]	71[c]	19	40	53	68[d]	67	67[e]	62	57[f]
Half-cystine	38	38	41	10	19	—	—	—	—	—	—
Glx	69[a]	90–92[b]	68–70[c]	28	44	38	46[d]	52	45[e]	59	42[f]
Gly	56	58–59	56–58	22	41	16	21	25	20	25	20
His	21	21–22	22	10	20	8	9	6	9	9	9
Ile	19	21–23	16–18	16	20	18	22	23	22	23	20
Leu	40	42–43	37–39	21	34	31	40	33	39	42	35
Lys	41	48–51	40–42	17	31	27	33	30	34	33	26
Met	8.5	7–8	8	5	8	3	3	1	4	4	4
Phe	17	19–20	15–18	9	14	13	15	12	15	15	14
Pro	65	71–75	67–68	16	29	17	20	19	21	24	21
Ser	44	49–51	42–48	22	35	21	24	22	26	27	24
Thr	54	56–58	55–58	19	32	25	30	27	28	31	26
Trp	20	21	19	5	10	1	1	—	1	2	2
Tyr	29	28–29	28–29	13	20	19	20	8	21	21	20
Val	43	44–46	40–42	11	23	19	23	26	23	26	20

[a] Asn + Gln = 79.　　　　　[c] Asn + Gln = 72–82.　　　　　[e] Asn + Gln = 48.
[b] Asn + Gln = 69–70.　　　[d] Asn + Gln = 61.　　　　　　[f] Asn + Gln = 34.

to these results, urokinase was supposed to be identical with the blood (or endothelium) activator which is excreted by the kidney (COLGAN et al., 1952; VON KAULLA and SWAN, 1958; SMYRNIOTIS et al., 1959; CELANDER and GUEST, 1960). However, in later studies no conformity was found between the fibrinolytic activities of blood and urine (FLETCHER et al., 1965). A plasminogen activator released from cultivated kidney cells showed corresponding properties and immunologic identity with urokinase (PAINTER and CHARLES, 1962; BERNIK and KWAAN, 1967, 1969; KUCINSKI et al., 1968; BARLOW and LAZER, 1972; BERNIK, 1973). Thus, urokinase is regarded to be a true kidney factor which is produced by the epithelial cells of the kidney tubules (LADEHOFF, 1960; PROKOPOWICZ et al., 1964; VIGORITO et al., 1965; KWAAN and FISCHER, 1965; MCCONNEL et al., 1966; EPSTEIN et al., 1968; TYMPANIDIS and ASTRUP, 1971). Urokinase and other plasminogen activating enzymes of the human organism seem to be closely related or identical proteins (for therapeutic uses of urokinase see chapter by DUCKERT in this volume).

c) Activators from Other Body Fluids

The release of a blood activator from the vascular endothelium and of a urine activator from the epithelium of the kidney tubules may represent examples of a general physiologic principle for the regulation of fibrinolytic activity in body fluids. Presumably, epithelial cells of tubular systems commonly produce and release those activators which are responsible for the dissolution of fibrin clots potentially formed here. In this way the free flow of body fluids is ensured. Plasminogen activators were found in human milk (ASTRUP and STERNDORFF, 1953), in tears (STORM, 1955), as well as in seminal fluid (von KAULLA and SHETTLES, 1953; LUNDQUIST et al., 1955), cerebrospinal fluid (MIHARA et al., 1969), saliva (ALBRECHTSEN and THAYSEN, 1955; SCHULTE and VORBAUER, 1965), and bile (OSHIBA et al., 1968). The latter activator ("bilokinase") was isolated in its purified form, and preliminary results on its amino-acid composition were published. In this respect and in respect to its kinetic and immunologic properties it is described as being different from urokinase (OSHIBA and ARIGA, 1975).

2. Tissue Activators

Factors with plasminogen activator activity were demonstrated in a great number of human and animal tissues (ASTRUP and PERMIN, 1947; PERMIN, 1950; ALBRECHTSEN, 1957 a, b, 1959; SANDBERG et al., 1963; ASTRUP, 1966; PERLEWITZ and MARKWARDT, 1969; GLAS and ASTRUP, 1970). High quantitative differences exist in the concentrations of these factors in the various tissues (Table 5). Generally, animal tissues were found to contain smaller amounts of activators than human tissues. Among human organs, testicles, liver, and spleen possess low activator contents, whereas uterus, suprarenal glands, lymphatic nodes, prostate, thyroid, lungs, and ovaries are activator-rich organs. The activity observed depends strongly on the functional state of the tissue. For a long time, studies on tissue activators were hampered, because these factors could not be obtained in a soluble state. Thus, preparation of highly purified activator proteins and investigations of their properties were impossible (ASTRUP and PERMIN, 1947; PERMIN, 1947; ASTRUP, 1951). Soluble preparations were obtained

Table 5. Fibrinolytic activity of human organs, material taken up to 8 hours post mortem

Organ	n	Diameters of lysis zones on fibrin plates after 6 h incubation at 37° C (mean values with standard deviation)	
		Explants (edge length 1 mm)	KSCN-extracts (0.02 ml)
Cerebrum	24	3.8 ± 2.2	7.2 ± 0.7
Cerebellum	20	3.2 ± 2.1	5.7 ± 2.9
Parotid	23	8.1 ± 2.5	9.3 ± 1.33
Masseter	22	9.1 ± 2.9	10.0 ± 2.1
Submandibular gland	21	6.8 ± 2.9	9.0 ± 1.2
Sublingual gland	22	8.4 ± 2.4	9.2 ± 1.2
Thyroid	29	7.1 ± 3.9	10.3 ± 2.0
Lungs	25	6.2 ± 4.2	9.2 ± 1.3
Myocardium	26	5.8 ± 3.7	8.0 ± 1.7
Pericardium	20	5.4 ± 1.7	9.3 ± 1.1
Stomach (cardia)	23	8.4 ± 3.5	11.8 ± 1.7
Stomach (fundus)	21	6.1 ± 2.5	11.2 ± 1.8
Stomach (pylorus)	20	8.0 ± 2.7	10.4 ± 1.2
Duodenum	28	8.2 ± 3.4	10.8 ± 2.4
Jejunum	25	6.5 ± 2.8	9.7 ± 1.8
Ileum	25	6.3 ± 4.1	9.6 ± 1.3
Colon	20	6.4 ± 2.7	8.5 ± 0.8
Rectum	20	6.4 ± 2.9	8.6 ± 1.5
Bladder	20	5.9 ± 2.2	9.2 ± 1.2
Kidneys	21	8.1 ± 3.1	9.7 ± 1.6
Suprarenals	28	8.5 ± 4.0	10.5 ± 1.4
Mammae	12	6.3 ± 2.3	8.5 ± 0.7
Uterus	13	5.8 ± 2.4	9.5 ± 1.2
Ovaries	11	6.7 ± 4.3	9.7 ± 0.6
Prostate	13	8.2 ± 3.4	9.8 ± 1.5
Testicle	16	0	0
Lymphatic node	20	7.0 ± 1.3	8.4 ± 0.8
Aorta	29	3.7 ± 2.7	6.2 ± 0.4
Vena cava	21	6.0 ± 2.3	10.2 ± 1.0
Liver	12	0	0
Spleen	14	0	0

by means of tissue extraction with concentrated KSCN-solution (ASTRUP and STAGE, 1952; ASTRUP and ALBRECHTSEN, 1957; ASTRUP et al., 1971), urea solution (BACHMANN and SHERRY, 1962; McCALL and KLINE, 1965) or acetate buffer, pH 4.2 (BACHMANN et al., 1964). By means of these procedures it became possible, on the one hand, to measure more precisely the activator content in different tissues and, on the other hand, to isolate these factors in a purified form. Purified preparations were obtained from pregnant pig ovaries (ASTRUP and KOK, 1965, 1970; KOK and ASTRUP, 1967, 1969), from pig heart (BACHMANN et al., 1964; McCALL and KLINE, 1965; RICKLI and ZAUGG, 1970; ANDREENKO and MIGALINA, 1971; HIJIKATA et al., 1974), from pig leukocytes (KOPITAR et al., 1974), from pig parotid glands (CARTWRIGHT, 1974), and from human erythrocytes (SEMAR et al., 1969).

The tissue activator from ovaries was obtained by acid precipitation of the KSCN tissue extract, reextraction of the precipitates with NH_4SCN and repeated precipitations by Zn^{2+} salts and by pH changes. Finally, the factor was isolated by gel filtration on Sephadex G-200 (KOK and ASTRUP, 1969; ASTRUP and KOK, 1970). The activator from pig heart was extracted by urea or acetate solutions and further purified by chromatographic and gel filtration procedures (BACHMANN et al., 1964; RICKLI and ZAUGG, 1970; HIJIKATA et al., 1974). These preparation techniques led to electrophoretically homogeneous products showing a molecular weight of 45000 (heart activator) and 50000–60000 (ovary activator), respectively. The activator from pig leukocytes was also obtained in an electrophoretically homogeneous form. It was prepared by chromatography on DEAE-cellulose, gel filtration on Sephadex G-100, chromatography on CM-cellulose and final preparative gel electrophoresis. The molecular weight was determined as 28000 to 30500 (KOPITAR et al., 1974). The activator from pig parotid glands was extracted by citrate buffer and purified mainly by salt precipitation and gel filtration procedures. The purified protein has a molecular weight of 20000 to 25000 (CARTWRIGHT, 1974).

Little is known about the molecular and enzymatic properties of these highly purified tissue activators. They activate plasminogen by cleaving the special arginyl-valine bond (ROBBINS et al., 1967) in the C-terminal part of the plasminogen molecule (see p. 23). Hydrolysis of synthetic substrates has not been observed up to now. Tissue activators are inhibited by amino acid analogues of lysine, by DFP, and by protein-like proteinase inhibitors (KOPITAR et al., 1974; HIJIKATA et al., 1974; CARTWRIGHT, 1974). As with urokinase, inhibition of tissue activators by TLCK was not observed (HIJIKATA et al., 1974). From these results it is believed that the tissue activators are also serine proteinases with trypsin-like substrate specificity and a narrowly restricted proteolytic activity towards plasminogen.

In spite of the reported differences in molecular weight the factors from various tissues do not seem to be distinct proteins. All tissue factors are assumed to be identical with the activator from the venous endothelium (TODD, 1959, 1964). This factor may also be extracted by KSCN-solutions and the fibrinolytic activity of various tissues seems to be related to the degree of vascularization (ASTRUP, 1966, 1967). Thus, a single tissue factor identical with the specific plasminogen activator of the system: vascular endothelium/blood might be postulated. Additionally, relationships may exist between this fibrinolytic activator and those from urine and other body fluids. An antiserum against highly purified urokinase showed cross-reactivity with tissue and endothelial activators (BERNIK et al., 1974). This result points to identity or close relationships between the various activator proteins. However, most scientists consider these factors to be biochemically different (COUGHLIN, 1966; KUCINSKI et al., 1968; ASTRUP and KOK, 1970, AOKI and VON KAULLA, 1971; OSHIBA and ARIGA, 1975).

The relations between the tissue activators described above and plasminogen activators contained in the lysosomal fractions of the cells of numerous tissues are not yet fully understood (LACK and ALI, 1964; ALI and LACK, 1965; ALI and EVANS, 1968; BEARD et al., 1968, 1969; ALI, 1970). Activators of that type, named "cytokinase," seem to represent true lysosomal enzymes, the significance of which for the fibrinolytic processes in the organism is not clear. The factor from rabbit kidney lysosomes was purified by chromatography on DEAE-cellulose. The isolated protein being approximately 70% pure, has a molecular weight of 50000, a sedimentation constant of $S°_{20,w} = 2.9–3.1$ and an isoelectric point of 8.6 (ALI and EVANS, 1968; ALI, 1970). It proved to be a plasminogen-activating enzyme which is inhibited by basic amino acids. Hydrolysis of synthetic substrates or other protein substrates has not been reported so far. The kinetics of plasminogen activation by cytokinase was investigated, and a Michaelis-constant of $K_m = 3.1 \cdot 10^{-5} M$ was determined (ALI, 1970).

In recent studies a specific plasminogen activator was shown to be produced by in vitro cultivated malignant mammalian cells (UNKELESS et al., 1974; QUIGLEY et al., 1974). The factor now isolated in a highly purified state proved to be a basic protein consisting of subunits linked together by disulfide bonds. It is inhibited by DFP and, therefore, seems to be a serine proteinase (CHRISTMAN and ACS, 1974).

3. Bacterial Activators

Plasminogen activators are produced and liberated into the culture medium by various bacteria. Among these factors the well-known streptokinase, a product of certain Streptococcus strains, is the most important one. In contrast to other plasminogen activators mentioned here, streptokinase does not act directly on the proenzyme, but forms a plasminogen-converting factor only in reaction with a special human blood plasma protein, "proactivator." In early investigations it was suggested that plasminogen activators of that type of action are also present in the human organism (LEWIS and FERGUSON, 1951; ASTRUP and STERNDORFF, 1956; DEUTSCH and ELSNER, 1959; KWAAN et al., 1960). However, the occurrence of those factors in human blood ("lysokinases") seems doubtful from the present point of view. Therefore, this indirect mechanism of plasminogen activation is now believed to be restricted to bacterial activators, and the term "lysokinases" is no longer used.

Bacterial activators cannot be strictly attributed to the factors of the fibrinolytic system. However, it seems reasonable to describe their biochemistry in this review, because streptokinase is the most frequently used plasminogen activator in experimental and therapeutic fibrinolysis. By studying its mechanism of action, important results have been accumulated on the biochemistry of the fibrinolytic process in toto.

a) Streptokinase

Streptokinase is a protein factor which is released into the culture medium by β-hemolytic streptococci of the group A (TILLET and GARNER, 1933; MILSTONE, 1941; CHRISTENSEN, 1945). After the therapeutic significance of streptokinase had become evident, numerous methods for the purification and isolation of the factor were elaborated. These procedures generally include separation of the culture medium from the microorganisms, adsorption of the active principle to silica gel or cellulose, and isolation of purified streptokinase by chromatographic or gel filtration techniques. In this way, highly purified homogeneous streptokinase preparations were obtained (DILLON and WANAMAKER, 1965; BLATT et al., 1964; DE RENZO et al., 1967b, TAYLOR and BOTTS, 1968, TOMAR, 1968).

Highly purified streptokinase behaves in immunoelectrophoresis like an α_2-globulin. During ultracentrifugation it is sedimented homogeneously showing a sedimentation constant of $S°_{20,w} = 3.2$ (DAVIES et al., 1964; TAYLOR and BOTTS, 1968). Some

Table 6. Physicochemical data on streptokinase

Molecular weight	47,000–49,000	DAVIES et al. (1964), DE RENZO et al. (1967b), TAYLOR and BOTTS (1968), MORGAN and HENSCHEN (1969)
	44,000	BROCKWAY and CASTELLINO (1974)
Specific activity (CHRISTENSEN units/mg protein)	90,000–100,000	DE RENZO et al. (1967b)
Sedimentation constant, $S_{20,w}^0$ (S)	3.2	DAVIES et al. (1964)
	3.03	BROCKWAY and CASTELLINO (1974)
Diffusion coefficient, $D_{20,w}^0$ (cm^2/g)	6.5×10^{-7}	DAVIES et al. (1964)
Partial specific volume, $\bar{V}$ (ml/g)	0.73–0.75	DAVIES et al. (1964), DE RENZO et al. (1967b), TAYLOR and BOTTS (1968)
Frictional ratio, f/f_0	1.4	DAVIES et al. (1964)
Isoelectric point (pH)	4.7	DE RENZO et al. (1967b)
Extinction coefficient, $E_{1\,cm}^{1\%}$, 280 nm	9.49	TAYLOR and BOTTS (1968)

physicochemical data on streptokinase are summarized in Table 6. The quantitative amino-acid composition (Table 4) was repeatedly investigated (SCHWICK, 1964; DE RENZO et al., 1967b; TAYLOR and BOTTS, 1968; BILINSKI et al., 1968; MORGAN and HENSCHEN, 1969; BROCKWAY and CASTELLINO, 1974). According to these results streptokinase is composed of amino acids only; it contains neither carbohydrate nor phosphorus. A relatively high amount of acidic amino acids was found. Most interestingly, cysteine is absent. Thus, the streptokinase molecule is not stabilized by disulfide bonds, a fact that is uncommon in the chemistry of proteins of this molecular size (more than 400 amino acids). The molecular weight calculated from the amino-acid composition amounts to approximately 48000. Only one N- and one C-terminal amino acid were demonstrated, indicating, that the streptokinase molecule consists of a single polypeptide chain. The N-terminal sequence was shown to be H$_2$N-Ile-Ala-Gly-Pro-Glu-Trp-Leu-Leu-Asp-Arg-Pro-Ser (HENSCHEN and MORGAN, 1969; BROCKWAY and CASTELLINO, 1974). The C-terminal amino acid is lysine (MORGAN and HENSCHEN, 1969). The protein is unstable at neutral pH values and almost insoluble at pH values below 5.0.

In contrast to earlier results (DE VAUX SAINT-CYR, 1962) streptokinase does not possess any enzymatic activity. It is neither a proteinase nor an esterase, and it is not inhibited by DFP (ROBERTS, 1963; BUCK and DE RENZO, 1964; DE RENZO et al., 1967a, 1967b). The sole biologic activity of streptokinase is its ability to convert human plasminogen (as opposed to most animal plasminogens) into plasmin (see p. 26ff). Streptokinase activity is measured in units established by CHRISTENSEN (1949). At present, streptokinase activity is mostly calibrated by comparing it with that of a WHO streptokinase standard (TAYLOR and TOMAR, 1970). (For pharmacology and clinical uses of streptokinase see KLÖCKING and VOGEL in this volume.)

b) Staphylokinase

Staphylokinase is a protein factor which is produced and released into the culture medium by strains of *Staphylococcus aureus* (LEWIS and FERGUSON, 1951; CLIFFTON and CANNAMELA, 1953; DAVIDSON, 1960a, 1960b). The factor was obtained in a highly purified state by salt precipitation of the bacteria-free culture medium, subsequent chromatography on CM-cellulose und alcohol fractionation. It has a molecular weight of 22 500 (LACK and GLANVILLE, 1970). In recent studies staphylokinase was separated by isoelectric focusing into three components with isoelectric points of 5.8, 6.2 and 6.8 (VESTERBERG and VESTERBERG, 1972).

The plasminogen activating effect is the only known biologic activity of staphylokinase. It does not hydrolyze ester or protein substrates (SWEET et al., 1965). Although it was shown that staphylokinase activates human and canine plasminogen in an enzymatic reaction, it is possible that the factor works via a streptokinase-like activation modus, since several animal plasminogens, especially bovine plasminogen, are not activated by it (DAVIDSON, 1960b; LACK and GLANVILLE, 1970). The plasmin formed by staphylokinase is not different from that produced by other activators (SORU, 1968).

III. Inhibitors

Blood plasma contains several proteins which inhibit plasmin and plasminogen activators. Because the activation products formed during fibrinolysis must be inactivated by physiologic pathways, these inhibitors can be regarded as factors belonging to the fibrinolytic system. However, they not only function as inhibitors of the active components of the fibrinolytic process but also inactivate a number of other proteolytic enzymes. With regard to this polyvalent action, these factors may be better characterized as components of a universally acting antiproteolytic protective system of the organism in blood plasma. Only the antiactivators may be regarded, at least in part, as specific inhibitors of the fibrinolytic system. Up to now, with the exception of a urokinase inhibitor, they have been insufficiently characterized (LAURITSEN, 1968; KAWANO et al., 1968, 1970, 1971). Moreover, the reversible complexing of plasmin to α_2-macroglobulin may be interpreted as a specific inhibitory mechanism of physiologic significance. This reversible inhibition is assumed to prevent plasmin from reacting with blood proteins, since the enzyme-inhibitor complex dissociates in the presence of fibrin, and thereby causes a specific transfer of the fibrinolytic enzyme to its physiologic substrate (AMBRUS and MARKUS, 1960; BACK et al. 1965). Recent investigations support the idea of such a mechanism (MÜLLERTZ, 1974).

For a detailed description of the plasmatic inhibitors see the article by MARKWARDT in this volume.

B. Mechanisms of the Fibrinolytic Process

I. Plasmin Formation (Plasminogen Activation)

The activation of the fibrinolytic enzyme, plasmin, from its inactive precursor, plasminogen, is a proteolytic process similar to the activating mechanism of other evolutionarily related serine proteinases. As demonstrated in the case of chymotrypsin, trypsin, and thrombin, the typical result of this mechanism is the proteolytic removal of peptide material from the N-terminal portion of the proenzyme molecule. As a result of this alteration the residual molecule undergoes extensive conformational changes. Thus, some amino-acid side chains although widely separated from each other within the primary structure, attain steric contact. Their cooperative action brings about substrate binding and catalytic effect. The N-terminal peptide is either released (trypsin, thrombin; diminution of the molecular size during activation), or else remains connected with the residual molecule by a disulfide bridge (chymotrypsin; both proenzyme and active enzyme possess the same molecular size).

It has not yet been fully established whether the release of a peptide is required for the activation of plasminogen. In earlier investigations plasminogen was shown to lose 25% of its nitrogen content during the activation process by releasing three polypeptides (RIFÉ and SHULMAN, 1963, 1964a, 1964b). These results were not confirmed in later studies using highly purified preparations of plasminogen, showing correspondingly that plasminogen and plasmin from both human and bovine sources possess nearly equivalent molecular weight (DAVIES et al., 1964; ROBBINS et al., 1965; CHAN and MERTZ, 1966c; HOEPFINGER and MERTZ, 1969). From the enzymatic activities of plasminogen activators relating to esters of basic amino acids, and from the competitive inhibitor effect of those esters in the process of plasminogen activation (see p. 15), it was suggested that plasmin formation is caused by hydrolysis of one or several arginyl or lysyl peptide bonds in the proenzyme molecule. This suggestion was confirmed with human and a number of animal plasminogens which were shown to gain plasmin activity after a single arginyl-valine peptide bond was split. By the hydrolysis of this "activation bond" the polypeptide chain of the plasminogen molecule is cut into two chains of different sizes (A- and B-chain; — see p. 11). Furthermore, this cleavage triggers conformational changes in the B-chain which result in the formation of the active center of the enzyme (ROBBINS et al., 1967; SUMMARIA et al., 1967a, 1967b, 1971b). Both chains remain connected with each other by a single disulfide bridge. Therefore, by analogy with the process of activation of chymotrypsinogen a peptide is not released. Activation by urokinase, streptokinase, and tissue activator, as well as by trypsin (see p. 26) proceeds in the same manner (SUMMARIA et al., 1967a).

However, this mechanism seems to represent only part of the reaction sequence in plasminogen activation. As was shown in recent investigations with human plasminogen, a peptide with a molecular weight of 6000–8000 becomes free in addition to the mentioned hydrolysis of the arginyl-valine activation bond (TAYLOR and BOTTS, 1968; BARLOW et al., 1969). In detailed studies on this subject by WIMAN and WALLÉN (1973) and RICKLI and OTAVSKY (1973) release of peptide material was observed only during the activation of native plasminogen (plasminogen A). According to WIMAN (1973), two peptides consisting of 63 and 5 amino-acid residues, respectively, are removed by the activator (urokinase) from the N-terminal part of

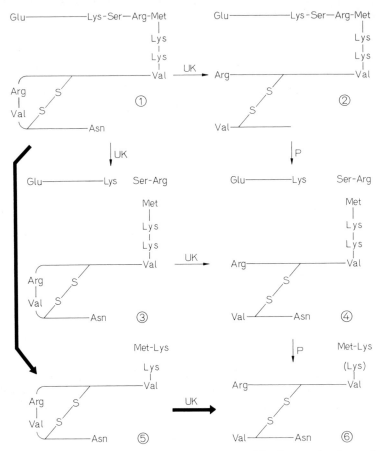

Figure 2. Molecular changes in plasminogen and plasmin resulting from activation and proteolytic alteration. ①: plasminogen A, ⑤: plasminogen B, ⑥: plasmin, ②, ③, ④: Intermediate activation products. As reported in the text, plasmin will be formed from plasminogen A via ①–③–④ (–⑥) or via ①–② (–④–⑥). The main route of plasmin formation seems to be activation of plasminogen B which forms primarily from plasminogen A by autolytic alteration. P: plasmin; Uk: urokinase

the molecule of native plasminogen. The amino-acid sequence of these peptides is revealed (see Table 2). The removal of these peptides leads to an enzymatically inactive intermediate activation product with N-terminal methionine which is subsequently activated to plasmin by hydrolysis of the activation bond previously noted. Plasmin with N-terminal methionine formed in this way, however, proved to be very transient in nature, because it is immediately autolytically altered. In this way, additional nine amino-acid residues are split off from the N-terminal part of Met-plasmin (WIMAN and WALLÉN, 1973, 1975c), yielding Lys-plasmin and later Val-plasmin (deslysyl-plasmin; see Table 2). Lys-plasmin possesses the same N-terminal sequence as proteolytically altered plasminogen (plasminogen B). The very detailed knowledge of the primary structure of the N-terminal part of the plasminogen molecule led to the deduction of the relationships between the different forms of human

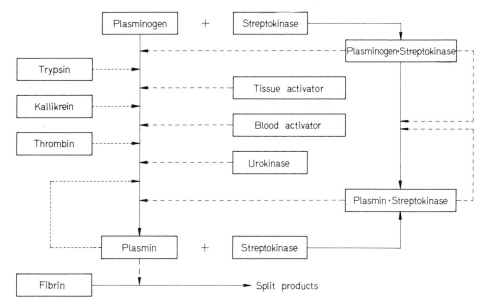

Figure 3. Scheme of the different possibilities of plasminogen activation. -- -→: action on (highly effective); ⋯⋯→: action on (slightly effective): ⟶: transformation into

plasminogen and plasmin on a molecular level (Fig. 2). On the basis of these data, the suggestion of ROBBINS et al. (1973 b) and SUMMARIA et al. (1975), that the formation of Lys-plasmin from plasminogen B should also be accompanied by peptide release, is improbable.

According to these findings on the mechanism of plasminogen activation, peptide release is considered to be an essential step which precedes the actual activation step. This consists of the cleavage of the arginyl-valine bond. Therefore, the peptides released were designated "activation peptides" (WIMAN, 1973) or better "pre-activation peptides" (WALTHER et al., 1974). With respect to the substantial conformational changes the proenzyme molecule undergoes after removal of these peptides, it seems reasonable to assume such an activation sequence (WIMAN, 1973; SJÖHOLM et al., 1973). The exposition of the arginyl-valine bond in question may be the result of these structural changes and a necessary prerequisite for the formation of active plasmin (McCLINTOCK et al., 1974). This suggestion is in accordance with the observation that plasminogen B is activated at a velocity approximately ten times higher than the native proenzyme is (CLAEYS and VERMYLEN, 1974; THORSEN and MÜLLERTZ, 1974).

In most recent experimental studies this activation sequence could not be confirmed. If the proteolytic activity of the plasmin formed during the activation process is carefully excluded by inactivation with the polyvalent proteinase inhibitor from bovine organs, the activation of native plasminogen yields plasmin still containing the "pre-activation peptide" sequence within its molecule (SODETZ et al., 1974; SODETZ and CASTELLINO, 1975; SUMMARIA et al., 1975). Therefore, it is conceivable that, in contrast to the activation mechanism reported above, the first and unique effect of plasminogen activators is the hydrolysis of the arginyl-valine activation bond, whereas the removal of N-terminal peptide material is a secondary effect due to the autolytic action of the formed plasmin. At present there is no uniform concept of the molecular mechanism of plasminogen activation (Fig. 2).

Because of their ability to hydrolyze arginyl bonds, proteolytic enzymes such as trypsin (LEWIS and FERGUSON, 1952, JACOBSSON, 1953; JACKSON and MERTZ, 1954; ALKJAERSIG et al., 1958b; SUMMARIA et al., 1967a), thrombin (ENGEL et al., 1966), kallikrein (COLMAN, 1969), and plasmin itself (ALKJAERSIG et al., 1958a), can produce plasmin from plasminogen. The activator effect of these enzymes is weak. They must be incubated with plasminogen for hours or days, and effective activation occurs only when proteolytic degradation of the formed plasmin is prevented, for example by glycerol (ALKJAERSIG et al., 1958a, 1958b). A scheme of the various pathways of plasminogen activation is given in Figure 3.

II. Formation of Activator (Mechanism of Action of Streptokinase)

Plasminogen activators as previously characterized are proteolytic enzymes which hydrolyze a single or a small number of peptide bonds in plasminogen in a very specific manner. In contrast, streptokinase does not act enzymatically, and therefore its activator activity is brought about by a different mechanism.

A second peculiarity of streptokinase action is its limited effect on the human proenzyme. Animal plasminogen can be activated only with difficulty or not at all. However, in the presence of small quantities of the human proenzyme all animal plasminogens become activated easily by streptokinase. In order to explain this behavior human plasminogen preparations were assumed to contain, in contrast to animal plasminogen preparations, a second proenzyme, proactivator. This entity was thought to form a complex with streptokinase possessing activator activity in a stoichiometric reaction. This complex represents a plasminogen activator which produces plasmin from all types of plasminogen similar to other specific activators (TROLL and SHERRY, 1955; MÜLLERTZ, 1955; LASSEN 1959a, 1959b). Thus, in reaction mixtures of human plasminogen and streptokinase two enzyme activities form, namely activator and plasmin.

Extensive work on the separation of a special proactivator molecule from human plasminogen was unsuccessful (HAGAN et al., 1960). However, it could be demonstrated that the plasmin contained in distinct quantities in all plasminogen preparations can fulfil the function of the postulated proactivator (ZYLBER et al., 1959; HAGAN et al., 1960; KLINE and FISHMAN, 1961b; BLATT et al., 1964; MARKUS and WERKHEISER, 1964; LING et al., 1965; HUMMEL et al., 1966; DE RENZO et al., 1967a; SUMMARIA et al., 1968; WULF and MERTZ, 1969). Plasmin can be transformed into activator quantitatively by addition of streptokinase. A complex possessing high activator activity forms between plasmin and streptokinase in a molecular ratio of 1:1 (LING et al., 1965, 1967; TS'AO and KLINE, 1969).

Besides plasmin, human plasminogen itself is able to form a complex with streptokinase in a molecular ratio of 1:1 (BAUMGARTEN and COLE, 1961; DAVIES et al., 1964; BARG et al., 1965; HUMMEL et al., 1966; RIMON et al., 1966; DE RENZO et al., 1967a; LING et al., 1967; BUCK et al., 1968; SUMMARIA et al., 1968; TS'AO and KLINE, 1969; TOMAR and TAYLOR, 1971). Primarily, it was not clear whether this complex

also possesses activator activity (GUTMAN and RIMON, 1964; WERKHEISER and MAR-
KUS, 1964; HUMMEL et al., 1966; RIMON et al., 1966; DE RENZO et al., 1967a; BUCK et
al., 1968) or is only an intermediate inactive reaction product appearing during the
formation of the true activator (streptokinase-plasmin complex) (LING et al., 1967;
SUMMARIA et al., 1968; TAYLOR and BOTTS, 1968; TS'AO and KLINE, 1969). For
methodical reasons this question can be answered only with difficulty because of the
transient nature of this complex, which was shown to be rapidly converted into the
streptokinase-plasmin complex (SUMMARIA et al., 1968, 1971a). Recently it was demonstrated that plasmin is formed easily from plasminogen preparations which are
free of plasmin traces or which were treated with DFP or other inhibitors in order to
inactivate accompanying plasmin (SUMMARIA et al., 1969; KLINE and TS'AO, 1971).
Accordingly, the presence of plasmin is not necessary for streptokinase action. Moreover, there is evidence that maximum activator activity is reached before traces of
plasmin have been formed and before the special arginyl-valine activation bond in
the plasminogen moiety of the streptokinase-plasminogen complex can be cleaved.
Therefore, the latter complex (but not the streptokinase-plasmin complex!) is the
primarily formed and acting activator in the interaction of plasminogen with streptokinase (MCCLINTOCK and BELL, 1971; REDDY and MARKUS, 1972, 1973, 1974;
SCHICK and CASTELLINO, 1973, 1974).

These data may be interpreted assuming the enzymatic activity of the streptokinase-plasminogen complex to be caused by conformational changes of the proenzyme molecule bound to streptokinase. Those structural changes leading to the
exposition of the active center in the proenzyme molecule by interaction with another protein effector alone, and without hydrolysis of an activation bond (generally
the absolute prerequisite for creating enzymatic activity) comprise a highly interesting phenomenon unique in the biochemistry of serine proteinases.

The primary activator, the streptokinase-plasminogen complex, activates plasminogen to plasmin and converts itself into the streptokinase-plasmin complex (see
Fig. 3).

These reactions are generally thought to proceed in a way in which each molecule
of the streptokinase-plasminogen complex converts a large number of free plasminogen molecules to plasmin or of other streptokinase-plasminogen complex molecules
to streptokinase-plasmin. Alternatively, direct formation of streptokinase-plasmin
and of plasmin from the streptokinase-plasminogen complex is suggested by KOSOW
(1975).

Recent work demonstrated that the streptokinase-plasmin complex is not the
final reaction product of streptokinase and plasminogen. It was shown rather, that
both the streptokinase and the plasmin moiety of the complex underly proteolytic
alterations. In any case, the degradation of streptokinase bound in the activator
complex seems to be an obligatorily occurring reaction (DE RENZO et al., 1967a;
TOMAR and TAYLOR, 1971; SUMMARIA et al., 1971a, 1974). Studying this process,
BROCKWAY and CASTELLINO (1974) found that a polypeptide with a molecular weight
of 8000–9000 is split off from the N-terminal part of native streptokinase.

The remainder of the molecule with a molecular weight of 35000–36000 forms
fully active activator complexes with human plasminogen and plasmin. Its amino-
acid composition was analyzed. The N-terminal sequence was found to be H_2N-Ser-
Lys-Pro-Phe-Ala-X-Asp-Ser-Gly-Ala-Met-Ser; the C-terminus is lysine as in native

streptokinase. Degradation products of streptokinase arise from the streptokinase-plasminogen complex. They can be demonstrated within seconds of mixing the reactants. Their appearance seems to reflect the formation of the enzymatically active center (SUMMARIA et al., 1974).

During prolonged incubation of activator complexes, streptokinase is degraded into small fragments which remain tightly bound to the plasmin moiety and can be released from it only in denaturing media (SUMMARIA et al., 1971a, 1974). Simultaneously, with the degradation of the streptokinase moiety of the complex, the plasmin portion also underlies proteolytic alterations. The fragments of streptokinase and plasmin, described by different authors, are only partially comparable. Recently, the degradation process of both proteins was re-investigated by McCLINTOCK et al. (1974). The reaction sequences depicted in this study do not correspond to those leading to the early-occurring streptokinase fragment reported by BROCKWAY and CASTELLINO (1974) and described previously.

Finally, those streptokinase degradation products described by TAYLOR and BEISSWENGER (1973) which were said to produce a direct enzymatic activation of animal plasminogens in the absence of human plasminogen or plasmin should be mentioned. In recent investigations (BROCKWAY and CASTELLINO, 1974; SCHICK and CASTELLINO, 1974; CHESTERMAN et al., 1974; REDDY and MARKUS, 1974; REDDY and KLINE, 1975) these interesting results have not been confirmed.

Highly contradictory results have been published about the ability of streptokinase to activate a broad spectrum of animal plasminogens. All reports agree on the fundamental difference between human and animal plasminogen. Even plasminogens from the highest primates are not as easily activated by streptokinase as the human proenzyme (McKEE et al., 1971). Different molecular parameters of the various plasminogens and plasmins, respectively, are believed to influence their reactivity toward streptokinase and in this way to cause the species differences observed. Furthermore, the velocity of fragmentation of plasminogen or plasmin-bound streptokinase also seems to be of importance. For instance, in the rabbit system, streptokinase was shown by SCHICK and CASTELLINO (1973) to form complexes only with plasminogen, while the bacterial protein in complexes with plasmin is degraded so rapidly that an effective activator cannot form.

The molecular structures of plasminogen and streptokinase which participate in the binding of both components are hardly known. Activator formation from human plasminogen and streptokinase takes place equally easily in the pH range of 4–10. Therefore, ε-amino groups of lysyl residues being fully protonated in this range are considered to contribute to complex formation (RIMON et al., 1966; HEIMBURGER, 1971). Streptokinase forms enzymatically inactive complexes with plasmin which was inactivated by DFP or other inhibitors. Those complexes are electrophoretically identical with normal plasmin-streptokinase complexes (SUMMARIA et al., 1968; REDDY and MARKUS, 1972; SCHICK and CASTELLINO, 1973). Therefore, groups of the active center do not seem to be involved in complex formation.

Up to now it is not absolutely clear whether the mechanism of action of streptokinase is restricted solely to the activator-complex pathway described in detail above. For instance, human plasminogen was found to be activated directly and apparently independently of the activator-complex mechanism under certain experimental conditions (KLINE and TS'AO, 1967, 1971; SUMMARIA et al., 1969). However, this mode of activation has become questionable after the detection of the clear-cut activator properties of the streptokinase-plasminogen complex. The reported "direct" action of streptokinase can now be explained fully by the complex mechanism, too. On the other hand, the existence in human plasma of distinct proactivator protein(s) different from plasminogen or plasmin cannot be completely excluded. The isolation of such factors was reported in recent years (TAKADA et al., 1970, 1972; YAMAMOTO and NAGAMATSU, 1971; OKAMOTO and YAMAMOTO, 1975).

The properties of the activators formed in the reactions of streptokinase with plasminogen or plasmin are well defined. Most investigations were undertaken with the streptokinase-plasmin complex. It is easily produced and isolated after mixture of the highly purified components (LING et al., 1967; Ts'AO and KLINE, 1969). According to the molecular size of the reactants it has a molecular weight of approximately 150000; however, especially in concentrated solutions, it tends to the formation of a dimer with a molecular weight of 308000. ε-Aminocaproic acid was shown to prevent this dimerization by its protein-desaggregating properties. The complex is stable at a temperature below 22° C. At 37° C it undergoes reversible dissociation. At pH values below 4, activator activity disappears. This property is used profitably for its removal from plasmin, which is not denatured under these conditions (TROLL and SHERRY, 1955; LING et al., 1967; BUCK et al., 1968; Ts'AO and KLINE, 1969).

A single enzymatically active center was determined per molecule of activator (SCHICK and CASTELLINO, 1973). This active center proved to be identical with the active center of the complex-bound plasmin (DE RENZO et al., 1967a; SUMMARIA et al., 1968; BUCK et al., 1968). The active center of the streptokinase-plasminogen complex is also formed in the plasminogen moiety and is presumably identical with the one forming after cleavage of the arginyl-valine activation bond (SCHICK and CASTELLINO, 1974; BROCKWAY and CASTELLINO, 1974). The activity of the streptokinase-plasmin complex is blocked by DFP and TLCK (SUMMARIA et al., 1968; BUCK et al., 1968). It was shown to cleave esters of the amino acids arginine, lysine, and histidine (MARKUS and AMBRUS, 1960; ROBERTS, 1960; KLINE and FISHMAN, 1961b; SHERRY et al., 1966; COLE and OLWIN, 1967; COLE, 1968; Ts'AO and KLINE, 1969; SCHICK and CASTELLINO, 1973). The streptokinase-plasminogen complex possesses an analogous esterolytic activity. Differences exist in the kinetics of hydrolysis of N^α-acetyl-L-lysine methyl ester by both activator complexes and by plasmin, respectively, as is summarized in Table 7 (REDDY and MARKUS, 1974).

According to these properties as well as to their mode of action towards plasminogen, i.e., cleavage of an arginyl bond, the activator complexes can be defined to be

Table 7. Kinetic constants for the hydrolysis of N^α-acetyl-L-lysine methyl ester by plasmin and activator complexes (according to REDDY and MARKUS, 1974)

Enzyme	K_m mM	Turnover number mol substrate/ nmol enzyme/h
Plasmin	7.48 ± 2.3	385
Streptokinase-plasminogen complex	7.47 ± 2.3	327
Streptokinase-plasmin complex	19.65 ± 7.6	1,105

(like plasmin) serine proteinases with trypsin-like substrate specificity. Corresponding to this assumption, both activators are inhibited by structure analogs of basic amino acids as well as by phenylguanidine and benzamidine derivatives (REDDY and MARKUS, 1972, LANDMANN, 1973; SCHICK and CASTELLINO, 1974). The conversion of the streptokinase-plasminogen complex into the streptokinase-plasmin complex is inhibited in the presence of high concentrations of lysine esters (REDDY and MARKUS, 1974). Both activators are inhibited to a different degree by the polyvalent proteinase inhibitor from bovine organs by forming ternary complexes between plasminogen/plasmin, streptokinase, and the inhibitor (TS'AO and KLINE, 1969; KLINE and TS'AO, 1971; REDDY and MARKUS, 1972, 1973, 1974). In contrast, neither activator is inhibited by soybean trypsin inhibitor. Because plasmin is inhibited by this protein, the quantitative determination of activator activity in the presence of plasmin by specific inhibition of the latter with that inhibitor becomes possible (KLINE and FISHMAN, 1961 b; SPRITZ and CAMERON, 1962; TS'AO and KLINE, 1969). Furthermore, the streptokinase-plasminogen complex is not inhibited by blood plasma antiplasmins (HEIMBURGER and SCHWICK, 1971).

The activators hydrolyze small molecular substrates at a velocity similar to that of plasmin (Table 7). However, in sharp contrast to plasmin, they attack casein, fibrinogen or fibrin, and other proteins extremely slowly (MARKUS and AMBRUS, 1960; KLINE and FISHMAN, 1961 b; LING et al., 1965; BARG et al., 1965; GAJEVSKI and MARKUS, 1968; TS'AO and KLINE, 1969; CLAEYS et al., 1971). The only protein substrate which is affected at a high cleavage rate is plasminogen, in which so far only the cleavage of the arginyl-valine bond was observed and not the release of peptides from the N-terminal part of the native protein. Thus, plasmin in a complex with streptokinase loses its general proteolytic efficacy in favor of a specific proteolytic activity towards plasminogen. This drastic alteration of the substrate specificity of plasmin may be caused by conformational changes of the enzyme in complex with streptokinase. It is suggested that the enzyme protein attains a special shape which is especially suited to react with the "activation bond" in the proenzyme molecule. Furthermore, the streptokinase moiety was assumed to improve the access of plasminogen molecules to the active center of the activator complex (BUCK and BOGGIANO, 1971). However, at present it is far from being understood why plasmin, by combining with streptokinase, is converted from an enzyme without or with only very low activator activity, into another one which is a potent activator. Progress is expected from investigations on the complexes by X-ray structure analysis (MCCLINTOCK et al., 1974).

III. Fibrin Dissolution

The biochemical mechanism of the fragmentation of the insoluble substrate fibrin into soluble split products by plasmin is not known in detail up to now. Recent studies on this subject were undertaken mainly with the aim of uncovering structural aspects of fibrin and gathering information about the localization of the covalent bonds formed in fibrin under the action of blood clotting factor XIII. They do not contribute essentially to clarifying the biochemistry of the remarkable process of the rapid and effective proteolytic liquefication of an insoluble protein. This process is of significance in physiology and pathology (CHEN and DOOLITTLE, 1971; FEDDERSEN and GORMSEN, 1971 a, b; GORMSEN and FEDDERSEN, 1972; PIZZA et al., 1973).

Table 8. Comparison of caseinolytic and fibrinolytic activity of plasmin and other proteolytic enzymes

	Equieffective enzyme concentrations		Quotient II./I.
	I. Caseinolysis	II. Fibrinolysis[a]	
Plasmin	0.5 casein units/ml	0.08 casein units/ml	0.16
Trypsin	15 µg/ml	10 µg/ml	0.67
Chymotrypsin	12 µg/ml	110 µg/ml	9.2
Subtilisin	15 µg/ml	60 µg/ml	4.0
Papain	500 µg/ml	2,000 µg/ml	4.0

[a] Enzyme concentration causing lysis of standard clots in 300 s; for experimental details see LANDMANN (1973).

In recent years data were accumulated which point to a special reactivity of plasmin toward its natural substrate, fibrin, presumably developed by evolutionary adaptation (HEIMBURGER, 1962; SCHWICK, 1967, WEINSTEIN and DOOLITTLE, 1972; LANDMANN, 1973). Other proteinases were clearly shown not to be able to attack the insoluble substrate as effectively as plasmin does (Table 8). The fibrinolytic enzyme provokes liquefication of fibrin already after having cleaved only four lysyl bonds per fibrin monomer unit. Trypsin, on the other hand, does not seem to be capable of discovering those "key bonds", which are thought to be of strategic significance for rapid fibrin dissolution. Trypsin was shown to cleave 12–14 lysine bonds and additionally 6 arginyl bonds per fibrin monomer unit before the fibrin network disrupts to soluble split products (WEINSTEIN and DOOLITTLE, 1972). There is evidence that a specific fibrinolytic activity of plasmin is brought about as a result of a special conformational change the enzyme undergoes in the presence of fibrin or fibrin monomer. Presumably, the antifibrinolytic ω-amino acids (see chapter by MARK-WARDT, in this volume) prevent the formation of that physiologically important structure (LANDMANN, 1973). In vivo a specific fibrinolytic effect may be produced additionally by the affinity of plasminogen for fibrinogen. Hereby, the proenzyme is enriched within fibrin deposits, and plasmin formed there can display its action in direct contact with the fibrin substrate.

Fibrin which is not stabilized by covalent bonds is formed when clotting factor XIII is absent or when this transpeptidatic enzyme is inhibited. Fibrin of that type seems to be dissolved by plasmin more easily than stabilized fibrin (LORAND and JACOBSEN, 1962; BRUNER-LORAND et al., 1966; GORMSEN et al., 1967; TYLER, 1969; HENDERSON and NUSSBAUM, 1969; FEDDERSEN and GORMSEN, 1971 b). This fact may be of pharmacologic consequence, because it encourages the search for effective factor XIII inhibitors (LORAND and NILSSON, 1972). These inhibitors are considered to facilitate fibrin dissolution, and thus it seems possible to achieve a therapeutic enhancement of the effectivity of the fibrinolytic system. A great number of inhibitors of the enzyme in question have been described. Up to now, they have been investigated only biochemically, but they did not attain therapeutic significance. Attempts have been made to develop an improved dissolution of fibrin clots in vivo by the physical effects of intravenously administered dextrane derivatives (TANGEN et al., 1972; WALLENBECK and TANGEN, 1975).

Final Remarks

As a result of extensive study in the past 30 years the biochemistry concerned with the factors of the fibrinolytic system and of the reactions provoked by them at a molecular level is now known in some depth. Certainly, for the protein chemist interesting questions in molecular biology of the factors and mechanisms have not yet been answered; their solution, however, seems above all to be a problem of material expense rather than of creative endeavor. The causal interconnections between the fibrinolytic system, on the one hand, and the blood coagulation, kallikrein-kinin, and complement systems, on the other, are at present little understood. It seems possible that uncontrolled interactions between the proteolytic reaction chains of the various systems may conceal key problems in some diseases which have been hitherto insufficiently known in their pathogenetic mechanism. Therefore, the pharmacologic and pharmaceutic interest in further work on the biochemistry of fibrinolysis and related processes remains active. At present, with the discovery and therapeutic use of fibrinolytic and antifibrinolytic agents, the most that could be expected from the elucidation of the biochemistry of the fibrinolytic process seems to have been reached. Furthermore, the present situation in the work on both classes of drugs, fibrinolytics and antifibrinolytics, permits the prognosis that the limits of their potential perspectives can be attained.

Note added in proof

In 1977 the complete amino-acid sequence of human plasmin(ogen) was clarified. The molecule consists of 790 amino-acid residues. The heavy chain (residues 1–560) includes the "preactivation peptide" sequence (1–68) as well as five "kringle" portions (83–161, 165–242, 255–333, 357–434, 461–540) showing extensive homology with each other and with two domains in prothrombin. The light chain (residues 561–790) possesses all binding sites for streptokinase. Removal of "preactivation peptides" is not an essential step in plasminogen activation. (SOTTRUP-JENSEN, L., T. E. PETERSEN, S. MAGNUSSON: Primary structure of plasminogen. Separation of two lysine-binding domains and one neoplasminogen (M w = 38 000). 11th FEBS Meeting, Abstract 856, Copenhagen 1977.)

Acknowledgements: The diligent assistance of Mrs. G. DIETZE and Miss W. GÜNTHER in preparing and checking the applied literature is gratefully acknowledged.

References

Abiko, Y., Iwamoto, M., Shimizu, M.: Plasminogen-plasmin system. II. Purification and properties of human plasmin. J. Biochem. (Tokyo) **64**, 751 (1968)

Abiko, Y., Iwamoto, M., Tomikawa, M.: Plasminogen-plasmin system. V. A stoichiometric equilibrium complex of plasminogen and synthetic inhibitor. Biochim. biophys. Acta (Amst.) **185**, 424 (1969)

Ablondi, F., Hagan, J. J.: Plasmin. In: The Enzymes, Vol. IV, New York-London: Academic Press 1960

Ablondi, F., Hagan, J. J., Philips, M., de Renzo, E. C.: Inhibition of plasmin, trypsin and the streptokinase-activated fibrinolytic system by ε-aminocaproic acid. Arch. Biochem. **82**, 153 (1959)

Albrechtsen, O. K.: The fibrinolytic activity of human tissues. Brit. J. Haemat. **3**, 284 (1957 a)

Albrechtsen, O. K.: The fibrinolytic activity of human tissues. Acta physiol. scand. **39**, 284 (1957 b)

Albrechtsen, O. K.: Fibrinolytic activity in the organism. Acta physiol. scand. **47**, Suppl. 165, 40 (1959)

Albrechtsen, O. K., Thaysen, J. H.: Fibrinolytic activity in human saliva. Acta physiol. scand. **35**, 138 (1955)

Ali, S. Y.: Tissue activator of plasminogen (cytokinase). In: Methods in enzymology, Vol. XIX: Proteolytic enzymes. New York-London: Academic Press 1970

Ali, S. Y., Evans, L.: Purification of rabbit kidney cytokinase and a comparison of its properties with human urokinase. Biochem. J. **107**, 293 (1968)

Ali, S. Y., Lack, C. H.: Studies on the tissue activator of plasminogen. Distribution of activator and proteolytic activity in the subcellular fractions of rabbit kidney. Biochem. J. **96**, 63 (1965)

Alkjaersig, N.: The purification and properties of human plasminogen. Biochem. J. **93**, 171 (1964)

Alkjaersig, N., Fletcher, A. P., Sherry, S.: The activation of human plasminogen. I. Spontaneous activation in glycerol. J. biol. Chem. **233**, 81 (1958 a)

Alkjaersig, N., Fletcher, A. P., Sherry, S.: The activation of human plasminogen. II. A kinetic study of activation with trypsin, urokinase, and streptokinase. J. biol. Chem. **233**, 86 (1958 b)

Ambrus, C. M., Ambrus, J. L., Roholt, O. A., Meyer, B. K., Shields, R. R.: Insolubilized activators of the fibrinolysin system. In vitro studies. J. Med. **3**, 270 (1972)

Ambrus, C. M., Markus, G.: Plasmin-antiplasmin complex as a reservoir of fibrinolytic enzymes. Amer. J. Physiol. **199**, 491 (1960)

Andreenko, G. V., Migalina, L. A.: Procedure for isolation and investigation of the characteristics of the tissue activator of plasminogen (profibrinolysin). Biokhimiya **36**, 685 (1971)

Aoki, N., Kaulla, K. N. von: Dissimilarity of human vascular plasminogen activator and human urokinase. J. Lab. clin. Med. **78**, 354 (1971)

Aoyagi, T., Miyata, S., Nanbo, M., Kojima, F., Matsuzaki, M., Ishizuka, M., Takeuchi, T., Umezawa, H.: Biological activities of leupeptins. J. Antibiot. (Tokyo) **22**, 558 (1969)

Aoyagi, T., Takeuchi, T., Matsuzaki, A., Kawamura, K., Kondo, S., Hamada, M., Maeda, K., Umezawa, H.: Leupeptins, new protease inhibitors from actinomycetes. J. Antibiot. (Tokyo) **22**, 283 (1969)

Astrup, T.: Fibrinokinase. Acta physiol. scand. **24**, 267 (1951)

Astrup, T.: Fibrinolysis in the organism. Blood **11**, 781 (1956)

Astrup, T.: Die Bedeutung der Fibrinolyse. Med. Grundlagenforsch. **2**, 197 (1959)

Astrup, T.: Tissue activators of plasminogen. Fed. Proc. **25**, 42 (1966)

Astrup, T.: Biologie des Plasmins. Thrombos. Diathes. haemorrh. (Stuttg.) Suppl. **22**, 5 (1967)

Astrup, T., Albrechtsen, O. K.: Estimation of the plasminogen activator and the trypsin inhibitor in animal and human tissue. Scand. J. clin. Lab. Invest. **9**, 233 (1957)

Astrup, T., Glas, P., Kok, P.: Assay of the plasminogen activator in tissues. In: Thrombosis and bleeding disorders. Theory and Methods. New York: Academic Press 1971

Astrup, T., Kok, P.: Preparation and purification of a plasminogen activator from porcine tissue. Thrombos. Diathes. haemorrh. (Stuttg.) **13**, 587 (1965)

Astrup, T., Kok, P.: Assay and preparation of a tissue activator. In: Methods in enzymology, Vol. XIX: Proteolytic enzymes. New York-London: Academic Press 1970

Astrup, T., Permin, P. M.: Fibrinolysis in the animal organism. Nature (Lond.) **159**, 681 (1947)

Astrup, T., Rosa, A. T.: A plasminogen proactivator-activator system in human blood effective in absence of Hageman factor. Thrombos. Res. **4**, 609 (1974)

Astrup, T., Stage, A.: Isolation of a soluble fibrinolytic activator from animal tissue. Nature (Lond.) **170**, 929 (1952)

Astrup, T., Sterndorff, I.: A fibrinolytic system in human milk. Proc. Soc. exp. Biol. (N.Y.) **84**, 605 (1953)

Astrup, T., Sterndorff, I.: Fibrinolysokinase activity in animal and human tissue. Acta physiol. scand. **37**, 40 (1956)

Astrup, T., Thorsen, S.: The physiology of fibrinolysis. Med. Clin. N. Amer. **56**, 153 (1972)

Bachmann, F. W., Fletcher, A. P., Alkjaersig, N., Sherry, S.: Partial purification and properties of the plasminogen activator from pig heart. Biochemistry **3**, 1578 (1964)

Bachmann, F. W., Sherry, S.: Purification and properties of plasminogen activator from pig heart. Fed. Proc. **22**, 562 (1962)

Back, N., Hiramoto, R., Ambrus, J. L.: Immunohistochemical study of thrombolytic mechanism. Blood **25**, 1028 (1965)

Ball, A. P., Silver, D., Day, E. D.: Plasminogen-fibrinogen complex formation as a prelude to fibrinogenolysis. Density-gradient ultracentrifugation study of radioiodinated systems involving urokinase, plasminogen, and fibrinogen. Thrombos. Diathes. haemorrh. (Stuttg.) **25**, 114 (1971)

Bang, N. U.: Physiology and biochemistry of fibrinolysis. In: Thrombosis and Bleeding Disorders, p. 292. New York: Academic Press 1971

Barg, W. F., Boggiano, E., de Renzo, E. C.: Interaction of streptokinase and human plasminogen. II. Starch gel electrophoretic demonstration of a reaction product with activator activity. J. biol. Chem. **240**, 2944 (1965)

Barlow, G. H., Lazer, L. V.: Characterization of the plasminogen activator isolated from human embryo kidney cells. Comparison with urokinase. Thrombos. Res. **1**, 201 (1972)

Barlow, G. H., Summaria, L., Robbins, K. C.: Molecular weight studies on human plasminogen and plasmin at the microgram level. J. biol. Chem. **244**, 1138 (1969)

Barnhart, M. I., Riddle, J. M.: Cellular localization of profibrinolysin (plasminogen). Blood **21**, 306 (1963)

Baumgarten, W., Cole, R. B.: Human plasminogen-streptokinase complex: The question of the existence of a separate activator entity. Thrombos. Diathes. haemorrh. (Stuttg.) **5**, 605 (1961)

Beard, E. L., Busuttil, R. W., Gottshalk, S. K.: Stress induced release of plasminogen activator from lysosomes. Thrombos. Diathes. haemorrh. (Stuttg.) **21**, 20 (1969)

Beard, E. L., Montuori, M. H., Danos, G. J.: Plasminogen activator activity of rat lysosomes. Proc. Soc. exp. Biol. (N. Y.) **129**, 804 (1968)

Berg, W.: Urokinase activation of plasminogen and spontaneous inactivation of the plasmin formed. A kinetic study. Thrombos. Diathes. haemorrh. (Stuttg.) **19**, 145 (1968)

Bernik, M. B.: Increased plasminogen activator (urokinase) in tissue culture after fibrin deposition. J. clin. Invest. **52**, 823 (1973)

Bernik, M. B., Kwaan, H. C.: Origin of fibrinolytic activity in cultures of the human kidney. J. Lab. clin. Med. **70**, 650 (1967)

Bernik, M. B., Kwaan, H. C.: Plasminogen activator activity in cultures from human tissues. An immunological and histochemical study. J. clin. Invest. **48**, 1740 (1969)

Bernik, M. B., White, W. F., Oller, E. P., Kwaan, H. C.: Immunologic identity of plasminogen activator in human urine, heart, blood vessels, and tissue culture. J. Lab. clin. Med. **84**, 546 (1974)

Bickford, A. F., Taylor, F. B., Sheena, R.: Inhibition of the fibrinogen-plasmin reaction by ω-aminocarboxylic acids and alkylamines. Biochim. biophys. Acta (Amst.) **92**, 328 (1964)

Bilinski, T., Loch, T., Zakrzewski, K.: Studies on streptokinase. Purification and some molecular properties. Acta biochim. pol. **15**, 123 (1968)

Birktoft, J. J., Blow, D. M., Henderson, R., Steitz, T. A.: The structure of α-chymotrypsin. Phil. Trans. B **257**, 67 (1970)

Blatt, W. F., Segal, H., Gray, J. L.: Purification of streptokinase and human plasmin and their interaction. Thrombos. Diathes. haemorrh. (Stuttg.) **11**, 393 (1964)

Blombäck, B., Blombäck, M.: Purification of human and bovine fibrinogen. Ark. Kemi **10**, 415 (1957)

Blombäck, B., Blombäck, M., Hessel, B., Iwanaga, S.: Structure of N-terminal fragments of fibrinogen and specificity of thrombin. Nature (Lond.) **215**, 1445 (1967)

Brockway, W. J., Castellino, F. J.: The mechanism of the inhibition of plasmin activity by ε-aminocaproic acid. J. biol. Chem. **246**, 4641 (1971)

Brockway, W. J., Castellino, F. J.: Measurement of the binding of antifibrinolytic amino acids to various plasminogens. Arch. Biochem. **151**, 194 (1972)

Brockway, W. J., Castellino, F. J.: A characterization of native streptokinase and altered streptokinase isolated from a human plasminogen activator complex. Biochemistry **13**, 1063 (1974)

Bruner-Lorand, J., Pilkington, T. R. E., Lorand, L.: Inhibitors of fibrin cross-linking: relevance for thrombolysis. Nature (Lond.) **210**, 1273 (1966)

Buck, F. F., Boggiano, E.: Interaction of streptokinase and human plasminogen. VI. Function of the streptokinase moiety in the activator complex. J. biol. Chem. **246**, 2091 (1971)

Buck, F. F., Hummel, B. C. W., de Renzo, E. C.: Interaction of streptokinase and human plasminogen. V. Studies on the nature and mechanism of formation of the enzymatic site of the activator complex. J. biol. Chem. **243**, 3648 (1968)

Buck, F. F., de Renzo, F. C.: Naphthyl-acetate-esterase activity of streptokinase preparations. Biochim. biophys. Acta (Amst.) **89**, 348 (1964)

Burges, R. A., Brammer, K. W., Coombes, J. D.: Molecular weight of urokinase. Nature (Lond.) **208**, 894 (1965)

Capet-Antonini, F. C., Grimard, M., Tamenasse, J.: Properties of two types of solid-phase urokinase preparations. Thrombos. Res. **2**, 479 (1973)

Cartwright, T.: Partial purification of a specific plasminogen activator from porcine parotid glands. Thrombos. Diathes. haemorrh. (Stuttg.) **31**, 403 (1974)

Castellino, F. J., Brockway, W. J., Thomas, J. K., Liao, H., Rawitch, A. B.: Rotational diffusion analysis of the conformational alterations produced in plasminogen by certain antifibrinolytic amino acids. Biochemistry **12**, 2787 (1973 a)

Castellino, F. J., Siefring, G. E., Sodetz, J. M., Bretthauer, R. K.: Amino terminal amino acid sequences and carbohydrate of the two major forms of rabbit plasminogen. Biochem. Biophys. Res. Commun. **53**, 845 (1973 b)

Celander, D. R., Guest, M. M.: The biochemistry and physiology of urokinase. Amer. J. Cardiol. **6**, 409 (1960)

Celander, D. R., Langlinais, R. P., Guest, M. M.: The application of foam technique to the partial purification of an urine activator of plasma profibrinolysin. Arch. Biochem. **55**, 286 (1955)

Chan, J. Y. S., Mertz, E. T.: Studies on plasminogen. IV. Alteration of bovine and human plasminogens during isolation. Canad. J. Biochem. **44**, 469 (1966 a)

Chan, J. Y. S., Mertz, E. T.: Studies on plasminogen. V. Purification of bovine and human plasminogens by Sephadex chromatography. Canad. J. Biochem. **44**, 475 (1966 b)

Chan, J. Y. S., Mertz, E. T.: Studies on plasminogen. VI. Activation products of bovine and human plasminogens. Canad. J. Biochem. **44**, 487 (1966 c)

Chase, T., Shaw, E.: Comparison of the esterase activities of trypsin, plasmin, and thrombin on guanidinobenzoate esters. Titration of the enzymes. Biochemistry **8**, 2212 (1969)

Chen, R., Doolittle, R. F.: γ-γ-Cross-linking sites in human and bovine fibrin. Biochemistry **10**, 4486 (1971)

Chesterman, C. N., Allington, M. J., Sharp, A. A.: Relation of plasminogen activator to fibrin. Nature (Lond.) **238**, 15 (1972)

Chesterman, C. N., Cederholm-Williams, S. A., Allington, M. J., Sharp, A. A.: The degradation of streptokinase during the production of plasminogen activator. Thrombos. Res. **5**, 413 (1974)

Christensen, L. R.: Streptococcal fibrinolysis: a proteolytic reaction due to a serum enzyme activated by streptococcal fibrinolysin. J. gen. Physiol. **28**, 363 (1945)

Christensen, L. R.: Methods for measuring the activity of components of the streptococcal fibrinolytic system, and streptococcal desoxyribonuclease. J. clin. Invest. **28**, 163 (1949)

Christensen, L. R., McLeod, C. M.: A proteolytic enzyme of serum: characterization, activation and reaction with inhibitors. J. gen. Physiol. **28**, 559 (1945)

Christensen, L. R., Smith, D. H.: Plasminogen purification by acid extraction. Proc. Soc. exp. Biol. (N. Y.) **74**, 840 (1950)

Christman, J. K., Acs, G.: Purification and characterization of a cellular fibrinolytic factor associated with oncogenic transformation: The plasminogen activator from SV-40-transformed hamster cells. Biochim. biophys. Acta (Amst.) **340**, 339 (1974)

Claeys, H., Amery, A., Verhaege, R.: Proteolytic activity of the activator produced by streptokinase in human plasma. Thrombos. Diathes. haemorrh. (Stuttg.) **26**, 88 (1971)

Claeys, H., Molla, A., Verstraete, M.: Conversion of the NH_2-terminal glutamic acid to NH_2-terminal lysine human plasminogen by plasmin. Thrombos. Res. **3**, 515 (1973)

Clayes, H., Vermylen, J.: Physico-chemical and proenzyme properties of NH_2-terminal glutamic acid and NH_2-terminal lysine human plasminogen. Biochim. biophys. Acta (Amst.) **342**, 351 (1974)

Cliffton, E. E., Cannamela, D. A.: Proteolytic and fibrinolytic activity of serum. Activation by streptokinase and staphylokinase indicating dissimilarities of enzymes. Blood **8**, 554 (1953)

Coats, E. A.: Comparative inhibition of thrombin, plasmin, trypsin, and complement by benzamidines using substituent constants and regression analysis. J. med. Chem. **16**, 1102 (1973)

Cole, E. R.: Hydrolysis of L-histidine methyl ester. II. Activity of various proteolytic enzymes with
special reference to activators of plasminogen. Thrombos. Diathes. haemorrh. (Stuttg.) **19**,
334 (1968)

Cole, E. R., Olwin, J. H.: Hydrolysis of L-histidine methyl ester by proteolytic enzymes with particular reference to thrombin and plasminogen activators. Thrombos. Diathes. haemorrh.
(Stuttg.) **18**, 304 (1967)

Colgan, J., Gates, E., Miller, L. L.: Serum and urinary fibrinolytic activity related to the hemorrhagic diathesis in irradiated dogs. J. exp. Med. **95**, 531 (1952)

Collen, D., de Mayer, L.: Molecular biology of human plasminogen. I. Physicochemical properties and microheterogeneity. Thrombos. Diathes. haemorrh. (Stuttg.) **34**, 396 (1975)

Collen, D., Verstraete, M.: Molecular biology of human plasminogen II. Metabolism in physiological and some pathological conditions in man. Thrombos. Diathes. haemorrh. (Stuttg.) **34**,
403 (1975)

Colman, R. W.: Activation of plasminogen by human plasma kallikrein. Biochem. biophys. Res.
Commun. **35**, 273 (1969)

Coughlin, W. R.: Circulating plasminogen activator. Ph. D. Thesis, Yale University, 1966

Dastre, A.: Fibrinolyse dans le sang. Arch. physiol. (Paris) **5**, 661 (1893)

Davidson, F. M.: The activation of plasminogen by staphylokinase: Comparison with streptokinase. Biochem. J. **76**, 56 (1960a)

Davidson, F. M.: Activation of plasminogen by staphylokinase. Nature (Lond.) **185**, 626 (1960b)

Davies, M. C., Englert, M. E.: Physical properties of highly purified human plasminogen. J. biol.
Chem. **235**, 1011 (1960)

Davies, M. C., Englert, M. E., de Renzo, E. C.: Interaction of streptokinase and human plasminogen. I. Combining of streptokinase and plasminogen observed in the ultracentrifuge under a
variety of experimental conditions. J. biol. Chem. **239**, 2651 (1964)

Delezenne, C., Pozerski, E.: Action du sèrum sanguin sur la gélatine, en présence du chloroforme.
C. R. Soc. Biol. (Paris) **55**, 327 (1903)

Denis, P. S.: Essai sur l'Application de la Chimie à l'Etude Physiologique du Sang de l'Homme, et
à l'Etude Physiologique, Hygienique et Thérapeutique des Maladies de Cette Humeur. Paris:
Bechet, Jr. 1838

Denys, J., de Marbaix, H.: Les peptonisations provoqués par le chloroforme. Cellule **5**, 197 (1889)

Derechin, M.: Purification of human plasminogen. Biochem. J. **82**, 241 (1962)

Derechin, M., Johnson, P., Szuchet, S.: Further studies with human plasminogen. Biochem. J. **84**,
336 (1962)

Deutsch, E., Elsner, P.: The mechanism of fibrinolysis induced by bacterial pyrogens. Thrombos.
Diathes. haemorrh. (Stuttg.) **3**, 286 (1959)

Deutsch, D. G., Mertz, E. T.: Plasminogen: purification from human plasma by affinity chromatography. Science **170**, 1095 (1970)

Deutsch, D. G., Mertz, E. T.: Activation of plasminogen with insoluble derivatives of urokinase. J.
Med. (Basel) **3**, 224 (1972)

Dillon, H. C., Jr., Wannamaker, L. W.: Physical and immunological differences among streptoki-
nases. J. exp. Med. **121**, 351 (1965)

Doleschel, W.: Isolierung einer dritten humanen Urokinase (S_0-Typ). Wien. klin. Wschr. **87**, 282
(1975)

Doleschel, W., Auerswald, W.: Determination of molecular weights of uroprotein fraction with
urokinase activity by means of molecular sieving. Med. Pharmacol. exp. (Basel) **16**, 225 (1967)

Duckert, F.: Urokinase. In: Current problems in clinical biochemistry. II: Enzymes in urine and
kidney. Bern-Stuttgart: Huber 1968

Engel, A., Alexander, B., Pechet, L.: Activation of trypsinogen and plasminogen by thrombin
preparations. Biochemistry **5**, 1543 (1966)

Epstein, M. D., Beller, F. K., Douglas, G. W.: Kidney tissue activator of fibrinolyses in relation to
pregnancy. Obstet. Gynec. **32**, 494 (1968)

Fearnley, G. R.: Fibrinolysis. London: Edward Arnold Publishers 1965

Fearnley, G. R., Ferguson, J.: Arteriovenous differences in natural fibrinolysis. Lancet 1957 II,
1040

Fearnley, G. R., Tweed, J. M.: An active fibrinolytic enzyme in plasma of normal people with observations on inhibition associated with the presence of calcium. Clin. Sci. **12**, 81 (1953)

Feddersen, C., Gormsen, J.: Plasmin digestion of stabilized and nonstabilized fibrin illustrated by immunoelectrophoresis and hemagglutination inhibition immunoassays. Scand. J. Haematol. **8**, 461 (1971a)

Feddersen, C., Gormsen, J.: Plasmin digestion of stabilized and nonstabilized fibrin illustrated by pH-stat titration and thrombelastography. Scand. J. clin. Lab. Invest. **27**, 195 (1971b)

Fletcher, A. P., Alkjaersig, N., Sherry, S.: The maintenance of a sustained thrombolytic state in man. I. Induction and effects. J. clin. Invest. **38**, 1096 (1959)

Fletcher, A. P., Alkjaersig, N., Sherry, S.: Pathogenesis of the coagulation defect developing during pathological plasma proteolytic ("fibrinolytic") states. I. The significance of fibrinogen proteolysis and circulating fibrinogen breakdown products. J. clin. Invest. **41**, 896 (1962)

Fletcher, A. P., Alkjaersig, N., Sherry, S., Genton, E., Hirsh, J., Bachmann, F.: The development of urokinase as a thrombolytic agent. Maintenance of a sustained thrombolytic state in man by its intravenous infusion. J. Lab. clin. Med. **65**, 713 (1965)

Gaffney, P. J., Brasher, M.: Subunit structure of the plasmin-induced degradation products of crosslinked fibrin. Biochim. biophys. Acta (Amst.) **295**, 308 (1973)

Gajewski, J., Markus, G.: A new method for plasminogen standardization. Thrombos. Diathes. haemorrh. (Stuttg.) **20**, 548 (1968)

Geratz, J. D.: Inhibition of thrombin, plasmin and plasminogen activation by amidino compounds. Thrombos. Diathes. haemorrh. (Stuttg.) **23**, 486 (1970)

Geratz, J. D.: Inhibition of coagulation and fibrinolysis by aromatic amidino compounds. Thrombos. Diathes. haemorrh. (Stuttg.) **25**, 391 (1971)

Geratz, J. D.: Kinetic aspects of the irreversible inhibition of trypsin and related enzymes by p-[m-(-m-fluorosulfonylphenylureido)-phenoxyethoxy]-benzamidine. FEBS-Letters **20**, 294 (1972)

Geratz, J. D.: Structure-activity relationships for the inhibition of plasmin and plasminogen activation by aromatic diamidines and a study of the effect of plasma proteins on the inhibition process. Thrombos. Diathes. haemorrh. (Stuttg.) **29**, 154 (1973)

Geratz, J. D., Cheng, M. C.-F.: The inhibition of urokinase by aromatic diamidines. Thrombos. Diathes. haemorrh. (Stuttg.) **33**, 230 (1975)

Glas, P., Astrup, T.: Thromboplastin and plasminogen activator in tissues of the rabbit. Amer. J. Physiol. **219**, 1140 (1970)

Gormsen, J., Feddersen, C.: Degradation of stabilized and nonstabilized fibrin clots by plasmin. Immunological study. Ann. N. Y. Acad. Sci. **202**, 329 (1972)

Gormsen, J., Fletcher, A. P., Alkjaersig, N., Sherry, S.: Enzymic lysis of plasma clots: The influence of fibrin stabilization on lysis rates. Arch. Biochem. **120**, 654 (1967)

Groskopf, W. R., Hsieh, B., Summaria, L., Robbins, K. C.: The specificity of human plasmin on the B-chain of oxidized bovine insulin. Biochim. biophys. Acta (Amst.) **168**, 376 (1968)

Groskopf, W. R., Hsieh, B., Summaria, L., Robbins, K. C.: Studies on the active center of human plasmin. The serine and histidine residue. J. biol. Chem. **244**, 359 (1969a)

Groskopf, W. R., Summaria, L., Robbins, K. C.: Studies on the active center of human plasmin. Partial amino acid sequence of a peptide containing the active center serine residue. J. biol. Chem. **244**, 3590 (1969b)

Guest, M. M., Celander, D. R.: Urokinase: physiologic activator of profibrinolysin. Tex. Rep. Biol. Med. **19**, 89 (1961)

Gutmann, M., Rimon, A.: Studies on the activator of plasminogen. II. The nature of the proactivator. Canad. J. Biochem. **42**, 1339 (1964)

Hagan, J. J., Ablondi, F. B., de Renzo, E. C.: Purification and biochemical properties of human plasminogen. J. biol. Chem. **235**, 1005 (1960)

Hartley, B. S.: Amino-acid sequence of bovine chymotrypsinogen A. Nature (Lond.) **201**, 1284 (1964)

Hartley, B. S.: Homologies in serine proteinases. Phil. Trans. B **257**, 77 (1970)

Hayes, M. L., Brethauer, R. K., Castellino, F. J.: Carbohydrate compositions of the rabbit plasminogen isoenzymes. Arch. Biochem. **171**, 651 (1975)

Heberlein, P. J., Barnhart, M. I.: Canine plasminogen: Purification and demonstration of multimolecular forms. Biochim. biophys. Acta (Amst.) **168**, 195 (1968)

Heimburger, N.: Neuere Erkenntnisse über den Mechanismus der Fibrinolyse unter besonderer Berücksichtigung der Fibrinagar-Elektrophorese. Behringwerk-Mitt. Heft **41**, 84 (1962)

Heimburger, N.: Basis mechanism of action of streptokinase and urokinase. Thrombos. Diathes. haemorrh. (Stuttg.), Suppl. **47**, 21 (1971)

Heimburger, N., Schwick, H. G.: Beitrag zur Charakterisierung des durch Streptokinase induzierten Aktivators. Arzneimittel-Forsch. **21**, 1439 (1971)

Henderson, K. W., Nußbaum, M.: Mechanism of enhanced streptokinase-induced clot lysis following in vitro Factor-XIII inactivation. Brit. J. Haemat. **17**, 445 (1969)

Henderson, R.: Structure of crystalline α-chymotrypsin. IV. The structure of indoleacryloyl-α-chymotrypsin and its relevance to the hydrolytic mechanism of the enzyme. J. molec. Biol. **54**, 341 (1970)

Henderson, R., Wright, C. S., Hess, G. P., Blow, D. M.: α-Chymotrypsin: What can we learn about catalysis from X-ray diffraction. Cold Spr. Harb. Symp. quant. Biol. **36**, 63 (1971)

Hijikata, A., Fujimoto, K., Kitaguchie, H., Okamoto, S.: Some properties of the tissue plasminogen activator from the pig heart. Thrombos. Res. **4**, 731 (1974)

Höpfinger, L. M., Mertz, E. T.: Studies on plasminogen. VII. Mechanism of activation of bovine plasminogen. Canad. J. Biochem. **47**, 909 (1969)

Hummel, B. C. W., Buck, F. F., de Renzo, E. C.: Interaction of streptokinase and human plasminogen. III. Plasmin and activator activities in reaction mixtures of streptokinase and human plasminogen or human plasmin of various molar ratios. J. biol. Chem. **241**, 347 (1966)

Iwamoto, M., Abiko, Y., Shimizu, M.: Plasminogen-plasmin system. III. Kinetics of plasminogen activation and inhibition of plasminogen-plasmin system by some synthetic inhibitors. J. Biochem. (Tokyo) **64**, 759 (1968)

Iwanaga, S., Wallén, P., Gröndahl, N. J., Henschen, A., Blombäck, B.: Isolation and characterization of N-terminal fragments obtained by plasmin digestion of human fibrinogen. Biochim. biophys. Acta (Amst.) **147**, 606 (1967)

Jackson, H. D., Mertz, E. T.: Activation of bovine plasminogen by trypsin. Proc. Soc. exp. Biol. (N. Y.) **86**, 827 (1954)

Jacobsson, K.: Activation of plasminogen with trypsin. Acta chem. scand. **7**, 430 (1953)

Johnson, A. J., Kline, D. L., Alkjaersig, N.: Assay methods and standard preparations for plasmin, plasminogen and urokinase in purified systems 1967–1968. Thrombos. Diathes. haemorrh. (Stuttg.) **21**, 259 (1969)

Kaulla, K. N. von: Urine adsorbate with fibrinolytic and thromboplastic properties. J. Lab. clin. Med. **44**, 944 (1954)

Kaulla, K. N. von: Methods for preparation of purified human thromboplastin and fibrinolysokinase from urine. Acta haematol. (Basel) **16**, 315 (1956a)

Kaulla, K. N. von: Extraction and concentration of thromboplastic material from human urine. Proc. Soc. exp. Biol. (N. Y.) **91**, 543 (1956b)

Kaulla, K. N. von, Shettles, L. B.: Relationship between human seminal fluid and the fibrinolytic system. Proc. Soc. exp. Biol. (N. Y.) **83**, 692 (1953)

Kaulla, K. N. von, Swan, H.: Clotting deviations in man during cardiac bypass; fibrinolysis and circulating anticoagulant. J. thorac. Cardiovasc. Surg. **36**, 519 (1958)

Kawano, T., Morimoto, K., Uemura, Y.: Urokinase inhibitor in human placenta. Nature (Lond.) **217**, 253 (1968)

Kawano, T., Morimoto, K., Uemura, Y.: Partial purification and properties of urokinase inhibitor from human placenta. J. Biochem. (Tokyo) **67**, 333 (1970)

Kawano, T., Uemura, Y.: Inhibition of tissue activator by urokinase inhibitor. Thrombos. Diathes. haemorrh. (Stuttg.) **25**, 129 (1971)

Kickhöfen, G., Struwe, F. E., Bramesfeld, B., Westphal, O.: Über einige Beobachtungen am Uropepsinogen und Plasminogen-Aktivator des menschlichen Urins. Biochem. Z. **330**, 467 (1958)

Kjeldgaard, N. O., Ploug, J.: Urokinase an activator of plasminogen from human urine. II. Mechanism of plasminogen activation. Biochim. biophys. Acta (Amst.) **24**, 283 (1957)

Kline, D. L.: The purification and crystallization of plasminogen (profibrinolysin). J. biol. Chem. **204**, 904 (1953)

Kline, D. L.: Caseinolytic techniques. In: Thrombosis and Bleeding Disorders. New York-London: Academic Press 1971

Kline, D. L., Fishman, J. B.: Improved procedure for the isolation of human plasminogen. J. biol. Chem. **236**, 3232 (1961 a)

Kline, D. L., Fihsman, J. B.: Proactivator function of human plasmin as shown by lysine esterase assay. J. biol. Chem. **236**, 2807 (1961 b)

Kline, D. L., Ts'ao, C.-H.: The direct activation of human plasminogen by streptokinase. Thrombos. Diathes. hacmorrh. (Stuttg.) **18**, 288 (1967)

Kline, D. L., Ts'ao, C.-H.: Activation of human plasminogen by streptokinase in absence of plasmin-SK activator. Amer. J. physiol. **220**, 440 (1971)

Kok, P., Astrup, T.: Some comparative studies on tissue activator and urokinase. Thrombos. Diathes. haemorrh. (Stuttg.) **18**, 294 (1967)

Kok, P., Astrup, T.: Isolation and purification of a tissue activator and its comparison with urokinase. Biochemistry **8**, 79 (1969)

Konttinen, Y. P.: Fibrinolysis. Chemistry, physiology, pathology and clinics. Tampere: Star 1968

Kopitar, M., Stegnar, M., Accetto, B., Lebez, D.: Isolation and characterization of plasminogen activator from pig leukocytes. Thrombos. Diathes. haemorrh. (Stuttg.) **31**, 72 (1974)

Kosow, D. P.: Kinetic mechanism of the activation of human plasminogen by streptokinase. Biochemistry **14**, 4459 (1975)

Kowalski, E., Kopeć, M., Latallo, Z., Rozkowski, S., Sendys, N.: On the occurrence of a plasminogen-like substance in human tissues. Blood **8**, 436 (1958)

Kowalski, E., Latallo, Z., Niewiarowski, S.: Untersuchungen über die Aktivierung des Plasminogens und die Inaktivierung des Plasmins. Folia haemat. (Lpz.) **75**, 225 (1957)

Krieger, M., Kay, L. M., Stroud, R. M.: Structure and specific binding of trypsin: Comparison of inhibited derivatives and a model for substrate binding. J. molec. Biol. **83**, 209 (1974)

Kucinski, C. S., Fletcher, A. P., Sherry, S.: Effect of urokinase antiserum on plasminogen activators: Demonstration of immunologic dissimilarity between plasma plasminogen activator and urokinase. J. clin. Invest. **47**, 1238 (1968)

Kwaan, H. C., Fischer, S.: Localization of fibrinolytic activity in kidney tissues. Fed. Proc. **24**, 387 (1965)

Kwaan, H. C., Lai, K. S., McFadzean, A. J. S.: Lysokinase activity in ascitic fluid. Lancet **1960 I**, 1327

Laake, K., Venneröd, A. M.: Factor XII-induced fibrinolysis: Studies on the separation of prekallikrein, plasminogen proactivator, and factor XI in human plasma. Thrombos. Res. **4**, 285 (1974)

Lack, C. H., Ali, S. Y.: Tissue activator of plasminogen. Nature (Lond.) **201**, 1030 (1964)

Lack, C. H., Glanville, K. L. A.: Staphylokinase. In: Methods in enzymology. XIX: Proteolytic enzymes. New York-London: Academic Press 1970

Ladehoff, A. A.: The content of plasminogen activator in the human urinary tract. Scand. J. clin. Lab. Invest. **12**, 136 (1960)

Landmann, H.: Vergleichende Untersuchungen über Antifibrinolytika. Folia haemat. (Lpz.) **87**, 106 (1967)

Landmann, H.: Synthetische Hemmstoffe des Plasmins. Haematologia (Budapest), Suppl. **1**, 169 (1970)

Landmann, H.: Studies on the mechanism of action of synthetic antifibrinolytics. A comparison with the action of derivatives of benzamidine on the fibrinolytic process. Thrombos. Diathes. haemorrh. (Stuttg.) **29**, 253 (1973)

Landmann, H., Markwardt, F.: Irreversible synthetische Inhibitoren der Urokinase. Experientia (Basel) **26**, 145 (1970)

Lassen, M.: The esterase activity of the fibrinolytic system. Biochem. J. **69**, 360 (1958)

Lassen, M.: Evidence of the different nature of human plasminogen and proactivator. Acta chem. scand. **13**, 1064 (1959 a)

Lassen, M.: The reaction between streptokinase and human plasma. Acta chem. scand. **13**, 1332 (1959 b)

Latallo, Z. S., Teisseyre, E.: Preliminary experience with a new chromogenic substrate in studies on blood coagulation and fibrinolysis. 9th FEBS-Meeting, Abstr. f 3 a 6, Budapest 1974

Lauritsen, O. S.: Urokinase inhibitor in human plasma. Scand. J. clin. Lab. Invest. **22**, 314 (1968)

Lesuk, A., Terminiello, L., Traver, J. H.: Crystalline human urokinase: Some properties. Science **147**, 880 (1965)

LesukA., Terminiello, L., Traver, J. H., Groff, J. L.: Biochemical and biophysical studies of human urokinase. Thrombos. Diathes. haemorrh. (Stuttg.) **18**, 293 (1967a)

Lesuk, A., Terminiello, L., Traver, J. H., Groff, J. L.: Proteolytic degradation of human urokinase to active fragments. Fed. Proc. **26**, 647 (1967b)

Lewis, J. H., Ferguson, J. H.: Activation of dog serum profibrinolysin by staphylokinase. Amer. J. Physiol. **166**, 594 (1951)

Lewis, J. H., Ferguson, J. H.: Activation of profibrinolysin by trypsin. Amer. J. Physiol. **170**, 636 (1952)

Ling, C.-M., Summaria, L., Robbins, K. C.: Mechanism of formation of bovine plasminogen activator from human plasmin. J. biol. Chem. **240**, 4213 (1965)

Ling, C.-M., Summaria, L., Robbins, K. C.: Isolation and characterization of bovine plasminogen activator from a human plasminogen-streptokinase mixture. J. biol. Chem. **242**, 1419 (1967)

Lorand, L., Condit, E. V.: Ester hydrolysis by urokinase. Biochemistry **4**, 265 (1965)

Lorand, L., Jacobsen, A.: Accelerated lysis of blood clots. Nature (Lond.) **195**, 911 (1962)

Lorand, L., Mozen, M. M.: Ester hydrolyzing activity of urokinase preparations. Nature (Lond.) **201**, 392 (1964)

Lorand, L., Nilsson, J. G. L.: Molecular approach for designing inhibitors to enzymes involved in blood clotting. In: Drug Design. III. New York-London: Academic Press 1971

Lundquist, F., Thorsteinson, T., Buus, O.: Purification and properties of some enzymes in human seminal plasma. Biochem. J. **59**, 59 (1955)

MacFarlane, R. G.: The development of ideas on fibrinolysis. Brit. med. Bull. **20**, 173 (1964)

MacFarlane, R. G., Pilling, J.: Fibrinolytic activity of normal urine. Nature (Lond.) **159**, 779 (1947)

Magnusson, S., Sottrup-Jensen, L., Claeys, H., Zajdel, M., Petersen, T. E.: Complete primary structure of prothrombin, partial primary structures of plasminogen and hirudin. 5th Congr. Int. Soc. Thromb. Haemostasis, Abstr. 200, Paris 1975a

Magnusson, S., Sottrup-Jensen, L., Claeys, H., Zajdel, M., Petersen, T. E.: Extensive sequence homology in the nonserine protease parts of prothrombin and plasminogen. A general structure common to large zymogens? 10th FEBS-Meeting. Abstr. 904, Paris 1975b

Marder, V. J., Sherry, S.: Fibrinolysis. In: Pathophysiology. Philadelphia: J. B. Lippincott 1972

Mares-Guia, M., Shaw, E.: Studies on the active center of trypsin. The binding of amidines and guanidines as models of substrate side chain. J. biol. Chem. **240**, 1579 (1965)

Markus, G., Ambrus, C. M.: On the formation of different types of plasmin by streptokinase activation. J. biol. Chem. **235**, 1673 (1960)

Markus, G., Werkheiser, W. C.: The interaction of streptokinase with plasminogen. I. Functional properties of the activated enzyme. J. biol. Chem. **239**, 2637 (1964)

Markwardt, F., Landmann, H.: Blutgerinnungshemmende Proteine, Peptide und Aminosäurederivate. In: Handbuch der experimentellen Pharmakologie, Vol. XXVII. Berlin-Heidelberg-New York: Springer 1971

Markwardt, F., Landmann, H., Klöcking, H.-P.: Fibrinolytika und Antifibrinolytika. Jena: Fischer 1972a

Markwardt, F., Landmann, H., Walsmann, P.: Comparative studies on the inhibition of trypsin, plasmin, and thrombin by derivatives of benzylamine and benzamidine. Europ. J. Biochem. **6**, 502 (1968)

Markwardt, F., Wagner, G., Walsmann, P., Horn, H., Stürzebecher, J.: Inhibition of trypsin and thrombin by amidinophenyl esters of aromatic carboxylic acids. Acta biol. med. germ. **28**, K 19 (1972b)

Markwardt, F., Walsmann, P., Landmann, H.: Hemmung der Thrombin-, Plasmin- und Trypsinwirkung durch Alkyl- und Alkoxybenzamidine. Pharmazie **25**, 551 (1970b)

Markwardt, F., Richter, M., Walsmann, P., Landmann, H.: The inhibition of trypsin, plasmin, and thrombin by benzyl 4-guanidino benzoate and 4'-nitrobenzyl 4-guanidinobenzoate. FEBS-Letters **8**, 170 (1970a)

Markwardt, F., Walsmann, P., Richter, M., Klöcking, H.-P., Drawert, J., Landmann, H.: Aminoalkylbenzolsulfofluoride als Fermentinhibitoren. Pharmazie **26**, 401 (1971)

Markwardt, F., Walsmann, P., Stürzebecher, J., Landmann, H., Wagner, G.: Synthetische Inhibitoren von Serinproteinasen. 1. Mitteilung: Über die Hemmung von Trypsin, Plasmin und Thrombin durch Ester der Amidino- und Guanidinobenzoesäure. Pharmazie **28**, 326 (1973)

McCall, D. C., Kline, D. L.: Mechanism of action and some properties of a tissue activator of plasminogen. Thrombos. Diathes. haemorrh. (Stuttg.) **14**, 116 (1965)

McClintock, D. K., Bell, P. H.: The mechanism of activation of human plasminogen by streptokinase. Biochem. Biophys. Res. Commun. **43**, 694 (1971)

McClintock, D. K., Englert, M. E., Dziobkowski, C., Snedeker, E. H., Bell, P. H.: Two distinct pathways of the streptokinase-mediated activation of highly purified human plasminogen. Biochemistry **13**, 5334 (1974)

McConnel, D., Johnston, J. G., Young, I., Holemans, R.: Localization of plasminogen activator in kidney. Lab. Invest. **15**, 980 (1966)

McKee, P. A., Lemmon, W. B., Hampton, J. W.: Streptokinase and urokinase activation of human, chimpanzee and baboon plasminogen. Thrombos. Diathes. haemorrh. (Stuttg.) **26**, 512 (1971)

Mihara, H., Fujii, T., Okamoto, S.: Fibrinolytic activity of cerebro-spinal fluid and the development of artificial cerebral haematomas in dogs. Thrombos. Diathes. haemorrh. (Stuttg.) **21**, 294 (1969)

Milstone, H.: A factor in normal human blood which participates in streptococcal fibrinolysis. J. Immunol. **42**, 109 (1941)

Morgan, F. J., Henschen, A.: The structure of streptokinase. I. Cyanogen bromide fragmentation, amino acid composition and partial amino acid sequences. Biochim. biophys. Acta (Amst.) **181**, 93 (1969)

Mosesson, W. M.: The preparation of human fibrinogen free of plasminogen. Biochim. biophys. Acta (Amst.) **57**, 204 (1962)

Mounter, L. A., Mounter, M. E.: The inhibition of hydrolytic enzymes by organophosphorous compounds. J. biol. Chem. **238**, 1079 (1963)

Mounter, L. A., Shipley, B. A.: The inhibition of plasmin by toxic phosphorous compounds. J. biol. Chem. **231**, 855 (1958)

Movat, H. Z., Burrowes, C. E., Soltay, M. J., Takeuchi, Y., Habal, F., Özge-Anwar, A. H.: Interrelation between the clotting, fibrinolytic, and kinin systems of human plasma. Protides Biol. Fluids, Proc. Colloq. **20**, 315 (1972)

Müllertz, S.: Formation and properties of the activator of plasminogen and of human and bovine plasmin. Biochem. J. **61**, 424 (1955)

Müllertz, S.: Mechanism of activation and effect of plasmin in blood. Acta physiol. Scand. **38**, Suppl. 130 (1956)

Müllertz, S.: Activation of plasminogen. Ann. N.Y. Acad. Sci. **68**, 38 (1957)

Müllertz, S.: Different molecular forms of plasminogen and plasmin produced by urokinase in human plasma and their relation to protease inhibitors and lysis of fibrinogen and fibrin. Biochem. J. **143**, 273 (1974)

Muramatu, M., Fujii, S.: Inhibitory effects of ω-guanidino acid esters on trypsin, plasmin, thrombin and plasma kallikrein. J. Biochem. (Tokyo) **64**, 807 (1968)

Muramatu, M., Fujii, S.: Inhibitory effects of ω-amino acid esters on the activity of trypsin, plasmin and thrombin. J. Biochem. (Tokyo) **65**, 17 (1969)

Muramatu, M., Fujii, S.: Inhibitory effects of ω-guanidino acid esters on trypsin, plasmin, plasma kallikrein and thrombin. Biochim. biophys. Acta (Amst.) **242**, 203 (1971)

Muramatu, M., Fujii, S.: Inhibitory effects of ω-guanidino acid esters on trypsin, plasmin, plasma kallikrein and thrombin. Biochim. biophys. Acta (Amst.) **268**, 221 (1972)

Muramatu, M., Hayakumo, Y., Fujii, S.: Synthetic inhibitors of trypsin, plasmin, and chymotrypsin. J. Biochem. (Tokyo) **62**, 408 (1967)

Muramatu, M., Hayakumo, Y., Onishi, T., Sato, T., Fujii, S.: Comparison of human plasmin formed by activation with trace and large amounts of streptokinase. J. Biochem. (Tokyo) **65**, 329 (1969)

Muramatu, M., Onishi, T., Makino, S., Fujii, S., Yamamura, Y.: Inhibition of caseinolytic activity of plasmin by various synthetic inhibitors. J. Biochem. (Tokyo) **57**, 402 (1965a)

Muramatu, M., Onishi, T., Makino, S., Fujii, S., Yamamura, Y.: Inhibition of fibrinolytic activity of plasmin by various synthetic inhibitors. J. Biochem. (Tokyo) **57**, 450 (1965b)

Nagamatsu, A., Hayashida, T.: Hydrolysis of lysine peptides by plasmin. Chem. pharm. Bull. **11**, 2680 (1974)

Nagamatsu, A., Okuma, T., Hayashida, T., Yamamura, Y.: Studies on antiplasminic agents. Chem. Pharm. Bull. **16**, 211 (1968)

Nagamatsu, A., Okuma, T., Watanabe, M., Yamamura, Y.: The inhibition of plasmin by some amino acid derivatives. J. Biochem. (Tokyo) **54**, 491 (1963)

Nagasawa, S., Suzuki, T.: The N-terminal sequence of the light chain derivative of bovine plasmin. Biochem. biophys. Res. Commun. **41**, 562 (1970)

Nanninga, L. B.: Rapid determination of profibrinolysin (plasminogen) in plasma. Thrombos. Diathes. haemorrh. (Stuttg.) **17**, 8 (1967)

Nanninga, L. B.: Molar concentrations of fibrinolytic components, especially free fibrinolysin, in vivo. Thrombos. Diathes. haemorrh. (Stuttg.) **33**, 244 (1975)

Nanninga, L. B., Guest, M. M.: Activity-pH relationship and Michaelis constants during activation of profibrinolysin and during fibrinogenolysis. Thrombos. Diathes. haemorrh. (Stuttg.) **19**, 492 (1968)

Nolf, P.: Contribution à l'étude de la coagulation du sang. (5e memoire) La fibrinolyse. Arch. int. Physiol. **6**, 306 (1908)

Ogston, D., Ogston, C. M., Ratnoff, O. D., Forbes, C. D.: Studies on a complex mechanism for the activation of plasminogen by kaolin and by chloroform. The participation of Hageman factor and additional cofactors. J. clin. Invest. **48**, 1786 (1969)

Okamoto, S., Hijikata, A., Kinjo, K., Kikumoto, R., Ohkubo, K., Tonomura, S., Tamao, Y.: A novel series of synthetic thrombin inhibitors having extremely potent and highly selective action. Kobe J. med. Sci. **21**, 43 (1975)

Okamoto, U., Yamamoto, J.: A smaller molecule Sk-reactive protein (plasminogen-proactivator) derived from the macromolecule of human plasma fraction I. 5th Congr. Int. Soc. Thromb. Haemostatis, Abstr. 11, Paris 1975

Okano, A., Inaoka, M., Funabashi, S., Iwamoto, M., Isoda, S., Moroi, R., Abiko, Y., Hirata, M.: Medicinal chemical studies on antiplasmin drugs. 4. Chemical modification of trans-4-aminomethylcyclohexanecarboxylic acid and its effect on antiplasmin activity. J. med. Chem. **15**, 247 (1972)

Oshiba, S., Ariga, T.: Purification and characterization of bilokinase, a biliary plasminogen activator. 5th Congr. Int. Soc. Thromb. Haemostasis, Abstr. 13, Paris 1975

Oshiba, S., Hata, S., Okamoto, S.: Plasminogen activator in mammalian bile. Jap. J. Physiol. **19**, 212 (1968)

Painter, R. H., Charles, A. F.: Characterization of a soluble plasminogen activator from kidney cell cultures. Amer. J. Physiol. **202**, 1125 (1962)

Paoni, N. F., Castellino, F. J.: Isolation of a low molecular weight form of plasminogen. Biochem. biophys. Res. Commun. **65**, 757 (1975)

Perlewitz, J., Markwardt, F.: Über die fibrinolytische Aktivität menschlicher Gewebe. Folia haemat. (Lpz.) **92**, 46 (1969)

Permin, P. M.: Properties of the fibrinokinase-fibrinolysin system. Nature (Lond.) **160**, 571 (1947)

Permin, P. M.: The fibrinolytic activator in animal tissue. Acta physiol. scand. **21**, 1959 (1950)

Petkov, D., Christova, E., Pojarlieff, I., Stambolieva, N.: Structure-activity relationship in the urokinase hydrolysis of α-N-acetyl-L-lysine anilides. Europ. J. Biochem. **51**, 25 (1975)

Pizza, S. V., Schwartz, M. L., Hill, R. L., McKee, P. A.: The effect of plasmin on the subunit structure of human fibrin. J. biol. Chem. **248**, 4574 (1973)

Ploug, J., Kjeldgaard, N. O.: Isolation of plasminogen activator (urokinase) from urine. Arch. Biochem. **62**, 500 (1956)

Ploug, J., Kjeldgaard, N. O.: Urokinase, an activator of plasminogen from human urine. I. Isolation and properties. Biochim. biophys. Acta (Amst.) **24**, 278 (1957)

Prokopowicz, J.: Purification of plasminogen from human granulocytes using DEAE-Sephadex column chromatography. Biochim. biophys. Acta (Amst.) **154**, 91 (1968)

Prokopowicz, J., Rejniak, L., Niewiarowski, S., Worowski, K.: Fibrinolytic activity of tissue sections of dog kidney. Thrombos. Diathes. haemorrh. (Stuttg.) **12**, 394 (1964)

Quigley, J. P., Ossowski, L., Reich, E.: Plasminogen, the serum proenzyme activated by factors from cells transformed by oncogenic viruses. J. biol. Chem. **249**, 4306 (1974)

Rabiner, S. F., Goldfine, I. C., Hart, A., Summaria, L., Robbins, K. C.: Radioimmunoassay of human plasminogen and plasmin. J. Lab. clin. Med. **74**, 265 (1969)

Reddy, K. N. N., Kline, D. L.: Requirement of human plasmin for streptokinase activation of bovine plasminogen. Thrombos. Res. **6**, 481 (1975)

Reddy, K. N. N., Markus, G.: Mechanism of activation of human plasminogen by streptokinase. Presence of active center in streptokinase-plasminogen complex. J. biol. Chem. **247**, 1683 (1972)

Reddy, K. N. N., Markus, G.: Further evidence for an active center in streptokinase-plasminogen complex; interaction with pancreatic trypsin inhibitor. Biochem. biophys. Res. Commun. **51**, 672 (1973)

Reddy, K. N. N., Markus, G.: Esterase activities in the zymogen moiety of the streptokinase-plasminogen complex. J. biol. Chem. **249**, 4851 (1974)

Remmert, L. F., Cohen, P.: Partial purification and properties of a proteolytic enzyme of human serum. J. biol. Chem. **181**, 431 (1949)

Renzo, E. C. de, Boggiano, E., Barg, W. F., Buck, F. F.: Interaction of streptokinase and human plasminogen. IV. Further gel electrophoretic studies on the combination of streptokinase with human plasminogen or human plasmin. J. biol. Chem. **242**, 2428 (1967a)

Renzo, E. C. de, Siiteri, P. K., Hutchings, B. L., Bell, P. H.: Preparation and certain properties of highly purified streptokinase. J. biol. Chem. **242**, 533 (1967b)

Rickli, E. E.: The activation mechanism of human plasminogen. Thrombos. Diathes. haemorrh. (Stuttg.) **34**, 386 (1975)

Rickli, E. E., Cuendet, P. A.: Isolation of plasmin-free human plasminogen with N-terminal glutamic acid. Biochim. biophys. Acta (Amst.) **250**, 447 (1971)

Rickli, E. E., Otavski, W. J.: Release of an N-terminal peptide from human plasminogen during activation with urokinase. Biochim. biophys. Acta (Amst.) **295**, 381 (1973)

Rickli, E. E., Zaugg, H.: Isolation and purification of highly enriched tissue plasminogen activator from pig heart. Thrombos. Diathes. haemorrh. (Stuttg.) **23**, 64 (1970)

Rifé, U., Shulman, S.: The streptokinase activation of human plasminogen. Direct analysis of the activation mixture. Thrombos. Diathes. haemorrh. (Stuttg.) **10**, 133 (1963)

Rifé, U., Shulman, S.: Molecular changes in activation of plasminogen. I. Release of peptide fragments. Biochim. biophys. Acta (Amst.) **86**, 317 (1964)

Rifé, U., Shulman, S.: Molecular changes in activation of plasminogen. II. Comparison of peptide liberations during incubation with and without streptokinase. Biochim. biophys. Acta (Amst.) **86**, 328 (1964)

Rimon, A., Shamash, J., Shapiro, B.: The plasmin inhibitor of human plasma. IV. Its action on plasmin, trypsin, chymotrypsin and thrombin. J. biol. Chem. **241**, 5102 (1966)

Robbins, K. C., Bernabe, P., Arzadon, L., Summaria, L.: The primary structure of human plasminogen. I. The NH_2-terminal sequences of human plasminogen and the S-carboxymethyl heavy (A) and light (B) chain derivatives of plasmin. J. biol. Chem. **247**, 6757 (1972)

Robbins, K. C., Bernabe, P., Arzadon, L., Summaria, L.: The primary structure of human plasminogen. II. The histidine loop of human plasmin. Light (B) chain active center histidine sequence. J. biol. Chem. **248**, 1631 (1973a)

Robbins, K. C., Bernabe, P., Arzadon, L., Summaria, L.: NH_2-terminal sequences of mammalian plasminogens and plasmin S-carboxymethyl heavy (A) and light (B) chain derivatives. A re-evaluation of the mechanism of activation of plasminogen. J. biol. Chem. **248**, 7242 (1973b)

Robbins, K. C., Ling, C. M., Elwyn, D., Barlow, G. H.: Further studies on the purification and characterization of human plasminogen and plasmin. J. Biol. Chem. **240**, 541 (1965)

Robbins, K. C., Summaria, L.: Purification of human plasminogen and plasmin by gel filtration and chromatography on diethylaminoethyl-Sephadex. J. biol. Chem. **238**, 952 (1963)

Robbins, K. C., Summaria, L.: Human plasminogen and plasmin. In: Methods in enzymology. Vol. XIX: Proteolytic enzymes. New York-London: Academic Press 1970

Robbins, K. C., Summaria, L.: Biochemistry of fibrinolysis. Thrombos. Diathes. haemorrh. (Stuttg.), Suppl. **47**, 9 (1971)

Robbins, K. C., Summaria, L., Hsieh, B., Shah, R. J.: The peptide chains of human plasmin. Mechanism of activation of human plasminogen to plasmin. J. biol. Chem. **242**, 2333 (1967)

Roberts, P. S.: Measurement of the rate of plasmin action on synthetic substrates. J. biol. Chem. **232**, 285 (1958)

Roberts, P. S.: The esterase activities of human plasmin during purification and subsequent activation by streptokinase or glycerol. J. biol. Chem. **235**, 2262 (1960)

Roberts, P. S.: The postulated acetyl esterase activity of streptokinase. Biochim. biophys. Acta (Amst.) **77**, 145 (1963)

Roberts, P. S., Burkat, R. K.: The stabilizing effect of neutral salts on plasmin. Biochim. biophys. Acta (Amst.) **113**, 193 (1966)

Ronwin, E.: Enzymatic properties of bovine plasmin preparations; evidence for similarity to but non-identity with trypsin. Canad. J. Biochem. **34**, 1169 (1956)

Rybak, M., Petakova, M.: Investigations of plasminogen and plasmin by immunoelectrophoresis on fibrin-agar plates. Detection of two plasminogens in human serum. Clin. chim. Acta **8**, 133 (1963)

Sahli, W.: Über das Vorkommen von Pepsin und Trypsin im normalen menschlichen Urin. Pflügers Arch. ges. Physiol. **36**, 209 (1885)

Sandberg, H., Rezai, M., Bangayan, T. T., Bellet, S., Feinberg, L. J., Hunter, S.: Organ distribution of fibrinolytic activity in man. J. Lab. clin. Med. **61**, 592 (1963)

Scheraga, H. A., Ehrenpreis, S., Sullivan, E.: Comparative kinetic behaviour of thrombin, plasmin, and trypsin toward synthetic substrates. Nature (Lond.) **182**, 461 (1958)

Schick, L. A., Castellino, F. J.: Interaction of streptokinase and rabbit plasminogen. Biochemistry **12**, 4315 (1973)

Schick, L. A., Castellino, F. J.: Direct evidence for the generation of an active site in the plasminogen moiety of the streptokinase-human plasminogen activator complex. Biochem. biophys. Res. Commun. **57**, 47 (1974)

Schmitz, A.: Über die Freilegung von aktivem Trypsin aus Blutplasma. Zweite Mitteilung. Zur Kenntnis des Plasma-Trypsin-Systems. Hoppe-Seylers Z. physiol. Chem. **250**, 37 (1937)

Schulte, W., Vorbauer, J.: Fibrinolytische Effekte beim Kontakt von Speichel und Blut. Dtsch. Zahn-, Mund- u. Kieferheilkd. **44**, 23 (1965)

Schwick, H. G.: Biochemie der Fibrinolyse. Behringwerk-Mitt. Heft **44**, 103 (1964)

Schwick, H. G.: Biochemie der Fibrinolyse. Thrombos. Diathes. haemorrh. (Stuttg.), Suppl. **22**, 27 (1967)

Schwick, H. G.: Entwicklungstendenzen immunologischer Methoden in der Klinik. Fresenius Z. analyt. Chem. **243**, 424 (1968)

Semar, M., Skoza, L., Johnson, A. J.: Partial purification and properties of a plasminogen activator from human erythrocytes. J. clin. Invest. **48**, 1777 (1969)

Sgouris, J. T., Inman, J. K., McCall, K. B.: The preparation of human urokinase. Amer. J. Cardiol. **6**, 406 (1960)

Sgouris, J. T., Storey, R. W., McCall, K. B., Anderson, H. D.: The purification, assay, sterilization, and removal of pyrogenicity of human urokinase. Vox Sang. (Basel) **7**, 739 (1962)

Sherry, S.: The fibrinolytic activity of streptokinase activated human plasmin. J. clin. Invest. **33**, 1054 (1954)

Sherry, S.: Present concept of the fibrinolytic mechanism. Scand. J. haemat. **7**, 70 (1965)

Sherry, S.: Fibrinolysis. Ann. Rev. Med. **19**, 247 (1968)

Sherry, S., Alkjaersig, N.: Studies on the activation of human plasminogen. J. clin. Invest. **35**, 735 (1956)

Sherry, S., Alkjaersig, N., Fletcher, A. P.: Assay of urokinase preparations with the synthetic substrate acetyl-L-lysine methyl ester. J. Lab. clin. Med. **64**, 145 (1964)

Sherry, S., Alkjaersig, N., Fletcher, A. P.: Comparative study of thrombin on substituted arginine and lysine esters. Amer. J. Physiol. **209**, 577 (1965)

Sherry, S., Alkjaersig, N., Fletcher, A. P.: Activity of plasmin and streptokinase activator on substituted arginine and lysine esters. Thrombos. Diathes. haemorrh. (Stuttg.) **18**, 18 (1966)

Sherry, S., Fletcher, A. P., Alkjaersig, N.: Fibrinolysis and fibrinolytic activity in man. Physiol. Rev. **39**, 343 (1959)

Siefring, G. E., Castellino, F. J.: The role of sialic acid in the determination of distinct properties of the isozymes of rabbit plasminogen. J. biol. Chem. **249**, 7742 (1974)

Silverstein, R. M.: The plasmin-catalyzed hydrolysis of N^{α}-cbz-L-lysine p-nitrophenyl ester. Thrombos. Res. **3**, 729 (1973)

Silverstein, R. M.: Determination of human plasminogen using N^{α}-CBZ[carbobenzyloxy]-L-lysine p-nitrophenyl ester as substrate. Analyt. Biochem. **65**, 500 (1975)

Sjöholm, I., Wiman, B., Wallén, P.: Studies on the conformational changes of plasminogen induced during activation to plasmin and by 6-aminohexanoic acid. Europ. J. Biochem. **39**, 471 (1973)

Slotta, K. H., Gonzales, J. D.: Native plasminogen. Biochemistry **3**, 285 (1964)

Slotta, K. H., Michel, H., Santos, B. G.: Comparative studies on native and acid treated plasminogens. Biochim. biophys. Acta (Amst.) **58**, 459 (1962)

Smillie, L. B., Furka, A., Nagabushan, N., Stevenson, K. J., Parkes, C. O.: Structure of chymotrypsinogen B compared with chymotrypsinogen A and trypsinogen. Nature (Lond.) **218**, 343 (1968)

Smyrniotis, F. E., Fletcher, A. P., Alkjaersig, N., Sherry, S.: Urokinase excretion in health and its alteration in certain disease states. Thrombos. Diathes. haemorrh. (Stuttg.) **3**, 257 (1959)

Sobel, G. W., Mohler, S. R., Jones, N. W., Dowdy, A. B. C., Guest, M. M.: Urokinase: an activator of plasma profibrinolysin extracted from urine. Amer. J. Physiol. **171**, 768 (1952)

Sodetz, J. M., Brockway, W. J., Castellino, F. J.: Multiplicity of rabbit plasminogen. Physical characterization. Biochemistry **11**, 4451 (1972)

Sodetz, J. M., Brockway, W. J., Mann, K. G., Castellino, F. J.: The mechanism of activation of rabbit plasminogen by urokinase. Lack of a preactivation peptide. Biochem. biophys. Res. Commun. **60**, 729 (1974)

Sodetz, J. M., Castellino, F. J.: A comparison of steady and presteady state kinetics of bovine and human plasmin. Biochemistry **11**, 3167 (1972)

Sodetz, J. M., Castellino, F. J.: The mechanism of activation of rabbit plasminogen by urokinase. J. biol. Chem. **250**, 3041 (1975)

Sottrup-Jensen, L., Zajdel, M., Claeys, H., Petersen, T. E., Magnusson, S.: Amino acid sequence of activation cleavage site in plasminogen: Homology with "pro" part of prothrombin. Proc. nat. Acad. Sci. (Wash.) **72**, 2577 (1975)

Soru, E.: Thin layer chromatography of staphylokinase activated human plasmin. Purification of human plasmin by serial molecular sieve chromatography on polyacrylamide. Rev. Roum. Biochimie **5**, 17 (1968)

Spritz, N., Cameron, D. J.: Streptokinase induced lysine-methyl-esterase activity of human euglobulin. Proc. Soc. exp. Biol. (N.Y.) **109**, 848 (1962)

Storm, O.: Fibrinolytic activity in human tears. Scand. J. clin. Lab. Invest. **7**, 55 (1955)

Stroud, R. M., Kay, L. M., Dickerson, R. E.: The structure of bovine trypsin: Electron density maps of the inhibited enzyme at 5 Å and at 2.7 Å resolution. J. molec. Biol. **83**, 185 (1974)

Stürzebecher, J., Markwardt, F., Richter, P., Wagner, G., Walsmann, P., Landmann, H.: Synthetische Inhibitoren von Serinproteinasen. 3. Mitteilung: Über die Hemmwirkung basisch substituierter Phenylcarbonsäureester gegenüber Trypsin, Plasmin und Thrombin. Pharmazie **29**, 337 (1974)

Summaria, L., Arzadon, L., Bernabe, P., Robbins, K. C.: Studies on the isolation of the multiple molecular forms of human plasminogen and plasmin by isoelectric focusing methods. J. biol. Chem. **247**, 4691 (1972)

Summaria, L., Arzadon, L., Bernabe, P., Robbins, K. C.: Isolation, characterization, and comparison of the S-carboxy methyl heavy (A) and light (B) chain derivatives of cat, dog, rabbit, and bovine plasmins. J. biol. Chem. **248**, 6522 (1973)

Summaria, L., Arzadon, L., Bernabe, P., Robbins, K. C.: The interaction of streptokinase with human, cat, dog, and rabbit plasminogen. The fragmentation of streptokinase in the equimolar plasminogen-streptokinase complexes. J. biol. Chem. **249**, 4760 (1974)

Summaria, L., Arzadon, L., Bernabe, P., Robbins, K. C.: The activation of plasminogen to plasmin in the presence of the plasmin inhibitor Trasylol. The preparation of plasmin with the same NH_2-terminal heavy (A) chain sequence as the parent zymogen. J. biol. Chem. **250**, 3988 (1975)

Summaria, L., Hsieh, B., Groskopf, W. R., Robbins, K. C.: Direct activation of human plasminogen by streptokinase. Proc. Soc. exp. Biol. (N.Y.) **130**, 737 (1969)

Summaria, L., Hsieh, B., Groskopf, W. R., Robbins, K. C., Barlow, G. H.: The isolation of the S-carboxymethyl β-(light)-chain derivative of human plasmin. The localization of the active site on the light chain. J. biol. Chem. **242**, 5046 (1967b)

Summaria, L., Hsieh, B., Robbins, K. C.: The specific mechanism of activation of human plasminogen to plasmin. J. biol. Chem. **242**, 4279 (1967a)

Summaria, L., Ling, C.-M., Groskopf, W. R., Robbins, K. C.: The active site of bovine plasminogen activator. Interaction of streptokinase with human plasminogen and plasmin. J. biol. Chem. **243**, 144 (1968)

Summaria, L., Robbins, K. C., Barlow, G. H.: Dissociation of the equimolar human plasmin-streptokinase complex. Partial characterization of the isolated plasmin and streptokinase moieties. J. biol. Chem. **246**, 2136 (1971 a)

Summaria, L., Robbins, K. C., Barlow, G. H.: Isolation and characterization of the S-carboxymethyl heavy chain derivative of human plasmin. J. biol. Chem. **246**, 2143 (1971 b)

Sweet, B., McNicol, G. P., Douglas, A. S.: In vitro studies of staphylokinase. Clin. Sci. **29**, 375 (1965)

Szczeklik, E., Orlowski, M., Szczeklik, A., Narczewska, B.: The activity of plasma, serum, thrombin, and plasmin toward synthetic trypsin substrates. Thrombos. Diathes. haemorrh. (Stuttg.) **19**, 99 (1968)

Takada, A., Takada, Y., Ambrus, J. L.: Streptokinase-activatable proactivator of human and bovine plasminogen. J. biol. Chem. **245**, 6389 (1970)

Takada, A., Takada, Y., Ambrus, J. L.: Proactivators in the fibrinolysin system. Thrombos. Diathes. haemorrh. (Stuttg.), Suppl. **47**, 37 (1971)

Takada, A., Takada, Y., Ambrus, J. L.: Further studies of plasminogen proactivator. Biochim. biophys. Acta (Amst.) **263**, 610 (1972)

Tangen, O., Wik, K. O., Almqvist, I. A. M., Arfors, K. E., Hint, H. C.: Effects of dextran on the structure and plasmin-induced lysis of human fibrin. Thrombos. Res. **1**, 487 (1972)

Taylor, F. B., Beisswenger, J. G.: Identification of modified streptokinase as the activator of bovine and human plasminogen. J. biol. Chem. **248**, 1127 (1973)

Taylor, F. B., Botts, J.: Purification and characterization of streptokinase with studies of streptokinase activation of plasminogen. Biochemistry **7**, 232 (1968)

Taylor, F. B., Tomar, R. H.: Streptokinase. In: Methods in enzymology. Vol. XIX: Proteolytic enzymes. New York-London: Academic Press 1970

Thorsen, S., Müllertz, S.: Rate of activation and electrophoretic mobility of unmodified and partially degraded plasminogen. Effects of 6-aminohexanoic acid and related compounds. Scand. J. clin. Lab. Invest. **34**, 167 (1974)

Tillett, W. S., Garner, R. L.: The fibrinolytic activity of hemolytic streptococci. J. exp. Med. **58**, 485 (1933)

Todd, A. S.: The histological localization of fibrinolytic activator. J. Path. Bact. **78**, 281 (1959)

Todd, A. S.: Localization of fibrinolytic activity in tissues. Brit. med. Bull. **20**, 210 (1964)

Tomar, R. H.: Streptokinase: preparation, comparison with streptococcal proteinase, and behavior as a trypsin substrate. Proc. Soc. exp. Biol. (N.Y.) **127**, 239 (1968)

Tomar, R. H., Taylor, F. B.: The streptokinase-human plasminogen activator complex. Composition and identity of a subcomponent with activator activity. Biochem. J. **125**, 793 (1971)

Troll, W., Sherry, S.: The activation of human plasminogen by streptokinase. J. biol. Chem. **213**, 881 (1955)

Troll, W., Sherry, S., Wachmann, J.: The action of plasmin on synthetic substrates. J. biol. Chem. **208**, 85 (1954)

Ts'ao, C. H., Kline, D. L.: Plasminogen activator by reaction of streptokinase with human plasminogen. J. appl. Physiol. **26**, 634 (1969)

Tyler, H. M.: Fibrin crosslinking demonstrated by thrombelastography. Thrombos. Diathes. haemorrh. (Stuttg.) **22**, 398 (1969)

Tympanidis, K., Astrup, T.: Fibrinolytic activity of epithelium of bladder of rat and man. J. Urol. (Baltimore) **105**, 214 (1971)

Umezawa, H.: Enzyme inhibitors of microbial origin. Baltimore: Univ. Press 1972

Unkeless, J., Danø, K., Kellerman, G. M., Reich, E.: Fibrinolysis associated with oncogenic transformation. Partial purification and characterization of the cell factor, a plasminogen activator. J. biol. Chem. **249**, 4295 (1974)

Vaux Saint-Cyr, C. de: Mise en évidence de constituants possédant une activité estérasique dans les préparations de streptokinase. C.R. Soc. Biol. (Paris) **254**, 3749 (1962)

Vesterberg, K., Vesterberg, O.: Staphylokinase. J. med. Microbiol. **5**, 441 (1972)

Vigorito, T. F., Celander, E., Celander, D. R.: The origin of urokinase. Fed. Proc. **24**, 512 (1965)

Vogel, R., Trautschold, I., Werle, E.: Natürliche Proteinasen-Inhibitoren. In: Biochemie und Klinik. Stuttgart: Thieme 1966

Wallén, P.: Studies on the purification of human plasminogen. I. The preparation of a partially purified human plasminogen with a low spontaneous proteolytic activity. Ark. Kemi **19**, 451 (1962 a)

Wallén, P.: Studies on the purification of human plasminogen. II. Further purification of human plasminogen on cellulose ion exchangers and by means of gel filtration on Sephadex. Ark. Kemi 19, 469 (1962b)

Wallén, P., Bergström, K.: Action of thrombin on plasmin digested fibrinogen. Acta chem. scand. 12, 574 (1958)

Wallén, P., Bergström, K.: Effect of lysine on the purification of human plasminogen on cellulose ion exchangers. Acta chem. scand. 13, 1464 (1959)

Wallén, P., Bergström, K.: Purification of human plasminogen on DEAE-cellulose. Acta chem. scand. 14, 217 (1960)

Wallén, P., Iwanaga, S.: Differences between plasmic and tryptic digests of human S-sulfo fibrinogen. Biochim. biophys. Acta (Amst.) 221, 20 (1968)

Wallén, P., Wiman, B.: Characterization of human plasminogen. I. On the relationship between different molecular forms of plasminogen demonstrated in plasma and found in purified preparations. Biochim. biophys. Acta (Amst.) 221, 20 (1970)

Wallén, P., Wiman, B.: Characterization of human plasminogen. II. Separation and partial characterization of different molecular forms of human plasminogen. Biochim. biophys. Acta (Amst.) 257, 122 (1972)

Wallenbeck, I.A.M., Tangen, O.: Lysis of fibrin formed in the presence of dextran and other macromolecules. Thrombos. Res. 6, 75 (1975)

Walsmann, P., Horn, H., Landmann, H., Markwardt, F., Stürzebecher, J., Wagner, G.: Synthetische Inhibitoren der Serinproteinasen. 5. Mitteilung: Über die Hemmung von Trypsin, Plasmin und Thrombin durch araliphatische Amidinoverbindungen mit Ätherstruktur sowie Ester der 3- und 4-Amidinophenoxyessigsäure. Pharmazie 30, 386 (1975)

Walsmann, P., Landmann, H., Markwardt, F., Stürzebecher, J., Vieweg, H., Wagner, G.: Synthetische Inhibitoren der Serinproteinasen. 3. Mitteilung: Über die Hemmwirkung substituierter Anilide der 3- und 4-Amidinobenzoesäuren und Amidinoanilide verschiedener Benzoe- und Benzolsulfonsäuren. Pharmazie 29, 405 (1974b)

Walsmann, P., Markwardt, F., Richter, P., Stürzebecher, J., Wagner, G., Landmann, H.: Synthetische Inhibitoren von Serinproteinasen. 2. Mitteilung: Über die Hemmung von Homologen der Amidinobenzoesäuren und ihrer Ester gegenüber Trypsin, Plasmin und Thrombin. Pharmazie 29, 333 (1974a)

Walther, P.J., Steinman, H.M., Hill, R.L., McKee, P.A.: Activation of human plasminogen by urokinase. J. biol. Chem. 249, 1173 (1974)

Walton, P.L.: The hydrolysis of α-N-acetylglycyl-L-lysine methyl ester by urokinase. Biochim. biophys. Acta (Amst.) 132, 104 (1967)

Warren, B.A.: Fibrinolytic activity of vascular endothelium. Brit. med. Bull. 20, 213 (1964)

Weinstein, M.J., Doolittle, R.F.: Differential specificities of thrombin, plasmin, and trypsin with regard to synthetic and natural substrates and inhibitors. Biochim. biophys. Acta (Amst.) 258, 577 (1972)

Werkheiser, W.C., Markus, G.: The interaction of streptokinase with human plasminogen. II. The kinetics of activation. J. biol. Chem. 239, 2644 (1964)

White, W.F., Barlow, G.H.: Urinary plasminogen activator (urokinase). In: Methods in enzymology, Vol. XIX: Proteolytic enzymes. New York-London: Academic Press 1970

White, W.F., Barlow, G.H., Mozen, M.M.: The isolation and characterization of plasminogen activators (urokinase) from human urine. Biochemistry 5, 2160 (1966)

Williams, J.R.B.: The fibrinolytic activity of urine. Brit. J. exp. Path. 32, 530 (1951)

Wiman, B.: Structure of the N-terminal fragment of human plasminogen obtained after cleavage with cyanogen bromide. Thrombos. Res. 1, 89 (1972)

Wiman, B.: Primary structure of peptides released during activation of human plasminogen by urokinase. Europ. J. Biochem. 39, 1 (1973)

Wiman, B., Wallén, P.: Activation of human plasminogen by an insoluble derivative of urokinase. Structural changes of plasminogen in the course of activation of plasmin and demonstration of a possible intermediate compound. Europ. J. Biochem. 36, 25 (1973)

Wiman, B., Wallén, P.: On the primary structure of human plasminogen and plasmin, cyanogen bromide fragments. 5th Congr. Int. Soc. Thromb. Haemostasis, Abstr. 109, Paris 1975a

Wiman, B., Wallén, P.: Amino acid sequence around the arginyl-valyl bond in plasminogen which is cleaved during the second step of the activation process. Thrombos. Res. 7, 239 (1975b)

Wiman, B., Wallén, P.: Structural relationship between "glutamic acid" and "lysine" forms of human plasminogen and their interaction with the NH_2-terminal activation peptide as studied by affinity chromatography. Europ. J. Biochem. **50**, 489 (1975c)

Wiman, B., Wallén, P.: On the primary structure of human plasminogen and plasmin. Purification and characterization of cyanogen-bromide fragments. Europ. J. Biochem. **57**, 387 (1975d)

Wiman, B., Wallén, P.: Amino-acid sequence of the cyanogen-bromide fragment from human plasminogen that forms the linkage between the plasmin chains. Europ. J. Biochem. **58**, 539 (1975e)

Wulf, R. J., Mertz, E. T.: Plasminogen VIII. Species specificity of streptokinase. Canad. J. Biochem. **47**, 927 (1969)

Yamamoto, J., Nagamatsu, Y.: Low molecular weight proactivator of plasminogen derived from the macromolecular one by lysine-Sepharose chromatography. Nippon Seirigaku Zasshi **36**, 176 (1974)

Zylber, J., Blatt, W. F., Jensen, H.: Mechanism of bovine plasminogen activation by human plasmin and streptokinase. Proc. Soc. exp. Biol. (N.Y.) **102**, 755 (1959)

Fibrinogen and Fibrin Formation

B. BLOMBÄCK

Introduction

Fibrinogen is defined as that protein in blood and tissue extract, which in the presence of thrombin is transformed into an insoluble product called fibrin. Fibrinogen exists in the blood plasma of all vertebrates and a protein similar in character to fibrinogen is found in many invertebrates. Accordingly, lobster lymph contains a protein which aggregates in the presence of tissue extract from the same species and thereby becomes insoluble.

It is generally accepted that the most important biological role of fibrinogen is that of a precursor to the thread-like material, fibrin, and that its most important function is that of a structural element in hemostatic blood clots formed at injured endothelium surfaces in the circulating system. This does not mean to say that the importance of fibrinogen is limited entirely to the hemostatic mechanisms in the organism. Evidence that fibrinogen/fibrin has other functions is suggested by the fact that only a small proportion of the circulating fibrinogen is necessary for an adequate hemostasis. Furthermore, investigations have been carried out which point to the fact that fibrinogen/fibrin could be of great importance in wound healing.

Fibrinogen belongs to a group of proteins whose concentration in blood increases markedly following infection. The latter situation has given rise to the suggestion that fibrinogen may play some role in the organism's defence against infection. The occurrence of a clotting protein in the hemocytes of the horseshoe crab (*Limulus polyphemus*) is in this connection interesting (SOLUM, 1973). This protein aggregates when in contact with bacteria endotoxin. It is possible that bacteria endotoxin activates coagulating enzymes in the hemocytes which then activate the aggregating protein. These findings provide a basis for the speculation that the fibrinogen in mammals has developed possibly from an ancestral protein, which is still preserved in invertebrates, where it is in readiness to prevent infection. Is the agglutination of staphylococci in the presence of mammalian fibrinogen a reminiscence of such an ancestral protein?

More than a hundred years have passed since DENIS DE COMMERCY and OLOF HAMMARSTEN carried out their pioneering studies of the isolation of fibrinogen from plasma and on its conversion into fibrin in the presence of thrombin. Our knowledge of the physico-chemical and molecular properties of fibrinogen has increased dramatically over the past hundred years. However, in spite of all the information at hand today, we can merely speculate as to how the fibrin fiber is built up of individual, activated fibrinogen units.

In what follows, I shall give a summarised description of the most important physico-chemical and chemical properties of fibrinogen, the molecular basis of its transformation to fibrin and finally its physiological importance in health and disease. The reader who requires a more detailed understanding of this subject is referred to the review work of SCHERAGA and LASKOWSKI (1957), BLOMBÄCK (1967), LAKI (1968), BLOMBÄCK and BLOMBÄCK (1972), DOOLITTLE (1973), and MURANO, G. (1974).

A. Physico-chemical Properties of Fibrinogen

Various physico-chemical properties of fibrinogen are presented in Table 1. Fibrinogen is a plasma protein of which more than 90% is amino acids. The amino acid composition is very similar in different species (CARTWRIGHT and KEKWICK, 1971; HENSCHEN and BLOMBÄCK, 1964). Approximately 4–5% of the weight is made up of covalently bound carbohydrate which in its turn is composed of neutral sugar, glusosamine and sialic acid. The molecule contains also small amounts of ester-linked phosphoric acid and sulphuric acid (cf. BLOMBÄCK, 1967).

On the basis of its diffusion and sedimentation properties, fibrinogen is estimated to have a molecular weight of 340000 (Table 1). Light scattering measurements have suggested a molecular weight of approximately the same value.

By quantitative determination of the NH_2-terminal amino acids of fibrinogen, it has been concluded that the molecule is a dimer (BLOMBÄCK and YAMASHINA, 1958). The two identical halves each consist of three polypeptide chains, $A\alpha$, $B\beta$, and γ, which are connected by disulphide bridges. The two half-molecules are also joined to each other via disulphide bridges (BLOMBÄCK and BLOMBÄCK, 1972; BLOMBÄCK et al., 1976). The molecule can be represented by the formula $(A\alpha, B\beta, \gamma)_2$. There is evidence suggesting that fibrinogen in circulating blood consists of a population of somewhat different molecules. By studying the solubility of fibrinogen in ethanol-water mixtures we can distinguish three types of fibrinogen: one with high, one with low, and one with intermediate solubility (BLOMBÄCK and BLOMBÄCK, 1957; MOSESSON et al., 1967). The fibrinogen having low solubility in ethanol-water has been shown to be associated with a cold-insoluble globulin in plasma (MOSESSON and UMFLEET, 1970). Whether the fibrinogen in this complex has properties different from those of the remaining plasma fibrinogen, has not as yet been investigated. The fibrinogen most used in investigations is that form which has intermediate solubility. Unless otherwise stated, this is the type of fibrinogen which is referred to here (corresponding to fraction I-4 according to BLOMBÄCK and BLOMBÄCK, 1957).

Table 1. Physico-chemical and chemical parameters of bovine fibrinogen

Molecular weight	340000	CASPARY and KEKWICK (1957)
Sedimentation coefficient (S^0_{20w})	7.9 − 8.0	
Diffusion coefficient (D^0_{20w})	$2.0 \times 10^{-7} cm^{2/s}$	
Specific viscosity ($[\eta]$)	0.25 dl/g	
Partial specific volume (v)	0.71 − 0.72	SCHERAGA and LASKOWSKI (1957)
Frictional ratio (f/f_0)	2.34	
Molecular volume	$2.86 \times 10^3 nm^3$	
Degree of hydration (g/g protein)	4	BACHMANN et al. (1975)
Extinction coefficient ($E^{1\%}_{280 nm}$)	16.25	BLOMBÄCK (1958)
Isoelectric point (IP)	5.5	SCHERAGA and LASKOWSKI (1957)
α-Helix content (%)	33	MIHALYI (1965)

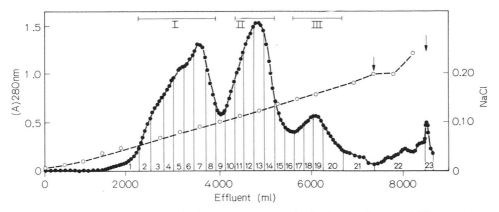

Fig. 1. Chromatogram of bovine fibrinogen on DEAE-Sephadex A 50. ●—●: UV-extinction; ○—○: NaCl concentration. The three fractions are indicated with roman numerals. (From MOSHER and BLOUT, 1973)

Fibrinogen having high solubility in ethanol-water has somewhat lower molecular weight. It probably arises as a consequence of plasmic degradation of fibrinogen as this process has been shown to give rise to products having high solubility (MOSESSON et al., 1967; MOSESSON et al., 1974). The carboxy-terminal of the A α-chain of fibrinogen is the first site of attack when the protein is degraded by plasmin; this is followed by degradation of the B β-chain. The γ-chain appears to be the most resistant to plasmic attack (MILLS and KARPATKIN, 1970; GAFFNEY and DOBOS, 1971; LY et al., 1974).

One cause of the heterogeneity of fibrinogen with regard to solubility may be the occurrence of degradation of the molecule during its circulation in the blood. This degradation is thought to take place primarily at the carboxy-terminal portion of the chains, but NH₂-terminal analysis of fibrinogen suggests that the heterogeneity may be explained, in part, by the occurrence of degradation at the NH₂-terminal portion of the peptide chains (BLOMBÄCK et al., 1966; LAHIRI and SHAINOFF, 1973). Another cause of heterogeneity is the existence of heterogeneity in the oligosaccharide residues which are bound to the peptide chains, or the difference in distribution of phosphate (GAFFNEY, 1971; BLOMBÄCK et al., 1972; BLOMBÄCK et al., 1973). The resulting charge heterogeneity is reflected in the chromatographic behavior of fibrinogen on DEAE-cellulose (FINLAYSSON and MOSESSON, 1963; MOSHER and BLOUT, 1973). According to MOSHER and BLOUT, fibrinogen is separated into three distinct fractions (Fig. 1). The separation in fractions is due to the occurrence of two different γ-chains in fibrinogen. The fibrinogen in the first fraction contains γ-chains of one type while the fibrinogen in the third fraction has γ-chains of another type. The intermediate fraction contains fibrinogen having γ-chains of both types. Nevertheless, MOSHER and BLOUT found that even fibrinogen in these chromatographically pure fractions was heterogenous. This superimposed heterogeneity appeared to be a consequence of differences in protein-bound phosphate. As a result of their experiments, MOSHER and BLOUT suggested that as many as 36 slightly different fibrinogen molecules could exist in any one individual.

What does an average fibrinogen molecule look like? Hydrodynamic measurements indicate that the fibrinogen molecule is a rod- or ellipsoid-shaped particle having a length of 400–500 Å and a length/width ratio of 5–10 (SCHERAGA and LASKOWSKI, 1957; BACHMANN et al., 1975). However, the interpretation of the hydrodynamic data is dependent on the degree of hydration of the molecule. Data presented in recent years indicate that the molecule may contain as much as 6 g of water per gram of protein (MARGUERIE and STUHRMANN, 1975). This extremely high degree of hydration suggests that the molecule is a swollen lattice-like structure and the shape may be more or less rod-like.

As with the hydrodynamic measurements, electron-microscopic investigations have failed to yield unambiguous results. HALL and SLAYTER (1959) found that the molecule was a structure made up of three consecutive spherical particles, bound together by a thread-like structure. KÖPPEL (1966, 1970) was unable to verify this structure but obtained instead pictures showing spherical particles which appeared to have the form of a pentagondodecahedron. KÖPPEL assumed that the chains of the protein were surface-orientated while the inside was filled with water. Using the freeze-etching technique, LEDERER (1973) and BACHMANN et al. (1975) have recently produced electron-microscopic pictures of a structure which is believed to represent the hydrated fibrinogen molecule. The idealized molecule takes the form of a cylinder with rounded ends. It has a length of 450 Å and a width of 90 Å. Irregular forms of the molecule were also observed. The form observed by BACHMANN et al. requires a high degree of hydration. Consequently the molecular volume of the hydrated molecule will be seven times greater than the "dry-volume" calculated solely from data of molecular weight and partial specific volume. By applying electron microscopy to a dry preparation of fibrinogen, a different picture of the molecule was produced, which was fairly consistent with the results of HALL and SLAYTER. Therefore, the model of HALL and SLAYTER may represent an artifact produced by dehydration of the native fibrinogen molecule. TOONEY and COHEN (1972) have recently crystallized a derivative of fibrinogen where a small portion of the carboxy-terminal region of the Aα-chain of the molecule has been cleaved off. The crystals were shown by electron microscopy to have an ordered structure where the unit cell had the dimensions, 90 Å × 450 Å, i.e., the same dimensions as BACHMANN et al. (1975), found for non-crystalline but hydrated fibrinogen molecules. STRYER et al. (1963) found in low-angle X-ray diffraction studies that the axial repeats in the hydrated fibrinogen molecules were 226 Å. This number may represent the length of each half-molecule in the dimer of 450 Å. This would then indicate that the half-molecules of fibrinogen are joined in the center of the rod-shaped particle demonstrated by BACHMANN et al.

B. Biochemical Properties of Fibrinogen

I. Subunits and Prosthetic Groups

Following sulphitolysis of the disulphide bridges, HENSCHEN (1963, 1964a) was able to isolate the polypeptide chains Aα, Bβ and γ of fibrinogen. Similar results have been achieved by other workers following carboxymethylation or oxidation of the disulphide bridges (Fig. 2). As only three types of chains could be demonstrated in

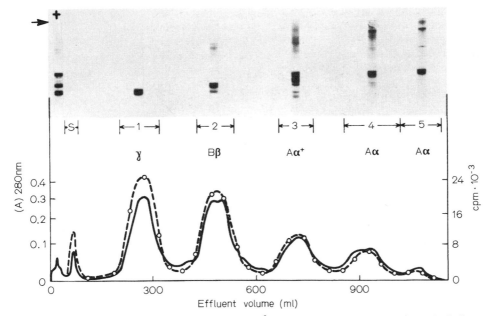

Fig. 2. Chromatogram of S-carboxymethylated (^{3}H) fibrinogen on carboxymethylcellullose. ——; extinction at 280 nm; ○—○; radioactivity. In the upper part of the diagram are inserted the polyacrylamide gel patterns of the fractions. (From MURANO, 1974)

these experiments and as the intact molecule has been shown by NH$_2$-terminal analysis to have six chains, it would appear that the molecule is composed of three polypeptide chains in a paired dimer. The amino acid composition of carboxy-methylated human fibrinogen and its isolated polypeptide chains is shown in Table 2. Polyacrylamide electrophoresis of the polypeptide chains in the presence of sodium dodecylsulphate, indicates molecular weights of: Aα, 64000, Bβ 57000 and γ 48000. These values are in good agreement with those obtained from sedimentation equilibrium studies. The molecular weight values for the chains provide a minimum of 170000 for a fibrinogen unit and so the molecular weight of 340000 attributed to the intact fibrinogen is satisfied by the formula (Aα, Bβ, γ)$_2$.

As one would expect from the observations carried out on intact fibrinogen, heterogeneity has been demonstrated to exist even in the isolated polypeptide chains of the molecule. MURANO (1974) mentions at least four variants of the Aα-chain having different chromatographic and/or electrophoretic mobility. Other authors mentioned above have also pointed out heterogeneity in the Aα- and Bβ-chains of fibrinogen. The heterogeneity of the Aα-chain, arising from plasmic degradation taking place in blood or during isolation, has already been mentioned. In the case of the γ-chain, the heterogeneity can be partially explained by heterogeneity present in the prosthetic carbohydrate groups which are bound to this chain in human fibrino-gen. The fact that differences exist also in the amino-acid compositions of the different γ-chains, suggests that possibly several types of genes are involved in the synthesis of γ-chains (HENSCHEN and EDMAN, 1972).

Table 2. Amino acid analysis of human fibrinogen and its isolated polypeptide chains. (From CARTWRIGHT and KEKWICK, 1971)

Amino acid	Mole per 10^5 protein or peptide			
	γ-chain	β (B)-chain	α (A)-chain	Native fibrinogen
Lysine	66.9	67.0	58.9	65.1 ± 1.0
Histidine	18.4	20.2	17.6	18.0 ± 0.2
Arginine	35.5	36.8	59.0	47.1 ± 0.4
Aspartic acid	108.1	119.1	106.3	106.5 ± 3.3
Threonine	51.9	45.5	60.5	53.2 ± 1.7
Serine	51.2	60.3	85.3	71.2 ± 5.0
Glutamic acid	104.7	113.8	99.2	99.4 ± 0.7
Proline	27.6	42.1	54.9	42.1 ± 1.4
Glycine	74.9	85.2	99.0	84.7 ± 3.6
Alanine	52.4	51.8	36.8	41.5 ± 0.9
Half-cystine	17.7	28.0	16.0	21.0 ± 0.4
Valine	38.2	44.9	44.8	40.0 ± 2.5
Methionine	16.9	27.9	16.7	18.9 ± 1.2
Isoleucine	37.7	35.6	39.2	36.0 ± 0.4
Leucine	55.2	54.3	50.4	54.2 ± 0.5
Tyrosine	40.4	38.2	17.8	29.6 ± 1.1

As mentioned previously, the prosthetic groups of fibrinogen consist of ester-bound phosphate and sulphate as well as carbohydrate. In the case of protein-bound phosphate in human fibrinogen, this is bound partially as serine phosphate in the NH_2-terminal portion of the Aα-chain (Aα 3 Ser) and is bound in other parts of the molecule which are, as yet, unlocalized (BLOMBÄCK et al., 1963, 1966). As Aα 3 Ser is only 30% phosphorylated, one could conclude that a significant degree of the heterogeneity between different molecules exists because of the extent of phosphorylation. Sulphate is bound as tyrosine-0-sulphate in the Bβ-chain in several animal species but such is not the case in humans, where a sulphated tyrosine residue is located in some other undefined region of the molecule (JEVONS, 1963; KRAJEWSKI and BLOMBÄCK, 1968).

The carbohydrate portion of human fibrinogen is bound to both the γ- and Bβ-chains, but also the Aα-chain has been reported to contain carbohydrate (for review see BLOMBÄCK, 1972). Considerable heterogeneity appears to exist within the structure of the carbohydrate chains themselves. The saccharide chains are generally composed of approximately ten monosaccharide residues; they are branched and built up of mannose, galactose, glucosamine, and sialic acid. Sialic acid and galactose are situated in the terminal position. The polysaccharide chain is linked to the polypeptide chain via an asparigine residue. These linking residues have been isolated in the form of 2-acetamide-1-N-4-L-aspartyl)-2-deoxy-β-D-glucosylamine (MESTER, 1969). In the γ-chain of human fibrinogen, the carbohydrate moiety is bound in this fashion to γ 52 Asn. In summary, we can say that the heterogeneity of fibrinogen is adequately explained by that heterogeneity which exists in its chains. As I briefly mentioned earlier, the heterogeneity may result from limited proteolytic degradation caused by exo- and endopeptidases, amidases and phosphatases. One can also imagine a situation where various amounts of carbohydrate and phosphorous have been incorporated into different molecules during biosynthesis or the production of genetically different molecules. In connection with the latter possibility, we know already that in one fibrinogen, fibrinogen Detroit, an amino acid substitution exists in the molecule's Aα-chain.

II. The Primary Structure

The elucidation of the complete primary structure of fibrinogen is a task which has demanded, and continues to demand, a great deal of effort.

Fibrinogen contains in its three chains approximately 3000 amino acids whose sequence is presently under investigation in several laboratories. In addition, the molecule contains 28–29 disulphide bridges (HENSCHEN, 1964b; HENSCHEN and BLOMBÄCK, 1964) the arrangement of which within the molecule is essential for an understanding of its covalent structure. When we have obtained sufficient insight into the primary structure of fibrinogen, we can understand better the function of the molecule, and even diseases where an abnormal function exists. However, a full understanding of this will probably not be provided by even an elucidation of the primary structure of the molecule. To be in this position, we require probably an elucidation of the tertiary structure by X-ray crystallography. In any event, the unravelling of the primary structure is a prerequisite so that we may solve the puzzle of the tertiary structure in a meaningful way.

In order to determine the amino-acid sequence of peptide chains which contain more than approximately 50 amino-acid residues, we usually require a breaking down of the chain by chemical agents or proteolytic enzymes. The amino-acid sequence is then determined after isolation of the fragments. The problem is then to place the fragment in its correct position within the chain structure. To be capable of doing this we must repeat the breaking down of the protein with an agent which produces fragments of a different type. When the amino-acid sequences of these have been determined, the two kinds of fragments are examined for similarities and in this way we can fit the fragments into the intact fibrinogen molecule. However, it can happen that degradation with two agents is not sufficient. No less than 10 such agents, including cyanogen bromide and proteolytic enzymes, have been used in determining the structure of fibrinogen. Nevertheless, two types of fragments have been of fundamental use in solving the task. The first type of fragment has been produced using *cyanogen bromide*, a chemical which reacts with methionine residues in a protein. Intramolecular rearrangement takes place during the reaction and the peptide bond between methionine and the amino-acid residue which follows, is cleaved. Methionine is converted into homoserine in the process. The advantage with that type of cleaving is that is gives rise to only negligible microheterogeneity. When the problem then arises of placing the CNBr fragments in the intact structure, use is made of fragments produced by cleaving with *plasmin*. The structures of these will form overlaps between different CNBr fragments and thereby facilitate the deduction of an unique amino-acid sequence for the intact chains.

1. CNBr Fragments

Cleavage of fibrinogen with CNBr produces some 30 fragments with molecular weights ranging from less than 2000 to up to 60000 (BLOMBÄCK et al., 1968a; GÅRDLUND et al., 1977). Several of these fragments have been isolated in pure form. Interest has been directed primarily towards those fragments which contain disulphide bridges (Table 3). The reason for this is that these bridges often play a decisive role in maintaining the conformation of the protein, and it can be supposed that the primary structure in the proximity of the disulphide bridges is also of importance in determining the protein's function. The largest CNBr fragment, having a molecular weight of 58000, is composed of NH_2-terminal fragments of fibrinogen's three chains (Aα, Bβ, and γ). This fragment, which represents approximately 16% of the entire molecule, contains approximately one-half of the disulphide bridges of the molecule and is given the name "NH_2-terminal disulphide knot" or N-DSK.

Following reduction and alkylation, the chain fragments of N-DSK have been isolated by gel filtration and chromatography. The Aα-chain fragment exists in three molecular forms. Apart from the common form, there is also a phosphorylated variant and a variant which is one amino acid shorter at the NH_2-terminal end of the chain fragment. The latter has probably arisen as a result of cleavage of fibrinogen in blood, in the presence of exopeptidases of the leucine aminopeptidase type. The phosphorylated variant may possibly be the primary product in synthesis, which after secretion from the cell is dephosphorylated in the presence of phosphatases. It has been demonstrated that phosphate bound to fibrinogen can be released by treating with alkaline phosphatase. The γ-chain of N-DSK also displays micro-heterogeneity which, as in the case of the intact γ-chain, is dependent on the heterogeneity in the polysaccharide bound to the peptide chain. The amino-acid sequence of the chains has been determined by stepwise degradation using Edman's phenyl isothiocyanate method (1970). Use was made of the intact chains, and fragments thereof obtained through fragmentation by several proteolytic enzymes.

The structure of the Aα-chain fragment is shown in Figure 3 (BLOMBÄCK et al., 1972). In the phosphorylated variant (AαP), the phosphoric acid is bound to serine in position 3 and in the variant (AαY), alanine is missing in position 1. Thrombin cleaves rapidly the bond between 16 Arg and 17 Gly in both N-DSK and the isolated Aα-chain fragments, releasing fibrinopeptide A (Aα 1–16). The bond between 19 Arg and 20 Val is cleaved at a much slower rate. It should be emphasized here that thrombin cleaves these same bonds in native fibrinogen, suggesting that the specific interaction between thrombin and fibrinogen is governed by a certain amino-acid sequence in the Aα-chain fragment of N-DSK. Kinetic measurements have corroborated this hypothesis (HOGG and BLOMBÄCK, 1974). Comparative studies of fibrinogen from various species have led to the suggestion that the amino-acid sequences corresponding to 5–19 and 45–49 in the Aα-chain of human fibrinogen have been selected during the course of biological evolution. It is therefore primarily among these residues where we must look for the cause of the affinity between thrombin and fibrinogen. In fibrinogen Detroit (BLOMBÄCK et al., 1968b) a mutation has taken place at position 19 in the Aα-chain where an arginine in normal fibrinogen has been replaced by serine (bracketed in Fig. 3). This mutation has taken place in the constant or invariable portion of the chain without having a measurable effect on the ability of

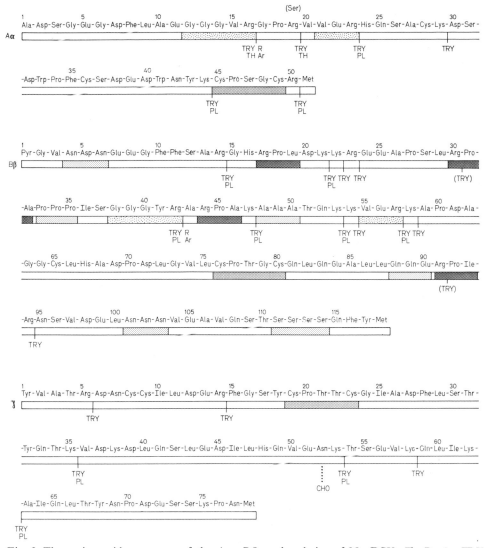

Fig. 3. The amino-acid sequences of the Aα-, Bβ- and γ-chains of N−DSK. *Th, R, Ar, TRY* and *PL:* positions of cleavage by thrombin, botroxobin, arvin, trypsin and plasmin. *CHO:* carbohydrate chain. (From HESSEL, B. Primary structure of human fibrinogen and fibrin. Thesis 1975. Chemistry Dept., Karolinska Institute, Stockholm, Sweden)

thrombin to release fibrinopeptide A, suggesting that the residue at position 19 does not play a role of any great importance in the binding of thrombin to its substrate (refer to the section on polymerization and fibrinogen in health and disease). Certain investigations have been carried out which support the hypothesis that at least residues 5–16 (i.e. the carboxy-terminal part of fibrinopeptide A) provide a binding site for thrombin (HOGG and BLOMBÄCK, 1978; SCHERAGA, 1977). This hypothesis is supported by the fact that synthetic peptide substrates having structures resembling that of fibrinopeptide A are cleaved by thrombin. Such a substrate is Bz-Phe-Val-Arg-paranitroanilide (BLOMBÄCK et al., 1969; SVENDSEN et al., 1972).

With regard to the effect of other enzymes on the Aα-chain, it has been shown that Botroxobin (an enzyme isolated from the venom of *Bothrops atrox*) cleaves the same bond as thrombin (HESSEL and BLOMBÄCK, 1971). On the other hand, Arvin (a clotting enzyme isolated from the venom of *Agkistrodon rhodostoma*), has a somewhat different specificity (see Fig. 3). However, it should be added that the most important site of cleavage is the same for all three enzymes, i.e. the 16 Arg–17 Gly bond. The cleavage at this position is fast and is related to the subsequent formation of fibrin.

The primary structure of the Bβ-chain of N-DSK is seen in Figure 3 (HESSEL et al., 1976). It consists of 118 amino-acid residues and as such, constitutes approximately one-fifth of the entire Bβ-chain. The primary structure was unravelled in a manner analogous to that used in the case of the Aα-chain. The Bβ-chain fragment contains some structures which warrant a closer discussion. One structural detail of interest is the presence of pyroglutamic acid in the NH$_2$-terminal position. This, in all probability, arises after the biosynthesis of the chain by ring closure taking place between the γ-carboxyl and α-amino groups of glutamine. Furthermore, repeating sequences of Arg-Pro-X are found along the length of the Bβ-chain, reminding us of Gly-Pro-X repetitions in collagen. It is possible that these repeated units are an indication of some special regularity in the secondary or tertiary structure of the chain. In the isolated Bβ-chain thrombin cleaves only slowly the 14 Arg–15 Gly bond with release of fibrinopeptide B. Both Botroxobin and Arvin release slowly fibrinopeptide B from the isolated Bβ-chain as well as causing a much slower cleavage of another bond. It is necessary to point out here that these enzymes cause practically no release of fibrinopeptide B from intact fibrinogen (see the chapter on fibrin formation).

The γ-chain fragment of N-DSK contains 78 amino-acid residues (BLOMBÄCK et al., 1973). The structure is represented in Figure 3. This fragment contains carbohydrate, which is bound to the β-amide group of asparigine in position 52. This is the only position of attachment of carbohydrate to the entire γ-chain. The carbohydrate portion consists of mannose, galactose, glucosamine and sialic acid. Galactose and/or sialic acid are the terminal residues in the carbohydrate chain which is branched (MÉSZÁROS and BLOMBÄCK, 1972). Because the carbohydrate chains in certain fibrinogen molecules have two sialic acid residues while others have one (or none), there exists a charge heterogeneity in the γ-chain fragment which can be seen in electrophoresis of not only the γ-chain of N-DSK but also in electrophoresis of the whole intact γ-chain.

2. Disulphide Bridges

The combined molecular weight of the three chain fragments of N-DSK was calculated to be 29000. As the molecular weight of N-DSK is 58000, it follows that this probably represents a dimeric structure of three pairs of chains (WOODS et al., 1972). The conclusion that N-DSK is a dimer implies also that the entire fibrinogen molecule has the same intrinsic structure.

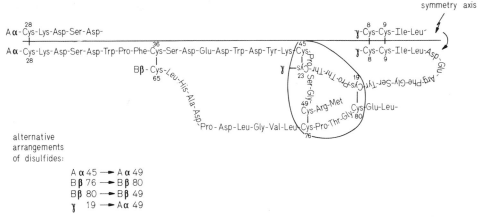

Fig. 4. The arrangement of the disulphide bridges in N−DSK. The disulphides in the circled region are the so-called labile disulphides, i.e. those found to take part in disulphide exchange. Alternative arrangements in this area are known to exist, see BLOMBÄCK, HESSEL, and HOGG (1976a)

The chains of N-DSK are obviously linked by disulphide bridges as these chains are liberated on reduction. In what follows I shall give a description of the arrangement of the disulphides in N-DSK. To obtain information about the arrangement of disulphides in a protein molecule, it is usual to cleave the intact protein with suitable enzymes and isolate thereafter fragments containing only one disulphide bridge. Following reduction of this disulphide bridge, the fragments thus produced are isolated and their structures are determined. By comparing the structures of the fragments with those of the chains in the protein one can determine how the disulphides are arranged in the intact structure. In the case of N-DSK, the cleavage was first performed using pepsin. As this did not produce fragments which were suitably small, the digestion was continued using trypsin and chymotrypsin at pH 6.5. The disulphide-containing fragments were then isolated by conventional methods, some being obtained in a pure form. After oxidation of the disulphide bridges in the latter, the fragments were repurified and their amino-acid compositions were determined. In this way, inferences could be made concerning the origin of respective fragments in chains of N-DSK, thus permitting deductions on the arrangement of the disulphides in the molecule.

The arrangement of disulphides is depicted in Figure 4 (BLOMBÄCK et al., 1976). As can be seen in this diagram, the two halves of the molecule are connected by symmetrical disulphide bridges in the Aα- and γ-chains. We have assumed that these disulphides have a two-fold symmetry. In Figure 4 it can also be seen that the three chains in each half-molecule are also linked by disulphide bridges. In this way a particularly compact knot is formed in the molecule (encircled in the diagram). It can be added here that disulphide exchange appears to take place in this area of the molecule. Proof of this lies in the fact that certain disulphide-containing peptides have been isolated which are not compatible with the structure shown in Figure 4. Instead, they suggest a different arrangement of these disulphide bridges (see inset in Fig. 4). Because of this, the disulphides in question have been given the name "labile"

Table 3. Fragments of fibrinogen obtained with cyanogen bromide and plasmin, K denotes the K value for the counter-current system: 2-butanol: 2% CF_3 COOH: 0.1% CH_3 COOH (2:1:1). (From GÅRDLUND et al., 1977)

	Moles per mole Fbg	Mol. wt.	Number of chains	Chain identity	S−S per mole Fbg	K
Cyanogen bromide fragments						
N − DSK	1	58 000	2 × 3	$A\alpha, B\beta, \gamma$	11	0.1
Hi2 − DSK	2	28 000	1	α	2	0.1
Hol − DSK	2	42 500	5	α, β, γ	12	6.2
Ho2 − DSK	2	7 000	1	β	2	3.0
Ho3 − DSK	2	7 000	2	γ	2	3.0
CNBr − 1	2	6 000	1	α	0	—
CNBr − 2	2	10 000	1	β	0	—
CNBr − 3	—	14 000	1	α	0	—
Plasmin fragments						
D	2	85 000 − 100 000	3	α, β, γ	15 − 16	—
E	1	50 000	2 × 3	$A\alpha, B\beta, \gamma$	11	—
PL − 1	2	50 000	1	α	2	—
PL − 2	2	20 000	1	α	0	—

disulphides. The exchange probably takes place during the isolation of the various disulphide-containing peptides.

Other CNBr fragments. The disulphide-containing peptides of the remaining CNBr fragments have all been isolated but their sequences have been only partially determined. The general properties of the fragments are given in Table 3. The number of disulphides in the various CNBr fragments of fibrinogen matches the 28–29 found in the molecule by HENSCHEN (1964 b). Besides N-DSK, no disulphide fragment from other parts of the molecule has been shown to contain symmetrical disulphides, suggesting that the half-molecules in fibrinogen are covalently linked only in the NH_2-terminal portion of the molecule.

Besides the above mentioned disulphide-containing fragments, a number of CNBr fragments have been isolated (Table 3) which have been shown to be of special importance since they provide overlaps with the fragments produced on degradation of the molecule with plasmin. Figure 5 shows how various CNBr fragments are arranged in the structure of fibrinogen.

3. Plasmin Fragments

Plasmin has an appreciably narrower specificity than trypsin when digesting fibrinogen. Consequently, plasmin cleaves approximately only half of those bonds which are cleaved by trypsin in S-sulpho fibrinogen (WALLÉN and IWANAGA, 1968). It can generally be said that plasmin, in comparison with trypsin, has a greater affinity for lysyl than for arginyl bonds. Plasmin rapidly cleaves bonds in the carboxy-terminal portion of the Aα-chain. On the other hand, bonds are also cleaved in both the NH_2- and carboxy-terminal portion of the Bβ-chain. Even the γ-chain is hydrolyzed by plasmin, but at a rate which is considerably slower than that for the other two chains

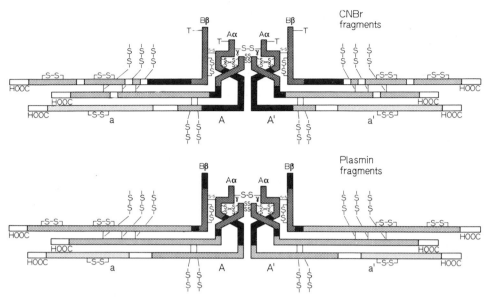

Fig. 5. Schematic representation of the fibrinogen molecule. *Upper half:* CNBr fragments inserted in the structure. *Dotted area:* N−DSK. *Filled black area:* CNBr-1-CNBr-3. *Criss-crossed area:* CNBr-fragments Ho1− and Ho2−DSK. *Striped area:* Hi2−DSK. *White area:* unknown structures. *T:* sites of cleavage by thrombin. *Lower half:* plasmin fragments inserted in the structure. *Dotted area:* Fragment E. *Filled black area:* regions of overlaps between CNBr and plasmin fragments. *Criss-crossed area:* Fragment D. *Striped area:* PL−1 containing the structure of PL−2. *White area:* unknown structures

(for review see DOOLITTLE, 1973; MURANO, 1974). The cleavage by plasmin follows a typical pattern which has been shown by, among others, MARDER et al. (1967, 1969). The cleavage taking place in the carboxy-terminal portion of the Aα-chain, and perhaps to a certain degree in the Bβ- and γ-chains, produces a group of fragments which is called X. If digestion is continued, a population of degradation products arises which is called Y. The final products of the digestion are the so-called core fragments, D and E, together with a number of smaller uncharacterized fragments (Table 3). Fragment Y is of interest, since it is produced from fragment X by splitting off of one molecule of fragment D per mole. Hence, fragment Y appears to be composed of one molecule of fragment E and one molecule of fragment D. Consequently, it is an intermediate arising from an unsymmetrical cleavage of fragment X. The positions of some plasmin fragments within the fibrinogen molecule are depicted in Figure 5. By comparing the upper and lower portions of the figure, it can be seen that fragment E has a considerable portion of its structure in common with N-DSK (KOWALSKA-LOTH et al., 1973). In contrast with N-DSK, fragment E is missing the first 53 amino-acid residues of the Bβ-chain and the carboxy-terminal portion of the γ-chain in N-DSK. Furthermore, fragment E has a somewhat longer Aα- and Bβ-chain than N-DSK. The latter discovery made possible the isolation of CNBr-fragments providing overlaps in the Aα- and Bβ-chains in fragment E and the corresponding chains in fragment D (schematically represented in Fig. 6). Fragment

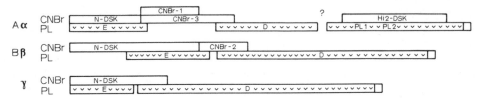

Fig. 6. Schematic representation showing the overlaps between CNBr and plasmin fragments in the three chains of fibrinogen. The principle fragment to which the chain fragments belong are indicated in the diagram

D is a monomeric unit. Since fibrinogen is a dimer, it follows that there must exist two fragments D per molecule of fibrinogen. Analysis of fragment D has shown that it can be related directly to the structures in N-DSK. Fragment D consists of three chains which have their respective origins in the Aα-, Bβ-, and γ-chain of the fibrinogen molecule (COLLEN et al., 1975). It has been found that the γ-chain of fragment D has structures in common with the carboxy-terminal portion of the γ-chain of N-DSK (Fig. 6). Furthermore, as mentioned before, a CNBr fragment has been isolated from the Bβ-chain, providing an overlap between this chain in fragment E and fragment D (Fig. 6) (BLOMBÄCK et al., 1976). A similar fragment from the Aα-chain forms an overlap between fragment E and the α-chain in fragment D. Thus it would appear that, apart from small carboxy-terminal fragments in the Bβ- and γ-chains, the principal chain structure of fibrinogen has been by and large completed (see Note added in proof). The structure of the carboxy-terminal of the Aα-chain remains somewhat unclear. A fragment of molecular weight 50000, released during the early phase of a plasmic digestion, constitutes most likely the carboxy-terminal portion of the chain and is situated probably in the immediate sequence following the α-chain of fragment D [Fig. 6 (HESSEL, 1975)]. However, no CNBr fragment has been found until now which provides an overlap between this plasmic fragment and the α-chain of fragment D.

Concerning the amino-acid sequence of the whole chains of fibrinogen HENSCHEN et al. (1976) have recently elucidated more than 75% of the amino-acid sequence for the γ-chain. This sequence for the NH_2-terminal residues present in N-DSK is in complete agreement with that found by us. For the other chains outside N-DSK much less detailed sequence data are available.

III. The Antigenic Structure of Fibrinogen and the Location of Epitopes and Other Structural Elements

NUSSENZWEIG et al. (1961) as well as MARDER et al. (1969) have used antisera raised against fibrinogen to show that the molecule has several antigenic determinants. Two of these determinants have their structural origin in fragment E and fragment D which arise from degradation of fibrinogen with plasmin. Fragments X and Y also

Since the preparation of this manuscript in 1975 additional information on the primary structure of the three chains of fibrinogen has been obtained. The readers is referred to the following articles DOOLITTLE et al. (1977), TAKAGI and DOOLITTLE (1975), LOTTSPEICH and HENSCHEN (1977), HENSCHEN et al. (1976).

have specific determinants and there also exist determinants which are unique for intact fibrinogen. By using antibodies which have been raised against fragments of fibrinogen, especially its CNBr fragments, one can elucidate the antigenic structure of the molecule as well as obtain information concerning the location of these determinants (or epitopes) in the three-dimensional structure. KUDRYK et al. (1974b) showed that the antigenic determinants in N-DSK were localized mainly in certain portions of this structure. Furthermore, it was shown that anti-N-DSK cross-reacted only to a small extent with intact fibrinogen and also only to a small extent with fragment E, the latter having a considerable portion of its structure in common with N-DSK. However, after cleavage with CNBr, fragment E reacted to the same extent as N-DSK. This would suggest that the antigenic determinants are not only buried in fibrinogen but also in fragment E. Fragment E, in comparison with N-DSK, has chain extensions on its Aα and Bβ chains. These extensions are removed on treatment with CNBr. One possibility is that the extensions are folded in such a way as to hide the epitopes in fragment E. Other interpretations of these results are also feasible but I shall not venture upon these in this connection. Results obtained from investigations using thioredoxin also indicate that certain structures of N-DSK are buried in the intact fibrinogen molecule. It has been shown that only 2 to 3 of the 11 disulphide bridges in N-DSK portion of fibrinogen are reduced by thioredoxin (BLOMBÄCK et al., 1974). In isolated N-DSK, all are reduced. It is interesting that the bonds which are reduced in intact fibrinogen constitute the symmetrical disulphides. The interchain disulphide bridges appear to be located in portions of the molecule which are hidden. Furthermore, NOSSEL et al. (1971) have demonstrated that the fibrinopeptide A determinants in fibrinogen are partially hidden. We, therefore, favour the idea that the disulphides which hold together the two half-molecules of fibrinogen are surface-exposed, but that they lie at the bottom of a cleft which is formed where the two half-molecules are united. In this cleft we find also the fibrinopeptide A structure—inaccessible to antibodies but not so to thrombin.

In general antibodies which have been raised against the hydrophobic structures of fibrinogen do not react with the intact fibrinogen molecule. Furthermore, the disulphide bridges in these are not available for reduction by thioredoxin in intact fibrinogen. We suppose, therefore, that the hydrophobic fragments lie hidden in the molecule. On the other hand, antibodies raised against hydrophilic structures in the molecule appear to be different. These antibodies react also with the intact fibrinogen molecule and the disulphide bridges in the structures are reduced by thioredoxin. Such a hydrophilic fragment is situated in the carboxy-terminal portion of the Aα-chain and is released from the molecule in the early phase of a plasmic digestion. In conclusion we can say that most of the disulphide bridges are buried in "core" structures in the molecule's interior. They are, without doubt, of great importance for maintaining the molecules' stability and as such are kept out of reach of the reducing system of the organism.

C. Fibrin—The Ordered Structure of Fibrinogen

I. Release of Fibrinopeptides

How the fibrinogen molecules are arranged in the ordered structure we know as the fibrin thread, continues to be a source of speculation. The fibrinogen-fibrin transformation takes place after removal of two acidic peptides from the NH_2-terminal portion of the Aα- and Bβ-chains. The molecular weight of the fibrinopeptides varies between 1500 and 3000, dependent on the species from which they have been isolated (for review see BLOMBÄCK, 1970). Dependent on their origin in the chains of fibrinogen, the peptides are denoted as either fibrinopeptide A or fibrinopeptide B. The release of these peptides is effected by hydrolytic cleavage, catalysed by thrombin. Thrombin is a trypsin-like enzyme which has a very narrow specificity toward protein substrates. Of the few hundred trypsin-sensitive bonds in fibrinogen, only four are cleaved by thrombin, two molecules of each fibrinopeptide being released from the fibrinogen dimer. Fibrinopeptide A is always released first (Fig. 7). After a lag phase, the release of fibrinopeptide B takes place.

II. Polymerization of Fibrin Monomers

Polymerization of the thrombin-activated fibrinogen molecules begins even before measurable amounts of fibrinopeptide B have been released. Fibrinopeptide A from various species shows a marked homology in its amino-acid sequence. This is especially true of the structure in close proximity to the thrombin-sensitive arginyl-glycyl bond (16 Arg–17 Gly in human fibrinogen) (Fig. 8). The structure of fibrinopeptide B has not been preserved to the same extent during evolution (Fig. 9). These facts may be an indication that thrombin has affinity primarily for structures in the Aα-chain,

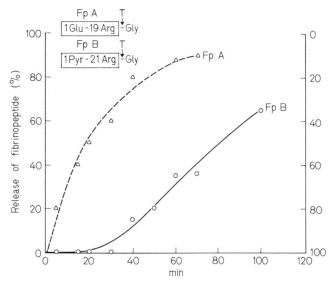

Fig. 7. Release of fibrinopeptides A and B from bovine fibrinogen after addition of thrombin. △- - -△: fibrinopeptide A ○—○: fibrinopeptide B. The susceptible bonds are shown in the upper part of the figure

which in its turn can explain the fast release of fibrinopeptide A. The specificity is dependent on a fairly limited amino-acid sequence associated with the cleaved bond. It would appear that all of the elements required for recognition by thrombin are present in the first 51 amino-acid residues of the Aα-chain (HOGG and BLOMBÄCK, 1974, 1976).

Concerning the polymerization mechanism, we have today experimental facts to support the following hypothesis. From a functional point of view the fibrinogen molecule has four domains—two in each half molecule. Let us call these domains A, A', a and a' (Fig. 5). The domains, A and A', are indeed structurally identical, but because the half-molecules in fibrinogen have a two-fold axis of symmetry in relation to one another, these halves will not appear identical. On viewing from any one direction, we see the polypeptide chains of one side of the molecule, while the corresponding chains of the other half of the molecule present their back sides. The same reasoning applies for the steric arrangement of a and a' which also are structurally identical.

This understanding of the molecule's symmetry is supported by chemical investigations which show clearly that the half-molecules are joined by three symmetrical disulphide bridges, one in the Aα-chain and two in the γ-chain. This in turn supports the hypothesis that there exists one twofold axis of symmetry, i.e. by turning the molecule through 180°, the new picture obtained can not be distinguished from the original.

In our model of the molecule, the release of the fibrinopeptides takes place in the domains A and A'. Through the release of fibrinopeptide A, a rearrangement or conformational change takes place in these domains, thereby exposing a structure or surface which is active in polymerization. The activated domains have the ability to take part in a binding interaction with the domains a and a', respectively, in another fibrinogen molecule or thrombin-activated fibrinogen molecule (i.e. fibrin monomer). The domains a and a' are capable of functioning even in fibrinogen as it circulated in blood, but as long as a specific activation of the domains A and A' has not taken place, there can be no polymerization and no clot formation. As each fibrinogen molecule consists of two half-molecules, each having two active domains, we can easily visualize how a fibrin thread can arise via "end-to-end" joining of an A or A' site in the NH$_2$-terminal portion of the molecule to an a or a' site in another molecule (Fig. 10). In this model each molecule in the fiber covers half of that molecule which precedes it.

I have previously mentioned that the thrombin-induced release of fibrinopeptide B takes place after a lag phase. This we have interpreted as arising from a conformational change which takes place in the molecule on the release of fibrinopeptide A. In this way, the fibrinopeptide B structure becomes accessible to thrombin. It is possible that here again a new binding region is uncovered, but for this we have as yet no experimental proof. If, however, this is the case, then we can denote these domains by B and B'. We can thus take it that there exist domains, complementary to B and B', in another part of the molecule and these we can denote by b and b'. Some evidence for the existence of such a binding domain is found in the fact that removal of only fibrinopeptide A by the snake venom enzyme, Botroxobin, gives rise to polymerization which is different from that which occurs when both fibrinopeptide A and B are released in the presence of thrombin. In the latter case, a polymer is formed which is

Fig. 8. Fibrinopeptide A

Amino acid positions (read left→right): 19 18 17 16 15 14 13 12 11 10 9 8 7 6 5 4 3 2 1. Residues in parentheses denote an undetermined order/composition. (Best-effort reading of a densely printed sequence-alignment figure.)

Order	Animal	Species	Sequence (position 19 → 1)
Primates	man	*Homo sapiens*	Ala–Asp–Ser–Gly–Glu–Gly–Asp–Phe–Leu–Ala–Glu–Gly–Gly–Gly–Val–Arg
	chimpanzee 1	*Pan troglodytes*	(Ala, Asx, Ser, Gly, Glx, Gly, Asx)–Phe–Leu–(Ala, Glx, Gly, Gly, Gly, Val) Arg
	green monkey 2	*Ceropithecus aethiops*	Ala–Asp–Thr–Gly–Glu–Gly–Asp–Phe–Leu–Ala–Glu–Gly–Gly–Val–Arg
	drill	*Mandrillus leucophaeus*	(Ala, Asx, Thr, Gly, Asx, Gly, Gly) Ile (Thr, Glx, Gly, Gly, Gly) Val–Arg
Rodentia	laboratory rat	*Rattus norvegicus*	Ala–Asp–Thr–Gly–Thr–Thr–Ser–Glu–Phe–Ile–(Asx, Glx, Gly, Ala, Gly, Ile, Arg)
	guinea pig	*Cavia porcellus*	Thr–Asp–Thr–Gly–Glu–Gly–Glu–Phe–Glu–Ala–Gly–Gly–Gly–Val–Arg
Lagomorpha	rabbit	*Oryctolagus cuniculus*	Val–Asp–Pro–Gly–Ser–Thr–Phe–Asp–Ala–Thr–Phe–Ile–Asp–Gly–Gly–Gly–Gly–Arg
Carnivora	dog, fox	*Canis familiaris, V. vulpes*	Thr–Asn–Ser–Lys–Gly–Glu–Glu–Phe–Ile–Ala–Glu–Gly–Gly–Gly–Val–Arg
	brown bear	*Ursus arctos*	Thr–Asp–Gly–Lys–Glu–Gly–Glu–Phe–Ile–Ala–(Gly, Gly, Val, Arg)
	cat	*Felis catus*	Gly–Asp–Val–Gln–Glu–Gly–Glu–Phe–Ile–Ala–Glu–Gly–Gly–Val–Arg
	grey seal	*Halichoerus grypus*	Thr–Asp–Thr–Lys–Glu–Thr–Glu–Phe–Ile–Ala–(Gly, Gly, Val, Arg)
	badger	*Meles meles*	Thr–Asp–Val–Lys–Glu–Gly–Glu–Phe–Ile–Ala–(Gly, Gly, Val, Arg)
	mink	*Mustela vison*	Thr–Asn–Val–Lys–Glu–Gly–Glu–Phe–Ile–Ala–(Gly, Gly, Gly, Arg)
Proboscoidea	indian elephant	*Elephas maximus*	Ala–Glu–Thr–Gln–Gly–Asp–Phe–Leu–(Glx, Glx, Gly, Gly, Val, Arg)
Perissodactyla	horse, mule 1	*Equus caballus*	Thr–Glu–Gly–Glu–Gly–Gly–Phe–Leu–His–Glu–Gly–Gly–Gly–Val–Arg
	donkey, mule 2	*Equus asinus*	Thr–Lys–Thr–Gly–Glu–Gly–Gly–Phe–Leu–Ser–Glu–Gly–Gly–(Gly, Val, Arg)
	zebra 1	*Equus quagga granti*	Thr–Lys–Thr–Gly–Glu–Gly–Gly–Phe–Leu–Ser–Glu–Gly–Gly–(Gly, Val, Arg)
	zebra 2		Thr–Lys–Thr–Gly–Glu–Gly–Gly–Phe–Leu–Ser–Glu–Gly–Gly–(Ala, Gly, Val, Arg)
Artiodactyla	ox	*Bos taurus*	Glu–Asp–Gly–Ser–Asp–Pro–Pro–Gly–Gly–Asp–Phe–Leu–Thr–Glu–Gly–Gly–Gly–Val–Arg
	european bison	*Bison bonasus*	Glu–Asp–Gly–Ser–Asp–Pro–Ser–Gly–Asp–Phe–Leu–Ala–Glu–Gly–Gly–Gly–Val–Arg
	cape buffalo	*Syncerus caffer*	Glu–Asp–Gly–Ser–Asp–Gly–Ser–Gly–Asp–Phe–Leu–(Ala, Glx, Gly, Gly, Gly, Val, Arg)
	water buffalo	*B. bubalus*	Gly–Asp–Gly–Ser–Asp–Ala–Val–Gly–Gly–Asp–Phe–Leu–(Ala, Glx, Gly, Gly, Gly, Val, Arg)
	mule deer	*Odocoileus hemionus*	Ser–Asp–Pro–Ala–Ser–Asp–Phe–Leu–(Leu, Ala, Glx, Gly, Gly, Gly, Val, Arg)
	red deer	*Cervus elaphus*	Ala–Asp–Gly–Ser–Asp–Pro–Ala–Ser–Asp–Phe–Leu–Ala–Glu–Gly–Gly–Gly–Val–Arg
	american elk	*Cervus canadensis*	(Ala, Asx, Gly, Ser, Asx, Pro, Ala, Ser)–Phe–(Leu, Ala, Glx, Gly, Gly, Gly, Val, Arg)
	sika deer	*Cervus nippon*	Ala–Asx–Gly–Ser–Asp–Pro–Ala–Ser–Glx–Phe–(Leu, Ala, Glx, Gly, Gly, Gly, Val, Arg)
	muntjak	*Muntiacus muntjak*	(Ala, Asx, Gly, Ser, Asx, Pro, Ala, Ser)–Phe–(Leu, Thr, Glx, Gly, Gly, Gly, Val, Arg)
	reindeer, european elk	*Rangifer tarandus, A. alces*	Ala–Asp–Gly–Ser–Asp–Pro–Ala–Gly–Phe–Leu–Ala–Glu–Gly–Gly–Gly–Val–Arg
	sheep, goat 3	*Ovis aries, Capra sp.*	Ala–Asp–Asp–Ser–Asp–Pro–Val–Gly–Gly–Asp–Phe–Leu–Ala–Glu–Gly–Gly–Gly–Val–Arg
	pronghorn	*Antilocapra americana*	Ala–Asp–Gly–Ser–Asp–Pro–Val–Gly–Ser–Asp–Phe–Leu–Pro–Ala–Gly–Gly–Gly–Gly–Arg
	pig, wild boar	*Sus scrofa*	Ala–Glu–Val–Gln–Asp–Lys–Asp–Phe–Leu–Ala–Glu–Gly–Gly–Gly–Val–Arg
	llama	*Lama glama*	Thr–Asp–Pro–Asp–Ala–Asp–Lys–Phe–Leu–Ala–Glu–Gly–Gly–Gly–Val–Arg
	vicuna	*Lama pacos vicugna*	(Thr, Asx, Pro, Ala, Ala, Asx)–Phe–(Leu, Ala, Glx, Gly, Gly, Gly, Val, Arg)
	camel	*Camelus bactrianus* / +*Camelus dromedaricus*	Thr–Asp–Pro–Asp–Ala–Asp–Glu–Phe–Leu–Ala–Glx–Phe–(Leu, Ala, Glx, Gly, Gly, Gly, Val, Arg)
Marsupalia	kangaroo	*Macropus sp.*	Thr–Lys–Asp–Pro–Ala–Asp–Asp–Lys–Thr–Phe–Ile–Ala–Glu–Gly–(Gly, Val, Arg)
	wombat	*Vombatus ursinus*	Thr–Lys–Thr–Gly–Gly–Ser–Thr–Phe–Ile–Ala–Glx–Phe–(Leu, Ala, Glx, Gly, Gly, Gly, Val, Arg)
Reptilia	stumpy tail lizard	*Trachydosaurus rugosus*	Glu–Asp–Thr–Gly–Thr–Thr–Gly–Asp–Glu–Gly–Gly–(His, Gly, Gly, Val, Arg)

Fig. 9. Fibrinopeptide B

Position numbers: 21 20 19 18 17 16 15 14 13 12 11 10 9 8 7 6 5 4 3 2 1

Group	Species	Sequence (positions 21 → 1)
Primates	Man 1	[Glu -Gly -Val -AsN -Asp -Glu -Glu -AsN -Glu -Glu -Gly -Phe -Phe -Ser -Ala -Arg
	Green monkey (*C. aeth.*)	-AsN -Glu -Glu -Gly -Leu -Phe -Gly -Ala -Arg
	Macaques (*Rh., Cyn.*)	-AsN -Glu -Glu -Ser -Pro -Phe -Ser -Gly -Arg
Artiodactyls	Ox	[Glu -Phe -Pro -Thr -Asp -Tyr -Asp -Glu -Glu -Gly -GlN -Asp -Glu -Glu -Arg -Pro -Lys -Val -Gly -Ala -Arg
	Bison	(Glu, Phe, Pro, Thr, Asp, Tyr, Asp, … Arg, Pro, Lys, Val, Gly, Ala, Arg)
	Red deer	(Glu, Ser, His, Thr, Asp, Tyr, Asp, … Lys, Val, Gly, Ala, Arg) (Ala -Lys)
	Reindeer	His -Glu -Leu -Ala -Asp -Tyr -Asp -Val -Leu -Asp -Ala -Arg (Leu, His, Leu, Asp, Ala, Ala, Arg)
	Sheep, Goat	-Gly -Tyr -Leu -Asp -Tyr -Asp -Glu -Val -His -Val -Ala -Arg (Lys, Val, Arg, Leu, Asp, Ala, Arg)
	Pig	-Ala -Ilu -Asp -Tyr -Asp -Glu -Arg -Pro -Lys -His -Val -Ala -Arg (–Lys, Val, Arg, Leu, Asp, Ala, Arg)
	Llama	-Ala -Thr -Asp -Tyr -Asp -Glu -Arg -Pro -Lys -Val -Leu -Ala -Arg
	Camel (*C. drom.*)	-Ala -Thr -Asp -Tyr -Asp -Glu -Arg -Pro -Lys -Val -Leu -Ala -Arg
Perissodactyls	Horse	-Leu -Asp -Tyr -Asp -His -Glu -Arg -Thr -Phe -Asp -Ala -Arg [Asp, Ala, Arg]
	Donkey	-Leu -Asp -Tyr -Asp -His -Glu -Arg -Thr -Phe -Asp -Ala -Arg (Val, Thr, Phe, Asp, Ala, Arg)
	Zebra	-Leu -Asp -Tyr -Asp -His -Gly -Arg -Lys -Val -Thr -Phe -Asp -Ala -Arg (Arg, Ala, Lys, Val, Thr, Phe, Asp, Ala, Arg)
Carnivores	Dog	-His -Tyr -Tyr -Asp -Asp -Ilu -Val -Ser -Thr -Val -Asp -Ala -Arg
	Fox	(Glu, Tyr, Tyr, Asp, Asp, Glu, Ilu, Val, Ser, Thr, Val, Asp, Ala, Arg) (Ilu, Ser, Leu, Ala, Arg)
	Cat	-Ilu -Asp -Tyr -Tyr -Asp -Arg -Asp -Val -Val -AsN -Ala -Arg (Thr, Val, Asp, Ala, Arg)
Rodents	Rat	-Ala -Thr -Thr -Asp -Ser -Asp -Lys -Val -Asp -Ser -Leu -Ala -Arg (Glu, Glu, Arg, Ilu, Val, Ser, Thr, Val, Asp, Ala, Arg)
Lagomorphs	Rabbit	-Ala -Asp -Asp -Tyr -Asp -Asp -Tyr -Glu -Val -Leu -Pro -Ala -Arg (Glu, Gly, Val, Gly, Lys, Ser, Ser, Val, Asp, Ala, Arg)
Marsupials	Kangaroo	-Ser -Phe -Asp -Tyr -Asp -Asp -Tyr -Gly (Glu, Gly, Gly, Val, Lys, Ser, Ser, Val, Asp, Ala, Arg)

Fig. 8. Fibrinopeptide A from different animal species. The amino-acid sequences have been elucidated by BLOMBÄCK (1970) and by Doolittle and co-workers (see DOOLITTLE, 1973). (Figs. 8 and 9 are from DAYHOFF, M.O.: Atlas of Protein Sequence and Structure. Washington, D.C.: National Biomedical Research Foundation, 1972, Vol. V, p. D. 87). Mule has equal amounts of horse and donkey fibrinopeptides. In zebra two types of fibrinopeptides has been found.
1. Chimpanzee, gorilla and orangutan fibrinopeptides are identical.
2. Green monkey, irus macaque, baboon and siamang fibrinopeptides are identical.
3. Ibex fibrinopeptides is identical to sheep and goat.
(Glu = pyrrolidone carboxylic acid)

Fig. 9. Fibrinopeptide B from different animal species. The amino-acid sequences have been elucidated by Blombäck and co-workers (see BLOMBÄCK, 1970) and by Doolittle and co-workers (see Doolittle, 1973) see below.
1. Chimpanzee and gorilla fibrinopeptides are identical.
(Glu = pyrrolidone carboxylic acid)

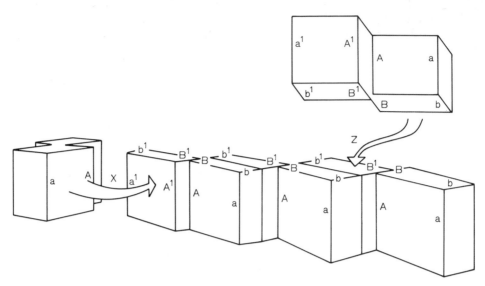

Fig. 10. Schematic representation of fibrin thread formation. In this model, rectangular boxes have been used as building units. These are joined in a double molecule having a twofold symmetry. The domains AA' − aa' are thought to be situated at the opposite ends on the broad sides of the boxes while the domains BB' − bb' are located at opposite ends of the narrow sides of the boxes. A polymer arises through "end-to-end" polymerization by the domain a or a' binding to the complementary domain A or A'(X). In a similar manner, "side-to-side" polymerization takes place, causing branching of the initial polymer by combining of the narrow sides of the boxes (Z). The arrows indicate the binding position of the units

appreciably more compact than that obtained in the presence of Botroxobin (LAU-RENT and BLOMBÄCK, 1958). It is obvious that if apart from the AA'–aa', even the BB'–bb' domains are active in polymer production, then the latter process would reinforce the fiber formed by only AA'–aa' interaction. The involvement of these domains (BB'–bb') also provides a simple means of branching the fibrin fiber and hence the construction of a intricate polymer network. In Figure 10 we can see one acceptable model of how these domains come together to operate in "end-to-end" and "side-to-side" polymerization. While I have chosen to use rectangular boxes in this model, the actual form is of no importance. We can extend the play with all these domains by allowing, as H. W. THOMAS in Cardiff (1970) has done, the succeeding activated dimer units to combine with the preceding ones at an angle of 120°. In such a way a protofibril is produced having a threefold screw symmetry. If we then consider that these protofibrils are linked, after activation of the BB'-domains, in a sixfold screw symmetry, then a polymer would be produced which is in good agreement with the results obtained through electron microscopic studies of the actual fibrin fiber. In the schematic model of the fibrin polymer which is shown in Figure 10, it has been assumed that all the domains have the same binding energy. Of course, it is also possible that this is not the case. It is just as likely that both negative and positive cooperative effects play a part and thereby change considerably the geometry of polymerization. Consequently, one can imagine the situation where the release of fibrinopeptide A with subsequent binding of the a or a' to one of the domains in N-DSK (e.g. A) changes the corresponding course of events in the other domain (e.g. A'). In this way the subsequent polymerization can be affected in a positive or negative manner causing a change in the geometry.

The experimental support for the ideas which I have attempted to substantiate above lies in several years of study of the chemical changes produced in the fibrinogen molecule in the presence of thrombin and other clotting enzymes (BLOMBÄCK and BLOMBÄCK, 1972). The localizing of the domains is based primarily on studies concerning the affinity between fragments of the fibrinogen molecule and various insoluble fibrinogen and fibrin derivatives (KUDRYK et al., 1973, 1974; YORK and BLOMBÄCK, 1976). If fibrinogen is covalently coupled to Sepharose and then activated with thrombin, the conjugate displays certain specific adsorption properties (HEENE and MATHIAS, 1973). This thrombin-activated, conjugated derivative adsorbs specifically fibrinogen from plasma. This conjugate has been shown to have the property to specifically adsorb fragment D from a plasmin digest of fibrinogen. Apparently, thrombin activation of the fibrinogen-Sepharose conjugate exposes structures which have the possibility of interacting with structures in fragment D. As even intact fibrinogen binds to the conjugate, we assume, that these structures are exposed in fibrinogen as it circulates in the blood. We have concluded from these investigations that the domains A and A' are capable of being activated by thrombin and that the complementary domains, a and a', are located in the fragment D portion of the molecule. Fragment D, which arises from plasmic digestion, consists of a population of molecules whose molecular weights vary from 80000 to 100000. It was demonstrated that only the high molecular weight form of fragment D (so called fragment D_s) had high affinity for the conjugate. In all probability, the differences between the various fragments D are to be found in the carboxy-terminal portions of the fragment D_s. These portions of fragment D_s may therefore be of particular importance for binding (COLLEN et al., 1975).

The question now arises as to where the domains A and A' are situated. Because these are activated by thrombin, it was natural to conclude that release of fibrinopeptide must be essential for their activation. It was therefore also reasonable to presume that the domains were located in the NH_2-terminal portion of the molecule. In an earlier chapter I have discussed the fragments which result from cleavage of fibrinogen with CNBr and plasmin. The NH_2-terminal fragment, N-DSK, was of special interest in this connection as it constitutes approximately 16% of the intact fibrinogen molecule. We conjugated this fragment with Sepharose and were able to show that this, like the fibrinogen-Sepharose conjugate, on activation with thrombin could specifically adsorb fibrinogen and even fragment D from plasmin-digested fibrinogen. As was expected, N-DSK in solution, on activation with thrombin, was shown to bind to the fibrinogen-Sepharose conjugate (YORK and BLOMBÄCK, 1976).

The structures in N-DSK which, directly or indirectly, are activated or exposed after activation with thrombin and which govern the interaction with fragment D, may be found in the first 43 NH_2-terminal amino-acid residues in the $B\beta$-chain and/ or the carboxy-terminal portion of the γ-chain. This is concluded from the fact that fragment E, which contains all of the structure of N-DSK except the above-mentioned amino-acid residues in the $B\beta$- and γ-fragments, does, after activation with thrombin, bind to the aa' domains only to a small extent. It is also likely that the amino-acid residue, Aα 19 Arg, is involved directly or indirectly in the interaction. The basis for this hypothesis is the fact that fibrinogen Detroit in which the positively charged argine residue has been replaced by a neutral amino-acid residue (serine), does not undergo polymerization in the presence of thrombin, in spite of the fact that the peptide bond between A' Arg and Aα 17 Gly is cleaved and fibrinopeptide A is released. In contrast to the situation in normal fibrinogen, fibrinopeptide B is only slowly released from fibrinogen Detroit (Blombäck and Blombäck, 1970). Apparently the mutation, Aα 19 Arg Gly, does not influence the primary substrate specificity of thrombin but rather the rearrangements which are necessary for the uncovering of the polymerization domains after release of fibrinopeptide A. Furthermore, one could postulate that this rearrangement is necessary so that the fibrinopeptide B portion of fibrinogen can be made available for hydrolysis by thrombin, thereby permitting exposure of the hypothetical polymerization domains BB'–bb'. Fibrinogen Detroit teaches us to make a clear distinction between the proteolytic activation caused by thrombin and the subsequent course of polymerization. Cleavage, in the presence of thrombin, under normal conditions only facilitates the secondary changes which are a *sine qua non* for polymerization.

There are, no doubt, structures in or around the symmetrical disulphide bridges which also play, directly or indirectly, a fundamental role in the structural integrity and function of the polymerization domains. Thus, it has been shown that thioredoxin-catalyzed reduction of the symmetrical disulphide bridges (Aα 28, γ 8 and/or 9) in the Aα- and γ-chains of fibrinogen, caused a total loss of the ability to form fibrin (Blombäck et al., 1974). This phenomenon cannot be ascribed to a change in the proteolytic activity of thrombin as the rate of release of fibrinopeptide A from the reduced fibrinogen is the same as that for the unreduced material (Hogg and Blombäck, 1974).

We consider that the conclusions concerning the polymerization of fibrinogen, drawn from the investigations using Sepharose conjugates to fibrinogen and N-DSK, are applicable also in the physiological state. This is found in the well known fact that fibrinolytic degradation products of fibrinogen, particularly the so-called early products including fragments X and Y and fragment D, inhibit the polymerization of fibrinogen. Furthermore, it is known that a pronounced bleeding tendency occurs in clinical states when the concentration of these degradation products is high. According to our theory, this is what one would expect. The presence in blood of fragment D or related fragments, causes the inhibition of the formation of a normal fibrin polymer by the interaction of these with the domains A and A' in the N-DSK portion of the fibrin monomers. Because these fragments most likely are monovalent, no further enlargement of the polymers can take place from the N-DSK end. Further, Bang (1964) has shown by electron microscopy that the fibrin network formed in the presence of fibrinogen degradation products has an appearance which deviates from the normal in that it was more fragile. However, the strongest support for our notion is given by findings with fibrinogen Detroit (Kudryk et al., 1976). In this it was demonstrated as was presumed in our model (see above), that the N-DSK portion of the molecule, after activation, had no ability to bind to the fragment D domain of normal fibrinogen. On the other hand, the fragment D portion of fibrinogen Detroit possesses normal binding properties. Consequently, the domain bearing the mutation has anomalous binding properties while the apparently normal struc-

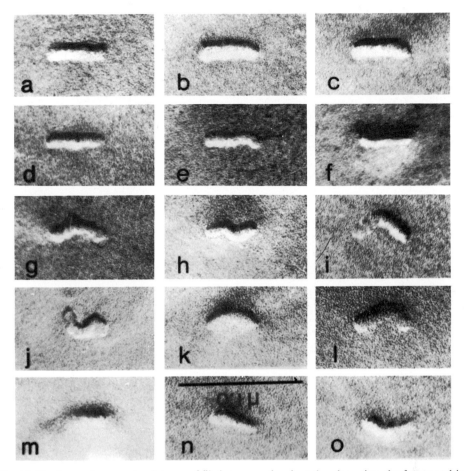

Fig. 11. Electron-microscopic pictures of fibrinogen molecules taken by using the freeze-etching technique. From BACHMANN et al., (1975). Photograph by courtesy of K. LEDERER

ture has normal binding properties. Knowing that patients with dysfibrinogenemia Detroit have a hemorrhagic diathesis and that their fibrinogen clots slowly in the presence of thrombin makes one think that there must exist a connection between mutation, defective binding properties, and defective hemostasis.

In our discussion of the location of the domains in the fibrinogen molecule, we have made use of that picture of the molecule which our chemical investigations have provided. This representation is, by necessity, linear. We can now ask ourselves: where are the domains situated in the tertiary structure of the molecule? If we accept that the electron microscopic pictures of BACHMANN et al. (Fig. 11) truly represent the native hydrated molecule, then we can already now come up with suggestions concerning the location of the domains, AA' and aa'. According to BACHMANN et al. the fibrinogen molecule probably has the form of a cylinder with rounded ends. If we carefully examine the enlargements of the various observed molecules, we find that several differ appreciably from the idealized picture (Fig. 11). One sees forms which

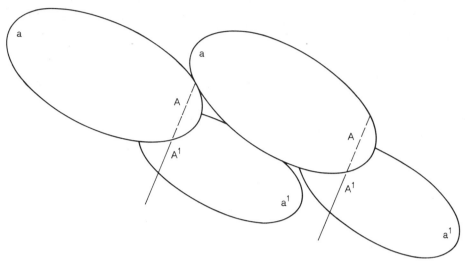

Fig. 12. Interpretation of the electron-microscopic pictures of the fibrinogen molecule. The drawing shows one projection of two molecules combined through the binding domains AA′—and aa′—when activated by thrombin. Each molecule consists of two half-molecules joined in a twofold symmetry by the symmetrical disulphides, creating clefts between the two half-molecules

appear to be puckered in the middle or are bent at the ends. The authors explained this by suggesting that the molecule has an appreciable flexibility. However, one could now interpret the electron microscopic pictures from another standpoint. The different forms may possibly represent various projections of a rigid molecule. In Figure 12, I have depicted our interpretation of how the half-molecules are joined to produce the molecular form which is observed by electron microscopy (BLOMBÄCK et al., 1976b). The puckered form (Fig. 11h) may represent a picture of a double molecule in which two rod-shaped half-molecules are linked in their NH_2-terminal ends so that they have a twofold axis of symmetry. Most of the pictures seen in Figure 11 will then fit a representation of the molecule in a projection which is more or less perpendicular to the former. The remaining forms which are seen in Figure 11 are either partially concealed or have forms (i and j) which are not consistent with our interpretation. In our interpretation of the electron microscopic pictures, the domains AA′ must be located in the central joining portion of the molecule. It may be that the domains, BB′–bb′, are located in the same parts of the molecule. In Figure 12, I have also ventured to show how two fibrinogen molecules are orientated when interaction takes place in the binding domains, AA′–aa′.

III. Stabilizing of the Fibrin Polymer

The fibrin polymer which is formed after activation with thrombin undergoes a secondary transformation through the introduction of covalent crosslinking between glutamine residues in one chain and lysine residues in another (DOOLITTLE, 1973; LORAND, 1972). In the initial phase of polymerization, these residues are brought

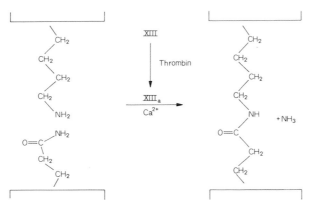

Fig. 13. Formation of ε-(γ-glotamyl) lysine crosslinks through condensation of glutamine and lysine side-chains. (Adopted from DOOLITTLE, 1973)

into juxtaposition. In the presence of activated transglutaminase (factor XIII) and calcium ions, condensation takes place between the γ-carbonyl group of glutamine and the amino group of lysine with release of ammonia (Fig. 13). Factor XIII is present in plasma and thrombocytes, where it exists as an inactive precursor and is activated by thrombin, probably by limited proteolysis. The stabilization entails crosslinking of the γ-chain in one molecule with the γ-chain in another. Even the α-chains undergo intermolecular crosslinking, but it is still unclear if the reaction mechanism is the same as that involving the γ-chains. The resulting stabilized fibrin is insoluble in urea solution and other solvents which dissolve non-stabilized fibrin.

D. Fibrinogen in Health and Disease

The normal fibrinogen concentration is 2–3 g/l plasma. Fibrinogen belongs to a group of "reactive proteins" and an increase in the blood level of fibrinogen can be seen in many conditions. In infection the fibrinogen level in blood increases markedly, this being the major cause of the increased red cell sedimentation rate seen in these conditions. In neoplastic diseases one sees just as often increased fibrinogen levels. Most typical is the very high fibrinogen concentration in hypernephromas even in the early state before metastasis has taken place. In post-operative states or after trauma, there is also generally an increase in the blood fibrinogen level.

It is probable that the increased fibrinogen levels are caused by increased synthesis. Increased synthesis can parallel an increased catabolism. However, turnover studies using ^{125}I-labeled fibrinogen can reveal such changes. If the catabolism increases by more than that of the synthetic capacity of the organism, the result is a drop in the blood fibrinogen level. Such an imbalance can arise in liver injury. Most common is the phenomenon in so-called intravascular coagulation. In this condition, fibrinogen catabolism increases because of the deposition of fibrin in the blood system and in the blood vessels. Uncontrolled activation of fibrinogen can take place on the invasion of substances into the blood which can activate prothrombin to thrombin. Intravascular coagulation is an extremely serious condition. It can arise as a complication in several diseases with different pathogeneses. It is found for example in abruptio placentae, after trauma, shock, hemolytic crisis, neoplasms, etc. The diagnosis is difficult. The fibrinogen concentration is low but need not necessarily be so. The concentration of other clotting factors is often reduced but one cannot describe common patterns. However, just recently we have been provided with a valuable tool for the diagnosis of intravascular coagulation. This is a radioimmunologic method for the measurement of fibrinopeptide A. As the release of fibrinopeptide A is a measure of the activation of the fibrinogen molecule, the level of this can reflect the thrombotic process and its intensity (NOSSEL et al., 1974). In intravascular coagulation we witness a substantial rise in the level of fibrinopeptide A (FPA). The FPA level is even increased in local thrombosis if the thrombosis is extensive.

In a rare, congenital disease, afibrinogenemia, there is an apparent lack of fibrinogen. These patients have a strong bleeding tendency. A thrombin-clotted protein can not be demonstrated in the blood. The presence of the protein cannot be demonstrated by immunologic means either. This does not of course mean that these patients are devoid of a fibrinogen-like protein. It is possible that an abnormal fibrinogen molecule is present but that this does not contain the antigenic determinants which are typical of normal fibrinogen. Congenital hypofibrinogenemia is not so uncommon. There exists hardly any increased bleeding tendency in such patients. It has been speculated that these patients may possibly be heterozygotes with regard to a afibrinogenemia trait.

During recent years, reports have appeared of patients who have a functionally defective fibrinogen. The condition is usually described by the term: dysfibrinogenemia. Up to now, some 20 families have been described as having this disorder. The most characteristic finding is a lengthening of the "thrombin time" of plasma. In other words, the time taken for coagulation of the plasma on addition of thrombin, is longer than normal. To distinguish these different types of abnormal fibrinogen from each other, they have been given the name of the town or district where the discovery was made. Most of the patients described were believed to be heterozygotes, having little or no hemostatic problem. Two members of a Black family in Detroit have been discovered to be homozygotes with regard to this abnormality. This fibrinogen, named fibrinogen Detroit, is inherited according to an auto-dominant pattern. The homozygotes have a severe bleeding diathesis, and unlike the heterozygotes, their plasma does not clot at all or very slowly in the presence of thrombin (MAMMEN et al., 1969; BLOMBÄCK et al., 1968 b).

Fibrinogen Detroit is an example of the dramatic consequences a genetically determined change in structure has for the function of a protein. The mutation (Aα 19 Arg→Ser) has occurred in the invariable portion of the structure, i.e. that portion which has been conserved during mammalian evolution. Evidently, this portion of the Aα-chain is critical for polymerization. However, this does not mean that the affinity shown by thrombin for this chain is necessarily lower than it is in normal fibrinogen. In fact, it has been demonstrated that fibrinopeptide A is released from fibrinogen Detroit and that the rate of release appears to be almost normal. Hence, we can suppose that the mutation brings about secondary changes in the conformation of fibrinogen so that the domains which are normally active in polymerization, remain dormant even after exposure to thrombin. In Figure 14 I have depicted how one could imagine the functional disorder to have arisen. Through a conformational

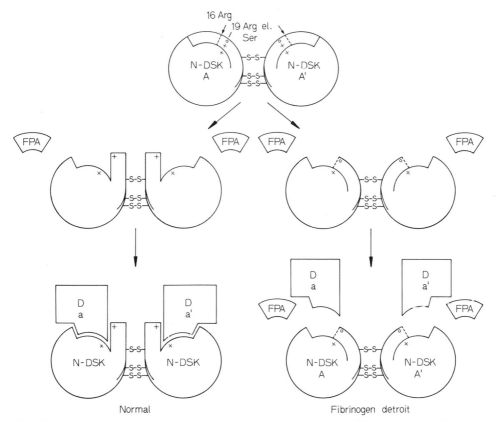

Fig. 14. Interaction between the polymerization sites in normal fibrinogen and fibrinogen Detroit. The figure shows a situation in which no conformational change occurs in the N – DSK domain of fibrinogen Detroit on release of fibrinopeptide A. *FPA*: fibrinopeptide A. *O*: denotes charge of neutral amino acid Aα19 Ser in fibrinogen Detroit

change, which takes place after the release of fibrinopeptide A, the polymerization domains in N-DSK (AA') and fragment D (aa') in two molecules combine in the normal situation. In fibrinogen Detroit, no conformational change takes place, or if it does, the change in conformation is not compatible with the combination of the two domains.

References

Bachmann, L., Schmitt-Fumian, W. W., Hammel, R., Lederer, K.: Size and shape of fibrinogen. I. Electron microscopy of the hydrated molecule. Makromol. Chem. **176**, 2603—2618 (1975)

Bang, N. U.: A molecular structural model of fibrin based on electron microscopy of fibrin polymerization. Thrombos. Diathes. haemorrh. (Stuttg.) Suppl. **13**, 73—80 (1964)

Blombäck, B.: On the properties of fibrinogen and fibrin. Ark. Kemi **12**, 99—113 (1958)

Blombäck, B.: Fibrinogen to fibrin transformation. In: Seegers, W. H. (Ed.): Blood Clotting Enzymology, pp. 143—215. New York: Academic Press Inc. 1967

Blombäck, B.: Carbohydrates in blood-clotting proteins. In: Gottschalk, A. (Ed.): Glycoproteins, their composition, structure and function. 5 Part B. pp. 1069—1081. Amsterdam: Elsevier Publ. Co. 1972

Blombäck, B.: Selectional trends in the structure of fibrinogen of different species. In Macfarlane, R. G. (Ed.): The haemostatic mechanism in man and other animals. No 27, pp. 167—187. Academic Press 1970

Blombäck, B., Blombäck, M.: Purification of human and bovine fibrinogen. Ark. Kemi 10, 415—443 (1957)

Blombäck, B., Blombäck, M.: Molecular defects and variants of fibrinogen. Nouv. Rev. franç. Hémat. 10, 671—678 (1970)

Blombäck, B., Blombäck, M.: The molecular structure of fibrinogen. Ann. N.Y. Acad. Sci. 202, 77—97 (1972)

Blombäck, B., Blombäck, M., Edman, P., Hessel, B.: Human fibrinopeptides; isolation, characterization, and structure. Biochim. biophys. Acta (Amst.) 115, 371—396 (1966)

Blombäck, B., Blombäck, M., Finkbeiner, W., Holmgren, A., Kowalska-Loth, B., Olovson, G.: Enzymatic reduction of disulfide bonds in fibrin-ogen by the thioredoxin system. I. Identification of reduced bonds and studies on reoxidation process. Thrombos. Res. 4, 55—75 (1974)

Blombäck, B., Blombäck, M., Henschen, A., Hessel, B., Iwanaga, S., Woods, K. R.: N-terminal disulphide knot of human fibrinogen. Nature (Lond.) 218, 130—134 (1968 a)

Blombäck, B., Blombäck, M., Olsson, P., Svendsen, L., Åberg, G.: Synthetic peptides with anticoagulant and vasodilating activity. Scand. J. clin. Lab. Invest. 24, Suppl. 107, 59—64 (1969)

Blombäck, B., Blombäck, M., Searle, J.: On the occurrence of phosphorus in fibrinogen. Biochim. biophys. Acta (Amst.) 74, 148—151 (1963)

Blombäck, B., Gröndahl, N. J., Hessel, B., Iwanaga, S., Wallén, P.: Primary structure of human fibrinogen and fibrin. II. Structural studies on NH_2-terminal part of γ-chain. J. biol. Chem. 248, 5806—5820 (1973)

Blombäck, B., Hessel, B., Hogg, D.: Disulfide bridges in NH_2-terminal part of human fibrinogen. Thrombos. Res. 8, 639—658 (1976 a)

Blombäck, B., Hessel, B., Iwanaga, S., Reuterby, J., Blombäck, M.: Primary structure of human fibrinogen and fibrin. I. Cleavage of fibrinogen with cyanogen bromide. Isolation and characterization of NH_2-terminal fragments of the α("A")-chain. J. biol. Chem. 247, 1496—1512 (1972)

Blombäck, B., Hogg, D. H., Gårdlung, B., Hessel, B., Kudryk, B.: Fibrinogen and fibrin formation. Thrombos. Res. Suppl. II, 329—346 (1976 b)

Blombäck, B., Yamashina, I.: On the N-terminal amino acids in fibrinogen and fibrin. Ark. Kemi 12, 299—319 (1958)

Blombäck, M., Blombäck, B., Mammen, E. F., Prasad, A. S.: Fibrinogen Detroit—a molecular defect in the N-terminal disulphide knot of human fibrinogen? Nature (Lond.) 218, 134—137 (1968 b)

Cartwright, T., Kekwick, R. G. O.: A comparative study of human, cow, pig, and sheep fibrinogen. Biochim. biophys. Acta (Amst.) 236, 550—562 (1971)

Caspary, E. A., Kekwick, R. A.: Some physicochemical properties of human fibrinogen. Biochem. J. 67, 41—48 (1957)

Collen, D., Kudryk, B., Hessel, B., Blombäck, B.: Primary structure of human fibrinogen and fibrin. III Isolation and partial characterization of chains of fragment D. J. biol. Chem. 250, 5808—5817 (1975)

Doolittle, R. F.: Structural aspects of the fibrinogen to fibrin conversion. Advanc. Protein Chem. 27, 1—109 (1973)

Doolittle, R. F., Cassman, K. G., Cottrell, B. A., Friezner, S. J., Hucko, J. T., Takagi, T.: Amino acid sequence studies on the α-chain of human fibrinogen. Characterization of 11 Cyanogen Bromide fragments. Biochemistry 16, 1703—1709 (1977)

Edman, P.: Sequence determination. In: Needleman, S. B. (Ed.): Protein sequence determination, pp. 211—255. Berlin-Heidelberg-New York: Springer 1970

Finlaysson, J. S., Mosesson, M. W.: Heterogeneity of human fibrinogen. Biochemistry 2, 42—46 (1963)

Gaffney, P. J.: Heterogeneity of human fibrinogen. Nature (Lond.) New Biol. 230, 54—56 (1971)

Gaffney, P. J., Dobos, P.: A structural aspect of human fibrinogen suggested by its plasmin degradation. FEBS Lett. **15**, 13—16 (1971)

Gårdlund, B., Hessel, B., Marguerie, G., Murano, G., Blombäck, B.: Primary structure of human fibrinogen. Characterization of disulfide containing cyanogenbromide fragments. European J. Biochem. **77**, 595—610 (1977)

Hall, C. E., Slayter, H. S.: The fibrinogen molecule: its size, shape and mode of polymerization. J. biophys. biochem. Cytol. **5**, 11—15 (1959)

Heene, D. L., Matthias, F. R.: Adsorption of fibrinogen derivatives on insolubilized fibrinogen and fibrinmonomer. Thrombos. Res. **2**, 137—154 (1973)

Henschen, A.: S-sulfo-derivatives of fibrinogen and fibrin: preparations and general properties. Ark. Kemi **22**, 1—28 (1963)

Henschen, A.: Peptide chains in S-sulfo-fibrinogen and S-sulfo-fibrin: isolation methods and general properties. Ark. Kemi **22**, 375—396 (1964a)

Henschen, A.: Number and reactivity of disulfide in fibrinogen and fibrin. Ark. Kemi **22**, 355—373 (1964b)

Henschen, A., Blombäck, B.: Amino acid composition of human and bovine fibrinogen and fibrin. Ark. Kemi **22**, 347—354 (1964)

Henschen, A., Edman, P.: Large scale preparation of S-carboxymethylated chains of human fibrin and fibrinogen and the occurrence of γ-chain variants. Biochim. biophys. Acta (Amst.) **263**, 351—367 (1972)

Henschen, A., Lottspeich, F., Sekita, T., Warbinek, R.: Amino acid sequence of human fibrin. Preliminary note on the order of peptides obtained by cleaving the γ-chain at the methionyl and arginyl bonds. Hoppe-Seylers Z. physiol. Chem. **357**, 605—608 (1976)

Hessel, B.: On the structure of the COOH-terminal part of the αA-chain of human fibrinogen. Thrombos. Res. **7**, 75—87 (1975)

Hessel, B., Blombäck, M.: The proteolytic action of the snake venom enzymes Arvin and Reptilase on N-terminal chain fragments of human fibrinogen. FEBS Letters **18**, 318—320 (1971)

Hessel, B., Makino, M., Iwanaga, S., Blombäck, B.: Primary structure of human fibrinogen and fibrin. Structural studies on NH$_2$-terminal part of Bβ-chain. In preparation 1978

Hogg, D. H., Blombäck, B.: The specificity of the fibrinogen-thrombin reaction. Thrombos. Res. **5**, 685—693 (1974)

Hogg, D. H., Blombäck, B.: The mechanism of the fibrinogen-thrombin reaction. Thrombos. Res. In press (1978)

Jevons, F. R.: Tyrosine O-sulphate in fibrinogen and fibrin. Biochem. J. **89**, 621—624 (1963)

Köppel, G.: Electron microscopic investigation of the shape of fibrinogen nodules: a model for certain proteins. Nature (Lond.) **212**, 1608—1609 (1966)

Köppel, G.: Morphology of the fibrinogen molecule. Thrombos. Diathes. haemorrh. (Stuttg.) Suppl. **39**, 71—73 (1970)

Kowalska-Loth, B., Gårdlund, B., Egberg, N., Blombäck, B.: Plasmic degradation products of human fibrinogen. II. Chemical and immunological relation between fragment E and N-DSK. Thrombos. Res. **2**, 423—450 (1973)

Krajewski, T., Blombäck, B.: The location of tyrosine-0-sulphate in fibrinopeptides. Acta chem. scand. **22**, 1339—1346 (1968)

Kudryk, B., Blombäck, B., Blombäck, M.: Fibrinogen Detroit. An abnormal fibrinogen with non-functional NH$_2$-terminal polymerization domain. Thrombosis Research **9**, 25—36 (1976)

Kudryk, B. J., Collen, D., Woods, K. R., Blombäck, B.: Evidence for localization of polymerization sites in fibrinogen. J. biol. Chem. **249**, 3322—3325 (1974a)

Kudryk, B., Reuterby, J., Blombäck, B.: Adsorption of plasmic fragment D to thrombin modified fibrinogen-Sepharose. Thrombos. Res. **2**, 297—304 (1973)

Kudryk, B., Reuterby, J., Blombäck, B.: Immunochemical studies on human fibrinogen and its fragments. Cross-reactivity of NH$_2$-terminal "disulfide knot" and related structures as determined by radioimmunoassay. Europ. J. Biochem. **46**, 141—147 (1974b)

Lahiri, B., Shainoff, J. R.: Fate of fibrinopeptides in the reaction between human plasmin and fibrinogen. Biochim. biophys. Acta (Amst.) **303**, 161—170 (1973)

Laki, K.: Fibrinogen. New York-London: Academic Press 1968

Laurent, T. C., Blombäck, B.: On the significance of the release of two different peptides from fibrinogen during clotting. Acta chem. scand. **12**, 1875—1877 (1958)

Lederer, K.: Physikalisch-chemische Strukturuntersuchungen des Fibrinogenmoleküls in Lösung. Technische Hochschule, Darmstadt (1973)

Lorand, L.: Fibrinoligase: The fibrin-stabilizing factor system of blood plasma. Ann. N.Y. Acad. Sci. **202**, 6—30 (1972)

Lottspeich, F., Henschen, A.: Amino acid sequence of human fibrinogen. Preliminary note on the peptides obtained by Cyanogen Bromide cleavage of the β-chain. Hoppe-Seyler's Z. Physiol. Chem. **358**, 1521—1524 (1977)

Ly, B., Kierulf, P., Arnesen, H.: Molecular aspects of the clottable proteins of human plasma during fibrinogenolysis. Thrombos. Res. **5**, 301—314 (1974)

Mammen, E. F., Prasad, A. S., Barnhart, M. I., Au, C. C.: Congenital dysfibrinogenemia: Fibrinogen Detroit. J. Clin. Invest. **48**, 235—249 (1969)

Marder, V. J., Shulman, N. R., Carroll, W. R.: The importance of intermediate degradation products of fibrinogen in fibrinolytic hemorrhage. Trans. Ass. Amer. Physicns **80**, 156—167 (1967)

Marder, W. J., Shulman, N. R., Carroll, W. R.: High molecular weight derivatives of human fibrinogen produced by plasmin. I. Physicochemical and immunological characterization. J. biol. Chem. **244**, 2111—2119 (1969)

Marguerie, G., Stuhrmann, H. B.: A neutron small-angle scattering study of bovine fibrinogen. J. Mol. Biol. **102**, 143—156 (1976)

Mester, L.: Structure and role of the carbohydrate fractions of glycoproteins implicated in blood coagulation. Bull. Soc. Chim. biol. (Paris) **51**, 635—648 (1969)

Mészáros, M., Blombäck, B.: Methylation analysis of carbohydrate moiety of γ-chain from human fibrinogen. Ann. Univ. Sci. Budapest. Rolando Eötvös Nominatae, Sect. Chim. **13**, 97—100 (1972)

Mihalyi, E.: Physicochemical studies of bovine fibrinogen. III. Optical rotation of the native and denatured molecule. Biochim. biophys. Acta (Amst.) **102**, 487—499 (1965)

Mills, D., Karpatkin, S.: Heterogeneity of human fibrinogen: possible relation to proteolysis by thrombin and plasmin as studied by SDS-polyacrylamide gel electrophoresis. Biochem. biophys. Res. Commun. **40**, 206—211 (1970)

Mosesson, M. W., Alkjaersig, N., Sweet, B., Sherry, S.: Human fibrinogen of relatively high solubility. Comparative biophysical, biochemical and biological studies with fibrinogen of lower solubility. Biochemistry **6**, 3279—3287 (1967)

Mosesson, M. W., Galanakis, D. K., Finlaysson, J. S.: Comparison of human plasma fibrinogen subfractions and early plasmic fibrinogen derivatives. J. biol. Chem. **249**, 4656—4664 (1974)

Mosesson, M. W., Umfleet, R. A.: The cold-insoluble globulin of human plasma. I. Purification, primary characterization, and relationship to fibrinogen and other cold-insoluble fraction components. J. biol. Chem. **245**, 5728—5736 (1970)

Mosher, D. F., Blout, E. R.: Heterogeneity of bovine fibrinogen and fibrin. J. biol. Chem. **248**, 6896—6903 (1973)

Murano, G.: The molecular structure of fibrinogen. Semin. Thrombos. Haemostas. **1**, July 1974

Nossel, H. L., Younger, L. R., Wilner, G. D., Procupez, T., Canfield, R. E., Butler, Jr., V. P.: Radioimmunoassay of human fibrinopeptide A. Proc. nat. Acad. Sci. (Wash.) **68**, 2350—2353 (1971)

Nossel, H. L., Yudelman, I., Canfield, R. E., Butler, Jr., W. P., Spanondis, K., Wilner, G. D., Qureshi, G. D.: Measurement of fibrinopeptide A in human blood. J. clin. Invest. **54**, 43—53 (1974)

Nussenzweig, V., Seligmann, M., Grabar, P.: Les produits de dégradation du fibrinogène humain par la plasmine. II. Etude immunologique: Mise en évidence d'anticorps anti-fibrinogene natif possédant des spécificités différentes. Ann. Inst. Pasteur **100**, 490—508 (1961)

Scheraga, H. A.: Active site mapping of thrombin. In: Lundlbad, R. L., Fenton, II. J. W. and Mann, K. G. (Eds.): Chemistry and Biology of Thrombin. Pp. 145—158. Michigan, U.S.A.: Ann Arbor Science Publishers, inc. 1977

Scheraga, H. A., Laskowski, Jr., M.: The fibrinogen-fibrin conversion. Advanc. Protein Chem. **12**, 1—131 (1957)

Solum, N. O.: The coagulogen of Limulus polyphemus hemocytes. A comparison of the clotted and non-clotted forms of the molecule. Thrombos. Res. **2**, 55—70 (1973)

Stryer, L., Cohen, C., Langridge, R.: Axial period of fibrinogen and fibrin. Nature (Lond.) **197**, 793—794 (1963)

Svendsen, L., Blombäck, B., Blombäck, M., Olsson, P. I.: Synthetic chromogenic substrates for determination of trypsin, thrombin and thrombin-like enzymes. Thrombos. Res. **1**, 267—278 (1972)

Takagi, T., Doolittle, R. F.: Amino acid sequence of the carboxy-terminal cyanogen bromide peptide of the human fibrinogen β-chain: Homology with the corresponding γ-chain peptide and presence in fragment D. Biochim. biophys. Acta **386**, 617—622 (1975)

Thomas, H. W.: Fibrous proteins: the polymerisation and gelation of fibrin. Personal communication (1970)

Tooney, N. M., Cohen, C.: Microcrystals of a modified fibrinogen. Nature (Lond.) **237**, 23—25 (1972)

Wallén, P., Iwanaga, S.: Differences between plasmic and tryptic digests of human S-sulfo-fibrinogen. Biochim. biophys. Acta (Amst.) **154**, 414—417 (1968)

Woods, K. R., Stephens Horowitz, M., Blombäck, B.: Effect of thrombin on the molecular weights of N-terminal fragments of human fibrinogen. Thrombosis Research **1**, 113—126 (1972)

York, L. L., Blombäck, B.: Interaction of fragments of fibrinogen with insolubilized fibrin monomers (activated fibrinogen). Thrombos. Res. **8**, 607—618 (1976)

Fibrinogen and Fibrin Degradation Products

M. Kopeć and Z. S. Latallo

Introduction

Degradation of fibrinogen as of many protein molecules may be brought about either by physical and/or chemical agents, heat, extreme pH changes, reduction of disulfide bridges, treatment with cyanogen bromide, etc., or by the action of various enzymes. Only enzymatic degradation will be taken into consideration here since the chemical one, closely related to studies on the structure of the fibrinogen molecule, is discussed below.

Fibrinogen, a glycoprotein of considerable size and internal diversity in structure, is susceptible to the action of a variety of enzymes. From the physiologic point of view and in practice most frequently encountered is its degradation by two major proteases of the blood-clotting system, namely thrombin and plasmin. Under physiologic conditions, both are present in blood almost exclusively in their precursor form. Hence, only traces of products of their action on fibrinogen could be found in the blood of normal subjects. In pathology, due to a common triggering mechanism, activation of both thrombin and plasmin occurs either simultaneously or in a subsequent manner. Usually, activation of the clotting system leading to the formation of thrombin precedes activation of plasmin but very often the effects of the second enzyme prevail. Depending on the extent of activation and time of its duration, variable quantities of products specific for either enzyme appear in circulating blood. This very fact creates an important aspect of our interest in products of fibrinogen degradation, since due to a potent inhibitory barrier it is hardly possible to detect active enzymes in blood. Although the biological half-life of the products is rather short, their quantitative assay allows for a fair, indirect measure of the extent of proteolytic reaction in vivo.

Another important aspect of our interest arises from the fact that a number of the products of fibrinogen degradation are not simply inert fragments but display various biological activities sometimes leading to very serious pathologic effects (for details and references concerning previous work, see KOWALSKI (1968).

A. Degradation of the Fibrinogen Molecule

I. Degradation by Thrombin

The action of thrombin on fibrinogen represents a very specific and limited proteolysis. This reaction is described in detail in the preceding chapter. Let us recall that the following degradation products are formed: fibrinopeptide A (FpA), intermediate fibrin monomer (fibrinogen deprived of fibrinopeptides A only), fibrinopeptide B (FpB), and fibrin monomer. In vivo the first appearing and perhaps prevailing products are fibrinopeptides A and intermediate fibrin monomer. It should be pointed out that both intermediate and final fibrin monomers are highly reactive molecules rapidly polymerizing to oligomers and polymers or forming complexes or copolymers with fibrinogen and some of its plasmic degradation products.

In addition, in plasma medium fibrin is exposed to the action of another enzyme-transglutaminase (fibrin-stabilizing factor, FSF, factor XIII), also activated by thrombin. As a result, the so-called stabilization of fibrin (or of its complexes) occurs. It consists in formation of intermolecular crosslinks between α–α and γ–γ chains (Buluk et al., 1961; Lorand et al., 1972).

Degradation of fibrinogen by thrombin leads, therefore, to formation of high molecular weight products which, due to their ability to polymerize and form complexes, largely exceed in their size the size of the original substrate. Since all these products are susceptible to plasmin action, a number of new substrates for this enzyme are formed. On the other hand, thrombin is able to attack not only fibrinogen but also some of its degradation products resulting from plasmin action.

II. Degradation by Plasmin

In contrast to thrombin, plasmin degrades fibrinogen much further. A very large number of studies on this subject has been performed. Appreciation of individual merits and detailed analysis of all the data concerning the sequence of events and biochemical characterization of the respective products would exceed the assigned space. The following description is based on more recent works (Fletcher et al., 1966; Budzynski et al., 1967; Marder et al., 1969; Dudek et al., 1970; Gaffney and Dobos, 1971; Mills, 1972; Pizzo et al., 1972b; Budzynski et al., 1974; Furlan et al., 1975a, b; Marder and Budzynski, 1975), and represents the prevailing opinion. The nomenclature applied is in accordance with the suggestions made by the Subcommittee on Nomenclature of the International Committee on Thrombosis and Hemostasis (Blombäck, 1976).

In the first step, the dimeric molecule of fibrinogen is attacked by plasmin symmetrically at both C-terminal ends of its α-chains. The N-terminal part of α-chains containing fibrinopeptide A remains intact. Simultaneously, but at a slower rate, the N-terminal of the Bβ-chains is attacked and a fragment with fibrinopeptide B removed. As a result, a number of high molecular weight products (HMW-FDP) closely resembling the parent molecule in their overall structure are produced. These very early intermediates, when exposed to thrombin, are still able to polymerize and form fibrin-like gel. The rate of polymerization is, however, considerably decreasing with the advance of degradation. During this stage, a number of smaller fragments are gradually split off and afterwards further degraded by plasmin to form eventually the main bulk of the low molecular weight fibrinogen degradation products (LMW-FDP).

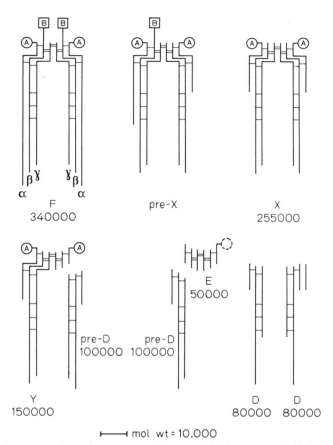

Fig. 1. Schematic presentation of consequent changes of fibrinogen molecule in the course of its degradation by plasmin. *A* and *B* represent respective fibrinopeptides located at the N-terminal ends of α- and β-chains. Distribution of disulphide bridges linking subunits and chains is only approximate. Intrachain disulphide bridges are not shown

Several names have been proposed for the HMW fragments formed at this stage. The smallest fragment in which the symmetrical structure and the ability to clot, although impaired, is still retained, is called fragment X. Its molecular weight is estimated to be about 250000 daltons. It has been proposed that until a more precise characteristic is provided, all preceding intermediates between intact fibrinogen and fragment X should be named pre-X fragments.

In the next, still early stage, a dramatic change seems to occur. It consists of an asymmetric cut through the three chains of one of the subunits of fibrinogen. As a result, the molecule of fragment X is broken into one monomeric fragment, called early D or pre-D of molecular size of about 100000 daltons containing the C-terminal parts of whatever is left from α- and β-chains and still intact γ-chain. The other fragment Y is asymmetric and contains three shorter and three longer remnants of the respective α-, β-, and γ-chains of fibrinogen. Its estimated size is about 155000 daltons. It still contains fibrinopeptides at the N-terminal parts of both α-chain remnants.

At the next stage, fragment Y is promptly cut through by plasmin and, as a result, two HMW fragments are formed. One is the second analogous monomeric fragment, pre-D, and comes from the C-terminal part of the fragment Y, whereas the other of about 50000 daltons represents the dimeric N-terminal part of the molecule. During or promptly after this event the latter-named fragment E, loses, but only partially, the fibrinopeptide A (BUDZYŃSKI et al., 1975).

Further degradation proceeds more slowly and results in formation of the final late FDP. These are two fragments, D, of about 80000 daltons each, one fragment E, and a large number of small LMW-FDP (TRIANTAPHYLLOPOULOS and TRIANTA-PHYLLOPOULOS, 1968).

The HMW-FDP (2 D + 1 E), representing about 65% of the mass of fibrinogen, if not denatured are apparently resistant to further digestion by plasmin (FURLAN et al., 1975a). Recently a fairly plasmin-resistant fragment H of about 20000 daltons has been isolated (HARFENIST and CANFIELD, 1975).

The above-described sequence of FDP formation is illustrated in Figure 1. As already stated, it is based on the prevailing opinion. It should be mentioned, however, that some authors hold a different view on this subject. PLOW and EDGINGTON (1974) postulate formation of two monomeric fragments E. This claim is based mainly on immunologic studies and does not withstand criticism when very solid data concerning the primary structure of fragment E and showing the existence of at least three intersubunit disulfide bridges are taken into account (KOWALSKA-LOTH et al., 1973).

A hypothesis on the formation of one dimeric fragment D (MOSESSON et al., 1973) is also difficult to accept. Structural studies on fragment D isolated at the late stage indicate that upon reduction of S-S bridges, the sum of the molecular weights of the three single-chain remnants of this fragment corresponds very well with the values of molecular weight obtained for the whole fragment by ultracentrifuge analysis (DU-DEK et al., 1970; GAFFNEY and DOBOS, 1971; PIZZO et al., 1972b; FURLAN et al., 1975a, b).

III. Degradation by Both Plasmin and Thrombin

Data presented above indicate that three species of HMW-FDP produced by plasmin, namely fragments X, Y, and E, contain fibrinopeptide A, and, therefore, are potential substrates for thrombin. In fact, the latter splits off fibrinopeptides from all three types of fragments (BUDZYNSKI et al., 1975). In case of fragment X (and all pre-X FDP) it results in spontaneous polymerization, whereas neither Y nor E treated with thrombin, do so. Some change in their reactivity occur, however (see below). All three are able to inhibit the thrombin action on fibrinogen.

Much more complicated is the reverse situation, when plasmin acts on the products of thrombin degradation of fibrinogen. Whereas fibrinopeptides appear to be resistant to plasmin digestion, the fibrin monomer and its derivatives are susceptible. Their rate of proteolysis and the products depend, however, upon the type of fibrin (INOUE et al., 1975).

Free fibrin monomer in solution appears to be degraded by plasmin at about the same rate as fibrinogen, and the products differ perhaps only by the absence of fibrinopeptides. Soluble complexes of fibrin, according to KONTTINEN et al. (1973), are even more susceptible to plasmin than fibrinogen.

The effect on fibrin polymer is rather difficult to evaluate. First, it depends on whether plasmin is generated inside the network of the fibrin clot or acts from outside the clot. Secondly, the quality of fibrin plays an important role. Fibrin polymer formed from intermediate fibrin monomers, e.g., fibrin obtained by treatment of fibrinogen with the thrombin-like enzyme, Reptilase (see below), appears to be more easily degraded than fibrin formed by thrombin (KOPEĊ et al., 1972; KWAAN and BARLOW, 1971; ZAJDEL et al., 1975). On the other hand, the rate of degradation of stabilized fibrin (cross-linked by transglutaminase) is lower than that of nonstabilized fibrin (McDONAGH et al., 1971).

Retraction of the clot and inclusion into the fibrin network of some blood proteins and cells as well as some other substances, e. g., dextran and histones (KOPEĊ et al., 1974), renders it even more resistant to plasmin.

The initial products of plasmic degradation of fibrin clots differ greatly from those of fibrinogen. These products are in fact fragments of polymers and their size is much larger than that of fibrinogen (BANG and CHANG, 1974). A fragment closely resembling fragment Y could be separated from the early stage digest of nonstabilized fibrin upon dissociation in urea (WEGRZYNOWICZ et al., 1971). Fragments D and E formed from this type of fibrin appear to differ slightly from those of fibrinogen (DUDEK et al., 1970; INOUE et al., 1975). In case of stabilized fibrin, fragment E appears to be similar to that from noncross-linked substrate, whereas instead of fragment D, a so-called double D fragment is formed (KOPEĊ et al., 1973; GAFFNEY and BRASHER, 1973; PIZZO et al., 1973a).

The latter has a molecular size of about 160000 daltons, i.e., twice that of fragment D. It is composed of three pairs of remnants of the respective α-, β-, and γ-chain and is cross-linked by the γ-chain.

IV. Degradation by Other Enzymes

1. Thrombin-like Enzymes

Besides thrombin, there exist a group of enzymes which also bring about a very limited degradation of fibrinogen. Such enzymes could be found in venoms of various species of snakes. Three are presently available in a highly purified form: Reptilase (Pentapharm, Basel) from two subspecies of Bothrops atrox (marajoensis and moojenii) used as laboratory reagent; Defibrase (Pentapharm, Basel) from B. moojenii; and Arvin (Ancrod) (Twyford, London) from Agkistrodon rhodostoma (subspecies not established). All these enzymes split off fibrinopeptides A only, although Arvin, after longer incubation, degrades also the α-chain of human fibrinogen (BLOMBÄCK, 1958; HOLLEMAN and COEN, 1970; MATTOCK and ESNOUF, 1971; PIZZO et al., 1972a). The resulting fibrin is in all cases more susceptible to plasmin than the thrombin fibrin (PIZZO et al., 1972a; ZAJDEL et al., 1975).

The enzyme from B. moojenii activates plasma transglutaminase (FSF), whereas that from B. marajoensis does not (McDONAGH and McDONAGH, 1973). The latter is, however, inactivated in vivo at a much higher rate than the former (Lopaciuk et al., 1974). Marked differences were found in the clotting activity of these enzymes on fibrinogen of various animal species (Wik et al., 1972).

Another very interesting enzyme has been isolated from the venom of *A. contortrix* (Herzig et al., 1970). This enzyme splits off fibrinopeptide B at a much higher rate than fibrinopeptide A. The intermediate fibrin monomer deprived of fibrinopeptide B does not polymerize.

A thrombin-like enzyme, called staphylothrombin or coagulase thrombin, is formed as a result of complexing of prothrombin with staphylocoagulase a protein produced by some strains of staphylococci (Tager, 1956; Soulier and Prou-Wartelle, 1967; Zajdel et al., 1976). Enzymes of various specificity are formed depending upon prothrombin species and bacterial strains (Zajdel, 1973).

2. Pancreatic Proteases

Trypsin, chymotrypsin, and elastase degrade fibrinogen rather extensively although in different ways, since they attack different peptide bonds. In case of trypsin, the initial attack consists in splitting off fibrinopeptides and formation of a fibrin-type derivative (Pechet and Alexander, 1962; Mihalyi and Godfrey, 1963).

This is a very transient phenomenon promptly followed by further degradation. At the early stage, all three enzymes produce some intermediate degradation products of fibrinogen endowed with similar anticlotting activity as the early plasmic FDP (Latallo et al., 1971a). Prolonged action of trypsin results in formation of a fragment D (Mihalyi and Godfrey, 1963). Exhaustive proteolysis appears to bring about further degradation than that by plasmin in all three cases. Still, even at this stage products produced by trypsin and elastase display anticlotting activity similar to the late plasmic FDP (Miller and Sanchez-Avalos, 1968; Latallo et al., 1971a).

3. Proteases from Other Sources

Highly purified proteases from *A. oryzae* (Brinase) and *A. ochraceus* (Ocrase) seem to be very similar in their properties and action (Roschlau and Ives, 1974; Töpfer and Piesche, 1974; Teisseyre et al., 1974).

Detailed studies on the degradation of fibrinogen and fibrin by Ocrase (Teisseyre et al., 1974) have shown the following. Similar to the above-discussed pancreatic proteases, Ocrase produces early FDP endowed with high anticlotting activity. As in case of plasmin, trypsin, and elastase, the late FDP obtained by exhaustive proteolysis of fibrinogen by Ocrase still display anticlotting activity, though lower than that of the early ones. The late products of Ocrase action were estimated to have a molecular weight of about 30000 daltons.

Pronase from *Streptomyces griseus* also gives at the early stage products resembling early plasmic FDP. Degradation proceeds very far. Final products are devoid of any anticlotting activity. More than 90% are peptides soluble in TCA (Latallo et al., 1971a).

Papain at the initial stage induces clot formation (Eagle and Harris, 1937), but longer incubation leads to further degradation.

Besides the above listed, many other enzymes are apparently capable of degrading fibrinogen. The action of the enzymes present in certain snake venoms, bacterias, and various cells and tissues should be explored properly, since some might play an important role in pathology. An interesting concept on the participation of leukocyte enzymes in fibrinogen catabolism has been recently put forward by PLOW and EDGINGTON (1975). The end products are structurally distinct from plasmic FDP and have a potent anticoagulant activity.

B. Biological Activities

I. Products of Thrombin Action

1. Fibrin Monomer

This HMW product of thrombin action is highly reactive. Under physiologic conditions, it polymerizes spontaneously very rapidly forming oligomers, intermediate polymers, and finally fully polymerized fibrin clot.

In the presence of an excess of fibrinogen, the reaction of fibrin polymerization is inhibited (LATALLO et al., 1962) and soluble complexes of fibrin monomer with fibrinogen are formed (SHAINOFF and PAGE, 1960). Formation of these complexes represents perhaps one of the major factors in prevention of fibrin deposition in the blood vessels. These complexes, in contrast to those formed from fibrin monomer and FDP (see below), are easily converted to fibrin polymer by further action of thrombin. Both types of complexes, also called soluble fibrin complexes (SFC), precipitate, forming fibrin-like structures under the influence of low molecular weight, basic proteins contained in blood and tissue cells, such as histones and lysozyme (KOPEĆ et al., 1970a). This "nonenzymatic clotting" may lead to the formation of fibrin-like deposits in pathologic states associated with cell destruction.

Soluble and polymerizing fibrin was shown to aggregate platelets (SOLUM, 1966; KOPEĆ et al., 1968; NIEWIAROWSKI et al., 1972). Fully polymerized fibrin does not have this ability.

During adhesion of platelets to partially polymerized fibrin, the release reaction occurs. It differs somewhat from that induced by thrombin or collagen.

The role of fibrin for the efficiency of hemostatic processes is well recognized. Its possible significance for spreading of bacteria and dissemination of neoplasms is also taken into consideration. These problems are somewhat beyond the scope of this chapter and therefore will not be discussed further.

2. Fibrinopeptide A and B (FpA, FpB)

FpA was shown to possess some ability to inhibit enzymatic action of thrombin, but only at relatively high concentrations (BLOMBÄCK, 1964).

FpB appears to induce a number of biological effects. First, FpB was found to potentiate the contractile effect of bradykinin on the rat uterus (GLADNER et al., 1963). Later, FpB was described to have the properties of a slow-acting vasoconstricting agent. At doses of $6 \times 10^{-3} + 8 \times 10^{-4}$ µmol FpB induced in rat a rise in blood pressure lasting considerably longer than the response to vasopressin or angiotensin.

The only substance approaching the duration of vasoactive effect of FpB appeared to be oxytocin (COLMAN et al., 1967). The following effects of FpB on lungs have been described: pulmonary hypertension, decrease in effective blood flow and compliance, increase in ventilation volume, and in the difference of arterial and alveolar P_{CO_2} (BAYLEY et al., 1967).

The recently discovered ability of FpB to enhance the ATP-ase activity and superprecipitation of myosin B might explain the effects of this peptide on smooth muscle (OSBAHR and CUSTODIO, 1975).

FpB was demonstrated to be a chemotactic agent. Leukocyte migration was induced by isolated FpB cleaved by thrombin as well as by the peptidic material cleaved from fibrinogen by the venom of *A. contortrix* but not by Reptilase or Arvin (KAY et al., 1974).

II. Products of Plasmin Action

1. Clottability

The ability to coagulate under the influence of thrombin is preserved in products pre-X and X, the rate of clotting declining from fibrinogen to X (FLETCHER et al., 1966).

2. Anticlotting Activity

In contrast to the above-mentioned products, consecutive fragments Y, D, and E do not coagulate. Their main biological effect consists in inhibiting conversion of fibrinogen into fibrin catalyzed by thrombin and thrombin-like enzymes. The name antithrombin VI has been applied to the whole mixture of FDP (NIEWIAROWSKI and KOWALSKI, 1958). Later it was recognized that the overall anticlotting effect of early FDP is much greater than that of late FDP. Purified fragment Y was shown to be the most active in this respect. The strongest anticlotting effect of FDP, formed at the early stages of proteolysis, has been ascribed to the fact that they inhibit the enzymatic as well as polymerization phase of clotting (KOWARZYK et al., 1961; LATALLO et al., 1964).

Therefore, attempts have been made to define the effect of various FDP fragments in terms of their thrombin and polymerization-inhibiting properties.

a) Inhibition of Thrombin

Studies in which at least partially purified fragments were used showed that Y and E are endowed with the ability to inhibit cleavage of fibrinopeptides catalyzed by thrombin (LARRIEU et al., 1972; KOPEC et al., 1972; ARNESEN, 1973). Partially purified Y decreased the rate of FpA release from fibrinogen containing tritium label in the region of this peptide. The number of N-terminal glycine residues appearing in fibrinogen due to fibrinopeptide cleavage by thrombin is diminished in the presence of fragment E. It remains to be established whether the antithrombin effect of Y and E depends exclusively on the presence of FpA in these molecules and hence on the competitive inhibition of its release from fibrinogen. No FDP fragments inhibit esterolytic activity of thrombin when TAME is used as a substrate (LARRIEU et al., 1972).

b) Inhibition of Fibrin Polymerization

Once formed, fibrin monomer polymerizes very fast under physiologic conditions (ionic strength, pH, and temperature). HMW-FDP appear to inhibit strongly fibrin polymerization (LIPINSKI et al., 1967). This phenomenon could be easily observed and evaluated by following changes in optical density accompanying fibrin polymerization in the presence or absence of FDP (LATALLO et al., 1962). Another quantitative way of evaluation consists in labeling fibrin monomer preparation with radioactive iodine and measuring the radioactivity remaining in solution (WEGRZYNOWICZ et al., 1971). In both cases, polymerization reaction is started by dilution of fibrin monomer dissolved in urea or sodium bromide with buffer. The results of such experiments clearly indicate that fragments X, Y, and D but not E are very potent inhibitors of fibrin polymerization. An assumption has been made that the underlying mechanism of this inhibition consists in formation of soluble complexes of fibrin monomer with the respective partner. Ultracentrifuge analysis of soluble fibrin provides strong evidence for the existence of its complexes with fibrinogen and early FDP (SASAKI et al., 1966; MARDER et al., 1969; WEGRZYNOWICZ et al., 1971).

In contrast to fibrin-fibrinogen and fibrin-fragment X (or pre-X) complexes, fibrin complexes with fragments Y and D are not clottable with thrombin. Solubility of complexed fibrin appears to be highly dependent upon concentration, temperature, pH, and ionic strength. The binding of fibrin monomer is due probably to the same forces acting in normal fibrin polymerization. The strength of association is, however, apparently different for various molecular partners. This perhaps explains an apparent discrepancy between the results described above and those obtained by the exclusion chromatography technique. The latter show that the heavy fractions eluted prior to fibrinogen and containing fibrin monomer component and fibrinogen (or fragment X) contain neither fragment D nor Y (SMITH and BANG, 1972; LATALLO et al., 1976).

A way to explain this discrepancy is to assume that the binding forces between fibrin monomer and fragments D or Y are relatively weak which results in constant rearrangement and eventually favors formation of some defective fibrin oligomers unable to polymerize further (LATALLO, 1976). At lower concentrations of FDP the fibrin clot is formed but its structure is different from normal fibrin. Hence it is called defective fibrin (BANG et al., 1962).

c) Inhibition of Thromboplastin Generation

The thromboplastin generation test (TGT) was also shown to be inhibited by FDP. (NIEWIAROWSKI et al., 1959). Interaction of FDP with platelets was postulated to contribute mainly to the inhibition of TGT on the basis of experiments in which particular components of the TGT system had been preincubated with FDP. Purified fragment E was later shown to be a very potent TGT inhibitor (LARRIEU et al., 1972).

3. Interference of FDP with Platelet Function

The digest of fibrinogen by plasmin was found to inhibit platelet aggregation, adhesion, and release reaction. FDP formed at early stages of proteolysis were, as shown by some authors, more active than the late FDP (KOWALSKI et al., 1964a; JERUSH-

Almy and Zucker, 1966). The absorbance of HMW-FDP on platelet surface was postulated as a possible mechanism of their interference with platelet aggregation (Kopec et al., 1966). Dialyzable LMW-FDP resulting from protracted proteolysis share the antiaggregating activity (Stachurska et al., 1970).

These in vitro effects are in agreement with the changes in platelet behaviour observed in vivo in dogs treated with streptokinase (Kowalski et al., 1964) or Reptilase (Olsson and Johnsson, 1972) as well as in patients defibrinated by Arvin (Prentice et al., 1969). The impairment of platelet function coincided with the accumulation of FDP and decline of the fibrinogen level in the circulating blood. The role of FDP for primary hemostasis was supported by the prolongation of the bleeding time observed in dogs after infusion of FDP (Kowalski et al., 1964a; Olsson and Johnsson, 1972). However, opinions concerning the significance of FDP for platelet function are still controversial. The concentrations of FDP, particularly of dialyzable ones, which definitely influence platelet reactions, are high and could hardly be expected to occur in in vivo conditions (Solum et al., 1973). Moreover, products of digestion of plasma clotting factor VIII by plasmin were recently described to be more potent as antiaggregating agent than FDP. Thus, factor VIII contaminants in fibrinogen preparations are suspected to be a major source of active fragments (Culasso et al., 1974).

4. Effects on Smooth Muscle, Heart, and Permeability of Biological Membranes

FDP appeared to induce a variety of effects on blood vessels, smooth muscle of various organs, and heart. These activities are connected with dialyzable LMW-FDP. At low concentrations, these peptides potentiate the contractile effects of bradykinin, kallidin, angiotensin, histamine, 5-hydroxytryptamine, acetyl-choline, adrenaline, and noradrenaline (Buluk and Małofiejew, 1969; Małofiejew, 1971). The following organs were studied: guinea-pig intestine, rat duodenum and uterus, and strips of rabbit aorta. At high concentrations, the same FDP induced an increased tonus of smooth muscle and a decline in sensitivity to the above-listed peptides and amines. The potentiation of bradykinin and angiotensin effects by FDP could also be demonstrated in in vivo experiments. It was suggested that in severe fibrinolytic states in humans, FDP can attain concentrations affecting smooth muscle reactivity. FDP derived from plasmic digestion of fibrin-free FpB induced quite similar effects; hence a possibility that FpB contributes mainly to the observed phenomena seems unprobable.

Recently, a well-defined biologically active decapeptide was isolated from the digest of fibrinogen by plasmin and later on synthesized by the solid phase method. This peptide, Ser-Gln-Leu-Gln-Glu-Ala-Pro-Leu-Glu-Lys, besides anticlotting activity, showed kinin-like properties. It induced a hypotensive effect in vivo in rats and a smooth muscle contraction in the strips of guinea-pig organs. Atropine, hyoscine, and tetrodotoxin remain without influence on the contractile activity of the studied decapeptide (Takaki et al., 1974).

Heart function is also affected by LMW-FDP. They were shown to accelerate the appearance of action potentials of rat heart atria (Małofiejew, 1971) and to induce a positive chronotropic effect (Buczko et al., 1975). The latter is possibly a cAMP-mediated reaction, as evidenced by enhancement of FDP action by theophylline and by detection of increased concentrations of c-AMP in the atrial strips.

Dialyzable FDP increase the permeability of capillaries of guinea-pig skin (MAŁOFIEJEW, 1971).

Of great interest for pharmacodynamics is another effect of LMW-FDP, i.e., their ability to change the distribution of some drugs in the mammalian organism.

FDP of this type were found to increase the level of some drugs in the brain of rat. FDP-induced rise in concentrations of amphetamine, caffeine, thiopental, and chloropromazine in brain, was associated with an enhancement of their pharmacologic effects (BUCZKO et al., 1973; BUCZKO and MONIUSZKO-JAKONIUK, 1975).

FDP of a molecular weight below 5000 daltons introduced into the lateral ventricle of the rat brain changed the behavior of these animals, depressing their activity (WIŚNIEWSKI et al., 1975).

5. Stimulation of Fibrinogen Biosynthesis

A pronounced increase in fibrinogen concentration was observed after infusion of fibrinogen digest or isolated fragment D. The stimulatory effect of FDP on fibrinogen synthesis was considered as a probable explanation for these results (BOCCI et al., 1974). However, when fibrinogen biosynthesis in rabbits was investigated by measurements of incorporation of ^{75}Se-methionine, the above assumption could not be confirmed. Administration of either fragment D or E remained without any influence on the rate of fibrinogen synthesis (OTIS and RAPAPORT, 1973).

6. Other Effects

Some other FDP effects of possible significance for hemostasis have been described, such as inhibition of prothrombin consumption (TRIANTAPHYLLOPOULOS et al., 1969) and inhibition of fibrin digestion by plasmin (NANNINGGA and GUEST, 1968). The latter observation disagrees with the results of others (MYŚLIWIEC et al., 1973).

C. Immunologic Properties of FDP

HMW-FDP derived from proteolysis of fibrinogen and fibrin by plasmin contain some antigenic determinants of the parent fibrinogen molecule[1]. Therefore, all these fragments can be visualized by immunoelectrophoretic technique with antifibrinogen antiserum. Fibrinogen diffuses poorly into the gel and gives, as immunoloelectrophoretic pattern, an arc close to the application point. Fragment X migrates slightly to the cathode while consecutive fragment Y shows slow anodic migration. The final D and E fragments migrate more rapidly to the cathode or anode, respectively, and give arcs close to antiserum due to their good diffusion into the agar gel (Fig. 2). Smaller peptides are not precipitated by presently available antisera.

Using Ouchterlony double diffusion technique, it has been shown that fragments X and Y are antigenically deficient, compared with fibrinogen, while D and E lack some fibrinogen determinants still present in fragments X and Y.

---

[1] For details and references concerning previous work, see MARDER (1968) and EDGINGTON and PLOW (1973).

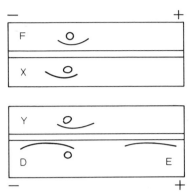

Fig. 2. Immunoelectrophoretic pattern of fibrinogen and HMW-FDP

Radioimmunoassay, consisting of determination of the ability of purified FDP fragments to compete with ^{125}I-fibrinogen in binding to antinative fibrinogen antibodies, allowed the quantitation of native fibrinogen antigenic determinants in FDP. Using this technique, progressive loss of these determinants, occurring in the following sequence $(X > Y > D > E)$ could be expressed in quantitative terms.

From these facts a conclusion of practical interest emerged, that immunologic assays in which antifibrinogen antiserum has been applied must differ in sensitivity to particular FDP fragments.

On the other hand, HMW-FDP exhibit specific differences in antigenic expression. Nussenzweig et al. (1961) found that fragments D and E possess distinct and independent antigenic determinants. Further studies with Ouchterlony technique confirmed this statement demonstrating the reaction of nonidentity of D and E fragments. Fragments X and Y yield the reaction of antigenic identity and both share some antigenic determinants of D and E.

Besides some antigens common to the parent fibrinogen molecule, D and E fragments contain antigenic determinants not expressed in the native fibrinogen. Exposure of amino acid sequences buried in the structure of intact fibrinogen, associated perhaps with the creation of new conformations, is considered to explain the appearance of the cleavage specific determinants in D and E. They are called Dneo or Eneo antigens (Edgington and Plow, 1973). The concept of neoantigens was derived from the finding that antisera obtained by immunization of rabbits with human fibrinogen retain the ability to react with the fragment used for immunization after absorption of the antiserum with fibrinogen. No cross-reactivity of Dneo and Eneo was detected. On the basis of these findings, specific radioimmunoassays of cleavage-associated neoantigens could be elaborated. With the use of these assays it has been established that fragment X and Y compete in similar degree as fragment D in the binding of ^{125}I-labeled D to anti-Dneo antiserum; hence it was concluded that either X or Y products contains about 1 mol of Dneo antigen and can be detected with similar efficiency as D by this radioimmunoassay. Somewhat different results were obtained in radioimmunoassay of Eneo antigen. The expression of this antigen was found to increase progressively in fragments resulting from more advanced proteolysis $X < Y < E$.

Moreover, in accordance with the described discrete differences in subunits, amino acid composition, and in vivo clearance of fragments D and E derived from fibrinogen and fibrin, the expression of distinct antigenic determinants could be detected in products from these two substrates. Antigenic differences are postulated to be strong enough to elaborate radioimmunoassays allowing discrimination of fibrinogen and fibrin-derived FDP.

Fibrinopeptide A is also sufficiently immunogenic to induce the production of anti-FpA antibodies. Antigenic determinants of FpA appeared to be species specific. (NOSSEL et al., 1971; BUDZYNSKI et al., 1975).

From the presented data, a conclusion can be drawn that recent progress achieved in studies on antigenic properties of fibrinogen derivatives creates a basis for development of assays, which can be not only helpful for investigations on the structure of fibrinogen and FDP but also offer an advantage for discrimination in patients' plasma of various types of fibrinogen degradation products depending on the enzyme involved and stage of proteolysis.

D. Detection and Quantitation of FDP

As already mentioned, fibrinolysis, either systemic or local, is activated concommitantly or subsequently to coagulation. Besides iatrogenic fibrinolytic states induced by infusion of streptokinase or urokinase, primary activation of fibrinolysis has not been proven in any human disease. Hence, the appearance of both thrombin and plasmin-derived fibrinogen degradation products should be expected in most patients with thrombotic and fibrinolytic states. Separate quantitation of products formed by each of these enzymes may be of considerable value for establishing the actual prevalence of intravascular coagulation or fibrinolysis. Therefore, in recent years the efforts of many workers were directed to the elaboration of two types of methods, firstly, specific assays which allow the quantitation and differentiation of various types of fibrinogen derivatives, secondly, simple and rapid bedside tests for frequent monitoring of patients in emergency situations (for recent review, see also NIEWIAROWSKI (1972).

I. Immunologic Assays

Detection of fibrinogen-related antigen (FR antigen) in serum constitutes the principle of most widely used immunologic techniques for determination of unclottable FDP. To avoid false positive results blood should be collected on plasmin inhibitors (EACA, Aprotinin, or soybean trypsin inhibitor) and all fibrinogen removed from the sample by addition of adequate amounts of thrombin.

Due to well-known species-dependent differences of fibrinogen antigenic properties, antiserum against human fibrinogen must be used for clinical studies and homologous antisera for experimentation in animals.. The sensitivity of FDP assay is commonly expressed as a minimum detectable amount of fibrinogen in micrograms (Table 1). Immunoelectrophoresis and immunodiffusion were applied for FDP studies in the conventional manner as well as in a combined way, e.g., the rocket method (LAURELL, 1966; NILEHN and NILSSON, 1964). These methods enable one to detect all HMW-FDP fragments and to evaluate their relative concentrations. Sensitivity of

Table 1. Sensitivity of immunoassays of FDP

Method	Minimum concentrations of detectable fibrinogen equivalents	Sensitivity to fragment
Immunoelectrophoresis	> 100 μg/ml	X, Y, D, E sensitivity can be increased by usage of specific antifragment antisera
Immunodiffusion	10–100 μg/ml	
Precipitation flocculation	5.0–40.0 μg/ml	X, Y, D, E,
Fitest	1.0–10.0 μg/ml	Mostly intact fibrinogen slight to X and Y
TRCHII	0.03–3.0 μg/ml	X, Y, D
Radioimmunoassays	0.08–2.0 ng/ml	

these techniques can be increased significantly by employing specific antisera against particular fragments.

The precipitation (flocculation) test consists of direct visual observation of the immunoprecipitate formed in the mixture of the examined sample with antifibrinogen antiserum. The test can be performed in cavity plates or capillary tubes (Ferreira and Murat, 1963; Stiehm and Trygstad, 1969).

In tanned red cell hemagglutination inhibition immunoassay (TRCHII: Merskey et al., 1969), tanned red cells coated with fibrinogen are used. The ability of the tested serum to neutralize agglutinating antibodies in antifibrinogen antiserum is a measure of FDP content. TRCHII is a two-step test; in the first, serial dilutions of examined samples are incubated with antifibrinogen antiserum; in the second, agglutination of red cells is estimated.

Paralelly, the hemagglutination inhibition titer of standard fibrinogen is determined and results are expressed as equivalents of micrograms of fibrinogen. The sensitivity of TRCHII is high, about twofold greater for X and Y fragments than for D while E is not detected at all (Marder et al., 1971). In normal sera FDP concentration determined by TRCHII was found to range from 1–4 μg/ml.

Allington (1971) applied latex particles coated with fibrinogen instead of tanned red cells in an analogous procedure. It appeared to be of similar sensitivity and the results of both tests correlated quite well.

In the Fitest the content of FDP is defined by establishing the highest dilution of tested serum which agglutinates latex particles coated with antifibrinogen antibodies. This test is mostly sensitive to intact fibrinogen. It reacts poorly even with fragments X and Y and not at all with D and E. Hence, the Fitest is considered of value for measuring fibrinogen content in the presence of FDP (Marder et al., 1971; Thomas et al., 1970).

II. Radioimmunoassay

The principle of these most sensitive and specific assays of FDP consists in determination of the ability of the tested material to compete with radioactively labeled FDP in the reaction with appropriate antiserum. ^{125}I-D, ^{125}I-E, and antisera against isolated fragments D or E, are mainly applied (GORDON et al., 1973; GORDON et al., 1975; EDGINGTON and PLOW, 1973). Employment of specific antisera against cleavage-associated neoantigens enables the quantitation of the sum of clottable and unclottable FDP in plasma.

Radioimmunoassays discriminating FDP derived from fibrinogen or fibrin have been also described (EDGINGTON and PLOW, 1973; CHEN and SHURLEY, 1975). These promising methods need further evaluation. Sensitivity of the presently available radioimmunoassays is in the order of single nanograms per milliliter, hence considerably higher than that of other tests for FDP quantitation.

Radioimmunoassay for FpA was also worked out and introduced to clinical studies. Preceding tyrosination of FpA was necessary for its labelling, since natural FpA does not contain residues to which radioactive iodine could be coupled. Using highly sensitive and specific FpA radioimmunoassay, this peptide was found to be present in plasma of healthy people in concentrations of 1–2 ng/ml (NOSSEL et al., 1975).

III. Staphylococcal Clumping Test (SC)

The principle of the SC test emerged from the observations that some strains of staphylococci in suspension are agglutinated by fibrinogen and its derivatives. This reaction depends on the presence of so-called clumping factor in the bacterial wall. It is a peptide distinct from staphylococcal coagulase.

The test consists of visual observation of agglutination in a mixture of equal volumes of staphylococcal suspension and serial dilutions of the tested serum. Comparison with standard fibrinogen preparation by titration-dilution technique enables the expression of the results in micrograms of fibrinogen (HAWIGER et al., 1970).

The SC test shows a similar sensitivity as TRCHII for fragments X and Y but is not sensitive to D and E products (MARDER et al., 1971). In sera of patients with various pathologic states a good agreement of the results was obtained using SC and TRCHII (MARDER et al., 1971; THOMAS et al., 1970).

Definite differences in reactivity of fibrinogens of various species in the SC test were discovered. Plasmas of the following mammals are able to clump staphylococci: echidna, wallaby, hedgehog, monkey, armadillo, rabbit, mouse, rat, porpoise, dog, cat, fox, raccoon, mink, seal, manatee, horse, pig, guanaco, and cow. In contrast, opossum, guinea-pig, elephant, sheep, and goat plasma appeared nonreactive (LEWIS and WILSON, 1973).

IV. Thrombin and Reptilase Time

Since FDP inhibit fibrinogen-fibrin conversion, determination of the thrombin clotting time of plasma was introduced as a screening test for evaluation of FDP content in blood (KOWALSKI et al., 1965).

In patients treated with heparin and thus showing a considerable prolongation of the thrombin time, this enzyme can be substituted by Reptilase (LATALLO et al., 1971 b). Coagulation induced by Reptilase is not influenced by heparin but shows equal sensitivity to FDP as thrombin-induced coagulation. When the fibrinogen level declines to very low values resulting in prolonged coagulation, thrombin or Reptilase time can be recorded in mixtures of equal volumes of patient and donor plasma.

Thrombin and Reptilase times are mostly sensitive to fragments X and Y from fibrinogen. Anticlotting activity of early products derived from fibrin and that of fragments D and E from both substrates is markedly lower.

Even fragments X and Y must be present in concentrations of above 25 μg/ml to prolong significantly the coagulation (Marder et al., 1971).

V. Detection of Soluble Fibrin Complexes

Detection of soluble fibrin complexes (SFC) is based on some of the characteristic features by which fibrin and SFC differ from fibrinogen.

The size of fibrin complexes considerably exceeds the size of the fibrinogen molecule. Hence, exclusion chromatography on agarose gel columns has been successfully applied for qualitative as well as quantitative assay of SFC (Fletcher and Alkjaersig, 1971, 1973; Bang et al., 1973a, b; Smith and Bang, 1972; La-tallo et al., 1976; Latallo, 1976). In principle, when a carefully calibrated column packed with Bio-Gel 5M is used, SFC elute prior to the fibrinogen peak and FDP behind. Analysis of the effluent fractions with the immunoassay for fibrinogen related antigen or by SC clumping test allows for detection of these threee major components. A computerized program making it possible for a semiquantitative analysis of SFC, fibrinogen, and HMW-FDP has been recently proposed by Alk-jaersig et al., 1973.

The difference in N-terminal amino acids between fibrinogen and fibrin has been used as a basis for SFC detection by Kierulf and Abildgaard (1971) and Kierulf (1973). The method consists in harvesting fibrinogen and fibrin from plasma by ethanol precipitation and comparing the amount of N-terminal glycine in the total precipitated fraction and in the clot and clot liquor resulting from treatment of this fraction with thrombin.

The ability of FSF (factor XIII) to incorporate ^{14}C-glycine ethyl ester preferentially into fibrin than into fibrinogen or FDP provided a principle of the method proposed by Kisker and Rush (1971).

Both methods seem to respresent a logical approach but are rather cumbersome, time-consuming, and need further clinical testing.

In contrast to the above-described tests there exist a number of simple tests based on the so-called paracoagulation phenomenon. This consists in formation of a fibrin gel, when SFC are subjected to the action of some physical or chemical agents (Kopec et al., 1960). Among others, cooling of plasma or addition of ethanol or protamine sulphate were applied for diagnostic purposes.

The assay for "cryofibrinogen" precipitating from plasma-containing SFC upon its storage at $+4°$ C, has been employed by several investigators (Korst and Kratochvil, 1955; McKee et al., 1963; Pindyck et al., 1970). All found a significantly high incidence of positive results in various pathologic states in which the presence of SFC in blood should be expected.

In the ethanol gelation test of Godal and Abildgaard (1966) precipitation of fibrin or rather its gelation is achieved within minutes at 20° C due to the change in dielectric constant of water by ethanol. Intact fibrinogen, if its concentration in plasma is not too high, remains in solution.

Addition of protamine sulphate (PS) to the plasma-containing SFC at 37° C appears to result in formation of complexes of PS with each of the components of SFC (i.e., fibrin, fibrinogen, and FDP). The gel is formed from fibrin or fibrin fragment X (deprived of FpA), whereas complexes of PS with fibrinogen or FDP remain in solution (LATALLO et al., 1971b; LATALLO, 1976). The assay of PS gelation, as described by KOPEC et al. (1970b), SEAMAN (1970), LATALLO et al. (1971c) is performed at 37° C using citrated plasma. It is less affected by high content of fibrinogen in plasma but otherwise gives similar results as ethanol gelation. More comparative studies on the two tests are needed.

The PS gelation test could be made semiquantitative by running it with serial dilutions of tested plasma (LATALLO et al., 1971c). Another approach to quantitation has been made by NIEWIAROWSKI and GUREWITCH (1971) with the employment of PS dilutions.

The test originally proposed by LIPINSKI and WOROWSKI (1968), in which optical density changes were measured upon addition of PS to oxalated plasma at room temperature is, according to our experience, unspecific and highly dependent on fibrinogen content.

More details concerning the conditions influencing fibrin gelation and the clinical experience with protamine and ethanol gelation can be found in recent reviews of BANG and CHANG (1974) and LATALLO (1976).

VI. Practical Value

Each of the above mentioned assays possesses some advantages and limitations. The most specific, differential, and extremely sensitive radioimmunoassays are at the early stage of their development and cannot be introduced easily to routine clinical practice.

TRCHII shows high sensitivity, but is rather complex and takes about 2 h to perform. In specialized centers TRCHII test is widely applied for clinical investigations and diagnoses not requiring urgency. TRCHII is successfully employed for quantitation of FDP in urine due to sensitivity of this assay to both early and late fragments.

Determination of FDP in urine is considered of interest for studies on pathogenic mechanisms of kidney diseases and practical evaluation of their severity (CLARKSON et al., 1971; HEDNER et al., 1974; EKBERG and PANDOLFI, 1975).

The staphylococcal clumping test is simple and rapid and its practical use is growing steadily. Its main limitation is a lack of sensitivity to fragments formed at later stages of fibrinogen digestion.

Immunoelectrophoresis, immunodiffusion, and their combinations belong to the tests of low sensitivity, giving semiquantitative results. They can be very helpful, however, in identifying FDP fragments appearing in blood, urine, and other biological fluids in various diseases.

The Fitest and recording of thrombin or Reptilase time are the most rapid and simple tests of the lowest sensitivity. Their value, however, should not be neglected for monitoring of severely bleeding patients and efficiency of treatment. The gelation tests with ethanol or protamine sulphate play an equally important role for fast diagnosis.

E. The Role of FDP in Clinical Practice

Studies on fibrinogen catabolism and on products of its intravascular proteolysis are of interest and practical value mainly for three serious clinical problems—for diagnosis of disseminated intravascular coagulation (DIC), for detection of prethrombotic states and thromboembolic incidents, and for control of thrombolytic therapy.

It should be realized that in general the biological half-life of the products of fibrinogen degradation is much shorter than that of fibrinogen. It ranges from minutes for FpA (NOSSEL et al., 1975) to a few hours for fragments D and E (CANTAZARO and EDGINGTON, 1974) in normal subjects. One should expect that these values might be drastically changed under pathological conditions.

DIC can be induced by a variety of pathogenic mechanisms still not completely understood. In its acute form DIC is often a life threatening complication, while chronic DIC belongs to the mechanisms of tissue damage in many pathologic states. DIC can be suspected on the basis of clinical symptoms but firm diagnosis and indications for specific treatment are established by laboratory studies.

The most acute DIC leading to so-called defibrination of patients is easily diagnosed by characteristic laboratory findings, i.e., unclottability of blood and plasma, or very prolonged and poor coagulation with thrombin due to partial or total disappearance of fibrinogen and accumulation of FDP, lowered levels of factor VIII and V, decreased platelet count, rapid dissolution of the clot formed from the euglobulin fraction of plasma. Even in these cases, as mentioned already, assays for products formed by thrombin and plasmin can be helpful for establishing the actual prevalence of coagulation or fibrinolysis and hence for rational treatment with either heparin or inhibitors of fibrinolysis.

Diagnosis of less acute and intense DIC is much more difficult, particularly when it develops in pathologic states associated with hyperfibrinogenemia and/or high platelet counts. In such cases, pronounced consumption of fibrinogen and platelets due to DIC can be manifested by a decrease to values near to the norm.

Detection of increased concentrations of plasmin-derived FDP was found helpful for diagnosis of deep vein thrombosis, particularly complicated by pulmonary embolism (RUCKLEY et al., 1970; TIBUTT et al., 1975). Quantitation of FpA in plasma by radioimmunoassay seems to be a promising procedure even for detection of threatening thrombosis (NOSSEL et al., 1975). Increased concentrations of FpA could be detected in some cases earlier than any other signs and symptoms (NOSSEL et al., 1975). During thrombolytic therapy with streptokinase or urokinase alone or combined with Defibrase or Arvin (LATALLO et al., 1974), frequent estimation of FDP in blood is helpful for evaluation of efficiency of treatment and for proper dosage of the thrombolytic drugs.

Preliminary results indicate a possible value of FDP determination in cerebrospinal fluid for diagnosis of inflammatory diseases of the central nervous system (MYŚLIWIEC and MYŚLIWIEC, 1973) and in amniotic fluid for prenatal diagnosis of congenital neural-tube anomalies (PURDIE et al., 1975).

Note added in proof

Since this chapter was submitted for publication an important and new area of FDP activity was discovered, namely, their immunosuppressive and chemotactic effects. LMW-FDP were shown to inhibit incorporation of ^{3}H-thymidine into human blood lymphocytes stimulated by phytohemagglutinin and to decrease the number of plaque forming cells in mouse spleen immunized with sheep red blood cells. LMW material inducing immunosuppression could be isolated from sera of patients with DIC in the course of malignancy.

It has been postulated that LMW-FDP might contribute to the impairment of immunological reactivity of patients with cancer (GIRMAN et al., 1976).

Another property of FDP which might be of significance for immunoinflammatory reaction consists in chemotaxis of fragments D and E for monocytes and of LMW-FDP for neutrophiles (RICHARDSON et al., 1976).

References

Alkjaersig, N., Roy, L., Fletcher, A. P.: Analysis of gel exclusion chromatographic data by chromatographic plate theory analysis: Application to plasma, fibrinogen chromatography. Thrombos. Res. **3**, 525—544 (1973)

Allington, M. J.: Detection of fibrinogen degradation products by a latex clumping method. Scand. J. Haemat. Suppl. **13**, 115—119 (1971)

Arnesen, H.: The effect of purified products D and E on the conversion of fibrinogen to fibrin as studied by N-terminal amino acid analysis. IVth Int. Congr. on Thrombosis and Haemostasis. Abstr. 253, Vienna 1973

Bang, N. U., Chang, M. L.: Soluble fibrin complexes. Semin. Thromb. Haemostas. **1**, 91—128 (1974)

Bang, N. U., Fletcher, A. P., Alkjaersig, N., Sherry, S.: Pathogenesis of the coagulation defect developing during pathological plasma proteolysis ("fibrinolytic") states. III. Demonstration of abnormal clot structure by electron microscopy. J. clin. Invest. **41**, 935—948 (1962)

Bang, N. U., Hansen, M. S., Smith, G. P., Latallo, Z. S., Chang, M. L., Mattler, L. E.: Molecular composition and biological properties of soluble fibrin polymers encountered in thrombotic states. Ser. haemat. **6**, 494—512 (1973a)

Bang, N. U., Hansen, M. S., Smith, G. P., Mosesson, M. W.: Properties of soluble fibrin polymers encountered in thrombotic states. Thrombos. Diathes. haemorrh. (Stuttg.) Suppl. **56**, 75—90 (1973b)

Bayley, T., Clement, J. A., Osbahr, A. J.: Pulmonary and circulatory effects of fibrinopeptides. Circulat. Res. **21**, 469—486 (1967)

Blombäck, B.: Studies on the action of thrombic enzymes on bovine fibrinogen as measured by N-terminal analysis. Ark. Kemi **12**, 321—335 (1958)

Blombäck, B.: Chemical aspects of fibrinogen and fibrin. Thrombos. Diathes. haemorrh. (Stuttg.) Suppl. **13**, 29—39 (1964)

Bocci, V., Conti, T., Muscettola, M., Pacini, A., Pessina, G. P.: Factors regulating plasma protein synthesis. IV. Influence of fragments D and E on plasma fibrinogen concentration. Thrombos. Diathes. haemorrh. (Stuttg.) **31**, 395—402 (1974)

Buczko, W., Franco, R., Bianchetti, G., Donati, M. B., de Gaetano, G.: Passive chronotropic effect of dialysable peptides derived from plasmin digestion of bovine fibrinogen preparations. Role of cyclic AMP. Vth Int. Congr. on Thrombosis and Haemostasis Abstr. 113, Paris 1975

Buczko, W., Moniuszko-Jakoniuk, J.: Influence of fibrinogen degradation products (FDP) on the central nervous system and on the effects of centrally acting drugs. Pharmacology **13**, 252—259 (1975)

Buczko, W., Wisniewski, K., Malinowska, L.: Effects of fibrinogen degradation products FDP on the action of certain centrally acting drugs. Thrombos. Res. **2**, 219—227 (1973)

Budzyński, A. Z., Marder, V. J., Shainoff, J. R.: Structure of plasmic degradation products of human fibrinogen. Fibrinopeptide and polypeptide chain analysis. J. biol. Chem. **249**, 2294—2302 (1974)

Budzyński, A. Z., Marder, V. J., Sherry, S.: Reaction of plasmic degradation products of fibrinogen in the radioimmunoassay of human fibrinopeptide A. Blood **45**, 757—768 (1975)

Budzyński, A. Z., Stahl, M., Kopeć, M., Latallo, Z. S., Wegrzynowicz, Z., Kowalski, E.: High molecular weight products of the late stage of fibrinogen proteolysis by plasmin and their structural relation to the fibrinogen molecule. Biochim. biophys. Acta (Amst.) **147**, 313—323 (1967)

Buluk, K., Januszko, T., Olbromski, J.: Conversion of fibrin to desmofibrin. Nature **191**, 1093—1094 (1961)

Buluk, K., Małofiejew, M.: The pharmacological properties of fibrinogen degradation products Brit. J. Pharmacol. **35**, 79—89 (1969)

Cantazaro, A. Z., Edgington, T. S.: The in vivo behaviour of the terminal derivatives of fibrinogen and fibrin cleaved by plasmin. J. Lab. clin. Med. **83**, 458—469 (1974)

Chen, J. P., Shurley, H. M.: A simple efficient production of neoantigen antisera against fibrinolytic degradation products: radioimmunoassay of fragment. E. Thromb. Res. **7**, 425—434 (1975)

Clarkson, A. R., MacDonald, M., Petrie, J. J. B., Casch, J. D., Robson, J. S.: Serum and urinary fibrin/fibrinogen degradation products in glomerulonephritis. Brit. med. J. **3**, 1—5 (1971)

Colman, R. W., Osbahr, A. J., Morris, R. E., Jr.: New vasoconstrictor, bovine peptide B released during blood coagulation. Nature (Lond.) **215**, 292—293 (1967)

Culasso, D. E., Donati, M. B., de Gaetano, G., Vermylen, J., Verstraete, M.: Inhibition of human platelet aggregation by plasmin digest of human and bovine fibrinogen preparations: role of contaminating factor VIII related material. Blood **44**, 169—175 (1974)

Dudek, G. A., Kłoczewiak, M., Budzyński, A. Z., Latallo, Z. S., Kopeć, M.: Characterization and comparison of macromolecular end products of fibrinogen and fibrin proteolysis by plasmin. Biochim. biophys. Acta (Amst.) **214**, 44—55 (1970)

Eagle, H., Harris, T. N.: Studies in blood coagulation. V. The coagulation of blood by proteolytic enzymes (Trypsin, papain). J. gen. Physiol. **20**, 453—551 (1937)

Edgington, T. S., Plow, E. F.: Functional molecular anatomy of fibrinogen: antibodies as biological probes of structure. Contemp. Top. molec. Immunol. **2**, 237—271 (1973)

Ekberg, M., Pandolfi, M.: Origin of urinary fibrin/fibrinogen degradation products in glomerulonephritis. Brit. med. J. **2**, 17—19 (1975)

Ferreira, H. C., Murat, L. G.: An immunological method for demonstrating fibrin degradation products in serum and its use in the diagnosis of fibrinolytic states. Brit. J. Haemat. **9**, 299—308 (1963)

Fletcher, A. P., Alkjaersig, N.: Blood hypercoagulability, intravascular coagulation and thrombosis. New diagnostic concepts. Thrombos. Diathes. haemorrh. (Stuttg.) Suppl. **45**, 389—394 (1971)

Fletcher, A. P., Alkjaersig, N.: Laboratory diagnosis of intravascular coagulation. In: Poller, L. (Ed.). Recent Advances in Thrombosis, pp 87—113. London: Livingston-Churchill 1973

Fletcher, A. P., Alkjaersig, N., Fisher, S., Sherry, S.: The proteolysis of fibrinogen by plasmin: the identification of thrombin-clottable fibrinogen derivatives which polymerize abnormally. J. Lab. clin. Med. **58**, 780—802 (1966)

Furlan, M., Kemp, G., Beck, E. A.: Plasmic degradation of human fibrinogen. III. Molecular model of the plasmin-resistant disulphide knot in monomeric fragment D. Biochim. biophys. Acta (Amst.) **400**, 95—111 (1975a)

Furlan, M., Seelicht, T., Beck, E. A.: Plasmic degradation of human fibrinogen. IV. Identification of subunit chain remnants in fragment Y. Biochim. biophys. Acta (Amst.) **400**, 112—120 (1975b)

Gaffney, P. J., Brasher, M.: Subunit structure of the plasmin-induced degradation products of crosslinked fibrin. Biochim. biophys. Acta (Amst.) **295**, 308—323 (1973)

Gaffney, P. J., Dobos, P.: A structural aspect of human fibrinogen suggested by its plasmin degradation. Febs Letters **15**, 13—17 (1971)

Gerrits, W. B.: Fibrinogen and its derivatives in intravascular coagulation. Neth. J. Med. **18**, 31—44 (1975)

Girman, G., Pees, H., Schwarze, G., Scheurlen, P. G.: Immunosuppression by micromolecular fibri-fibrinogen degradation products in cancer. Nature **259**, 399—401 (1976)

Gladner, J. A., Murtaugh, P. A., Fole, J. E., Laki, K.: Nature of peptides released by thrombin. Ann. N. Y. Acad. Sci. **104**, 47—52 (1963)

Godal, H. C., Abildgaard, U.: Gelation of soluble fibrin in plasma by ethanol. Scand. J. Haemat. **3**, 342—350 (1966)

Gordon, Y. B., Martin, M. J., Landon, J., Chard, T.: The development of radioimmunoassays for fibrinogen degradation products: fragment D and E. Brit. J. Haemat. **29**, 109—119 (1975)

Gordon, Y. B., Meneill, A. T., Martin, M. J., Chard, T.: Specific and sensitive determination of fi-brinogen degradation products by radioimmunoassay. Lancet **1973 II**, 1168—1170

Hall, C. L., Pejhan, N., Terry, J. M., Blainey, J. D.: Urinary fibrin-fibrinogen degradation products in nephrotic syndrome. Brit. med. J. **1**, 419—422 (1975)

Harfenist, E. I., Canfield, R.: Degradation of fibrinogen by plasmin. Isolation of an early cleavage product. Biochemistry **14**, 1410—1417 (1975)

Hawiger, J., Niewiarowski, S., Gurewitch, V., Thomas, D. P.: Measurement of fibrinogen degrada-tion products in serum by staphylococcal clumping test. J. Lab. clin. Med. **75**, 93—108 (1970)

Hedner, U., Ekberg, M., Nilsson, M. I.: Urinary fibrin/fibrinogen degradation products (FDP) and glomerulonephritis. Acta med. scand. **195**, 81—85 (1974)

Herzig, R. H., Ratnoff, O. D., Schainoff, J. R.: Studies on a procoagulant fraction of southern cop-perhead snake venom: the preferential release of fibrinopeptide B. J. Lab. clin. Med. **76**, 451—465 (1970)

Holleman, W. H., Coen, C. J.: Characterization of peptides released from human fibrinogen by Arvin. Biochim. biophys. Acta (Amst.) **200**, 587—589 (1970)

Inoue, N., Moroi, M., Yamasaki, M.: Plasmin degradation of bovine fibrinogen and non-cross-linked fibrins in solution and in gel form. Biochim. biophys. Acta **400**, 322—333 (1975)

Jerushalmy, Z., Zucker, M. B.: Some effects of fibrinogen degradation products (FDP) on blood platelets. Thrombos. Diathes. haemorrh. (Stuttg.) **15**, 413—419 (1966)

Kay, A., B., Pepper, D. S., McKenzie, R.: The identification of fibrinopeptide B as a chemotactic agent derived from human fibrinogen. Brit. J. Haemat. **27**, 669—677 (1974)

Kierulf, P.: Studies on soluble fibrin in plasma. II. N-terminal analysis of a modified fraction I (Cohn) from patients plasma. Scand. J. clin. Lab. Invest. **31, 32**, 37—42 (1973)

Kierulf, P., Abildgaard, U.: Studies on soluble fibrin in plasma. I. N-Terminal analysis of a modified fraction I (Cohn) from normal and thrombin-incubated plasma. Scand. J. clin. Lab. Invest. **28**, 231—240 (1971)

Kisker, C. T., Rush, R.: Detection of intravascular coagulation. J. clin. Invest. **50**, 2235—2241 (1971)

Konttinen, Y. P., Lalla, M. L. T., Torunen, O.: Preferential degradation of soluble fibrin monomers in streptokinase-activated plasma. Thrombos. Diathes. haemorrh. (Stuttg.) **30**, 403—413 (1973)

Kopeć, M., Budzyński, A., Stachurska, J., Wegrzynowicz, Z., Kowalski, E.: Studies on the mecha-nism of interference by fibrinogen degradation products (FDP) with the platelet function. Role of fibrinogen in the platelet atmosphere. Thrombos. Diathes. haemorrh. (Stuttg.) **15**, 476—490 (1966)

Kopeć, M., Kowalski, E., Stachurska, J.: Studies on paracoagulation. Role of antithrombin VI. Thrombos. Diathes. haemorrh. (Stuttg.) **5**, 285—295 (1960)

Kopeć, M., Teisseyre, E., Dudek-Wojciechowska, G., Kłoczewiak, M., Pankiewicz, A., Latal-lo, Z. S.: Studies on the "Double D" fragment from stabilized bovine fibrin. Thrombos. Res. **2**, 283—291 (1973)

Kopeć, M., Wegrzynowicz, Z., Budzyński, A. Z., Latallo, Z. S., Lipinski, B., Kowalski, E.: Interac-tion of fibrinogen degradation products (FDP) with platelets. Exp. Biol. Med. **3**, 73—81 (1968)

Kopeć, M., Wegrzynowicz, Z., Kłoczewiak, M., Latallo, Z. S.: Antithrombin action of fibrinogen degradation products (FDP). Folia haemat. (Lpz.) **98**, 417—425 (1972)

Kopeć, M., Wegrzynowicz, Z., Latallo, Z. S.: Precipitation of soluble complexes of fibrin mon-omer (SFMC) by cellular basic proteins and the antagonistic effect of sulphonated mucopo-lysaccharides. Proc. Soc. exp. Biol. (N. Y.) **135**, 579—675 (1970)

Kopeć, M., Wegrzynowicz, Z., Latallo, Z. S.: Soluble fibrin complexes and a new specific test for their detection. Thrombos. Diathes. haemorrh. (Stuttg.) Suppl. **39**, 219—238 (1970 b)

Kopeć, M., Wegrzynowicz, Z., Zajdel, M., Sawecka, J., Szumiel, I.: Effects of histones and dextran on some properties of fibrin, particularly on its susceptibility to plasmin. Thrombos. Res. **5**, 359—374 (1974)

Korst, D. R., Kratochvil, C. H.: "Cryofibrinogen" in a case of lung neoplasm associated with thrombophlebitis migrans. Blood **10**, 945—953 (1955)

Kowalska-Loth, B., Gårdlund, B., Egberg, N., Blombäck, B.: Plasmic degradation products of human fibrinogen. I. Chemical and immunological relation between Fragment E and N-DSK. Thrombos. Res. **2**, 423—450 (1973)

Kowalski, E.: Fibrinogen derivatives and their biological activities. Semin. Haemat. **1**, 45—59 (1968)

Kowalski, E., Budzyński, A. Z., Kopeć, M., Latallo, Z., Lipiński, B., Wegrzynowicz, Z.: Studies on the molecular pathology and pathogenesis of bleeding in severe fibrinolytic states in dogs. Thrombos. Diathes. haemorrh. (Stuttg.) **10**, 406—423 (1964 b)

Kowalski, E., Budzyński, A. Z., Kopeć, M., Latallo, Z. S., Lipiński, B., Wegrzynowicz, Z.: Circulation fibrinogen degradation products FDP in dog blood after intravenous thrombin influsion. Thrombos. Diathes. haemorrh. (Stuttg.) **13**, 12—24 (1965)

Kowalski, E., Kopeć, M., Wegrzynowicz, Z.: Influence of fibrinogen degradation products (FDP) on platelet aggregation, adhesiveness and viscous metamorphosis. Thrombos. Diathes. haemorrh. (Stuttg.) **10**, 406—423 (1964)

Kowarzyk, H., Głogowska, J., Szymik, S.: The enzymatic action of thrombin and the physical phase of fibrin clotting. Arch. Immunol. Ter. dosw. **9**, 341—355 (1961)

Kwaan, H. C., Barlow, G. H.: The mechanism of action of Arvin and Reptilase. Thrombos. Diathes. haemorrh. (Stuttg.) Suppl. **47**, 361—369 (1971)

Larrieu, M. J., Rigollot, C., Marder, V. J.: Comparative effects of fibrinogen degradation fragments D and E on coagulation. Brit. J. Haematol. **22**, 719—733 (1972)

Latallo, Z. S.: Formation and detection of fibrinogen derived complexes. Thrombos. Haemost. (1976) in press

Latallo, Z. S., Budzyński, A. Z., Lipiński, B., Kowalski, E.: Inhibition of thrombin and of fibrin polymerization. Two activities derived from plasmin-digested fibrinogen. Nature (Lond.) **203**, 1184—1185 (1964)

Latallo, Z. S., Lopaciuk, S., Meissner, J.: A combined treatment with defibrase and streptokinase. In: Aktuelle Probleme in der Angiologie: Defibrinierung mit thrombinähnlichen Schlangengiftenzymen, Vol XXVI, pp. 181—190. Bern-Stuttgart-Vienna: Huber 1974

Latallo, Z. S., Fletcher, A. P., Alkjaersig, N., Sherry, S.: Inhibition of fibrin polymerization by fibrinogen proteolysis products. Amer. J. Physiol. **202**, 681—686 (1962)

Latallo, Z. S., Mattler, L. E., Bang, N. U., Hansen, M. S., Chang, M. I.: Analysis of soluble fibrin complexes by agarose gel chromatography and protamine sulfate gelation. Biochim. biophys. Acta (Amst.) **420**, 69—80 (1976)

Latallo, Z. S., Teisseyre, E.: Evaluation of Reptilase R and thrombin clotting time in the presence of fibrinogen degradation products and heparin. Scand. J. Haemat. Suppl. **13**, 261—266 (1971)

Latallo, Z. S., Teisseyre, E., Wegrzynowicz, Z., Kopeć, M.: Effect of various proteolytic enzymes on fibrinogen. Folia haemat. (Lpz.) **95**, 158—166 (1971 a)

Latallo, Z. S., Wegrzynowicz, Z., Budzyński, A. Z., Kopeć, M.: Effect of protamine sulphate on the solubility of fibrinogen, its derivatives and other plasma proteins. Scand. J. Haemat. Suppl. **13**, 151—162 (1971 b)

Latallo, Z. S., Wegrzynowicz, Z., Teisseyre, E., Kopeć, M.: Simple and rapid evaluation of the intravascular coagulation and fibrinolytic states by application of protamine sulphate and Reptilase R. Scand. J. Haemat. Suppl. **13**, 387—388 (1971 c)

Laurell, C. B.: Quantitative estimation of proteins by electrophoresis in agarose containing antibodies. Analyt. Biochem. **15**, 45—52 (1966)

Lewis, J. H., Wilson, J. H.: Variations in abilities of animal fibrinogens to clump staphylococci. Thrombos. Res. **3**, 419—424 (1973)

Lipiński, B., Wegrzynowicz, Z., Budzyński, A., Kopeć, M., Latallo, Z. S., Kowalski, E.: Soluble unclottable complexes formed in the presence of fibrinogen degradation products (FDP) during the fibrinogen fibrin conversion and their potential significance in pathology. Thrombos. Diathes. haemorrh. (Stuttg.) **17**, 65—77 (1967)

Lipiński, B., Worowski, K.: Detection of soluble fibrin monomer complexes in blood by means of protamine sulphate. Thrombos. Diathes. haemorrh. (Stuttg.) **20**, 44—49 (1968)

Lopaciuk, S., Ziemski, M., Latallo, Z. S.: Unpublished data (1974)

Lorand, L., Chenoweth, D., Gray, A.: Titration of the acceptor cross-linking sites in fibrin. Ann. N. Y. Acad. Sci. **202**, 155—171 (1972)

Małofiejew, M: The biological and pharmacological properties of some fibrinogen degradation products. Scand. J. Haemat. Suppl. **13**, 303—308 (1971)

Marder, V. J.: Immunologic structure of fibrinogen and its plasmin degradation products: theoretical and clinical considerations. In: Laki, K. (Ed.): Fibrinogen, New York: Marcel Dekker 1968

Marder, V. J., Budzyński, A. Z.: Data for defining fibrinogen and its plasmic degradation products. Thrombos. Diathes. haemorrh. **33**, 199—207 (1975)

Marder, V. J., Matchett, M. O., Sherry, S.: Detection of serum fibrinogen degradation products. Comparison of six techniques using purified products and application in clinical studies. Amer. J. Med. **51**, 71—82 (1971)

Marder, V. J., Shulman, N. R., Carroll, W. R.: High molecular weight derivatives of human fibrinogen produced by plasmin. I. Physicochemical and immunological characterization. J. biol. Chem. **244**, 2111—2119 (1969)

Mattock, P., Esnouf, M. D., Differences in the subunit structure of human fibrin formed by the action of Arvin, reptilase and thrombin. Nature (Lond.) New Biol. **233**, 277—279 (1971)

McDonagh, J., McDonagh, R.: Activation of human plasma factor XIII. IVth. Int. Congr. Thrombosis and Haemostasis. Abstr. 155. June 12—22, Vienna 1973

McDonagh, R. P., Jr., McDonagh, J., Duckert, F.: The influence of fibrin cross-linking on the kinetics of urokinase-induced clot lysis. Brit. J. Haemat. 21, 323—332 (1971)

McKee, P. A., Kalbfleisch, J. M., Bird, R. M.: Incidence and significance of cryofibrinogenemia. J. Lab. clin. Med. **61**, 203—210 (1963)

Merskey, C., Lalezart, P., Johnson, A. J.: A rapid, simple, sensitive method for measuring fibrinolytic split products in human serum. Proc. Soc. exp. Biol. (N. Y.) **131**, 871—875 (1969)

Mihalyi, E., Godfrey, J. E.: Digestion of fibrinogen by trypsin. I. Kinetic studies of the reaction. Biochim. biophys. Acta (Amst.) **67**, 73—87 (1963)

Miller, S. P., Sanchez-Avalos, J.: Degradation of fibrinogen by proteolytic enzymes. II. Effect of the products on coagulation. Thrombos. Diathes. haemorrh. (Stuttg.) **20**, 15—22 (1968)

Mills, D. A.: Molecular mode for the proteolysis of human fibrinogen by plasmin. Biochim. biophys. Acta (Amst.) **263**, 619—630 (1972)

Mosesson, M. W., Finlayson, J. S., Galankis, D. K.: The essential convalent structure of human fibrinogen evinced by analysis of derivatives formed during plasmic hydrolysis. J. biol. Chem. **249**, 7913—7922 (1973)

Myśliwiec, B., Mysliwiec, M.: Studies on fibrinogen degradation products in cerebrospinal fluid in children. Pediat. pol. **48**, 1223—1227 (1973)

Myśliwiec, M., Arnesen, H., Godal, H. C.: The effect of fibrinogen degradation products on plasmin activity. Thrombos. Diathes. haemorrh. **29**, 592—597 (1973)

Nanninga, L. B., Guest, M. M.: Antifibrinolytic action of anticoagulant split products of fibrinogen. Thrombos. Diathes. haemorrh. (Stuttg.) **19**, 526—532 (1968)

Niewiarowski, S.: Detection of fibrinogen derivatives in plasma and in serum and its significance in the diagnosis of intravascular coagulation. XXII Congrès national d'anesthésie. Paris 67—84 (1975)

Niewiarowski, S., Gurewitch, V.: Laboratory identification of intravascular coagulation: The SDPS test for the detection of fibrin monomer and fibrin degradation products. J. Lab. clin. Med. **77**, 665—676 (1971)

Niewiarowski, S., Kowalski, E.: Un nouvel anticoagulant dérivé du fibrinogène. Rev. Hémat. **13**, 320—328 (1958)

Niewiarowski, S., Latallo, Z. S., Stachurska, J.: Apparation d'un inhibiteur da la thrombinoplastin formation au cours de la protéolyse du fibrinogène. Rev. Hémat. **14**, 118—128 (1959)

Niewiarowski, S., Regoeczi, E., Stewart, G. J., Senyi, A. F., Mustard, J. F.: Platelet interaction with polymerizing fibrin. J. clin. Invest. **51**, 685—700 (1972)

Niléhn, J. E.: Separation and estimation of split products of fibrinogen and fibrin in human serum. Thrombos. Diathes. haemorrh. (Stuttg.) **18**, 487—498 (1967)

Niléhn, J. E., Nilsson, I. M.: Demonstration of fibrinolytic split products in human serum by an immunological method in spontaneous and induced fibrinolytic states. Scand. J. Haemat. **1**, 313—330 (1964)

Nossel, H. L., Butler, V. P., Jr., Canfield, R. E., Yudelman, I., Spanodis, K., Soland, T.: Potential use of fibrinopeptide A measurements in the diagnosis and management of thrombosis. Thrombos. Diathes. haemorrh. (Stuttg.) **33**, 426—434 (1975)

Nossel, H. L., Younger, R., Wilner, G. D., Procupez, T., Canfield, R. E., Butler, V. P., Jr.: Radioimmunoassay of fibrinopeptide A. Proc. nat. Acad. Sci. (Wash.) **68**, 2350—2353 (1971)

Nussenzweig, V., Seligman, M., Grabar, P.: Les produits de dégradation du fibrinogène par la plasmine. II Etude immunologique: mise en évidence d'anticorps antifibrinogène natif possédant des spécifités différentes. Ann. Inst. Pasteur **100**, 490—508 (1961)

Olsson, P. I., Johnsson, H.: Interference of acetyl salicylic acid, heparin and fibrinogen degradation products in haemostasis of Reptilase-defibrinated dogs. Thrombos. Res. **1**, 135—146 (1972)

Osbahr, A. J., Custodio, R.: Action of peptide B from bovine fibrinogen on ATPase activity and superprecipitation of myosin B. Amer. J. Physiol. **228**, 488—495 (1975)

Otis, P. T., Rapaport, S. I.: Effects of FDPs/fibrinogen degradation products (DE) and (XY) on fibrinogen synthesis in rabbits. IVth Int. Congr. on Thrombosis and Haemostasis. Abstr. 254, Vienna 1973

Pechet, L., Alexander, B.: The effect of certain proteolytic enzymes on the thrombin-fibrinogen interaction. Biochemistry **1**, 875—883 (1962)

Pindyck, L., Lichtman, H., Kohl, S.: Cryofibrinogenemia in women using oral contraceptives. Lancet **1970 I**, 51—53

Pizzo, S. V., Schwartz, M. L., Hill, R. L., McKee, P. A.: Mechanism of Ancrod anticoagulation. A. direct proteolytic effect on fibrin. J. clin. Invest. **51**, 2841—2850 (1972a)

Pizzo, S. V., Schwartz, M. L., Hill, R. L., McKee, P. A.: The effect of plasmin on the subunit structure of human fibrinogen. J. biol. Chem. **247**, 636—645 (1972b)

Pizzo, S. V., Schwartz, M. L., Hill, R. L., McKee, P. A.: The effect of plasmin on the subunit structure of human fibrin. J. biol. Chem. **248**, 4574—4583 (1973a)

Pizzo, S. V., Taylor, Jr., L. M., Schwartz, M. L., Hill, R. L., McKee, P. A.: Subunit structure of fragment D from fibrinogen and crosslinked fibrin. J. biol. Chem. **248**, 4584—4590 (1973b)

Plow, E. F., Edgington, T. S.: The number of D and E regions in the fibrinogen molecule. Proc. nat. Acad. Sci. (Wash.) **71**, 158—162 (1974)

Plow, E. F., Edgington, T. S.: An alternative pathway for fibrinolysis. I. The cleavage of fibrinogen by leukocyte proteases at physiologic pH. J. clin. Invest. **56**, 30—38 (1975)

Prentice, C. R. M., Turpie, A. G. G., Hassanein, A. A., McNicol, G. P.: Changes in platelet behaviour during Arvin therapy. Lancet **1969 I**, 644—647

Purdie, D. W., Edgrar, W., Howie, P. W., Porbes, C. D., Prentice, C. R. M.: Raised amniotic-fluid FDP in fetal neural-tube anomalies. Lancet **1975 I**, 1013—1014

Richardson, D. L., Pepper, D. S., Kay, A. B.: Chemotaxis for human monocytes by fibrinogen derived peptides. Brit. J. Haematol. **32**, 507—513 (1976)

Roschlau, W. H. E., Ives, D. A. J.: Review of the biochemistry and coagulation physiology of Brinolase (fibrinolytic enzyme from *Aspergillus oryzae*). Folia haemat. (Lpz.) **101**, 22—37 (1974)

Ruckley, C. V., Das, P. C., Leitch, A. G., Donaldson, W. A., Redpath, A. T., Scott, P., Casch, J. D.: Serum fibrin-fibrinogen degradation products associated with postoperative pulmonary embolus and venous thrombosis. Brit. med. J. **4**, 395—398 (1970)

Sasaki, T., Page, I. H., Shainoff, J. R.: Stable complex of fibrinogen and fibrin. Science **152**, 1069—1071 (1966)

Seaman, A. J.: The recognition of intravascular clotting: The plasma protamine paracoagulation test. Arch. intern. Med. **125**, 1016—1021 (1970)

Shainoff, J. R., Page, I. H.: Cofibrin and fibrin intermediates as indicator of thrombin activity in vivo. Circulat. Res. **8**, 1013—1022 (1960)

Smith, G. F., Bang, N. U.: Formation of soluble fibrin polymers. Fibrinogen degradation fragments D and E fail to form soluble complexes with fibrin monomer. Biochemistry **11**, 2958—2966 (1972)

Solum, N. O.: Platelet aggregation during fibrin polymerization. Scand. UJ. clin. Lab. Invest. **18**, 577—587 (1966)

Solum, N. O., Rigollot, C., Budzyński, A. Z., Marder, V. J.: A quantitative evaluation of the inhibition of platelet aggregation by low molecular weight degradation products of fibrinogen. Brit. J. Haemat. **24**, 419—434 (1973)

Soulier, J. P., Prou-Wartelle, O.: Study of thrombin coagulase. Thrombos. Diathes. haemorrh. (Stuttg.) **17**, 321—334 (1967)

Stachurska, J., Latallo, Z. S., Kopeć, M.: Inhibition of platelet aggregation by dialysable fibrinogen degradation products (FDP). Thrombos. Diathes. haemorrh. (Stuttg.) **23**, 91—98 (1970)

Stiehm, R. E., Trygstad, C. W.: Split products of fibrin in human renal diseases. Amer. J. Med. **46**, 774—786 (1969)

Tager, M.: Studies on the nature and purification of coagulase reacting factor and its relation to prothrombin. J. Med. **104**, 675—686 (1956)

Takaki, A., Yamaguchi, T., Ohsato, K.: Kinin-like activities of the synthetic low molecular weight fragment of fibrinogen degradation products. Thrombos. Diathes. haemorrh. (Stuttg.) **32**, 350—355 (1974)

Teisseyre, E., Latallo, Z. S., Kopeć, M.: Studies on the proteolysis of fibrinogen and fibrin by *Aspergillus ochraceus* enzyme as compared to the action of plasmin. Folia haemat. (Lpz.) **101**, 99—110 (1974)

Thomas, D. P., Niewiarowski, S., Myers, A. R., Bloch, K. J., Colman, R. W.: Four methods for detecting fibrinogen degradation products in patients with various diseases. New Engl. J. Med. **283**, 663—668 (1970)

Tibutt, D. A., Chesterman, C. N., Allington, M. J., Willims, E. W., Faulkner, T.: Measurement of fibrinogen-fibrin-related antigen in serum as aid to diagnosis of deep vein thrombosis in our patients. Brit. med. J. **1**, 367—369 (1975)

Töpfer, H., Piesche, K.: Charakterisierung einer alkalischen Protease aus *Aspergillus ocharaceus*. Folia haemat. (Lpz.) **101**, 91—98 (1974)

Triantaphyllopoulos, D. C., Chen, C., Triantaphyllopoulos, E.: Nature of the inhibition of prothrombin consumption by lysed fibrinogen. Brit. J. Haemat. **16**, 589—598 (1969)

Triantaphyllopoulos, E., Triantaphyllopoulos, D. C.: Fibrinogenolysis: the micromolecular derivatives. Brit. J. Haemat. **15**, 337—343 (1968)

Wegrzynowicz, Z., Kopeć, M., Latallo, Z. S.: Formation of soluble fibrin complexes and some factors affecting their solubility. Scand. J. Haemat. Suppl. **13**, 49—59 (1971)

Wik, K. O., Tangen, O., McKenzie, F. N.: Blood clotting activity of Reptilase and bovine thrombin in vitro: A comparative study of seven different species. Brit. J. Haemat. **23**, 37—45 (1972)

Wiśniewski, K., Buczko, W., Moniuszko-Jakoniuk, J.: The effect of the products of fibrinogen digestion by plasmin (P-FDP) on the central nervous system. Acta neurobiol. exp. **35**, 275—283 (1975)

Zajdel, M.: Ph. D. thesis (1973)

Zajdel, M., Wegrzynowicz, Z. Sawecka, J., Jeliaszewicz, J., Pulverer, G.: Mechanism of action of staphylocoagulase. IIIrd Int. Symp. on Staphylococci. Stuttgart: Fischer (in press)

Zajdel, M., Wegrzynowicz, Z., Sawecka, J., Kopec, M.: Subunits and susceptibility of fibrins formed from bovine fibrinogen by Arvin, Reptilase, thrombin and staphylothrombin. Thrombos. Res. **6**, 337—344 (1975)

The Measurement of Fibrinolytic Activities

I. M. Nilsson, U. Hedner and M. Pandolfi

Introduction

Fibrinolysis is the proteolytic activity arising in the circulating blood on activation of the fibrinolytic system. Activation of fibrinolysis is brought about by various activators and results in the conversion of plasminogen to plasmin. Plasminogen activators occur naturally in most body tissues (tissue activator), in the circulating blood (blood activator), in urine (urokinase), and in some other body fluids.

Tissue activator. As early as 1947, Astrup and Permin showed that the *fibrinolytic activity* of *tissues* was due to an activator of fibrinolysis. This tissue activator has been related to the microsomes of the cells (Nakahara and Celander, 1968) and to the lysozymes (Lack and Ali, 1964). Astrup and coworkers (Albrechtsen, 1959; Astrup, 1966) have published extensive studies on the tissue activator. They have demonstrated that the tissue activator can be extracted from the tissues with strong solutions of potassium thiocyanate (2 M KSCN) and that the activator is thermostable (70–100° C) and is stable at acid pH.

The location of fibrinolytic activity in the tissues has been facilitated by Todd's histochemical method (Todd, 1959). It is now known (Astrup, 1966; Pandolfi et al., 1969) that the tissue activator is related chiefly to structures of the endothelial cells of the capillaries. A direct correlation has been found between the fibrinolytic activity of a tissue specimen and its content of vascularized connective tissue. The exact chemical nature of tissue activator is not yet known.

Kok and Astrup (1969, 1972) isolated plasminogen activator from hog ovaries with extraction methods and gel filtration and estimated the molecular weight to be about 60000. They believed it to be different from urokinase. Thorsen and Astrup (1974) have recently shown that tissue activator and urokinase differ in their reaction to inhibitors.

The distribution of tissue plasminogen activator in human and in animal tissues has been investigated with the extraction method as well as the histochemical method (see Astrup, 1966; Pandolfi, 1969). Most human tissues have been found to contain plasminogen activator. The highest concentrations occur in the uterus, adrenals, lymph nodes, prostate, meninges, and thyroid. Little or no activity has been found in the liver and the placenta, and only low activity in the renal cortex.

Blood activator. Much suggests that the fibrinolytic activity in the blood is derived from activators produced in the endothelium of small vessels and that the activators are continuously presented to the bloodstream (Fearnley, 1965; Nilsson and Pandolfi, 1970; Cash, 1975a). Åstedt et al. (1971a) and Åstedt and Pandolfi (1972) have produced evidence, also in tissue culture, that these activators are synthetized by vascular endothelium and are continuously released from the cells into the culture medium. The blood activator is labile (MÜLLERTZ, 1957). A labile plasminogen activator immunologically different from urokinase has been obtained by postmortem infusion of vessels with saline. This activator is probably identical with the blood activator (AOKI and VON KAULLA, 1971a, b). The molecular weight of this vascular activator, as estimated by gel filtration, was about 65000. However, using a different perfusion fluid, AUERSWALD et al. (1971) concluded that, although the maximal activity appeared to reside in the molecular weight region of 61000, this unit might represent a dimer made up of units with a molecular weight of 30500.

The spontaneous fibrinolytic activity in the blood is normally low, owing partly to the influence of inhibitors. The fibrinolytic activity of blood can be enhanced by a variety of stimuli, such as physical exercise, emotion, surgical operations, electric shock, pneumoencephalography, pyrogens, and venous occlusion. Many components, such as epinephrine, nicotinic acid, histamine, acetylcholine, vasopressin, and several other vasoactive drugs, enhance the fibrinolytic activity of the blood (see NILSSON and PANDOLFI, 1970; CASH, 1972; NILSSON, 1975). The vasoactive drugs have no such effect on blood in vitro. The mechanism responsible for the release of the activators from the vessel walls to the bloodstream is not known. It has been suggested that different stimuli causing quick changes in the calibers of the blood vessels, such as injection of vasoactive drugs, enhance the release of the activators from the vessel walls into the bloodstream (HOLEMANS, 1965; NILSSON and PANDOLFI, 1970). The mediator of the physiologic response may in part be catecholamines (see CASH, 1975a). Anyhow, unlike the spontaneous fibrinolytic activity, the activity demonstrable after the above-mentioned stimuli is so elevated as to permit measurement of intra- and interindividual differences. It is, above all, epinephrine, vasopressin, exercise, and venous occlusion of the limbs that have been used for estimating the fibrinolytic capacity of a given person.

The physiologic function of the activators must be to dissolve fibrin precipitates and to maintain the patency of blood vessels and urinary pathways and excretory ducts.

An increase of fibrinolytic activity in blood and tissues leads to bleeding. A decrease in fibrinolytic activators is followed by impairment of the dissolution of fibrin precipitates and thrombosis.

It is evident from the above considerations that if one is to assess the fibrinolytic activity in the body and tissues, one should, when possible, determine:

1. The spontaneous fibrinolytic activity of blood
2. The fibrinolytic response to various stimuli known to enhance the release of activators from the vessel walls into the bloodstream
3. The plasminogen activator content of vessel walls and tissues
4. Release of fibrinolytic agents from tissue culture

A. Methods for Measuring the Spontaneous Fibrinolytic Activity of Blood

The fibrinolytic activity in blood is a result of the effect of both fibrinolytic activators and inhibitors. To obtain a more specific measure of the fibrinolytic activators various methods have been elaborated in which the inhibitory effect is claimed to have been eliminated. The inhibitor activity has thus been diminished by dilution of plasma, by denaturation (treatment with chloroform or acetone), or by fractionation of plasma (euglobulin precipitation). The inhibitor activity is not completely extinguished (LAURITSEN, 1969; KLUFT and BRAKMAN, 1975). The tests and determinations most widely used for measuring the fibrinolytic activator activity in blood are:

1. Whole blood lysis test
2. Euglobulin clot lysis test
3. Diluted blood clot lysis time
4. Fibrin plate method
5. Fibrin degradation products (FDP)

I. Whole Blood Lysis Test

This is not a sensitive method for activator assay, but it can be used to get a rough estimation of the fibrinolytic activity in blood (NILSSON, 1974). Whole blood (2–3 ml) is collected in a tube and 0.5 ml thrombin (300 NIH units/ml) is added immediately to accelerate coagulation. The clot is incubated at $37°$ C (water bath) and the time necessary for the clot to dissolve is noted.

Normal value: the clot is not dissolved within 24 h. *Severe fibrinolysis* results in the dissolution of the clot within 5–10 min and *moderate fibrinolysis* within 1–2 h.

The method cannot be used for demonstrating abnormally low fibrinolytic activity.

II. Euglobulin Clot Lysis Test

This is a suitable screening test for routine use and clinical practice. In our experience the euglobulin lysis test does not give such accurate information on the fibrinolytic activity in the circulating blood as the fibrin plate method, but it is very valuable for quickly assessing whether the fibrinolytic activity is increased.

It derives from an observation by MILSTONE (1941) that the plasma euglobulin fraction contains a "lytic factor." In this test, diluted plasma is acidified. Acetic acid or exposure to CO_2 have been used for acidification and with comparable results. The euglobulin fraction contains the plasminogen, plasmin, fibrinogen, and fibrinolytic activators, while most of the fibrinolytic inhibitors remain in the supernatant. The euglobulin fraction is dissolved in buffer and coagulated with thrombin, and the time necessary for the clot to dissolve is noted. Normally, this time is shorter than that for whole blood because the major part of the fibrinolytic inhibitors is not precipitated together with the euglobulin fractions.

Factors influencing the method. The amounts of inhibitors coprecipitated with the euglobulin fraction have been shown to vary with the (1) *pH* and the (2) *dilution of the plasma* (KLUFT and BRAKMAN, 1975). The same authors found that $C\bar{1}$-Inactivator was precipitated in considerable amounts (up to 80–100%) in the euglobulin fraction especially at a low pH and a low ionic strength. Only traces of α_1-antitrypsin and α_2-macroglobulin were found. It is therefore recommended to use plasma diluted 1:10 to secure an appropriate ionic strength and a pH of 5.9–6.0 for euglobulin precipitation to avoid the coprecipitation of $C\bar{1}$-Inactivator.

The fibrinolytic activators are labile. The blood should be tested as soon as possible after it has been obtained. Both the (3) *interval between the withdrawal of the blood before centrifugation* and (4) the *interval between centrifugation and the performance of the test* are important for obtaining reliable results. The former interval should not exceed 30 min and the latter, not 2 h (SAMAMA et al., 1975). (5) The *type of anticoagulant* used can influence the method (BLIX, 1961). Euglobulin clots from oxalated plasma and heparinized plasma lyse less readily than euglobulin clots from citrated plasma. A standardized procedure is therefore absolutely necessary.

Performance. The test is performed on platelet-poor citrated plasma (9 parts of blood + 1 part of 3.8% sodium citrate) separated by centrifugation at 2000 g for 20 min within 30 min of collection. After centrifugation the plasma is sucked off and tested immediately (no storage or freezing of the plasma).

To 1 ml of the citrated plasma is added 9 ml of 0.025% acetic acid. pH should be 5.9–6.0. The tube is inverted and allowed to stand for 10 min at $+4°$ C. Afterwards it is centrifuged at 2000 g for 5 min, the supernatant is separated off, and the precipitate is dissolved in 1 ml of 0.01 M saline barbital buffer (OWREN, 1947) (containing 0.74% NaCl, pH 7.38, ionic strength 0.15). After incubation for 10 min at 37° C, 0.5 ml of a thrombin solution (2 NIH U/ml) is added and the stopwatch is started. A clot is formed, and the time necessary for it to dissolve is noted. An automatic clot lysis recorder can be used (Medicon UK Ltd).

Normal value: > 150 min. If fibrinolysis is severe, the dissolution time will be short (at most 30 min). Trasylol and heparin are not precipitated in the euglobulin fraction (SAMAMA et al., 1975). The test can therefore be used in patients receiving heparin treatment.

The dissolution time will be short if the fibrinogen is low (< 0.5 g/l). This is because the patient's own fibrinogen is used as the substrate. If the fibrinogen content is extremely small or nil, the test can be repeated by addition of a standard amount of fibrinogen to the plasma.

By careful reading of long lysis times (with an automatic lysis recorder) it is possible to detect abnormally low fibrinolytic activity.

Since fibrinolytic activity is proportional to the reciprocal of the lysis time (SHERRY and ALKJAERSIG, 1957), the results can also be expressed as units of activity calculated according to MCNICOL et al. (1963), whereby the reciprocal of a lysis time of 300 min is taken as unity.

It should be pointed out that the euglobulin lysis time is an artificial test system and primarily an activator-plasmin assay (JOHNSON et al., 1966). The resulting fibrinolytic activity in vitro does not necessarily reflect fibrinolysis in vivo.

III. Dilute Clot Lysis Time Methods

1. Dilute Whole Blood Clot Lysis Time

For determining fibrinolytic activator activity, FEARNLEY et al. (1957) described a dilution method for determining the lysis time of clots made from blood or plasma diluted 1:10 in phosphate buffer at pH 7.4 and then clotted with thrombin. The samples are incubated at 37° C and lysis times are recorded. Dilution decreases the activity of the plasma fibrinolytic inhibitors to a greater extent than that of the activators, and this is believed to explain why the test is more sensitive and shorter than the whole blood lysis time. The method usually gives lysis times 3 times as long as the euglobulin clot lysis test method.

The dilute whole blood clot lysis time is performed on whole blood collected without anticoagulant in order to decrease the delay between collection of the blood and performance of the test. The reading of the results has, however, been claimed to be difficult, especially at low fibrinogen levels (SAMAMA et al., 1975).

EACA and AMCA remain in the supernatant after euglobulin fractionation and the in vivo effect of these drugs is therefore diminished in the euglobulin clot lysis test. A test performed on whole blood should be preferred for estimation of the in vivo fibrinolytic activity in patients treated with these drugs (SAMAMA et al., 1975).

Performance. Blood is collected in a plastic tube and aliquots of 0.2 ml are rapidly pipetted into glass tubes containing 1.7 ml phosphate buffer (9.47 g $Na_2HPO_4 + 3.02$ g KH_2PO_4, pH 7.4) and 0.1 ml thrombin (50 NIH U/ml). After thorough mixing the tubes are placed at $+37°$ C. The time required for complete disappearance of the clot is recorded.

A modification of the method has been described by CHOHAN et al. (1975). Sodium acetate buffer, 0.12 M, pH 7.4, is used as diluent instead of phosphate buffer. This buffer was shown to be more effective in accelerating lysis than phosphate buffer of similar pH and molarity. The uniformity of the clot is maintained throughout the digestion in sodium acetate buffer and the end point of lysis is characteristically marked by abrupt and sharply defined disintegration. Sodium acetate buffer in addition shortens the lysis times.

Normal value: lysis times > 5 h (phosphate buffer). Results of less than 2 h usually denote an increased fibrinolytic activity.

The dilute whole blood clot lysis time technique has been used mainly for the estimation of blood fibrinolytic activity of physiologic degree and in serial determinations in patients who are receiving drugs for raising or lowering the fibrinolytic activity of their blood. It is not the method of choice for determining pathologic fibrinolysis (except in patients treated with EACA, AMCA). The long incubation periods involve a considerable source of error (growth of bacteria, unsatisfactory observation, etc).

2. Schneider's Test

Schneiders' test has been recommended as a screening method for determining fibrinolysis in acute situations. The degree of fibrinolysis is judged from the dissolution times of clots prepared from citrated plasma in various dilutions at 37° C. The test can also be used as a quick method for determining fibrinogen. The lowest plasma concentration in which a clot is formed after addition of thrombin is a semiquantitative measure of the amount of fibrinogen in the plasma (fibrin titer). For determination of the fibrin titer it is recommended to use citrated plasma obtained with addition of about 10 mg EACA/ml blood. Pooled plasma from normal persons is used as reference for determination of fibrinolysis as well as of the fibrin titer.

Performance. Two series of seven glass tubes are set up in two rows. To the first tubes of the two rows containing 1.8 ml 0.9% NaCl is added 0.2 ml citrated plasma from the patient and 0.2 ml of the control plasma, respectively. NaCl 1 ml 0.9%, is pipetted into all the other tubes. The dilution series are then set up by transferring 1 ml from tube 1 to tube 2 and then 1 ml from tube 2 to tube 3, etc. The dilutions in the different rows will then be 1:10, 1:20, 1:40, 1:80, 1:160, 1:320, 1:640. The tubes are placed in a water bath at 37° C and 0.1 ml thrombin (50 NIH U/ml; if the patient has received heparin, 300 NIH U/ml) is then added to each tube, the tubes are inverted, and stopwatches are started. The clots are inspected after 15, 60, and 120 min. The last tube in the series made with plasma with added EACA in which a clot appears within 15 min denotes the fibrin titer. The fibrin titer is reported as the dilution number. The state of the clots after 15, 60, and 120 min is noted as follows:

+ = firm clot
(+) = clot
(−) = clot floating free
− = no clot.

In the presence of fibrinolysis the clots in the patient's plasma (without EACA) will be dissolved more quickly than in normal plasma.

Normal values for fibrin titer: clot occurs in dilutions up to 1:80–1:320.

IV. Fibrin Plate Method

The fibrin plate method is a sensitive and accurate tool for measuring fibrinolytic activity. It can measure plasminogen activator activity and plasmin activity together or separately. The method was suggested by the observation that when placed on a fibrin film fragments of certain tissues lysed varying amounts of fibrin (PERMIN, 1949). The principle of the method is simple: a drop of a solution is placed on the surface of a layer of fibrin in a Petri dish, the plate is then incubated, and the fibrinolytic activity is calculated from the area of the lysed zone. Since its first description (ASTRUP and MÜLLERTZ, 1952) the method has been extensively used for measuring the fibrinolytic activity of blood (plasma), physiologic fluids, extracts of tissues, chromatographic fractions, etc. The method can be adapted to assay plasmi-

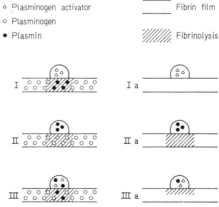

Fig. 1. When fibrin rich in plasminogen is used as substrate *(left)*, fibrinolysis is effected by solutions containing plasminogen activator *(I)*, plasmin *(II)* or both *(III)*. Plasminogen activator causes no lysis of plasminogen-free fibrin *(Ia)*, whereas plasmin (or other proteases) does *(IIa)*; mixtures of plasmin and activators induce lysis to an extent proportional to plasmin content of mixture *(IIIa)*

nogen (BRAKMAN, 1967) and fibrinolytic inhibitors. Since the fibrin used as substrate is usually contaminated with plasminogen, the dissolution of the fibrin can be caused either by plasminogen activator or by plasmin (or other proteases) or by both. Screening of the active agent can be done by running parallel assays with plasmino-gen-free fibrin as substrate. Figure 1 shows various possible combinations of test solution and substrate with the resulting fibrinolysis.

Since 1962 we at the Coagulation Laboratory, Malmö, use the fibrin plate method as modified by NILSSON and OLOW (1962).

Reagents

Fibrinogen. Human fibrinogen (Kabi) grade L is prepared according to the glycine method of BLOMBÄCK and BLOMBÄCK (1956). The human fibrinogen is diluted to *0.15%* in Tris buffer with ph 7.8 and μ 0.15.

Preparation of Tris buffer:

Base: 1.82% Trishydroxymethyl aminomethane in 0.9% NaCl

Salt: 3.64 g Trishydroxymethyl aminomethane, 30 ml 1.0 N HCl, aq. dest. ad 200 ml.

To obtain Tris buffer with pH 7.8, mix: 36 ml Tris base + 64 ml Tris salt. In this solution the ionic strength is 0.3. Therefore an equal volume of distilled water is added before using it for diluting the fibrinogen solution.

Plasminogen-free bovine fibrinogen can be obtained from Poviet Produktion, Oss, Holland.

Thrombin. Topostasin (Roche) (contamined with plasminogen) is used for the activator assay. One ampoule of Topostasin Roche (which contains 3000 NIH U thrombin) is diluted in 10 ml distilled water. This solution is diluted with 0.9% NaCl to give a final thrombin concentration of 20 NIH U/ml. The thrombin solution should be prepared on the same day as the plates.

Plasminogen-free thrombin for plasmin assay can be obtained from Leo, Copen-hagen.

Urokinase. Urokinase Leo (Copenhagen).

Plates. We use circular plates of special plexiglass with an outer and inner diame-ter of 13.3 and 12.0 cm, respectively (Fig. 2). These plates have an absolutely plane bottom and can be piled up on each other so that the bottom of one dish can serve as the lid of the underlying dish to prevent the fibrin from drying during incubation.

Preparation of the plates. A fibrin film is obtained by mixing in the plate, 0.3 ml of thrombin with 28.0 ml 0.15% fibrinogen. To secure rapid and homogeneous inter-mixture of the solutions it is advisable first to deposit the above amount of thrombin on the plate and thereafter the fibrinogen solution with the use of a pipette with a large distal opening so that it can be emptied in a few seconds. The plate is after-wards gently tilted to secure proper intermixture of the thrombin and fibrinogen and then left in a perfectly horizontal position for 30 min, during which a fibrin film approximately 0.25 cm thick is formed. *Plasminogen-free plates* are obtained in the same way using plasminogen-free thrombin and fibrinogen; alternatively, plasmino-gen can be destroyed by heating according to LASSEN (1952). According to the method of LASSEN, plasminogen-rich fibrin plates are incubated in a thermostat at 85° C for 45 min. An inconvenience of this procedure is the denaturation of the fibrin molecule.

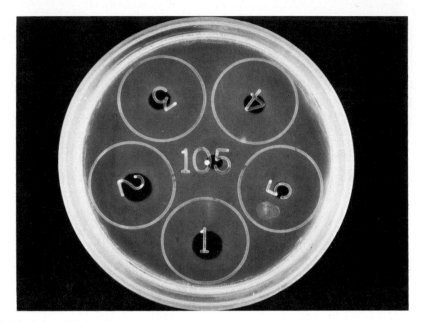

Fig. 2. Plexiglass dish for fibrin plate method

Testing procedure and reading of the results. Undiluted citrated plasma and resuspended euglobulin precipitate (see above) from plasma are used as test solutions for the assay of patients. It is very important that the plasma samples under examination be placed on the plates within at most 30 min of collection of the blood sample, because the activator is labile. The sample should not be frozen, because freezing and thawing leads to a marked loss of activity. The solution to be tested is deposited on the fibrin film in aliquots of 0.03 ml in triplicate. A 0.1–0.2 ml pipette or, more suitably, a constriction pipette is used. Each of our plates has a code number engraved on the bottom and five rings (numbered 1–5) within which the drops of the test solution are to be deposited (Fig. 2). Thereafter, the plates are carefully transferred to a thermostat with horizontal shelves and kept there at 37° C for 18 h. The plates are then examined and the areas of the lysed zones are noted. We measure two perpendicular main diameters, multiply them and express the areas of lysis in mm^2.

To check the sensitivity of the plates and to ascertain whether determinations made on different days are comparable, a standard preparation is tested on the plates every day. The standard preparation may consist of urokinase. Urokinase solutions with 25, 12.5, 6.75, 3.13, 1.57 Ploug U/ml are placed on the plates in the same way as the other samples.

Normal blood values (52 volunteers of both sexes, aged 20–53):

Plasminogen-rich plates (unheated plates). *Citrated plasma:* The activity varied between 10–40 mm^2 (95% confidence interval 3–12 mm^2). *Euglobulin precipitate:* The activity varied between 40–140 mm^2 (95% confidence interval 60–81 mm^2).

Plasminogen-free (or heated) plates. Normally plasminogen-free plates show no activity.

The precision of the fibrin plate method is high. The standard deviation is 13% for values above 50 mm^2 (ROBERTSON et al., 1972b). The detection limit is extremely low, e.g., 0.3 ng x 10^{-14} mol of trypsin can be detected (HAVERKATE and BRAKMAN, 1975).

Judging from our experience, the fibrin plate method is an accurate, reproducible, and sensitive method for the assay of plasminogen activator activity and of plasmin activity. It is useful both in routine clinical work and in basic research. A disadvantage is the long incubation time before results are available.

V. Determination of Fibrin/Fibrinogen Degradation Products (FDP)

Most methods available for determining FDP have an immunologic basis. If an antiserum against fibrinogen is used, the determination will include not only all FDP with antigenic sites in common with that of fibrinogen, i.e., high molecular weight degradation products (HMWDP or X- and Y-products) and D- and E-products, but also fibrinogen. FDP must therefore be measured in serum to avoid the influence of undigested fibrinogen. FDP are retained in the clot (NILÉHN, 1967), for which reason the serum values are lower than those in circulating blood. It has been shown (ARNESEN et al., 1973) that lowering of the pH to 6.3 will result in a higher FDP value.

In all FDP methods it is important to add thrombin to the blood to make sure that coagulation has been complete and all fibrinogen has been removed.

It is also important that the blood be collected in tubes containing an inhibitor of fibrinolysis such as EACA, AMCA, or Trasylol. Otherwise plasminogen in the samples may be activated, with too high a value as a result.

The methods most widely used are:

1. Tanned Red Cell Hemagglutination Inhibition Immunoassay (TRCHII)

This method was introduced by MERSKEY (MERSKEY et al., 1966). The serum to be tested is incubated with a highly diluted antifibrinogen serum. Afterwards fibrinogen-coated red blood cells (0-blood/cells) are added (MERSKEY et al., 1971). The degree of inhibition of aggregation is a measure of the amount of FDP. Normal citrated plasma with a known fibrinogen content is used as a standard. The method has been automated (MERSKEY et al., 1972). It measures concentrations down to about 0.5 μg/ml. The method is sensitive and fairly quick (2–6 h). It does not measure E-products, and it is not very sensitive to D-products, especially if the D-products are the only antigen (RAYNER et al., 1969; BOUMA, 1971).

For detailed description of the manual method the reader is referred to MERSKEY et al. (1969) and for the Auto-Analyzer assay to MERSKEY et al. (1972).

2. Latex Agglutination Tests

Both direct and indirect latex agglutination assays have been described.

In the *direct latex agglutination test* the latex particles are coated with γ-globulin isolated from antifibrinogen serum (MELLIGER, 1970) or with a mixture of antibodies to D- and E-products (Thrombo-Wellcotest) (HULME and PITCHER, 1973).

Serum or urine + antifibrinogen
incubation 5 min

0.1 ml of serum antifibrinogen mixture
+ 0.1 ml fibrinogen - coated latex

Sample rocked for 2 min

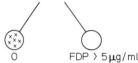

O   FDP ⟩ 5 μg/ml

Fig. 3. Agglutination-inhibition assay of FDP

The Thrombo-Wellcotest has been shown to be very sensitive to later fragments (CASH et al., 1973; DONATI et al., 1973), while the reactivity to clottable fibrinogen derivatives and HMWDP is relatively poor. The method measures fibrinogen down to 2–5 μg/ml.

An *indirect latex agglutination inhibition assay has* been described by ALLINGTON (1971), DONATI et al. (1973), and SVANBERG et al. (1974). In this method the latex particles are coated with fibrinogen. The serum or urine samples are incubated with antifibrinogen serum. Any FDP in the sample are neutralized by the antiserum, and addition of fibrinogen-coated latex particles is not followed by any agglutination. *Performance of indirect latex agglutination inhibition assay.* The reagents (fibrinogen-coated latex suspension, antifibrinogen serum, positive and negative control sera) are lyophilized and supplied in a kit (Splitax) manufactured by AB Kabi (Stockholm, Sweden). Before use the reagents are reconstituted in 1 ml of distilled water. The antifibrinogen serum concentration is adjusted to the fibrinogen-coated latex suspension in the same kit in such a way as to inhibit agglutination at a level of 10 μg/ml of FDP.

Serum or urine, 0.1 ml, is incubated with 0.1 ml antifibrinogen serum. After incubation of the mixture at room temperature for 4 min, 0.1 ml of it is placed on a black glass plate and 0.1 ml of the fibrinogen-coated latex suspension is added. The glass plate is then rocked gently for 2 min, after which it is inspected for agglutination. Control sera should be tested simultaneously in order to facilitate evaluation of the samples.

Agglutination is inhibited if the samples contain > 10 μg FDP/ml (Fig. 3).

The sensitivity of the test can be adjusted by changing the concentration of the antifibrinogen serum used.

The latex agglutination inhibition assay determines mainly the HMWDP and is less sensitive to the fragments D and E (DONATI et al., 1973).

3. Immunochemical Method According to NILÉHN (1967)

Principle. This method is based on the rocket method of LAURELL (1966), according to which a glass plate is covered with agarose gel containing specific antibodies against D-product. The samples are applied in the gel and on high voltage electrophoresis they are forced into the gel. Rocket-shaped precipitates form and their heights are proportional to the amount of antigen in the sample.

Reagents

1. *Barbital buffer.* 0.07 M, pH 8.6, containing 2 mM calcium lactate.

2. *Agarose solution.* 1.0 g of agarose (Miles-Seravac, Berks, England) is dissolved in 100 ml of barbital buffer and heated to 100° C. When the solution is quite clear and homogeneous, it is cooled to 45–48° C in a thermostatically controlled water bath.

3. *Washing fluid.* Acetic acid-methanol-water in proportions 1:5:5.

4. Amido black. 1.0 g amido black is dissolved in 500 ml of gently heated (50–60° C) washing fluid. This is followed by filtration.

5. 0.9% NaCl.

6. ε-aminocaproic acid (EACA) in substance supplied by AB Kabi (Epsikapron).

7. Tris buffer 0.07 M pH 7.8.

8. High molecular weight degradation products (HMWDP). These products are prepared by allowing human plasmin (25 CTA U plasmin/100 ml 1% human fibrinogen solution) to digest human fibrinogen for 20 min at 37° C, after which they are separated on DEAE-cellulose.

The fractions with the highest extinction values are pooled and concentrated in collodium membrane. The protein content is determined with Kjeldahl's method, after which the solution is diluted with Tris buffer to a concentration of 1.0 g/100 ml protein.

Human fibrinogen can be used as standard instead of HMWDP.

9. Antiserum against the D-product is obtained by immunizing rabbits with D-product, which is prepared by allowing human plasmin (25 CTA U/100 ml 1% fibrinogen solution) to digest human fibrinogen for 8 h at room temperature. The mixture is then fractionated on DEAE-cellulose (phosphate buffer; 750 ml 0.01 M and 600 ml 0.03 M KH_2PO_4). The highest peak is produced by D-product and the lowest and last by E-product. The fractions containing D-product are pooled and concentrated. A solution of D-product containing 10–15 mg protein/ml is emulsified with an equal volume of Freund's complete adjuvant and injected s.c. into rabbits weighing 2.5–3.0 kg. Of this mixture, each rabbit is given two injections à 4 ml at an interval of 3 weeks. The antiserum is adsorbed with normal serum and tested for specificity to D-product and high molecular weight degradation products.

Also commercially available antiserum to human fibrinogen can be used.

10. Antiserum to the E-product is obtained by immunizing rabbits with E-product, prepared by digesting human fibrinogen by human plasmin (25 CTA U/ml 1% fibrinogen solution) for 8 h. The fibrinogen digest is then heated (56° C for 30 min) to denature the D-product. The next step consists of ion exchange chromatography on DEAE-cellulose in phosphate buffer, 750 ml 0.01 M, and 600 ml 0.03 M KH_2PO_4. The fractions containing the E-product are pooled and concentrated.

Apparatus

    1. Glass plates $1.0 \times 205 \times 110$ mm
    2. Plastic frames 1.0 and 1.5 mm thick
    3. Electrophoresis apparatus of plexiglass (according to JOHANSSON, 1972)
    4. Transformer. Voltage aggregate (150—350 V max. 600 mA)
    5. Filter paper Whatman No. 3

6. Blotting paper

7. Paper clips (width 6.5 cm) "Bulldog"

8. Two punches with an outer diameter of 3.0 and 4.0 mm, respectively, with a ground inner wall

Sampling. Venous blood is collected in tubes containing EACA in substance (about 25 mg/3 ml blood) and thrombin (30 NIH U to 3 ml blood). The sample is then allowed to stand for 2 h at room temperature and then centrifuged for 20 min at 2000 g, after which the serum is pipetted off and frozen until used.

Performance. Agarose plates are obtained by pouring fluid 1% agarose (50–60° C) containing antiserum against D-product (usually in a concentration of 1:100) into the space between two glass plates held together with a 1.0-mm-thick triangular plastic frame and gripped by clips. After 15 min at +4° C the covering glass plate is removed by pressing it in over a 2.0-mm-thick glass plate, whose edge holds back the bottom plate and the frame. Holes containing 5 µl are punched 7.5 mm apart. The serum or urine samples (5 µl) are then deposited in the holes as soon as possible and a standard solution of high molecular weight degradation products (HMWDP) or human fibrinogen in concentrations of 200 µg/ml, 100 µg/ml, 50 µg/ml, 25 µg/ml, and 12.5 µg/ml in Tris buffer (pH 7.8) are used. The antibody concentration in the gel must be checked for each new batch of antiserum and should be such that the peaks of the standard solution in the middle (50 µg/ml) are 2–3 cm high.

The glass plate is then placed on the cooled electrophoresis unit and connected to the firm agarose bridges (1.5%) or paper bridges, which are placed in the electrode vessels by means of 1.5% agarose gel strips or wet paper strips. Electrophoresis (20 V/cm) is run for 5 h.

Afterwards the plate is taken off, and the plastic frame is removed and placed overnight in 0.9% NaCl. The following day the gel is covered with a thin filter paper moistened with water and dried by covering it with several layers of soft paper and placing it in front of a hot-air fan. The plate is stained in amido black and afterwards the plate is decolorized in washing fluid (acetic acid-methanol-water 1:5:5).

Calculation. The peak heights of the samples are measured and the amount of antigen is calculated by comparison with the standard.

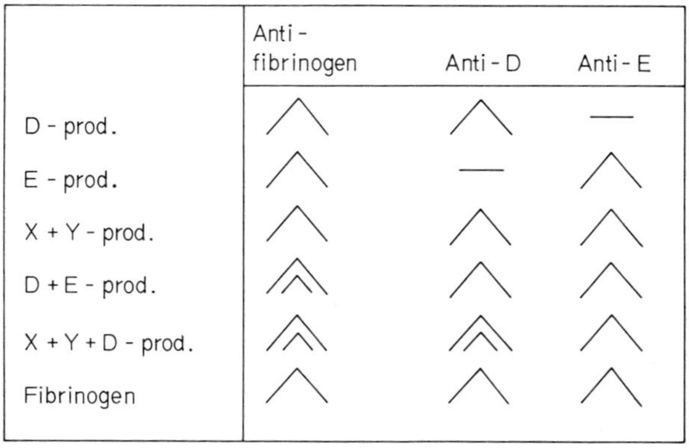

Fig. 4. Different types of FDP and fibrinogen producing single or double peaks against anti-fibrinogen, anti-D-fraction, and anti-E-fraction

The method has been modified and can now *type FDP in serum and urine* (BOUMA et al., 1971). Agarose plates containing antifibrinogen serum, anti-D serum, or anti-E serum, respectively, are prepared. Fibrinogen is used as standard for all the plates. The appearance of single or double peaks produced with the different antisera reveals the types of FDP, and their concentrations can be measured. In doubtful cases the type can be decided by addition of fibrinogen, HMWDP, and D- or E-products, respectively, to the sample (Fig. 4). Addition of a substance identical with that already present will increase the height of the peak. If the substance added is not identical, it will produce a separate peak.

Normally, no FDP can be demonstrated in serum or urine with this method, which determines FDP down to a level of 5 µg/ml. Increased amounts of FDP in serum occur in conditions associated with degradation of fibrin/fibrinogen.

The conditions most often associated with an increase in FDP are as follows:

a) Malignant Diseases

FDP were found in 60% of 346 patients with various forms of cancer in different stages (HEDNER and NILSSON, 1971; CARLSSON, 1973) and were found to vary in concentration with the vascular involvement of the tumour (CARLSSON and LINELL, 1973). Of patients with ovarian carcinoma, 82% were found to have FDP in the serum (ÅSTEDT et al., 1971b). No FDP were found in patients with benign ovarian tumors. After successful surgery and radiotherapy the FDP disappeared, but reappeared in association with recurrences of the tumor.

b) Renal Diseases

FDP in serum have been found to occur most often in *acute renal failure* (WARDLE and TAYLOR, 1968; HEDNER and NILSSON, 1971). The FDP concentration varies with the activity of the disease (BRAUN and MERRILL, 1268; LARSSON et al., 1971a, b; CLARKSON et al., 1971) and is therefore a valuable indicator of the course of the disease and the effect of therapy (STIEHM et al., 1971; LARSSON et al., 1971b). In *chronic uremia* FDP are more often demonstrable in urine than in serum (RAYNER et al., 1969; BRIGGS et al., 1972). In series of 76 patients, FDP were found in the serum in 37% and in unconcentrated urine in 39% (HEDNER and NILSSON, 1971). Here, too, the FDP concentration varied with the activity of the disease.

FDP have been demonstrated predominantly in the proliferative types of glomerulonephritis (CLARKSON et al., 1971; HEDNER et al., 1974) and have been found to be correlated with the extent of fibrin deposits in the kidney (STIEHM and TRYGSTAD, 1969; CLARKSON et al., 1971).

FDP in serum as well as in urine are common in patients with *hemolytic-uremic syndrome* (LUKE et al., 1970; KATZ et al., 1971; EKBERG et al., 1974).

After *renal transplantation* FDP occur in the serum in the postoperative course. Urinary FDP are, however, more informative in these cases. The occurrence of FDP in the unconcentrated urine more than 2 weeks after the transplantation is strong evidence of some complication, such as rejection or a disease in the transplant (CARLSSON et al., 1970; EKBERG et al., 1976a).

c) Conditions Associated with Abnormal Proteolysis

In the presence of endothelial damage, substances activating the coagulation system (thromboplastic material) as well as those activating the fibrinolytic system may be released into the circulation. Conditions with severe tissue destruction or endothelial damage such as *septicemia, burns, multiple fractures* are therefore often associated with signs of abnormal proteolysis with secondary degradation of fibrin/fibrinogen. FDP are therefore increased in such conditions (HEDNER and NILSSON, 1971; SKÅNSBERG et al., 1974).

Abnormal proteolysis has also been observed during pregnancy in women with a history of repeated late miscarriages probably due to placental insufficiency. In such women increased amounts of FDP are an early precursor of a complication of pregnancy. Signs of an activated coagulation system with a secondary fibrinolysis predominate in these cases (NILSSON et al., 1975).

Abnormal proteolysis due to other proteolytic enzymes, such as leukocyte proteases, has recently been reported (SCHMIDT et al., 1975). Such proteolysis resulting in degradation of fibrinogen and of certain other coagulation factors (f V, f XIII) has been demonstrated in a patient with a panniculitis of Weber-Christian's type (HENRIKSSON et al., 1975a) and in patients with Henoch-Schönlein's purpura (HENRIKSSON et al., 1975b). As a result of fibrin/fibrinogen degradation the FDP levels found in these patients were high.

4. Radioimmunoassay for Determination of FDP

Radioimmunochemical assays have been widely used in the estimation of minute amounts of various substances. Because of the high sensitivity of such a system to even small differences in structure and conformation of the molecules it is important to define and carefully study the various steps of the assay.

Radioimmunoassay techniques are used for FDP determination for two reasons: (1) to increase the sensitivity for detecting FDP, which is of value in determination of urinary FDP in early glomerulonephritis or for assessing the prognosis of a renal transplant (HEDNER et al., 1974; EKBERG et al., 1976b); and (2) to make it possible to determine FDP as the D- or E-products in plasma without interaction of fibrinogen. This is based on the fact that new antigenic sites are exposed during the breakdown of fibrin/fibrinogen. Such cleavage specific neoantigens are localized in the D-fragment as well as in the E-fragment and are distinct from those of the native D- or E-fragments. These neoantigenic sites are claimed to be present in the intact fibrinogen molecule, in a sterically hindered site, and are exposed after plasmin cleavage (PLOW et al., 1971; PLOW and EDGINGTON, 1972, 1973; CHEN and SHURLEY, 1975). In addition, characteristic differences between the neoantigenic sites present on the fibrinogen cleavage products and those found on the fibrin cleavage fragments have been demonstrated (PLOW and EDGINGTON, 1973). This makes it possible to distinguish between fragments obtained after plasmin degradation of fibrinogen and such obtained from degradation of fibrin. This makes a discrimination between conditions associated with primary fibrinolysis with predominantly fibrinogenolysis and conditions primarily associated with deposition of fibrin with secondary fibrinolysis possible. Fibrinogen degradation products obtained after the action of other proteolytic enzymes can also be distinguished from the plasmin degradation products if antisera against specific neoantigenic sites made available after such degradation, are used (PLOW et al., 1971; PLOW and EDGINGTON 1972; CHEN and SHURLEY, 1975).

Principle. D-product is obtained by plasmin degradation of human fibrinogen and purification on DEAE-cellulose chromatography. The purified D-product is then labeled with ^{125}I by means of the lactoperoxidase method (THORELL and JOHANSSON, 1971), the iodine monochloride technique (MCFARLANE, 1956) or chloramine-T oxidation (HUNTER and GREENWOOD, 1962; MCCONAHEY and DIXON, 1966).

Antiserum against the D-product ist raised in rabbits. Specific antisera against the neoantigenic sites of D-product can be obtained by repeated adsorption of the antiserum against D-product with human fibrinogen.

In the assay the labeled D-fragments are incubated with the antiserum and the sample to be tested. FDP present in the sample compete with the labeled D-products for the antiserum. The antibody-bound antigen is then separated from the free antigen by precipitation by ammonium sulphate on sodium sulphate, adsorption of the free antigen onto insoluble substance, double antibody precipitation or solid phase techniques, in which antibody is coupled to the surface. The bound radioactivity can be assessed from the precipitate or by supernatant counting. Three controls are necessary:

1. Control of *total counts added*. Normal serum is added to the labeled antigen, and the unlabeled antigen and the sample are replaced by buffer.

2. *Precipitation control* to correct for nonspecific precipitation of the labeled antigen. The precipitating antiserum is added to the labeled antigen. The unlabeled antigen and the sample are replaced by buffer.

The values of controls a) and b) should have identical results.

3. Control for *evaluating the integrity of the labeled antigen*. Trichloracetic acid (TCA) is added instead of the antiserum. All proteins are precipitated by the TCA, and the radioactivity of the supernatant is a measure of the unbound radioactivity.

At our laboratory a radioimmunoassay has been used for demonstrating FDP in urine from patients with early glomerulonephritis and in the evaluation of the prognosis of the renal graft (EKBERG et al., 1976b). Urinary FDP from such patients consist mostly of high molecular weight degradation products (HMWDP), but also small amounts of the end products, D- and E-fragments (BOUMA et al., 1971; HEDNER, 1973). To make the method more specific and to avoid interference of various binding properties of the antiserum against the D-product used, all FDP in the urine were broken down to end degradation products and determined as D-products.

Performance. Pretreatment of the urine samples. To 1 ml morning urine are added 0.1 mg plasminogen (AB Kabi, Stockholm, Sweden, 25 CTA U/mg protein) and 100 IU streptokinase (Kabikinase, AB Kabi, Stockholm, Sweden, 250000 IU/ampoule). After incubation for 30 min at 37° C the urine samples are diluted to 1:10 (Tris-HCl buffer 0,05 M, pH 7.5 containing 2.5 g/l of bovine albumin from Armour Pharmaceutical Co., Eastborne, England, and 1.0 g/l of sodium azide = assay buffer).

To 200 µl of the pretreated urine or standard D-product (250, 125, 62.5, 31.2, 15.6, 7.8, 3.9, and 1.9 µg/l) are added: 200 µl labeled D-product (0.2 mg/200 µl assay buffer) and 200 µl antiserum against D-product.

Controls a) and b) are run simultaneously. All samples are set up in triplicate. The samples are thoroughly mixed in a vibra mixer and incubated over night at +4°C. The antibody-bound and free portion of labeled D-product are then separated by the double antibody technique. According to this technique, 50 µl goat antirabbit gamma globulin serum and 50 µl normal rabbit serum in dil 1:10 are added to the samples and after incubation for 1 h the tubes are centrifuged at 2000 g for 15 min. The supernatants are discarded and the radioactivity of the precipitate is measured.

The titer of the *antiserum* (prepared according to Nilehn, 1967) is determined by adding 0.2 ng labeled D-product in 200 µl assay buffer (Tris-HCl-buffer containing bovine albumin and sodium azide) to 200 µl antiserum in dilutions ranging from 1:1000 to 1:2000000. After incubation at +4° C for 24 h the antibody-bound and free portion of the labeled D-product are separated as described above. The dilution at which 200 µl binds 50% of the added labeled D-product is given as the titer of the antiserum (1:500000 for our anti-D-serum). For our purpose (covering a concentration interval up to about 250 ng/ml) a dilution of this antiserum of 1:250000 was found to be optimal.

It is important to ascertain the specificity of the antiserum used. Different fibrinogen-related substances, such as the different types of FDP, react in a different way with antiserum because of their variable immunoreactivity. In our system all the urinary FDP are broken down to end degradation products and are determined as D-products against an antiserum raised against purified products derived from fibrinogen. This increased the specificity of the test. It must be checked that the antiserum does not cross-react with E-products.

Calculation and evaluation of the result. The results are expressed in ng FDP/mg creatinine. Normal range: 13–85 ng/mg creatinine. Increased values were found in early glomerulonephritis as well as in chronic rejection of renal grafts.

Gross hematuria will give artificially high levels. Microscopic hematuria does not influence the values.

B. Fibrinolytic Response to Stimuli, With Special Reference to Venous Occlusion Test

In order to measure the fibrinolytic capacity of a person, different stimuli have been used, such as exercise, injection of nicotinic acid, epinephrine, vasopresssin, and venous occlusion of the limbs, known to enhance the release of plasminogen activators into the bloodstream. It has been found that a certain group of individuals fail to release, or release only very small amounts of plasminogen activator on stimulation with a standardized stimulus (see Nilsson, 1975; Cash, 1975a, b; Åberg and Nilsson, 1975). These individuals have been called poor responders.

As for *nicotinic acid*, the high percentage of poor responders among volunteers and the long period of nonresponsiveness after such an injection makes the use of nicotinic acid i.v. unsuitable as a routine method for assessing the fibrinolytic capacity (Robertson, 1971).

Exercise and adrenaline have been used particularly by Cash and his group for elucidating the fibrinolytic response (Cash and Allan, 1967; Cash and Woodfield, 1967; Cash and McGill, 1969; Cash et al., 1970). The stimuli have been standardized, and reproducible results have been obtained. There is a highly significant positive correlation between the response to exercise and to adrenaline i.v. It is possible to isolate a group of constantly poor responders. In several clinical conditions, however, it is not possible to use exercise or adrenaline. *Venous occlusion* of the limbs is another method for measuring the fibrinolytic response or capacity. The findings of NILSSON and PANDOLFI (1970) have produced evidence that in venous stasis increased blood fibrinolysis is due to the release of plasminogen activators from the vessel wall. At the Coagulation Laboratory in Malmö we have for several years elaborated a standardized method for estimating the fibrinolytic capacity in a given person, as judged from the local response of the fibrinolytic activity to venous occlusion of the limbs. It is a rather simple method and without potential side-effects, which makes it suitable for routine clinical practice. We have now used the method for several years.

Venous Occlusion Test

Variables. Different variables capable of influencing the results have been investigated (ROBERTSON et al., 1972a, b, c). In an investigation to ascertain whether the arms or the legs are the more suitable for studying the fibrinolytic response to venous occlusion, it was found that the fibrinolytic activity of the blood obtained from the occluded arm was 3–4 times higher than that from the occluded leg. Venous occlusion was induced by application of a sphygmomanometer cuff, wrapped around the upper arm or the thigh for 20 min and inflated to a level midway between the systolic and diastolic pressure. The correlation between the local fibrinolytic activity induced by venous occlusion of the upper limbs varied closely with that of the legs. For this reason it is, as a rule, sufficient, especially in routine clinical work, to examine only the arms, where the response is stronger and the technique simpler.

The local fibrinolytic response in the arms varies with the occlusive pressure being highest with a pressure between the systolic and diastolic blood pressure and with the site of venous puncture blood from an antecubital vein showing the highest activity, and with duration of occlusion, the activity increasing significantly for up to 25 min. There is no systematic difference in the response of the fibrinolytic activity with side after venous occlusion. In the individual case, however, the difference with side can be rather large. The mean fibrinolytic activity of both arms is therefore a better measure of an individual's fibrinolytic capacity. Reassay after an interval of 1 day shows no significant change in normal individuals in the response of the fibrinolytic activity. Repeated assays on the same day may give falling values.

In order to obtain reproducible results with the venous occlusion test it must be performed by a strictly standardized technique.

Performance. 1. The examination is carried out with the person supine on the examination table. The weight and length of the patient should be recorded. Blood samples (5 ml citrated blood) are drawn from an antecubital vein before venous occlusion. These blood samples should be taken either without or with the help of a tourniquet that had been applied for less than 1 min.

2. Sphygmomanometer cuffs are wrapped around the upper arms and inflated to a pressure midway between the systolic and diastolic blood pressure for 20 min. Blood samples (5 ml citrated blood) are collected from an antecubital vein before deflating the cuffs.

3. The blood samples are immediately centrifuged at 2000 g for 20 min. The plasma is sucked off with a siliconized drop-pipette and transferred to plastic tubes.

The plasma is then immediately (no freezing or storage at room temperature) prepared for determination of the fibrinolytic activity on fibrin plates. It has proved sufficient to measure the fibrinolytic activity of resuspended euglobulin precipitate on unheated fibrin plates. A highly significant correlation has thus been found between the values noted for citrated plasma and resuspended euglobulin precipitate. The fibrinolytic activity of citrated plasma after venous occlusion is about two-thirds that of resuspended euglobulin precipitate. Bovine or human plasminogen-rich fibrinogen can be used for preparation of the fibrin plates (see above under fibrin plates).

4. The fibrinolytic capacity of an individual is expressed as the mean fibrinolytic activity in the blood obtained after venous occlusion of both arms at the same time.

5. Repeated investigations of the same subject are desirable to obtain more representative values.

Normal values. The lower limit of the normal range of the fibrinolytic activity after venous occlusion depends on the type of fibrinogen used for preparation of the fibrin plates. Each laboratory must determine its own normal range. In Malmö the following normal levels have been found: *Bovine fibrin plates* (bovine fibrinogen grade A, AB Kabi). The control material consisted of 118 volunteers of both sexes (aged 18—50). The percentile values of the fibrinolytic activity in resuspended euglobulin precipitate after venous occlusion of the arms, i.e., (left arm + right arm)/2, were: 5% value 158 mm^2 (95% confidence interval 88—169 mm^2). 10% value 173 mm^2 (95% confidence interval 158—199 mm^2). *Human fibrin plates* (human fibrinogen AB Kabi). The control material consisted of 52 volunteers of both sexes (aged 20—53) 5% value 345 mm^2 (95% confidence interval 313–377 mm^2).

Poor responders. The fibrinolytic capacity, as estimated from the effect of venous occlusion of the arms, has been studied in various conditions.

Patients with recurrent venous thrombosis show a low response to venous occlusion of the arms in 38% (ISACSON and NILSSON, 1972; NILSSON, 1977). During pregnancy the response to venous occlusion decreases markedly (ÅSTEDT et al., 1970).

In patients with Takayasu's disease the fibrinolytic response to venous occlusion is poor or absent (ISACSON et al., 1971).

In diabetics the mean fibrinolytic response to venous occlusion is significantly lower than in nondiabetics, and the frequency of poor responders is about 6 times as high as in nondiabetics (ALMÉR and NILSSON, 1975).

Obese patients have a significantly lower mean fibrinolytic response to venous occlusion than nonobese subjects (ALMÉR and NILSSON, 1975).

Patients with primary carbohydrate-induced hypertriglyceridemia have been found to have impaired response to venous occlusion (SPÖTTL et al., 1969).

C. The Fibrin Slide Method (Todd's Method)

This histochemical film technique for demonstrating fibrinolytic activity in tissue was described by TODD in 1959. With this method it was possible to demonstrate the site of strong fibrinolytic (plasminogen activator) activity in the endothelium of certain blood vessels. Investigation of fetal and diseased tissues (see PANDOLFI, 1972) revealed a wide variation in the distribution and strength of fibrinolytic activity and suggested different functions of plasminogen activator in health and in disease. It was

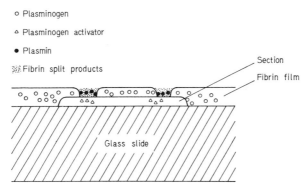

Fig. 5. Principle of histochemical method for determination of plasminogen activator content of tissue slices

mainly this method that made it possible to detect an association between a low fibrinolytic activity of the vessel wall and venous thrombosis (ISACSON and NILSSON, 1972), an observation lending support to the assumed antithrombotic role played by the fibrinolytic system.

Principle. The principle of the method is shown in Figure 5. A frozen section of tissue is incubated in contact with a fibrin film, rich in plasminogen. During incubation the plasminogen activators present in the section transform the plasminogen contained in the adjacent fibrin into plasmin with consequent focal lysis. Staining reveals fibrinolysis as white gaps in the fibrin film at the site of active structures of the section. By using parallel tests with fibrinogen not contaminated with plasminogen it is possible to exclude the possibility of lysis caused by agents other than activators of plasminogen.

Materials

Tissues. Tissue plasminogen activator is a very stable enzyme and no observable decrease in activity occurs within about 24 h after death. Cadaveric material can therefore be used. The specimens are quickly frozen with conventional methods for histochemistry. Sections are cut on a cryostat microtome. The optimal thickness of the sections is 6–8 μ (PANDOLFI et al., 1972). The slides can be stored up to 6 days at −20° C without any appreciable loss of fibrinolytic activity.

Biopsy specimen of vessel. For investigation of the plasminogen activator activity in *vein walls* a biopsy specimen is obtained from the distal part of a hand vein, a 0.5–1.0-cm-long segment, under local anesthesia (0.5% Carbocain). The specimen is quickly frozen. For investigation of *arteries* a segment of the temporal artery is excised under local anesthesia.

Fibrinogen. Plasminogen-rich human or bovine fibrinogen can be used. Phosphate buffer (i.e., Sörensen's phosphate buffer, pH 7.8 and ionic strength 0.15), prepared as indicated in Geigy's Scientific Tables 197 is recommended for dilution. Phosphate buffer increases the sensitivity of the fibrin to fibrinolytic activators and makes it especially useful for the fibrin slide technique, in which a very high sensitivity of the substrate is desirable. We generally use bovine fibrinogen prepared according to Brakman's modification (1967) of Astrup and Müllertz (1952) double ammonium sulphate precipitation method. The fibrinogen concentration may vary between 0.75 to 2.0% without any appreciable effect on the results; we generally use 1.0%.

Plasminogen-free fibrinogen can be obtained by absorbing plasminogen with bentonite according to Brakman (1965) or by precipitating it with its antibody according to Ohlsson (1969). A suitable commercially available plasminogen-free fibrinogen is that produced by Poviet (Poviet Produkten, Oss, Holland).

Thrombin. A suitable thrombin preparation is Topostasin Roche 20 NIH units/ml unbuffered 0.15 M NaCl. Plasminogen-free thrombin must be used for clotting plasminogen-free fibrinogen. A suitable commercially available preparation is that produced by Leo, Copenhagen.

Fibrin film. A good fibrin film can be obtained by mixing 60 μl of fibrinogen solution with 10 μl of thrombin and spreading the mixture over an area of 10 cm². In this way a fibrin film 70 μm thick is obtained. The thickness of the film can be increased to more than 0.2 mm. The film is usually prepared on the surface of the section. In doing so it is advisable to let the slide dry at room temperature for some minutes in order to facilitate the adhesion of the section to the glass. Alternatively, the section can be collected on a previously prepared fibrin film, but may then sometimes be difficult to collect from the blade.

Incubation temperature. A temperature of + 37° C is advisable. Lower temperatures can also be used, but then the incubation period must be extended. The distribution of the fibrinolytic activator does not vary with the incubation temperature.

Evaluation of the strength of the fibrinolytic activity. Like other histochemical techniques, the fibrin slide method can identify the structures containing the enzyme, but it is less useful for comparing the enzymic activity of different specimens. Kwaan and Astrup's (1967) introduction of the "focal lysis time" (shortest incubation time to produce lysis) as a measure of the activity implied a praiseworthy advance. We (Pandolfi et al., 1972) have tried to find a more sensitive and precise method of quantitation by assessing the strength of the fibrinolytic activity not only on the basis of the focal lysis time, but also of the size and shape of lytic areas. We prepared a series of slides for each specimen and incubated them for progressively increasing lengths of time. To each slide were then allotted 1 point for small punctate area of lysis in the majority of the sections, 2 points for larger, confluent areas of lysis, and 3 for massive fibrin digestion; 1.5 and 2.5 points were allotted for intermediate degrees of lysis, 1–2 and 2–3, respectively. The sum of the points scored by each set of slides was taken as a direct measure of the fibrinolytic activity of the specimen. This assay method has proved useful in comparison of the fibrinolytic activity of human veins of arms and legs in healthy persons and patients with thrombosis (Pandolfi et al., 1967, 1968, 1969). The same principle, but modified, has been used by other authors to assess the fibrinolytic activity of veins (Constantini et al., 1969a, b) and of the prostate (Kester, 1969).

In order to assess the precision of the method one examiner studied 496 fibrin slides of superficial limb veins on two occasions, the second 3 months after the first: 11.8% of the evaluations varied by half a grade, 3.2% by a whole grade, and only 0.006% by one grade and a half. The accuracy of the method cannot be calculated owing to lack of reference, in this case cells with a known amount of enzyme. Since the strength of the fibrinolytic activity is expressed by a sum of scores based on an arbitrary scale, the comparison of the activity of different groups of specimens requires the use of a rank-sum test.

Normal values for vein walls. The normal range of plasminogen activator activity depends upon the type of fibrinogen used for preparation of the fibrin plates. Each laboratory must establish its normal range. In Malmö the following normal levels have been found with use of bovine fibrinogen prepared according to BRAKMAN (1967). The control material consisted of 60 healthy volunteers, 31 women, and 29 men, with an average age of 37.0 years (range 17–70 years). Normal range was 6.0–10.0 arbitrary units. Median value 7.5.

In arm veins the plasminogen activator activity is 3–4 times higher than that in leg veins. A close correlation between the activator content of the veins and arteries has been found in diabetics (ALMÉR et al., 1975).

Abnormal values in veins. A significantly decreased activator content has been found in 159 of 289 patients with recurrent idiopathic venous thrombosis (ISACSON and NILSSON, 1972; NILSSON, 1977).

In pregnancy the plasminogen activator in the vein walls is moderately decreased (ÅSTEDT et al., 1970). The plasminogen activator activity of the vessel walls is significantly more often low in diabetics than in nondiabetics (ALMÉR and NILSSON, 1975). The plasminogen activator activity of the vessel walls is significantly more often low in obese than in nonobese subjects (ALMÉR and JANZON, 1975).

D. Release of Fibrinolytic Agents from Tissue Cultures ("Culture with Clot" Method)

Observation of fibrinolytic activity in tissue cultures prompted the first studies on tissue fibrinolysis (FISCHER, 1925; SANTESSON, 1935). In recent years attention has again been focused on the fibrinolytic properties on tissue culture as a tool for studying the mechanism of release of fibrinolytic agents from the cells. A method has recently been devised in which organ explants are cultured in the presence of standard clots (ÅSTEDT et al., 1971a). The advantage of this method is that fibrinolytic activators can exert their clot-dissolving action as soon as they are released into the medium, i.e., before they are inactivated (ÅSTEDT and PANDOLFI, 1972). The amount of fibrinolytic agents released is indirectly assessed by immunochemically assaying the fibrin degradation products (FDP) accumulating in the culture medium. In this way the method is less sensitive to fluctuation in the rate of release of fibrinolytic agents; the presence of substrates (plasminogen and plasmin) will limit the action of inhibitory substances possibly released together with the activators. The principle of the method is illustrated in Figure 6. PANDOLFI et al. (1974) have recently described a modification of the method in which the degree of fibrinolysis can be directly observed and determination of FDP is therefore unnecessary.

Tissues. Preparation of the culture system. Any human or animal tissue can be used. Since cultures have to be made in chemically defined media—the presence of serum interferes with fibrinolysis—embryonic and other less differentiated tissues, such as neoplastic tissue, are most suitable.

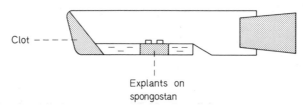

Fig. 6. Diagram of culture system

Tissue fragments are washed in the culture medium selected—we use Parker 199 (SBL, Stockholm) culture medium—and divided into pieces about 1 mm across. These explants are then placed on slices of gel foam (Spongostan, Ferrosan, Malmö), as a rule, three explants per slice. The slices of gel foam with the explants are placed in Leighton tubes (two slices in each tube) containing a clot formed by previous deposition in the tube of 1 ml 1% human fibrinogen (AB Kabi, Stockholm) and 0.04 ml thrombin (Topostasin Roche, 75 NIH U/ml) in unbuffered saline. One ml of the culture medium, Parker 199, is then added. Care is taken to avoid contact between the sponge slices and the standard clot. As controls, gel foam slices without explants are placed in similarly prepared Leighton tubes.

Determination of fibrin degradation products (FDP). During culture the fibrin of the clot undergoes progressive dissolution. After some days of culture the lysed areas become macroscopically visible as a notch in the fibrin clot at the site of contact with the culture medium. The amount of fibrin dissolved is calculated from the concentration of FDP in the culture medium. For this purpose small aliquots of culture medium are collected every 12 or 24 h with a capillary pipette. FDP are determined by the immunochemical method of Niléhn (1967) described above.

Control of culture survival and sterility. Explants are fixed in Bouin's solution and examined with conventional histologic methods. In doubtful cases the sterility of the cultures must be checked by culture for bacteria.

Modification—Direct observation of fibrinolytic activity. Leighton tubes without preformed fibrin clots are used. The procedure is the same as that described above but with the exception that a 4-cm-long glass tube (outer diameter 3 mm, inner 1.5 mm) open at one end is inserted in the Leighton tube containing a mixture of 1% human plasminogen-rich fibrinogen (AB Kabi) and a minimal amount of bovine thrombin (Topostasin Roche, 7.5 NIH U/ml 0.15 M NaCl) resulting in a cylinder of fibrin in the tube. During culture of active tissues there, the fibrin cylinder undergoes progressive dissolution starting from the open end of the glass tube (Fig. 7). The lysed zone can be measured under a dissecting microscope with an ordinary graduated ruler. The lysis measured in this way varies linearly with the amount of FDP in the medium.

Comments. The fibrin clot in the system undergoes spontaneous dissolution on the 4th day of culture. It is therefore advisable to run control systems without tissue explants. Very active tissue cultures are kidney (probably mainly because of the production of urokinase), meninges, lung, etc., while low or nonactive cultures are those of spleen, placenta, and other tissues known to be fibrinolytically inactive by the fibrin slide method.

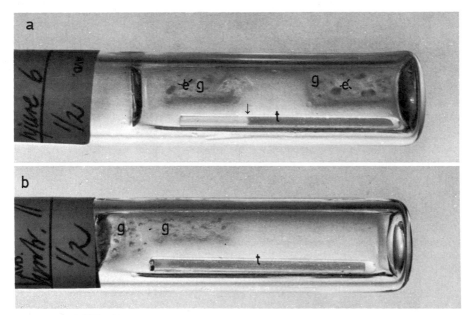

Fig. 7. Culture system. Two Leighton tubes photographed from above. In *a* (culture of kidney) slices of gel foam *(g)* support kidney explants *(e)*. Two-thirds of fibrin contained in glass tube *(t)* has been digested. *Arrow* points to limit between medium filling tube and undigested fibrin. In *b* (control, i.e., only slices of gel foam) no lysis has occurred and glass tube is completely filled with undigested fibrin.

The method can be used for assay of fibrinolytic inhibitors released by such tissues as placenta, decidua, or thymus. In the study of such tissues a fibrinolytic agent (urokinase, plasmin) is added to the culture medium of the system and the inhibitory effect of the added tissue is measured.

Death of the explants results in arrest of the lysis.

References

Åberg,M., Nilsson,I.M.: Fibrinolytic response to venous occlusion and vasopressin in health and thrombotic disease. In: Davidson,I.F., Samama,M.M., Desnoyers,P.C. (Eds.): Progress in chemical fibrinolysis and thrombolysis, pp. 121—129. New York: Raven Press 1975

Åstedt,B., Isacson,S., Nilsson,I.M., Pandolfi,M.: Fibrinolytic activity of veins during pregnancy. Acta obstet. gynec. scand. **49**, 171—173 (1970)

Åstedt,B., Pandolfi,M.: On release and synthesis of fibrinolytic activators in human organ culture. Rev. Europ. Etud. clin. Biol. **17**, 261—267 (1972)

Åstedt,B., Pandolfi,M., Nilsson,I.M.: Quantitation of fibrinolytic agents released in tissue culture. Experientia (Basel) **27**, 358—359 (1971a)

Åstedt,B., Svanberg,L., Nilsson,I.M.: Fibrin degradation products and ovarian tumours. Brit. med. J. **1971 IV**b, 458—459 (1971b)

Albrechtsen,O.K.: Fibrinolytic activity in the organism. Acta physiol. scand. **47**, Suppl. 165 (1959)

Allington,M.J.: Detection of fibrin(ogen) degradation products by a latex clumping method. Scand. J. Haemat. Suppl. **13**, 115—119 (1971)

Almér,L.-O., Janzon,L.: Low vascular fibrinolytic activity in obesity. Thrombos. Res. **6**, 171—175 (1975)

Almér,L.-O., Nilsson,I.M.: On fibrinolysis in diabetes mellitus. Acta med. scand. **198**, 101—106 (1975)

Almér,L.-O., Pandolfi,M., Åberg,M.: The plasminogen activator activity of arteries and veins in diabetes mellitus. Thrombos. Res. **6**, 177—182 (1975)

Aoki,N., Kaulla,K.N., von: The extraction of vascular plasminogen activator from human cadavers and a description of some of its properties. Amer. J. clin. Path. **55**, 171—179 (1971a)

Aoki,N., Kaulla,K.N., von: Dissimilarity of human vascular plasminogen activator and human urokinase. J. Lab. clin. Med. **78**, 354—362 (1971b)

Arnesen,H., Ly,B., Ödegård,O.R.: Improved quantitation of serum FDP after coagulation at low pH. Thrombos. Res. **3**, 643—655 (1973)

Astrup,T.: Tissue activators of plasminogen. Fed. Proc. **25**, 42—51 (1966)

Astrup,T., Müllertz,S.: The fibrin plate method for estimating fibrinolytic activity. Arch. Biochem. **40**, 346—351 (1952)

Astrup,T., Permin,P.M.: Fibrinolysis in the animal organism. Nature (Lond.) **159**, 681—682 (1947)

Auerswald,W., Binder,B., Doleschel,W.: "Angiokinase"—molecular weights of proteins representing a perivascular plasminogen activator. Thrombos. Diathes. haemorrh. (Stuttg.) **26**, 411—413 (1971)

Blix,S.: Studies on the fibrinolytic system in the euglobulin fraction of human plasma. A. A methodological study. B. Application of the methods. Scand. J. clin. Lab. Invest. **13** (Suppl. 58), 3—19 (1961)

Blombäck,B., Blombäck,M.: Purification of human and bovine fibrinogen. Ark. Kemi **10**, 415—443 (1956)

Bouma,B.N.: The results of a comparison of the tanned red cell hemagglutination inhibition immuno-assay with an immunochemical method for the determination of split products. Scand. J. Haemat. Suppl. **13**, 111—114 (1971)

Bouma,B.N., Hedner,U., Nilsson,I.M.: Typing of fibrinogen degradation products in urine in various clinical disorders. Scand. J. clin. Lab. Invest. **27**, 331—335 (1971)

Brakman,P.: Bovine fibrinogen without detectable plasminogen. Analyt. Biochem. **11**, 149—152 (1965)

Brakman,P.: Fibrinolysis. A standardized fibrin plate method, and a fibrinolytic assay of plasminogen. Amsterdam: Scheltema and Holkema 1967

Braun,W.E., Merrill,J.P.: Urine fibrinogen fragments in human renal allografts. New Engl. J. Med. **278**, 1366—1371 (1968)

Briggs,J.D., Prentice,C.R.M., Hutton,M.M., Kennedy,A.C., McNicol,G.P.: Serum and urine fibrinogen-fibrin-related antigen (F.R.-antigen) levels in renal disease. Brit. med. J. **1972 IV**, 82—85

Carlsson,S.: Fibrinogen degradation products in serum from patients with cancer. Acta chir. scand. **139**, 499—502 (1973)

Carlsson,S., Hedner,U., Nilsson,I.M., Bergentz,S.-E., Ljungqvist,U.: Kidney transplantation and fibrinolytic split products in serum and urine. Transplantation **10**, 366—371 (1970)

Carlsson,S., Linell,F.: Fibrinolytic degradation products in serum and urine in patients with renal cancer. Scand. J. Urol. Nephrol. **7**, 43—49 (1973)

Cash,J.: Platelets, fibrinolysis and stress. In: Brinkhous,K. (Ed.): Thrombosis: risk factors and diagnostic approaches, pp. 93—104. New York: Schattauer 1972

Cash,J.: Physiological aspects of fibrinolysis. In: Kaulla,K.N. von, Davidson,J.F. (Eds.): Synthetic fibrinolytic thrombolytic agents, pp. 5—19. Springfield, Ill.: Thomas 1975a

Cash,J.: Neurohumoral pathways associated with the release of plasminogen activator in man. In: Davidson,J.F., Samama,M.M., Desnoyers,P.C. (Eds.): Progress in chemical fibrinolysis and thrombolysis, pp. 97—107. New York: Raven Press 1975b

Cash,J.D., Allan,A.G.E.: The fibrinolytic response to moderate exercise and intravenous adrenaline in the same subjects. Brit. J. Haemat. **13**, 376—383 (1967)

Cash,J.D., Hoq,M.S., Cunningham,M., Anderton,J.L.: Rapid latex-screening test for urine FDP. Lancet **1973I**, 153—154

Cash, J. D., McGill, R. C.: Fibrinolytic response to moderate exercise in young male diabetics and non-diabetics. J. clin. Path. **22**, 32—35 (1969)

Cash, J. D., Woodfield, D. G.: Fibrinolytic response to moderate, exhaustive und prolonged exercise in normal subjetcs. Nature (Lond.) **215**, 628—630 (1967)

Cash, J. D., Woodfield, D. G., Allan, A. G. E.: Adrenergic mechanisms in the systemic plasminogen activator response to adrenaline in man. Brit. J. Haemat. **18**, 487—494 (1970)

Chen, J. P., Shurley, H. M.: A simple efficient production of neoantigenic antisera against fibrinolytic degradation products: radioimmunoassay of fragment E. Thrombos. Res. **7**, 425—434 (1975)

Chohan, I. S., Vermylen, J., Singh, I., Balakrishnan, K., Verstraete, M.: Sodium acetate buffer—A diluent of choice in the clot lysis time technique. Thrombos. Diathes. haemorrh. (Stuttg.) **33**, 226—229 (1975)

Clarkson, A. R., MacDonald, M. K., Petrie, J. J. B., Cash, J. D., Robson, J. S.: Serum and urinary fibrin/fibrinogen degradation products in glomerulonephritis. Brit. med. J. **1971 III**, 447—451

Constantini, R., Spöttl, F., Holzknecht, F., Braunsteiner, H.: On the role of the stable plasminogen activator of the venous wall in occlusion induced fibrinolytic states. Thrombos. Diathes. haemorrh. (Stuttg.) **22**, 544—550 (1969a)

Constantini, R., Spöttl, F., Holzknecht, F., Herbst, M., Braunsteiner, H.: On the plasminogen activator content of forearm-veins in patients with primary "carbohydrate-induced" hypertriglyceridemia. Coagulation **2**, 361—365 (1969b)

Donati, M. B., Semeraro, N., Vermylen, J.: Detection of fibrinogen antigens with two latex techniques applied to urine concentrates. J. clin. Path. **26**, 760—763 (1973)

Egbring, R., Schmidt, W., Havemann, K.: Possible destruction of factor I and XIII by leucocyte proteases in acute leukaemia. IVth Int. Congr. Thromb. and Haemostasis. Vienna, June 19—22 (1973)

Ekberg, M., Bergentz, S.-E., Hedner, U., Nilsson, I. M.: The determination of fibrinolytic degradation products in concentrated urine after renal transplantation. Scand. J. Urol. Nephrol. **10**, 56—62 (1976a)

Ekberg, M., Nilsson, I. M., Hedner, U., Larsson, I., Nosslin, B.: Determination of urinary fibrin/fibrinogen degradation products by radioimmunoassay. Scand. J. clin. Lab. Invest. **36**, 453—459 (1976b)

Ekberg, M., Nilsson, I. M., Denneberg, T.: Coagulation studies in hemolytic uremic syndrome and thrombotic thrombocytopenic purpura. Acta med. scand. **196**, 373—382 (1974)

Fearnley, G. R.: Fibrinolysis. London: Edward Arnold 1965

Fearnley, G. R., Balmforth, G., Fearnley, E.: Evidence of a diurnal fibrinolytic rhythm; with a simple method of measuring natural fibrinolysis. Clin. Sci. **16**, 645—650 (1957)

Fischer, A.: Beitrag zur Biologie der Gewebezellen. Arch. Entwickl.-Mech. Org. **104**, 210—261 (1925)

Haverkate, F., Brakman, P.: Fibrin plate assay. In: Davidson, J. F., Samama, M. M., Desnoyers, P. C. (Eds.): Progress in chemical fibrinolysis and thrombolysis, pp. 151—159. New York: Raven Press 1975

Hedner, U.: Urinary fibrin/fibrinogen degradation products (FDP) in renal diseases and during thrombolytic therapy. Scand. J. clin. Lab. Invest. **32**, 175—182 (1973)

Hedner, U., Ekberg, M., Nilsson, I. M.: Urinary fibrin/fibrinogen degradation products (FDP) and glomerulonephritis. Acta. med. scand. **195**, 81—85 (1974)

Hedner, U., Nilsson, I. M.: Clinical experience with determination of fibrinogen degradation products. Acta med. scand. **189**, 471—477 (1971)

Henriksson, P., Hedner, U., Nilsson, I. M., Nilsson, P.-G.: Generalized proteolysis in a young woman with Weber-Christian disease (nodular nonsuppurative panniculitis). Scand. J. Haemat. **14**, 355—360 (1975a)

Henriksson, P., Nilsson, I. M., Hedner, U.: Factor XIII in Henoch-Schönlein's purpura. Vth Congr. Int. Soc. on Thrombosis and Haemostasis. Paris, July 21—26, **522**, (1975b)

Holemans, R.: Enhancement of fibrinolysis in the dog by injection of vasoactive drugs. Amer. J. Physiol. **208**, 511—520 (1965)

Hulme, B., Pitcher, P. M.: Rapid latex-screening test for detection of fibrin/fibrinogen degradation products in urine after renal transplantation. Lancet **1973 I**, 6—8

Hunter,W.M., Greenwood,F.C.: Preparation of iodine-131 labelled human growth hormone of high specific activity. Nature (Lond.) **194**, 495—496 (1962)

Isacson,S., Nilsson,I.M.: Defective fibrinolysis in blood and vein walls in recurrent "idiopathic" venous thrombosis. Acta chir. scand. **138**, 313—319 (1972)

Isacson,S., Nilsson,I.M., Berg,B., Karlefors,T., Ursing,B.: Coagulation and fibrinolysis in young female arteritis. Acta med. scand. **190**, 179—183 (1971)

Johansson,B.G.: Agarose gel electrophoresis. Scand. J. clin. Lab. Invest. **29** (Suppl. 124), 7—19 (1972)

Johnson,A.J., Tse,A., Skoza,L.: Variation in assays of standard SK and plasmin preparations: evidence for and effect of variability in plasmins, plasminogen, and fibrinogen. Fed. Proc. **25**, 34—41 (1966)

Katz,J., Lurie,A., Kaplan,B.S., Krawitz,S., Metz,J.: Coagulation findings in the haemolytic-uremic syndrome of infancy: similarity to hyperacute renal allograft rejection. J. Pediat. **78**, 426—434 (1971)

Kester,R.C.: Plasminogen activator in the human prostate. J. clin. Path. **22**, 442—446 (1969)

Kluft,C., Brakman,P.: Effect of Flufenamate on euglobulin fibrinolysis: Involvement of C_1 Inactivator. In: Davidson,J.F., Samama,M.M., Desnoyers,P.C. (Eds.). Progress in chemical fibrinolysis and thrombolysis. pp. 375—381. New York: Raven Press 1975

Kok,P., Astrup,T.: Isolation and purification of a tissue plasminogen activator and its comparison with urokinase. Biochemistry **8**, 79—86 (1969)

Kok,P., Astrup,T.: Differentiation between plasminogen activators by means of epsilon-amino-caproic acid. Thrombos. Diathes. haemorrh. (Stuttg.) **27**, 77—87 (1972)

Kwaan,H.C., Astrup,T.: Demonstration of cellular fibrinolytic activity by the histochemical fibrin slide technique. Lab. Invest. **17**, 140—145 (1967)

Lack,C.H., Ali,Y.S.: Tissue activator of plasminogen. Nature (Lond.) **201**, 1030—1031 (1964)

Larsson,S.O., Hedner,U., Nilsson,I.M.: On fibrinolytic split products in serum and urine in uraemia. Scand. J. Urol. Nephrol. **5**, 234—242 (1971 a)

Larsson,S.O., Lindergård,B., Henriksson,H., Hedner,U., Nilsson,I.M.: A case of acute glomerulonephritis and severe uraemia treated with heparin and corticosteroids. Scand. J. Urol. Nephrol. **5**, 291—296 (1971 b)

Lassen,M.: Heat denaturation of plasminogen in the fibrin plate method. Acta physiol. scand. **27**, 371—376 (1952)

Laurell,C.B.: Quantitative estimation of proteins by electrophoresis in agarose gel containing antibodies. Analyt. Biochem. **15**, 45—52 (1966)

Lauritsen,O.S.: Inhibition of plasminogen activation and plasmin activity after euglobulin precipitation and acidification of plasma. Scand. J. clin. Lab. Invest. **23**, 121—218 (1969)

Luke,R.G., Siegel,R.R., Talbert,W., Holland,N.: Heparin treatment for post-partum renal failure with microangiopathic haemolytic anaemia. Lancet **1970 II**. 750—752

McConahey,P., Dixon,F.: A method of trace iodination of proteins for immunologic studies. Int. Arch. Allergy **29**, 185—189 (1966)

McFarlane,A.S.: Labelling of plasma proteins with radioactive iodine. Biochem. J. **62**, 135—143 (1956)

McNicol,G.P., Gale,S.B., Douglas,A.S.: In vitro and in vivo studies of a preparation of urokinase. Brit. med. J. **1963 I**, 909—915

Melliger,E.J.: Detection of fibrinogen degradation products by use of antibody coated latex particles. Thrombos. Diathes. haemorrh. (Stuttg.) **23**, 211—227 (1970)

Merskey,C., Johnson,A.J., Lalezari,P.: Increase in fibrinogen and fibrin-related antigen in human serum due to in vitro lysis of fibrin by thrombin. J. clin. Invest. **51**, 903—911 (1972)

Merskey,C., Kleiner,G.J., Johnson,A.J.: Quantitative estimation of split products of fibrinogen in human serum, relation to diagnosis and treatment. Blood **28** (No 1), 1—18 (1966)

Merskey,C., Lalezari,P., Johnson,A.J.: A rapid, simple, sensitive method for measuring fibrinolytic split products in human serum. Proc. Soc. exp. Biol. (N.Y.) **131**, 871—875 (1969)

Merskey,C., Lalezari,P., Johnson,A.J.: Tanned red cell hemagglutination inhibition immunoassay for fibrinogen-fibrin-related antigen in human serum. Scand. J. Haemat. Suppl. **13**, 83—85 (1971)

Milstone,H.: A factor in normal human blood which participates in streptococcal fibrinolysis. J. Immunol. **42**, 109 (1941)

Müllertz, S.: Activation of plasminogen. Ann. N. Y. Acad. Sci. **28**, 38—52 (1957)

Nakahara, M., Celander, D. R.: Properties of microsomal activator of profibrinolysin found in bovine and porcine heart muscle. Thrombos. Diathes. haemorrh. (Stuttg.) **19**, 483—491 (1968)

Nilehn, J.-E.: Separation and estimation of "split products" of fibrinogen and fibrin in human serum. Thrombos. Diathes. haemorrh. (Stuttg.) **18**, 487—498 (1967)

Nilsson, I. M.: Haemorrhagic and Thrombotic Diseases. London: Wiley and Sons 1974

Nilsson, I. M.: Methods for assessment of fibrinolytic activator activity. In: Kaulla, K. N., von, Davidson, J. F. (Eds.): Synthetic fibrinolytic thrombolytic agents, pp. 20—49. Springfield, Ill.: Charles C. Thomas 1975

Nilsson, I. M.: Coagulation, fibrinolysis and venous thrombosis. Triangle **16**, 19—27 (1977)

Nilsson, I. M., Hedner, U., Åstedt, B., Gennser, G., Jacobson, L., Holmberg, L., Ohrlander, S.: Intravascular coagulation in pregnancy—treatment with heparin. Acta obstet. gynec. scand. **53**, 491—496 (1975)

Nilsson, I. M., Olow, B.: Fibrinolysis induced by streptokinase in man. Acta chir. scand. **123**, 247—266 (1962)

Nilsson, I. M., Pandolfi, M.: Fibrinolytic response of the vascular wall. Thrombos. Diathes. haemorrh. (Stuttg.) **40**, 231—242 (1970)

Ohlsson, K.: Preparation of human fibrinogen free from plasminogen by an immunochemical method. Clin. chim. Acta **25**, 221—224 (1969)

Owren, P. A.: The coagulation of blood; investigations on a new clotting factor. Acta med. scand. Suppl **194** (1947).

Pandolfi, M.: Studies on fibrinolysis in some tissues and in aqueous humor. Thesis. Lund: Berlingska Boktryckeriet 1969

Pandolfi, M.: Histochemistry and assay of plasminogen activator(s). Rev. Europ. Etud. clin. Biol. **17** (No. 3), 254—260 (1972)

Pandolfi, M., Bjernstad, A., Nilsson, I. M.: Technical remarks on the microscopical demonstration of tissue plasminogen activator. Thrombos. Diathes. haemorrh. (Stuttg.) **27**, 88—98 (1972)

Pandolfi, M., Isacson, S., Nilsson, I. M.: Low fibrinolytic activity in the walls of veins in patients with thrombosis. Acta med. scand. **186**, 1—5 (1969)

Pandolfi, M., Nilsson, I. M., Robertson, B., Isacson, S.: Fibrinolytic activity of human veins. Lancet **1967 II**, 127—128

Pandolfi, M., Robertson, B., Isacson, S., Nilsson, I. M.: Fibrinolytic activity of human veins in arms and legs. Thrombos. Diathes. haemorrh. (Stuttg.) **20**, 247—256 (1968)

Pandolfi, M., Åstedt, B., Nilsson, I. M.: Direct observation of fibrinolysis in tissue culture. Thrombos. Diathes. haemorrh. (Stuttg.) **31**, 415—419 (1974)

Permin, P. M.: Undersøgelser over fibrinolytiske enzymer. Thesis. University of Copenhagen (1949)

Plow, E., Edgington, T. S.: Molecular events responsible for modulation of neoantigenic expression: the cleavage-associated neoantigen of fibrinogen. Proc. nat. Acad. Sci. (Wash.) **69**, 208—212 (1972)

Plow, E., Edgington, T. S.: Immunobiology of fibrinogen. Emergence of neoantigenic expressions during physiologic cleavage in vitro and in vivo. J. clin. Invest. **52**, 273—282 (1973)

Plow, E. F., Hougie, C., Edgington, T. S.: Neoantigenic expressions engendered by plasmin cleavage of fibrinogen. J. Immunol. **117**, 1496—1500 (1971)

Rayner, H., Paraskevas, F., Israels, L. G., Israels, E. D.: Fibrinogen breakdown products: Identification and assay in serum and urine. J. Lab. Clin. Med. **74**, 586—596 (1969)

Robertson, B. R.: Effect of nicotinic acid on fibrinolytic activity in health, in thrombotic disease and in liver cirrhosis. Acta chir. scand. **137**, 643—648 (1971)

Robertson, B. R., Pandolfi, M., Nilsson, I. M.: Response of local fibrinolytic activity to venous occlusion of arms and legs in healthy volunteers. Acta chir. scand. **138**, 437—440 (1972a)

Robertson, B. R., Pandolfi, M., Nilsson, I. M.: "Fibrinolytic capacity" of healthy volunteers as estimated from effect of venous occlusion of arms. Acta chir. scand. **138**, 429—436 (1972b)

Robertson, B. R., Pandolfi, M., Nilsson, I. M.: "Fibrinolytic capacity" in healthy volunteers at different ages as studied by standardized venous occlusion of arms and legs. Acta med. scand. **191**, 199—202 (1972c)

Samama, M., Conard, J., Bara, L.: Euglobulin and other clot lysis methods. Postgraduate course and workshop. Progress in fibrinolysis. European Thrombosis Research Organization. Fondazione Giovanni Lorenzini, Milan, March 6—8 (1975)

Santesson, L.: Characteristics of epithelial mouse tumour cells in vitro and tumour structures in vivo. A comparative study. Acta path. microbiol. scand. Suppl. **24** (1935)

Schmidt, W., Egbring, R., Havemann, K.: Effect of elastase-like and chymotrypsin-like neutral proteases from human granulocytes on isolated clotting factors. Thrombos. Res. **6**, 315—326 (1975)

Sherry, S., Alkjaersig, N.: A study of the fibrinolytic enzyme of human plasma. Thrombos. Diathes. haemorrh. (Stuttg.) **1**, 264—288 (1957)

Skånsberg, P., Cronberg, S., Nilsson, I. M.: The occurrence and significance of fibrin/fibrinogen degradation products (FDP) in acute infections. Scand. J. infect. Dis. **6**, 197—203 (1974)

Spöttl, F., Holzknecht, F., Braunsteiner, H.: Enhancement of the fibrinolytic activity by venous occlusion in patients with primary carbohydrate-induced hypertriglyceridemia. Acta haemat. (Basel) **41**, 154—161 (1969)

Stiehm, E. R., Kuplic, L. S., Ueling, D. T.: Urinary fibrin split products in human renal disease. J. Lab. clin. Med. **77**, 843—852 (1971)

Stiehm, E. R., Trygstad, C. W.: Split products of fibrin in human renal disease. Amer. J. Med. **46**, 774—786 (1969)

Svanberg, L., Hedner, U., Åstedt, B.: Value of determination of FDP during pregnancy by immunochemical and latex agglutination inhibition methods. Acta obstet. gynec. scand. **53**, 81—83 (1974)

Thorell, J., Johansson, B. G.: Enzymatic iodination of polypeptides with ^{125}I to high specific activity. Biochim. biophys. Acta (Amst.) **251**, 363—369 (1971)

Thorsen, S., Astrup, T.: Substrate composition and the effect of ε-aminocaproic acid on tissue plasminogen activator and urokinase-induced fibrinolysis. Thrombos. Diathes. haemorrh. (Stuttg.) **32**, 306—324 (1974)

Todd, A. S.: The histological localisation of fibrinolysin activator. J. Path. Bact. **78**, 281—283 (1959)

Wardle, E. N., Taylor, G.: Fibrin breakdown products and fibrinolysis in renal disease. J. clin. Path. **21**, 140—146 (1968)

Activators of Fibrinolysis

Biochemistry of Streptokinase

F. B. TAYLOR, JR., and P. C. COMP

Introduction

Streptokinase (SK), an extracellular protein produced by various strains of strepto-cocci, is capable of converting human plasminogen to plasmin. Its capacity to cause lysis of blood clots was first described by TILLET and GARNER in 1933. This effect was thought to be due to direct enzymatic action on the fibrin of these clots. However, MILSTONE, in 1941, demonstrated that streptokinase achieved its effect through acti-vation of a plasma protein. Thus the proenzyme and enzyme forms of this plasma protein were given the names plasminogen and plasmin, respectively, and the bacterial extract was given the name streptokinase. As of now, plasminogen and plasmin are the only substrates with which SK is known to react. Evidence indicates that a 1:1 molar complex of streptokinase and plasminogen or plasmin is formed producing an "activator complex" which then converts free (uncomplexed) plasminogen to plasmin. Activator activity may be defined in terms of its ability to convert bovine and guinea pig plasminogens to plasmin directly. Plasminogen, plasmin and strepto-kinase alone are unable to carry out this conversion. Activator is further characterized by its ability to cause lysis on unheated but not heated beef fibrin agar plates, the fact it is not inhibited by soy bean trypsin inhibitor, and its ability to convert guinea pig plasminogen to plasmin in the casein guinea pig serum assay.

The binding of streptokinase to plasminogen is thought to induce a conforma-tional change in plasminogen exposing a catalytic site which in turn acts on other plasminogen molecules to convert them to plasmin (DAVIES et al., 1964; MARKUS and WERKHEISER, 1964). Since this interaction of SK and plasminogen is of biologic and biochemical interest, we will describe: 1. assays of streptokinase activity, 2. puri-fication of streptokinase, 3. physical properties of SK and 4. current concepts of the mode of SK-plasminogen interaction.

A. Assays of Streptokinase Activity

All of the assays described below detect the presence of streptokinase indirectly through its capacity to activate plasminogen to plasmin. Plasmin then hydrolyzes an indicator substrate such as a fibrin clot, casein, or synthetic substrate. The rate of hydrolysis of the substrate is a function of the amount of plasmin formed from the proenzyme, and, within the limits described, this plasmin formation in turn is di-rectly related to the amount of SK present.

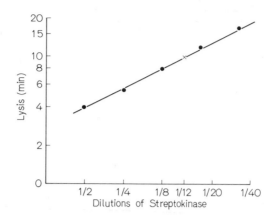

Fig. 1

I. Clot Lysis Assay

The assay used for standardization of commercial SK preparations is that of CHRISTENSEN (1949). It involves the determination of the smallest amount of streptokinase that will cause lysis of a standard fibrin clot in 10 min. One-tenth ml of serial dilutions of streptokinase in gelatin buffer, 0.8 ml of standard human "fibrinogen" solution (which also contains plasminogen), and 0.1 ml of thrombin solution (described below) are mixed and placed in a water bath at 37° C. The fibrinogen clots in 1 min or less. The clots then lyse because the SK activates the plasminogen contaminating the fibrinogen reagent. The lysis times of the clots in the series are followed up to 20 min. The lysis time of each dilution of SK is plotted against the reciprocal of that dilution on log-log paper (Fig. 1). A straight line can be drawn through the points beginning with the shortest lysis time (1.5–2 min) and extending to the longest lysis time (20–30 min). Above and below these points the curve is not linear and therefore cannot be used for purposes of calculation. The upper limit of the curve is determined by the amount of substrate (fibrin) relative to active enzyme (plasmin). However, it also should be noted that the upper limit is influenced by the fact that high concentrations of SK combine with plasminogen or plasmin to form an activator complex which has a lower affinity for fibrin than does plasmin. This assay of clot lysis can detect the presence of nanogram quantities of streptokinase.

Under the above conditions, one unit is that amount of SK which will lyse a standard clot in 10 min as determined by interpolation of the lysis time curve. A sample assay and calculation is a follows: One-tenth ml aliquots of undiluted, 1:2, 1:4, 1:8, 1:16, and 1:32 dilutions of streptokinase are added to the system as described above and lysis time recorded. Figure 1 shows the log plot of the lysis time vs. the dilutions. Employing the above definition of 1 unit of SK activity together with interpolation of this plot, the units of SK per ml or per mg protein in a sample containing an unknown amount of SK can be calculated by recording the lysis time for a given dilution or concentration of SK and using the following equation:

$$\frac{\text{Lysis time (min)}}{10 \text{ min}} \times (\text{dilution factor}) \times (10, \text{volume correction to 1 ml of SK} \tag{1}$$

$$\text{sample being assayed}) = \text{U of SK/ml of sample being assayed}$$

Interpolating along the plotted graph in Figure 1, one sees that a 1:12 dilution of the material containing an unknown amount of SK lysed a standard clot in 10 min. By definition then, 0.1 ml of a 1:12 dilution of this unknown contains 1 SK U. Therefore, the material assayed contained 120 SK U/ml:

$$\frac{10 \text{ min}}{10 \text{ min}} \times (12\text{-fold dilution}) (10) = 120 \text{ U/ml} \tag{2}$$

The WHO-Expert Committee on Biological Standardization used this clot lysis assay to establish an international standard for SK based on assay of aliquots of a 6 g lot (No. 48035-154) of an impure but stable preparation of SK provided by Lederle Laboratories (1965). One international unit (that amount of the SK standard described above which would lyse a clot in 10 min) was found to be equivalent to 0.002090 mg of this material.

The reagents for this assay are as follows:

1. Fibrinogen (containing human plasminogen). Cohn fraction I lyophilized and stored at 4° C is made into a 0.25% solution wt/vol with borate saline buffer on the day of the study.
   2. Thrombin. Lyophilized bovine thrombin (10000 NIH U, Parke-Davis) is made into a solution containing 1 NIH U thrombin activity per 0.1 ml with borate saline buffer on the day of the study.
   3. Lyophilized standard and test sample. SK diluted in gelatin buffer on the day of the study.
   4. Buffers: Borate Saline: Sodium borate hydrated, 7 g, Sodium chloride, 9 g, Boric acid, 11.1 g, Distilled water, 1000 ml, HCl, 5 N, to pH 7.4.
   Gelatin Buffer: Gelatin, 5 g dissolved in a small amount of warm water, NaCl, 10 g, KH_2PO_4, 13.6 g, make up to 1000 with distilled water, NaOH, 1 ON, to pH 7.4.
   Individual aliquots of these reagents can be prepared beforehand and stored at −60° C. However, neither the fibrinogen nor thrombin can be frozen and thawed more than once without affecting solubility and activity.
   Alternative reagents which are used less often are as follows: 0.7 ml of a 0.25% solution of highly purified fibrinogen (95% clottable) in phosphate buffer (pH 7.4, 0.1 M), 0.1 ml containing 1 casein U of highly purified plasminogen, 0.1 ml of 10 U/ml of bovine thrombin, and 0.1 ml of the SK to be tested, all in the same buffer. These reagents, though more difficult to prepare, can yield results which are more consistent than those obtained when the fibrinogen in the Cohn I fraction of plasma is used.
   This clot lysis assay is useful because it allows: (1) a comparatively simple determination of relative SK activities within a given laboratory; and (2) an approximation of specific activities of SK for biological purposes.
   However, the difficulty with such an assay for use in more rigorous biochemical studies is alluded to in the report on the establishment of the international unit of SK where a range of 2150 to 3886 Christensen units or 970 to 5093 British units was recorded by different laboratories (1965). This wide range is due to the fact that this assay requires subjective determination of the end point and the use of three biological products, fibrinogen, plasminogen and SK. As with most biologicals, lot-to-lot

variability, instability, and contamination by inhibitors multiply problems of standardization. This difficulty has been obviated in part by preparation of large batches of crude fibrinogen (plus plasminogen) for use solely in standardizing successive batches of SK. However, unless all laboratories have access to the same batch of SK or crude fibrinogen, more rigorous direct comparison of the various SK preparations is not possible. Other assays which have been employed for determinations of SK activity include the fibrin plate assay (Astrup and Müllertz, 1952) and the casein assay (Johnson et al., 1964).

II. Lysine Methyl Ester Assay

Synthetic esters instead of fibrinogen have been employed as substrates to define more rigorously the specific activity of SK (Roberts, 1960; Taylor and Botts, 1968). The following is a description of an assay for SK activity using lysine methyl ester (LMe) which utilizes plasminogen of known specific activity. It involves the addition of streptokinase to highly purified human plasminogen of known specific activity and assaying the rate of hydrolysis of a stable synthetic substrate (LMe).

In this assay 0.200 mg of plasminogen (20 casein U/mg protein) in 0.25 ml 0.001 N HCl is activated by 0.25 ml of the SK test sample in Tris buffer with 0.5 ml of 0.08 M LMe (obtained from Mann Research Co., N.Y., N.Y.) in Tris buffer (final pH 7.4) at 37° C. At the end of the desired time interval (usually 30 min), 2 ml of 1:1 mixture of reagents I and II (described below) are added to the above reaction mixture. The samples are then allowed to stand 2 min, followed by the addition of 1 ml reagent III (described below). After at least 30 min and not more than 24 h, the samples are centrifuged at 1000 g for 10 min to remove the precipitate. To 4 ml of reagent IV (described below) 1 ml of the supernatant is added and the color of the samples is read at 525 nm within 2 min. Control samples include LMe alone (0.5 ml) plus buffer (0.5 ml), and LMe (0.5 ml) plus plasminogen (0.25 ml) plus buffer (0.25 ml).

In defining the activity of SK by esterolysis, it is necessary to do so indirectly in terms of the amount of plasmin activity generated by the SK conversion of plasminogen to plasmin. Therefore, for each batch or lot of SK a standard curve is drawn of the change in optical density (mol of LMe hydrolyzed) per minute by the activated plasminogen (i.e., plasmin, 4 casein U/0.2 mg) vs. the concentration of SK in micrograms per milliliter of assay solution (Fig. 2). The explanation of the upper and lower limits of such a plot is the same as that given previously for the clot lysis assay. The specific activity of the plasmin used must be constant from assay to assay and this should be approximately 20 casein U/mg protein as determined by casein assay (to be described below). In order that the activity of different lots or batches of SK can be compared under the conditions described above, SK activity is expressed in units. One unit of SK activity is arbitrarily defined as 1×10^{-9} mol LMe hydrolyzed $\min^{-1}$, mg N^{-1} SK by 0.200 mg of plasmin (4 casein U/0.2 mg)

$$\frac{U \text{ of SK activity}}{\text{mg N of SK}} = \frac{(\Delta OD \text{ during } 30 \text{ min}) (2.79 \times 10^-) (10^3)}{(30 \text{ min}) (\text{No. mg N}) (1 \times 10^{-9})} \tag{3}$$

where: ΔOD is the difference in optical density at 525 nm between the test sample and control buffer and control plasminogen samples after the 30-min period of

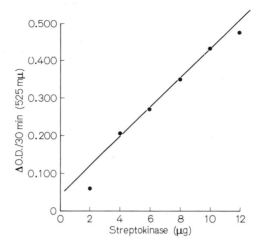

Fig. 2

incubation. In this way, spontaneous hydrolysis of LMe as well as hydrolysis by plasmin contamination of plasminogen are taken into account; ε-2.79×10^{-8} is the molar extinction coefficient for assay of LMe products; 10^3 is the factor which converts the OD reading to OD units; 30 min is the time interval during which the reaction took place; No. mg N is the total number of mg of nitrogen in the SK being assayed; 1×10^{-9} is the mol of LMe hydrolyzed chosen arbitrarily to represent 1 U of SK activity. A sample assay and calculations are as follows: 2, 4, 6, 8, 10, and 12 µg of SK (per 0.25 ml) are added to the plasminogen-LMe system as described above and the change in OD recorded. Figure 2 shows a plot of ΔOD (LMe hydrolyzed) vs. micrograms of SK. Given the above conditions and definition of 1 U to SK activity, the number of units of SK activity in 10 µg of SK is given by recording the ΔOD which corresponds to 10 µg and performing the following calculations:

$$\frac{\text{U of SK activity}}{\text{mg N of SK}} = \frac{(0.433)\,(2.79 \times 10^{-8})}{(30)\,(0.0015)\,(1 \times 10^{-9})} = 2.6 \times 10^5 \text{SK}^{(10)} \qquad (4)$$

The reagents for this assay are as follows:

Reagent I:
   $NH_2OH \cdot HCl$, 4 M
   139.5 g/500 ml, distilled H_2O filtered and stored at 4° C
Reagent II:
   NaOH, 7 M
   280 g/1000 ml distilled H_2O
Reagent III:
   12% TCA in 50% concentrated HCl. The TCA is hydrophilic. Therefore, it must be dried under vacuum with P_2O_5 and then weighed.
Reagent IV:
   $FeCl_3$, 0.11 M in approx. 0.04 M HCl
   29 g $FeCl_3$ in 1000 ml of H_2O, pH adjusted to 1.2 with HCl.

To check that these reagents give the proper pH when mixed, add 1 ml of re-agents I, II, and III to 1 ml of water or buffer in which the sample is to be dissolved, and determine the pH. It should be 1.2 or slightly less. Then add 1 ml of the I, II and III mixture to 1 ml of reagent IV. The pH of this must be 1.2 ± 0.1. The pH is critical in production of color. If it is too high, a precipitate forms. If it is too low, the color fades too rapidly.

The LMe assay may represent a useful more quantitative alternative to the Christensen or fibrin clot assays because: (1) the end point does not vary from laboratory to laboratory: (2) multiple points in a single determination may be made; (3) standardization of the substrate LMe is far easier than for fibrin or fibrinogen; (4) the plasminogen must be added as a separate entity with less possibility of plasmi-nogen or plasmin or their inhibitors contaminating the substrate as is the case when fibrinogen is used.

III. Casein Assay

To 1 ml of 4% casein prepared as described by DERECHIN (1962), add 1 ml of plasmi-nogen solution (borate saline buffer, pH 7.4). Then add 0.1 ml of SK (200 U) in the same buffer. Control samples consist of casein (1 ml) plus buffer (1 ml), and casein (1 ml) plus plasminogen (1 ml). Allow to incubate at $37°$ C for 30 min and then add 3 ml of 1 M PCA (or 12% TCA). Allow the system to sit in the cold for 60 min. Filter through Whatman No. 4 filter paper. Read the filtrate at 280 nm. Employing this assay, a standard curye relating ΔOD to the amount of plasmin (in units) in the system can be constructed in the same manner as has been described in the assays of SK activity. Given the limits of the system described by this curve, a unit of plasmin activity has been defined. One unit (casein units) of plasmin activity has been defined as that activity which releases 450 μg of TCA-soluble tyrosine (from casein) per milliliter of sample per hour (REMMERT and COHEN, 1949).

$$\text{Casein U/ml} = \frac{(\Delta\text{OD}) \,(150 \text{ μg tyrosine}) \,(2) \,(5) \,(\text{correction to 1 ml of plasmin})}{450 \text{ μg of tyrosine}} \tag{5}$$

where ΔOD is the difference in absorbances at 280 nm between the sample and the control plasminogen sample incubated for the same length of time, 150 μg of tyrosine is equal to 0.001 OD reading; 2 is the correction from 30 min to 60 min; and 5 represents the final volume in ml of the solution, including the PCA. The correction to 1 ml in this case is 1 since 1 ml of plasmin as described here is used in the assay. From this the specific activity of a plasmin preparation may by obtained.

$$\text{Casein U/mg N} = \frac{\text{casein U/ml}}{\text{mg N/ml}} \tag{6}$$

IV. NPGB Burst Assay

The active site titrant p-nitrophenyl-p-guanidinobenzoate (NPGB) has been em-ployed for various serine proteases including plasmin (CHASE and SHAW, 1969). McCLINTOCK and BELL (1971) and REDDY and MARKUS (1972) have employed the compound to assay plasmin and activator complex. The assays depend on the acylation of the active serine of the plasmin and the release of the p-nitrophenol which is detected colorimetrically. Some difficulty arises with the assay when the relatively poorly soluble lys-plasminogen (soluble to 1 mg/ml) not the native glu-plasminogen (10 mg/ml) is used.

B. Preparation of Streptokinase

Crude streptokinase-streptodornase (SK-SD) is usually prepared from cultures of β-hemolytic streptococci of group C, in a manner similar to that described by CHRISTENSEN (1947). Large amounts of crude SK-SD are distributed under the trade name Varidase. Although the crude SK-SD can be and is prepared in individual laboratories, the above preparation has been used as a starting material for preparation of purified SK.

I. Preparation of High Purity Streptokinase

Several satisfactory methods of SK purification have been published by DE RENZO et al. (1967 b), TAYLOR and BOTTS (1968), and TOMAR (1968).

1. The first of these methods was described by DE RENZO et al. (1967 b) for the Lederle Co., under U.S. patent 3,226,304. They describe in detail four different procedures for preparing the crude starting material. They then describe further purification procedures employing either DEAE-cellulose chromatography or density-gradient electrophoresis. Both these later procedures yield SK of high purity with an approximate specific activity of 600–700 Christensen U/µg N.

2. The second of these methods was developed simultaneously in our laboratory (TAYLOR and BOTTS, 1968). The details are as follows:

Approximately 100 mg of SK is dissolved in 3 ml of 0.10 M NaCl—0.01 M Tris buffer (pH 8.5) and dialyzed for 48 h at 4° C against two changes of 2 l volumes of the same buffer. This material is then adsorbed and fractionated on DEAE-Sephadex A-50 at 4° C employing a linear NaCl-Tris gradient. The DEAE-Sephadex A-50 has a binding capacity of 3.5 ± 0.5 mEq/g. Lots (5–10 g) of the DEAE-Sephadex are washed 9 times with 1 l volumes of 0.1 M NaCl-0.01 M Tris buffer (pH 8.5) and allowed to equilibrate with this buffer over 3 days after a final adjustment of the pH of the slurry to pH 8.5 with 0.1 N HCl. This is packed into a 45×3 cm column by gravity (at a flow rate of 20 ml/h). The total bed volume is 250 ml. The linear gradient is formed by using two 300 ml Erlenmeyer flasks (level with each other and open to the atmosphere) that are connected in series to each other and the column. These two flasks are connected at their bases by tubing and hence to the column by a 1/8-in. diameter polyethylene tube and plug. The first flask contains 250 ml of a 0.5 M NaCl-0.01 M Tris solution that runs into the second flask (mixing flask) which contains 0.1 M NaCl-0.01 M Tris. The thoroughly mixed solutions are then delivered into the top of the column by gravity feed at a rate of 20 ml/h. The total elution volume is 500 ml collected in 2–3 ml aliquots by a GME Model T 15^2 fraction collector. The protein concentration is determined by absorbance measurements in 1-cm quartz cells at 280 nm with a

Beckman DB spectrophotometer. The effluent containing SK is pooled and dialyzed for 48 h at 4° C against three changes of 3 l volumes of 0.001 M phosphate and 0.3 M NaCl at pH 7.4. This dialyzate is then filtered through G-100 Sephadex gel at 4° C at a flow rate of 20 ml/h. The Sephadex G-100 as a dry powder is suspended in a sufficient amount of phosphate buffer (0.001 M phosphate-0.03 M NaCl at pH 7.4) and stored for 72 h to assure complete swelling. The fines were removed by several decantations and the gel is packed into a 45 × 3 cm column. The total bed volume is 250 ml and the void volume is 32 ml as determined with blue dextran. The strepto-kinase is pooled, concentrated by ultrafiltration, and stored in 2 ml volumes at −60° C.

Rechromatography of the effluent from the G-100 (containing SK) on DEAE (Sephadex) is frequently necessary in order to complete the separation of γ-globulins which are closely associated with streptokinase. The final product has an approximate specific activity of 600–800 Christensen units per microgram nitrogen or 2.5×10^5 SK-LMe units. This represents a 10- to 11-fold increase in specific activity and is close to the results obtained by others (Fletcher and Johnson, 1957; Blatt et al., 1966; DeRenzo et al., 1967b).

3. The third of these methods described by Tomar (1968) involves a precipitation of SK from the starting material with 40–50% ammonium sulfate resulting in a 2- to 3-fold increase in specific activity together with a concentration of the material for subsequent variable gradient chromatography on DEAE-cellulose. The simple $(NH_2)_2SO_4$ step was originally described by Fletcher and Johnson (1957) and Johanson (1957) and represents the most simple single batch procedure for preparing SK from Varidase described to date.

Dillon and Wanamaker (1965) in a comparative study have described the separation and partial purification of SK from both Group C and Group A, β-hemolytic streptococci employing methods similar to those described above. Finally, it should be noted that Blatt et al. (1966) have also reported preparations of SK of the same order of purity.

II. Affinity Column Preparation of Streptokinase

We have developed, in our laboratory, a method of streptokinase purification employing affinity chromatography to gel bound plasmin inhibited with diisopropyl-fluorophosphate (DFP). Batches of plasminogen are isolated from outdated plasma treated with 0.01 M DFP by the method of Deutsch and Mertz (1970), modified to include an initial wash of the agarose-lysine column containing the plasminogen with 10^{-4} M EDTA in 0.1 M PO_4 buffer (pH 7.4) to remove nonspecifically bound plasma proteins. This is followed by an extensive wash with 0.3 M PO_4 buffer (pH 7.4). Lysine (0.2 M) elution buffer is used and the lysine is removed from the plasminogen using a Sephadex G-25 column in 0.2 M NaCl-0.1 M PO_4 pH 7.4 buffer at 4° C.

The plasminogen is then reacted with streptokinase in a 30:1 molar ratio for 60 min at 37° C to produce plasmin and the plasmin is then inhibited by the addition of DFP to a final concentration of 10^{-2} M. The plasmin is allowed to react with the DFP for 2 h at 25° C and then for 16 h at 4° C. The inhibited plasmin is bound to agarose using 1.5 g CnBr per 10 ml gel.

After being mixed at 4° C for 48 h, 0.01 M ethanolamine is used to block unreacted sites and finally unbound plasmin is eluted with 0.1 M PO_4 pH 7.4. Approximately 95% of the plasmin is bound.

Crude SK (Lederle, Varidase) is dialyzed against the same buffer and then mixed with the gel for 18 h at 4° C. Nonspecifically bound protein is removed by washing with 0.1 M NaCl-0.1 M PO_4 pH 7.4. The bound streptokinase is then eluted with 0.1 M citrate buffer pH 3.0.

This purification produces streptokinase without contaminating bands on gel electrophoresis and mobility unchanged from the SK in the starting material; the SK has a single N-terminal amino acid isoleucine. The SK is fully active. Yields up to 90% have been obtained. The SK to plasmin molar binding ratio has a maximum of 0.8.

C. Physical Properties of Streptokinase

The physical and chemical properties of streptokinase as reported in 1967 by DE RENZO et al. and BOTTS, 1968), are almost identical. Its molecular weight as determined by equilibrium sedimentation is between 47000 (DERENZO et al., 1967b) and 49000 (TAYLOR and BOTTS, 1968). Its partial specific volume as determined by pyknometry and calculation from amino acid analysis data is (DERENZO et al., 1967b) 0.75 and 0.73 (TAYLOR and BOTTS, 1968) and its specific viscosity as determined by measurement with an Ostwald type viscometer with an outflow time for water of 70 s at 37° C is 0.10 (TAYLOR and BOTTS, 1968). The isoelectric point of SK is 4.7

Table 1. Recovery of amino acids and ammonia in acid hydrolyzates of purified Streptokinase

Amino acid residue	Amount recovered in hydrolyzates at	
	23 h	48 h
	(mμmol/μg of nitrogen)	
Asp	8.16	8.09
Thr	3.48	3.36
Ser	3.72	2.34
Glu	5.54	5.76
Pro	2.45	2.53
Gly	2.55	2.50
Ala	2.83	2.80
Val	2.80	2.82
Met	0.28	0.28
Ile	2.86	2.66
Leu	5.01	4.97
Tyr	2.35	2.43
Phe	1.90	1.84
NH_3	6.50	8.63
Lys	4.08	4.01
His	1.08	1.00
Arg	2.51	2.57

(DeRenzo et al., 1967b), and it migrates on gel electrophoresis as an α-globulin (Taylor andBotts, 1968). Chemical analysis of streptokinase reveals a hexose and hexosamine content of less than 0.2 g/100 l and 0.1 g/100 l respectively (Taylor and Botts, 1968). No lipids are present, the nitrogen content is 14.5% (Taylor and Botts, 1968). From this, an extinction coefficient $E_{1cm}^{1\%}$ of 9.49 was determined (Taylor and Botts, 1968). Optical rotatory dispersion studies suggest that the helix content is 10–12% as determined from the depth of the trough of the Cotton effect (Taylor and Botts, 1968).

Table 1 shows the results of amino acid analysis (Taylor and Botts, 1968). Morgan and Henschen (1969) have obtained five cyanogen bromide fragments from streptokinase. The N-terminal sequence they found of isoleu-ala-glu- was confirmed in our laboratory.

D. Mechanism of Streptokinase Activity

The mode of action of SK on plasminogen and/or plasmin as assayed above remains to be fully elucidated. However, the following facts are known.

1. In 1961 Kline and Fishman presented evidence that increasing amounts of SK reacted directly with preformed plasmin to form a complex. This complex in turn had an increased affinity for certain synthetic substrates (i.e., LMe) and a decreased affinity for certain protein substrates (i.e., casein). This plasmin-SK mixture (complex) was termed "activator" because: 1) it was an efficient activator of bovine plasminogen to plasmin, whereas SK or plasmin alone was not; and 2) it was an effective activator of human plasminogen, whereas plasmin alone was not.

They also observed that the original plasmin activity could be recovered from this SK-plasmin mixture (activator complex) by exposure to pH 2.5 for 1 h. Upon readjusting the pH to 7.4 and reassay of this mixture on casein and LMe, the original affinity of plasmin for casein was restored along with the corresponding decrease of affinity of the mixture for LMe. Thus, the activity of the SK-plasmin "activator" complex had been transformed back to the activity of plasmin alone. From these studies in which large amounts of SK and plasmin were used, it was assumed that activation of plasminogen by small amounts of SK was mediated through its reaction with similarly small amounts of plasmin (1% or less of which is often associated with plasminogen). The two proteins complexed to form the activator just described, which, in turn, initiated further conversion of plasminogen to plasmin.

2. In 1964, the actual physical existence of such a complex was demonstrated by Davis et al. They showed that as a 1:1 to 1:2 molar ratio of streptokinase relative to plasmin (or plasminogen) was approached, a complex was formed which sedimented faster in the ultracentrifuge than either of the two components alone. It was postulated, but not shown, that this was activator. Later DeRenzo et al. (1967a) of this same group, demonstrated this same complex by starch gel electrophoresis. They also demonstrated that it had activator activity as defined by its capacity to convert bovine plasminogen to plasmin.

In recent years (1971–1974) the generation and location of the active site in the plasminogen-streptokinase complex has been explored extensively, with the active site titrant nitrophenol-guanidino-benzoate (NPGB). This agent blocks these sites by acylation as soon as they are formed. MCCLINTOCK and BELL (1971) and REDDY and MARKUS (1972) demonstrated that when the activator complex is formed, an NPGB titratable active site is exposed before any proteolytic cleavage of either streptokinase or plasminogen occurs. They also demonstrated that the SK-plasminogen complex was fully capable of activating plasminogen. However, the SK-plasminogen complex has lower activity when tested on synthetic substrates than did the SK-plasmin complex (REDDY and MARKUS, 1974).

Labeling of the active site of the SK-plasminogen activator complex with ^{32}-P-DFP demonstrated that the activator complex has a single DFP sensitive residue. It was postulated that the site was identical to the active site serine of plasmin. SCHICK and CASTELLINO (1974), using ^{14}C-labeled NPGB, demonstrated that the active site of the SK-plasminogen complex was indeed located on the plasminogen component of the complex and was in all probability identical to the plasmin active site.

These data suggest that both plasminogen and plasmin, while complexed to SK, can effectively convert free plasminogen to plasmin, and that both activator and the plasmin activity probably originate from the same active site. It is likely that the differing specificity of activator vs. plasmin is due to a conformational change induced by SK.

In addition to the opening of an active site on plasminogen, formation of plasminogen-streptokinase complex is followed immediately by an ordered sequence of proteolytic cleavages affecting both the plasminogen and SK moieties. The breakdown of the components of the complex has been studied by isolation of products at various intervals of time following formation of the SK-plasminogen complex using gel electrophoresis.

In the case of the plasminogen component of the complex, TAYLOR and BOTTS (1968) demonstrated that the conversion of plasminogen to plasmin involved the formation of an 8000 molecular weight fragment. Further work has demonstrated that this initial fragment is cut from the glu-N-terminal of plasminogen and leaves a lys-N-terminal (WIMAN and WALLÉN, 1973; WALTHER et al., 1974). A second step produces a heavy and light chain which are held together by disulfide bonds.

In the case of SK-plasminogen complexes formed wherein all the plasminogen molecules are saturated with SK (i.e., SK-plasminogen activator complex) the degradation of plasminogen and degradation of the plasminogen moiety occurs in a different sequence with formation of heavy and light chains *before* the initial 8000 molecular weight peptide is produced (MCCLINTOCK et al., 1974). In the case of the streptokinase component of the complex, it has been shown that the degradation of streptokinase involves a number of steps. TAYLOR and BEISSWENGER (1973) isolated an early breakdown product from the complex with a molecular weight of 40000 which appeared within the first 2 min following complex formation. BROCKWAY and CASTELLINO (1974) found a partially degraded fragment of 36000 molecular weight at the end of 5 min. Both these findings are consistent with the scheme for SK breakdown proposed by MCCLINTOCK et al. (1974) wherein SK goes from its native weight of 47000 to 43000 and then to 37000 by sequential cleavages.

References

Astrup,T., Müllertz,S.: Fibrin plate method for estimating fibrinolytic activity. Arch. Biochem.
    40, 346 (1952)
Bangham,D.R., Walton,P.L.: The international standard for streptokinase-streptodornase. Bull.
    Wld Hlth Org. **33**, 235 (1965)
Blatt,W.F., Segal,H., Gray,J.L.: Purification of streptokinase and human plasmin and their
    interaction. Thrombos. Diathes. haemorrh. (Stuttg.) **11**, 393 (1966)
Brockway,W.J., Castellino,F.,J.: A characterization of native streptokinase and altered strepto-
    kinase isolated from a human plasminogen activator complex. Biochemistry **13**, 2063 (1974)
Chase,T.Jr., Shaw,E.: Comparison of esterase activities of trypsin, plasmin and thrombin on
    guanidinobenzoate esters. Titration of the enzymes. Biochemistry **8**, 2212 (1969)
Christensen,L.R.: Protamine purification of streptokinase and effect of pH and temperature on
    reversible inactivation. J. gen. Physiol. **30**, 465 (1947)
Christensen,L.R.: Methods for measuring activity of components of streptococcal fibrinolytic
    system, and streptococcal desoxyribonuclease. J. clin. Invest. **28**, 1963 (1949)
Davies,M., Englert,M., DeRenzo,E.: Interaction of streptokinase and human plasminogen. I.
    Combining of streptokinase and plasminogen observed in the ultracentrifuge under a variety
    of experimental conditions. J. biol. Chem. **239**, 2651 (1964)
Derechin,M.: Hydrolysis of some casein fractions with plasmin. Biochemistry **82**, 42 (1962)
DeRenzo,E.C., Boggiano,E., Barg,W.F., Buck,F.F.: Interaction of streptokinase and human
    plasminogen. IV. Further gel electrophoretic studies on the combination of streptokinase
    with human plasminogen or human plasmin. J. biol. Chem. **242**, 2428, (1967a).
DeRenzo,E.C., Siiteri,P.K., Hutching,B.L., Bell,P.H.: Preparation and certain properties of
    highly purified streptokinase. J. biol. Chem. **242**, 533 (1967b)
Deutsch,D.G., Mertz,E.T.: Plasminogen: purification from human plasma by affinity chroma-
    tography. Science **170**, 1095 (1970)
Dillon,H.C., Wanamaker,L.W.: Physical and immunological differences among streptokinase. J.
    exp. Med. **121**, 351 (1965)
Fletcher,A.P., Johnson,A.J.: Methods employed for purification of streptokinase. Proc. Soc. exp.
    Biol. (N.Y.) **94**, 233 (1957)
Johnson,A.J., McCarty,W.R., Tillet,W.S., Tse,A.O., Skoza,L., Newman,J.. Semar,M.:
    Blood coagulation, hemorrhage and thrombosis, p. 449, New York: Grune and Stratton
    1964
Kline,D.L., Fishman,J.B.: Improved procedure for the isolation of human plasminogen. J. biol.
    Chem. **236**, 2807 (1961)
Markus,G., Werkheiser,W.: The interaction of streptokinase with plasminogen. I. Functional
    properties of the activated enzyme. J. biol. Chem. **239**, 2637 (1964)
McClintock,D.K., Bell,P.H.: The mechanism of activation of human plasminogen by streptoki-
    nase. Biochem. biophys. Res. Commun. **43**, 694 (1971)
McClintock,D.K., Englert,M.E., Dziobkowski,C., Snedeker,E.K., Bell,P.H.: Two distinct path-
    ways of the streptokinase mediated activation of highly purified human plasminogen. Bio-
    chemistry **13**, 5334 (1974)
Milstone,H.: Factor in normal human blood which participates in streptococcal fibrinolysis. J.
    Immunol. **42**, 109 (1941)
Morgan,F.J., Henschen,A.: The structure of streptokinase. I. Cyanogen bromide fragmentation,
    amino acid composition and partial amino acid sequences. Biochim. biophys. Acta (Amst.)
    181, 93 (1969)
Reddy,K.N.N., Markus,G.: Mechanism of activation of human plasminogen by streptokinase.
    Presence of active center in streptokinase-plasminogen complex. J. biol. Chem. **247**, 1683
    (1972)
Reddy,K.N.N., Markus,G.: Esterase activities in the zymogen moiety of the streptokinase-
    plasminogen complex. J. biol. Chem. **249**, 4851 (1974)
Remmert,F.L., Cohen,P.O.: Partial purification and properties of proteolytic enzyme of human
    serum. J. biol. Chem. **181**, 431 (1949)
Roberts,P.S.: The esterase activities of human plasmin during purification and subsequent acti-
    vation by streptokinase or glycerol. J. biol. Chem. **235**, 2262 (1960)

Schick, L. A., Castellino, F. J.: Direct evidence for the generation of an active site in the plasminogen moiety of the streptokinase-human plasminogen activator complex. Biochem. Biophys. Res. Commun. **57**, 47 (1974)

Summaria, L., Ling, C., Groskopf, W. R., Robbins, K. C.: The active site of bovine plasminogen activator. Interaction of streptokinase with human plasminogen and plasmin. J. biol. Chem. **243**, 144 (1968)

Taylor, F. B., Beisswenger, J. G.: Identification of modified streptokinase as the activator of bovine and human plasminogen. J. biol. Chem. **248**, 1127 (1973)

Taylor, F. B., Botts, J.: Purification and characterization of streptokinase with studies of streptokinase activation of plasminogen. Biochemistry **7**, 232 (1968)

Tillett, W. S., Garner, R. L.: Fibrinolytic activity of hemolytic streptococci. J. exp. Med. **58**, 485 (1933)

Tomar, R. H.: Streptokinase: preparation, comparison with streptococcal proteinase, and behavior as a trypsin substrate. Proc. Soc. exp. Biol. (N. Y.) **127**, 239 (1968)

Walther, P. J., Steinman, H. M., Hill, R. L., McKee, P. A.: Activation of human plasminogen by urokinase. Partial characterization of pre-activation peptide. J. biol. Chem. **249**, 1173 (1974)

Wiman, B., and Wallén, P.: Activation of human plasminogen by an insoluble derivative of urokinase. Structural changes of plasminogen in the course of activation to plasmin and demonstration of a possible intermediate compound. Europ. J. Biochem. **36**, 25 (1973)

Pharmacology of Streptokinase

H.-P. KLÖCKING

A. Characteristics and Requirements for Pharmacological Examination

As early as 1933, β-hemolytic streptococci were found to secrete into the culture medium a substance able to dissolve fibrin clots (TILLET and GARNER, 1933). Since this substance, now known as streptokinase, represented a potential thrombolytic agent, the possibility of its use in human therapy attracted growing interest. In the early sixties, following extensive studies in this field, streptokinase was isolated in a highly purified form that was suitable for therapeutic use (for review see MARK-WARDT et al., 1972; BROGDEN et al., 1973).

Prior to clinical use of streptokinase, however, animal experiments had to be designed for the determination of toxicity, pharmacodynamics, pharmacokinetics, and thrombolytic action of a variety of preparations. Because of the mode of action and the protein character of the agent, the pharmacotoxicological examination of streptokinase preparations required that certain criteria be observed and taken into consideration, such as the variability of reaction of the fibrinolytic system of experimental animals, the formation of plasminogen activator, the formation of antistreptokinase, and the generation of pyrogenic substances.

I. Selection of Experimental Animals

The activation of the fibrinolytic system by streptokinase varies between different animal species (Table 1). In addition to human plasminogen, streptokinase also activates plasminogen of dog, rabbit, cat, and monkey. In contrast to the action of streptokinase in human blood, rabbits are able to form activator only by interaction of streptokinase with rabbit plasminogen and not with rabbit plasmin. Plasminogen of rat, mouse, guinea pig, hamster, pig, sheep, cattle, and horse is not activated by streptokinase alone. However, plasminogen from these animals can be activated after the addition of small amounts of human plasminogen (in purified form, or as human plasma or human serum) (Fig. 1).

The activation of bovine plasminogen by the streptokinase-human plasminogen complex (SHERRY, 1954; ABLONDI and HAGAN, 1957; KLINE and FISHMAN, 1964; LING et al., 1967) depends on the presence of small amounts of human plasmin, as was demonstrated by REDDY and KLINE (1975). Plasminogen of frog, fish and turkey (and other wild and domestic birds) is not activated by streptokinase either alone or with the addition of human plasminogen (NIEWIAROWSKI and LATALLO, 1959). There is no evidence of a fibrinolytic mechanism in the blood of reptiles (HAWKEY, 1970).

Table 1. Response of various animal plasminogens to
activation with streptokinase

Species	Activation	References
Dog	+	1, 3, 4, 7, 10, 13, 18, 24
Rabbit	+	2, 4, 7, 11, 13, 19, 22
Cat	+	1, 8, 9, 13, 17, 18, 24
Monkey	+	1, 4, 6, 15, 18, 24
Rat	−	17, 18, 24
Mouse	−	14, 18
Guinea pig	−	5, 16, 18
Hamster	−	18
Pig	−	18, 24
Sheep	−	18, 23, 24
Cattle	−	12, 17, 18, 20, 21
Horse	−	10, 18

1. BAILLIE and SIM, 1971
2. CHATTOPADHYAY and CLIFFTON, 1965
3. CLIFFTON and CANNAMELA, 1953
4. CLIFFTON and DOWNIE, 1950
5. GEIGER, 1952
6. HAMPTON and MATTHEWS, 1966
7. HAYASHI and MAEKAWA, 1954
8. HIEMEYER and RASCHE, 1966
9. HIEMEYER and RASCHE, 1967
10. IRFAN, 1968
11. JOHNSON and TILLET, 1952
12. KLINE and FISHMAN, 1957
13. KLÖCKING and MARKWARDT, 1969
14. MARTIN et al., 1965
15. McKEE et al., 1971
16. MEYER, 1957
17. MOHLER et al., 1958
18. NIEWIAROWSKI and LATALLO, 1959
19. SCHICK and CASTELLINO, 1973
20. SHERRY, 1954
21. SHERRY and ALKJAERSIG, 1957
22. SODETZ et al., 1972
23. WARREN, 1964
24. WULF and MERTZ, 1969

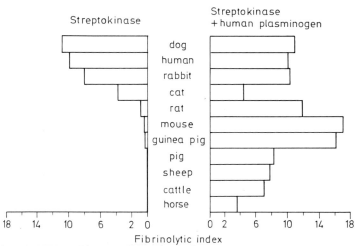

Fig. 1. Activation of the fibrinolytic system in animal plasma by streptokinase or streptokinase + human plasminogen. The fibrinolytic activity is expressed as fibrinolytic index $\left(F = \dfrac{1000}{t}; \text{lysis time in sec}\right)$

WULF and MERTZ (1969) divided the commonly used animals into three groups according to the degree of plasminogen activation by streptokinase: a) animals whose plasminogen is activated with small amounts of streptokinase (cat, monkey), b) animals requiring large amounts of streptokinase (dog, rabbit), c) animals whose plasminogen cannot be activated with streptokinase (cattle, sheep, mouse, rat).

In the past, the poor activation of animal plasminogen by streptokinase was thought to be due to the absence of proactivator in different animal species (ASTRUP, 1956; MÜLLERTZ, 1956). According to more recent findings, however, this poor activation is believed to be caused by a lack of complex formation between streptokinase and animal plasminogen (DOLESCHEL and AUERSWALD, 1967), or by the instability of animal plasminogen activator complexes (SCHICK and CASTELLINO, 1973). Obviously, the inhibitor level in plasma also plays a role. The content of plasmin inhibitors in the serum of alligators, guinea pigs, rats, pigs, and goats is very high, but it is very low in horse serum (GUEST et al., 1948; BLIX, 1964; CLIFFTON and MOOTSE, 1967). In recognition of the above-mentioned characteristics, therefore, only rabbits, dogs, cats and monkeys are likely to be suitable for experimental investigations of streptokinase.

II. Formation of Plasminogen Activator

The amount of plasmin formed by the action of streptokinase depends upon the streptokinase/plasminogen ratio (MARKWARDT et al., 1972). According to the mechanisms described (see p.146), the plasminogen in blood is converted in dependence on the streptokinase dose: at low and medium doses into plasmin and plasminogen activator, at high doses only into plasminogen activator. The fibrinolytic activity resulting from increasing concentrations of streptokinase runs through a maximum (Fig. 2) (MARKWARDT et al., 1976). When estimated by means of lysis time, the

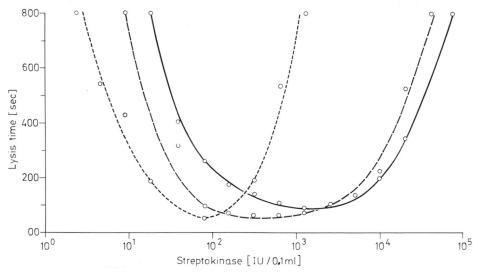

Fig. 2. Dependence of lysis time (plasma lysis test; human [- - -], dog [- - -], rabbit [———] plasma) on the streptokinase concentration (MARKWARDT et al., 1976)

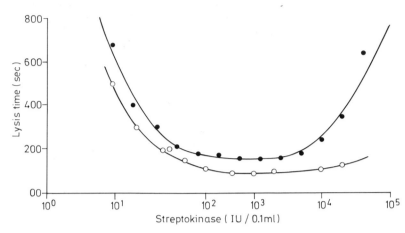

Fig. 3. Dependence of lysis times (plasma lysis test; rat [○], horse [●] plasma +5% of human serum each) on the streptokinase concentration (KLÖCKING, 1976b)

activity reaches its maximum at 100–500 IU streptokinase/ml rabbit plasma and 500–2500 IU streptokinase/ml dog plasma. Further increases in streptokinase concentration cause the fibrinolytic activity to decrease again (Fig. 2). In rat or horse plasma (Fig. 3) such activation curves are obtained only when 5% of human serum is added as human plasminogen source (KLÖCKING, 1976b; MARKWARDT et al., 1976).

III. Formation of Antistreptokinase

One year after the fibrinolytic action of streptokinase had been discovered (TILLET and GARNER, 1933), TILLET et al. (1934) described the inhibition of streptokinase by antibodies. Antibodies against streptokinase were found to form following streptococcal infection, or after treatment with streptokinase. They neutralize administered streptokinase by inactive complex formation. Such fibrinolytically inactive streptokinase-antibody complexes are very rapidly eliminated from the circulation (FLETCHER et al., 1958). The precipitating antibodies against streptokinase were shown to be antibodies of the IgG class (SPÖTTL and KAISER, 1974). In rabbits, the loss of efficacy from binding to streptokinase antibodies may amount to 20% of an administered dose (KLÖCKING et al., 1975); in dogs it amounts on average to 275 Christensen units streptokinase/ml plasma (TSAPOGAS et al., 1962). After repeated daily single intravenous streptokinase doses, as used for the dissolution of experimentally produced thrombi, a demonstrable increase in the antistreptokinase titer was observed in rabbits six days after the first administration (Fig. 4) (KLÖCKING and MARKWARDT, 1976). Also in rabbits, subcutaneous injection twice weekly of 50000 units of streptokinase in Freund's adjuvant produced an antistreptokinase titer of up to 11400. When given streptokinase, rabbits immunized in this way showed a clear rise in body temperature. The onset of fever could not be prevented by pretreatment with high-titer gammaglobulin, antihistaminic agents (pheniramine), or hydrocortisone (RONNEBERGER, 1975). After neutralization of the streptokinase antibodies by streptokinase, additional streptokinase doses did not produce fever. Besides the fact

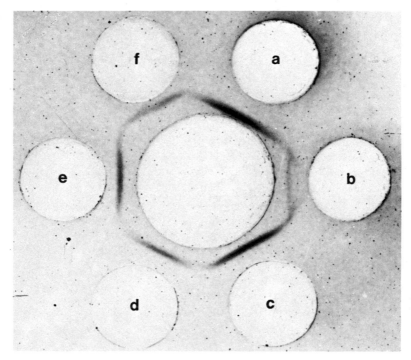

Fig. 4. Demonstration of antistreptokinase after administration of 30000 IU streptokinase/kg/day in rabbits over 6 days. 10 μl antigen solution (= 100 IU streptokinase) was pipetted into the central well and 30 μl serum each into the surrounding wells; *a* undiluted; *b* 1:2; *c* 1:4; *d* 1:8; *e* 1:16; *f* 1:32 (Klöcking and Markwardt, 1976)

that the fibrinolytic action of streptokinase depends on the level of prevailing antistreptokinase titers, the antigen-antibody reaction may in itself impair the effect of streptokinase on plasminogen activation.

IV. Formation of Pyrogenic Substances

As was demonstrated in studies on thrombolysis with streptokinase in rabbits, the dissolution of fibrin thrombi may be accompanied by formation of pyrogenic substances, leading to a rise in body temperature (Ronneberger, 1975). The results of conventional pyrogen tests might thus be distorted by the appearance of pyrogens in the course of streptokinase infusions.

B. Toxicity

The characteristics described above (A. I–IV) for the action of streptokinase in animals make it clear that only those species whose plasminogen is activated by streptokinase (rabbit, cat, dog, monkey) are suitable for toxicological examinations of the agent. The determination of acute toxicity in mice and rats does not represent the actual streptokinase action, because their plasminogen is not activated by streptokinase. When these animals are used for toxicological examinations, only the presence of toxic impurities in a given streptokinase preparation can be detected. Therefore, toxicological examinations should be performed in animals whose plasminogen responds to activation by streptokinase. Subacute or chronic administration cannot be utilized because of the antigen-antibody reaction (KLÖCKING and MARKWARDT, 1976). Streptokinase possesses a relatively low acute toxicity (TADOKORO et al., 1960; KLÖCKING, 1976a). After intravenous administration of the streptokinase preparation Awelysin, the acute toxicity (LD_{50}) was 3.7 g/kg in mice, and more than 2 g/kg in rats. This corresponds to a streptokinase dose of 6 000 000 IU/kg, or 1000 times the usual therapeutic dose (MARKWARDT and KLÖCKING, 1976). After intravenous injection of the streptokinase preparation Varidase the acute LD_{50} in mice was 4 789 000 units/kg, and after subcutaneous administration 16 450 000 units/kg. Oral doses of 18 750 000 units/kg were survived by mice. After administration of higher doses histological alterations were observed in the liver and kidneys (TADOKORO et al., 1960). Toxicological examinations of Awelysin in rhesus monkeys revealed that 10 times the therapeutic dose was tolerated without perceptible side effects (MARKWARDT and KLÖCKING, 1976).

C. Pharmacodynamics

The fibrinolytic action of streptokinase has been thoroughly investigated, but little is known about its general pharmacological effects.

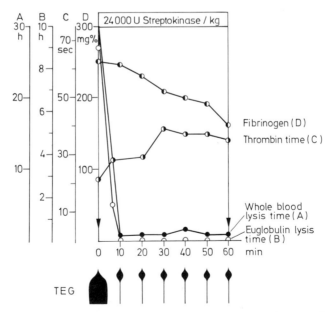

Fig. 5. Production of a hyperfibrinolytic state by streptokinase infusion (400 IU/kg/min) to rabbits; *A* whole blood lysis time in h (●); *B* euglobulin lysis time in h (○); *C* thrombin time in sec (◐); *D* fibrinogen in mg/100 ml (◑); *TEG* thrombelastograms from native blood (MARKWARDT et al., 1972)

I. Fibrinolytic Effect

Streptokinase owes its existence to its fibrinolytic efficacy. The relationship between streptokinase doses and fibrinolytic activity is shown in Figure 2. Fibrinolytic activity in blood was induced by streptokinase infusion to rabbits (MILLER et al., 1959; CHATTOPADHYAY and CLIFFTON, 1965; MARKWARDT and KLÖCKING, 1965 and 1966; KLÖCKING and MARKWARDT, 1969), cats (MOOTSE et al., 1965; HIEMEYER and RASCHE, 1966), dogs (TAYLOR et al., 1963), and monkeys (GROSS et al., 1960). Extensive fibrinolysis was produced in rabbits by intravenous infusion of 400 units streptokinase/kg/min over a period of 60 min (Fig. 5). Whole blood and euglobulin lysis times were shortened, the fibrinogen level was decreased, and the thrombin time was prolonged. Induced lysis can also be estimated by thrombelastograms of whole blood (KLÖCKING and MARKWARDT, 1969). Streptokinase administered to rabbits was found to cause a marked potentiation of thrombin-mediated platelet aggregation (Fig. 6), most probably resulting from the action of fibrinogen degradation products (GUREWICH and THOMAS, 1970).

II. Effects on Smooth Muscle, Heart and Circulation

In anesthetized dogs and rabbits, intravenous administration of up to 200000 IU streptokinase/kg (preparation Awelysin) had no effect on blood pressure and respiration (KLÖCKING, 1976a). Administration of 650000–6250000 units streptokinase/kg (preparation Varidase) produced accelerated respiration and a rise in blood pressure. These effects could not be prevented by vagotomy or administration of benzoylimidazoline (TADOKORO et al., 1960). On the isolated guinea-pig heart in a Langendorff preparation, the addition of streptokinase did not influence the positive inotropic effect of histamine (FISCHER, 1969).

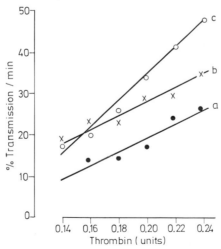

Fig. 6. Aggregation of platelet-rich plasma measured by the initial rate of change per minute of light transmission with increasing doses of thrombin. Blood samples taken *a* before, *b* 45 min after and *c* 15 min after administration of streptokinase. Each point represents the mean reading from the rabbits which showed a potentiating effect following administration of streptokinase (GUREWICH and THOMAS, 1970)

Besides its fibrinolytic effect, streptokinase is thought to possess antianaphylactic properties (FISCHER, 1969). In the isolated guinea-pig ileum, streptokinase inhibited the histamine action in a dose-dependent manner. Two hundred units of streptokinase reduced histamine-induced contractions by about 50%; after administration of 800 units the inhibition was about 100%, whereas 3200 units produced insensitivity of the ileum to histamine for a prolonged period. However, streptokinase did not influence the effects of other smooth muscle-stimulating substances, such as acetylcholine and bradykinin.

Since plasmin converts the kallikreinogen of plasma into kallikrein (LEVIS, 1958; BACK et al., 1963; EISEN, 1963; VOGT, 1964; BULUK et al., 1965; HAUSTEIN and MARKWARDT, 1965), kinins are liberated during streptokinase infusion (LEGER et al., 1960; EISEN, 1963; FISCHER and UDERMANN, 1970). This was believed to cause the fall in blood pressure observed in patients undergoing streptokinase therapy (FISCHER and UDERMANN, 1970). However, kinin liberation is dependent on the streptokinase dose. Low doses generated a large amount of plasmin and strong kinin liberation, whereas high doses produced a proteolytically ineffective activator which appeared to be unable to liberate kinin (FISCHER and UDERMANN, 1970).

Collagenolytic effects of streptokinase in rats have been described (SCHMALISCH, 1968). According to these studies, streptokinase is believed to cause cleavage of tropocollagen.

D. Pharmacokinetics

The study of the thrombolytic effect of streptokinase preparations requires an understanding of its pharmacokinetics. The course of the blood level is of special importance, since blood is both the transport organ and the site of action. Investigations of the pharmacokinetics of streptokinase with native and with ^{131}I- or ^{99m}Tc-labeled streptokinase have been carried out in rabbits (LUDWIG, 1966; KLÖCKING et al., 1975), cats (RASCHE et al., 1969), dogs (BACK et al., 1961; COATES et al., 1973 and 1975; GOODMAN et al., 1973; SOM et al., 1975), mice (COATES et al., 1973 and 1975; SOM et al., 1975), and rats (LUDWIG, 1966).

I. Native Streptokinase

Blood levels of streptokinase after intravenous administration can be monitored indirectly by determination of the fibrinolytic activity of the blood, i.e., by measuring the lysis time in plasma samples (MARKWARDT and KLÖCKING, 1976). After intravenous injection of 30000 IU streptokinase/kg to rabbits, lysis time shortened to 10 min with a return to the pretreatment value (>24 h) (Fig. 7). An effective level necessary for thrombolysis was maintained for a longer period by a single priming dose followed by intravenous infusion (KLÖCKING et al., 1975).

II. Radiolabeled Streptokinase

The curves of the effective fibrinolytic blood level are of importance for therapeutic purposes, but they give no information about the actual streptokinase concentrations. To obtain information about the amount and fate of streptokinase in blood and several organs, ^{131}I- and ^{99m}Tc-streptokinase was used.

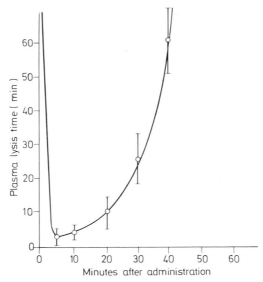

Fig. 7. Course of fibrinolytic activity in rabbit plasma (plasma lysis test) following i.v. administration of 30000 IU streptokinase/kg (MARKWARDT and KLÖCKING, 1976)

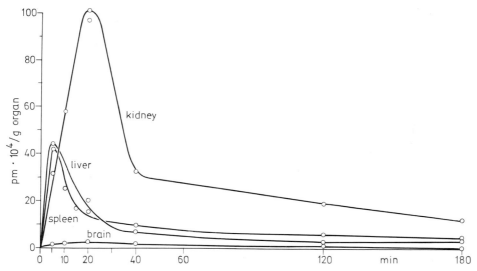

Fig. 8. Course of distribution of radioactivity following intravenous administration of 50 µCi ^{131}I-streptokinase/kg in rabbits (KLÖCKING et al., 1975)

Rabbit: After intravenous injection of ^{131}I-streptokinase a biphasic exponential decrease in radioactivity was measured in the blood. After rapid distribution elimination proceeded, with a half-life of 300 min. In the liver and kidneys a transient accumulation of radioactivity occurred (Fig. 8). The activity reached a maximum in the liver after 4 min and in the kidneys after 20 min. Thereafter, an increased excretion of radioactivity in the urine was observed, attaining 45% at 24 h and consisting mainly of fibrinolytically inactive low-molecular-weight fragments. The biliary excretion of streptokinase amounted to about 0.05% of the administered radioactivity, and this was found also in the feces (KLÖCKING et al., 1975). Studies on the distribution of ^{131}I-streptokinase in pregnant rabbits showed a transient accumulation of radioactivity in the spleen, the thyroid, and the uterine wall. Streptokinase does not readily cross the placental barrier. However, when 50 times the therapeutic dose of streptokinase was given, 10% of streptokinase circulating in the blood of the pregnant animal was found in the fetus (LUDWIG, 1966), indicating dose-dependency.

Cat: After intravenous injection of ^{131}I-streptokinase to cats, the radioactivity in the blood declined sharply. After 10–20 min only 50% of the initial activity (as measured 3 min after injection) was found. The activity detected in the urine after 4 h was equal to 13% of the administered dose. At this time, none of the organs investigated (thyroid, kidneys, liver, lungs, spleen, heart, aorta, and muscle) contained streptokinase (RASCHE et al., 1969).

Dog: After intravenous injection of ^{131}I-streptokinase to dogs the plasma clearance exhibited a biphasic course with half-lives of 15–20 min for the rapid phase and 160–200 min for the slow phase. The clearance of the protein-bound radioactivity also occurred in two phases, with half-lives of 20–25 min for the rapid phase and 60–80 min for the slow phase, which represents 30% of the total radioactivity. Four hours after administration, 70% of the plasma radioactivity was found as free iodide. In the liver, the radioactivity reached a maximum 1 h after administration (COATES et al., 1975). GOODMAN (1973) reported a half-life of 90 min for the blood clearance of ^{131}I-streptokinase. Four hours after administration, 27% of the administered dose was excreted in the urine (SOM et al., 1975).

Mouse: Studies on the distribution of ^{131}I-streptokinase in mouse organs showed an early accumulation of radioactivity in the liver (COATES et al., 1973 and 1975). In contrast to the decrease in radioactivity in blood and liver, a remarkable increase was observed in stomach and intestine (COATES et al., 1975; SOM et al., 1975). No accumulation of radioactivity occurred in the gastrointestinal tract when ^{99m}Tc-streptokinase was used. This is explained by the different metabolic fate of differently labeled compounds (SOM et al., 1975). One hour after administration 7% of the given dose was excreted in the urine (SOM et al., 1975).

Rat: In rats, only the permeability of the placental barrier to streptokinase was investigated (LUDWIG, 1966), and it was shown that the placenta of rats was not readily crossed by streptokinase.

E. Thrombolytic Effect

To detect the thrombolytic effect of streptokinase, the dissolution of induced intravascular clots was studied in animal experiments (for review see SCHMIDT, 1963; SCHMUTZLER and KOLLER, 1965). Rabbits, cats and dogs were the animals most often used, but in special cases monkeys, guinea pigs, and mice were used. To produce thrombi, the vessel walls were irritated mechanically, electrically or chemically, or thromboplastic substances were injected (for production of experimental thrombosis see HENRY, 1962; JOHNSON, 1965). Attempts were made to dissolve with streptokinase a variety of thrombi in venous vessel segments, in arterial vessel segments, as well as diffuse microthrombi (Table 2). Thrombolysis was followed by macroscopic

Table 2. Animal experiments on the thrombolytic effect of streptokinase

Type of thrombus	Localization	Animal	Induction of thrombus	Monitoring of thrombus formation and of lysis	Streptokinase preparation	Dosage	Result	References
Venous clotting thrombus	External jugular vein	Rabbit	Stasis + thrombin injection (300 NIH-U) into an isolated segment	Visual inspection	Kabikinase (AB Kabi, Stockholm)	Infusion of 125000 or 250000 units over 180 min	Reduction of thrombus	SAILER and EBER, 1963
Venous clotting thrombus	External jugular vein	Rabbit	Stasis + thrombin injection (80 NIH-U) into an isolated segment	Measurement of the length of thrombus	Streptase (Behringwerke AG, Marburg/Lahn)	40 injections (1250 units each) over 2 days, or 20 injections (500 units each) over 2 days	Total lysis in 25% of the animals at both doses, thrombus reduction in 30% of the animals at lower dose, in 45% of the animals at higher dose	SANDRITTER et al, 1964
Venous clotting thrombus	Marginal ear vein	Rabbit	Stasis + thrombin injection (90 NIH-U) (for method see JESTÄDT and SCHLÜTER, 1964)	Visual inspection and continuous recording of the rectal temperature	Streptase (Behringwerke AG, Marburg/Lahn)	Daily infusion of 2000 units/kg over 360 min for 3 days	Total lysis and rise in body temperature between 2nd and 3rd days after thrombus induction in 66% of the animals	RONNEBERGER, 1975
Venous clotting thrombus	Jugular vein	Dog	Injection of dog blood + thrombin into an isolated segment	Determination of the volume of thrombus	Streptase (Behringwerke AG, Marburg/Lahn)	Local infusion of 90000–100000 units over 90–100 min	No significant difference from the control	EGEBLAD and BERTELSEN, 1969
Venous clotting thrombus	Jugular vein	Rat	Injection of human serum + stasis of an isolated segment	Visual inspection	Awelysin (VEB Arznei-mittelwerk Dresden)	Daily infusion of 2000 units/kg over 360 min for 3 days	Total lysis in 100% of the animals	MARKWARDT et al, 1976

Table 2 (continued)

Type of thrombus	Localization	Animal	Induction of thrombus	Monitoring of thrombus formation and of lysis	Streptokinase preparation	Dosage	Result	References
Venous clotting thrombus	Ear vein	Mouse	Stasis + current provocation (1.25 mA, 5 min); injection of human plasma (0.01 ml/g mouse) before induction of thrombus	Vital microscopic observation	Streptase (Behringwerke AG, Marburg/Lahn)	Hourly injection of 750 units/ml blood volume over 8 h	Total lysis in 85% of the animals	MARTIN et al., 1965
Venous deposition thrombus	Medial or marginal ear vein	Rabbit	Injury of the intima by sodium morrhuate	Trans-illumination	Varidase (Lederle Laboratories, Division of American Cyanamid Company)	Infusion of 35000–40000 units/kg/h over 8 h	Total lysis in 76% of the animals, partial lysis in 16% of the animals	JOHNSON and TILLET, 1952
Venous deposition thrombus	External jugular vein	Rabbit	Injury of the intima by Varicocid + stasis of a segment	Angiography	Awelysin (VEB Arzneimittelwerk Dresden); Kabikinase (Deutsche Kabi GmbH, München)	Initial dose 30000 units/kg i.v. and infusion of 400 units/kg/min over 180 min	Total lysis in 80% of the animals	MARKWARDT et al., 1976
Arterial clotting thrombus	Femoral artery	Dog	Stasis + thromboplastin injection into an isolated segment	Presence of pulse, histological examination	Varidase (Lederle Laboratories, Division of American Cyanamid Company)	250000 units i.v.	Total lysis in 50% of the animals	SHERRY et al., 1954
Arterial clotting thrombus	Femoral artery	Dog	Stasis + injection of homologous serum	Inspection, palpation, and arteriography	Kinalysin (Merck, Sharp & Dohme Ltd.)	Intraarterial infusion of 100000–200000 units over 180 min	Total lysis in 16–66% of the animals, partial lysis in 33–66% of the animals	TSAPOGAS et al., 1962

Thrombus	Animal	Thrombus production	Examination	Streptokinase	Dose	Result	Reference
Arterial clotting thrombus	Dog	Stasis + injection of homologous serum	Inspection, palpation, and arteriography		Intraarterial infusion of 25000–200000 units	Total lysis in 85% of the animals	TSAPOGAS, 1964
Arterial deposition thrombus	Dog	Electrical provocation (10 mA, 15 min)	Arteriography	Awelysin (VEB Arzneimittelwerk Dresden); Kabikinase (Deutsche Kabi GmbH, München)	Initial dose 96000 units/kg i.v. and infusion of 1200 units/kg/min over 180 min	Total lysis in 100% of the animals	MARKWARDT et al., 1976
Arterial deposition thrombus	Rabbit	Injury caused by insertion of a silk suture	Histological examination	Kabikinase (AB Kabi, Stockholm)	Infusion of 40000 units/h over 3 h	Total lysis in 80% of the animals	JØRGENSEN et al., 1971
Arterial deposition thrombus	Rabbit	Electrical provocation (5 mA, 3 min)	Rheography	Awelysin (VEB Arzneimittelwerk Dresden); Kabikinase (Deutsche Kabi GmbH, München)	Initial dose 30000 units/kg i.v. and infusion of 1200 units/kg/min over 80 min	Total lysis in 100% of the animals	MARKWARDT et al., 1976
Arterial deposition thrombus	Rat	Electrical provocation (5 mA, 3 min)	Rheography	Kabikinase (Deutsche Kabi GmbH, München)	Initial dose 13000 units/kg i.v. and infusion of 2500 units/kg/min over 50 min. Administration of 1.3 ml human citrated plasma/kg before streptokinase	Total lysis in 100% of the animals	MARKWARDT et al., 1976
Pulmonary embolus	Dog	^{131}I-labeled fibrin clot inserted via the inferior vena cava into circulation as pulmonary embolus	Determination of the weight of embolus, scintillation scanning	Varidase (Lederle Laboratories, Division of American Cyanamid Company)	Infusion of 450000 units over 6.5 h	Embolus reduced to 79% of initial weight	HUME et al., 1960

Table 2 (continued)

Type of thrombus	Localization	Animal	Induction of thrombus	Monitoring of thrombus formation and of lysis	Streptokinase preparation	Dosage	Result	References
Pulmonary embolus	Lungs	Dog	^{131}I-labeled fibrin clot inserted via the inferior vena cava into circulation as pulmonary embolus	Scintillation scanning	Varidase (Lederle Laboratories, Division of American Cyanamid Company); Streptokinase B (Merck, Sharp & Dohme)	Varidase: initial dose 5000 units i.v. and infusion of 10000 units/h over 6 h. Streptokinase B: infusion of 37000 units over 2 h and of 12000 units/h over 4 h; 3 h later infusion of 37000 units over 1 h and 12000 units/h over 13 h	No complete lysis	HUME, 1961
Pulmonary embolus	Lungs	Dog	^{131}I-labeled fibrin clot inserted via the inferior vena cava into circulation as pulmonary embolus	Determination of the weight of embolus	Streptokinase (Travenol Laboratories); Varidase (Lederle Laboratories, Division of American Cyanamid Company)	Injection (half of infusion dose, i.v.) and infusion of 100, 200, 300, or 400 units Travenol/ml plasma into the pulmonary artery, or 100, 200, 300, 400, or 500 units Varidase/ml plasma into the inferior vena cava over 5 h	Complete lysis in each group	HUME, 1964

Pulmonary embolus	Rabbit	Release of 1 or 2 blood clots produced in vitro into the lungs via the jugular vein	Determination of the weight of embolus	Streptokinase (Hoechst Pharmaceutical Company, Cincinnati, Ohio)	2000 units/kg i.v.	Significant acceleration of thrombolysis	GUREWICH and THOMAS, 1970
Pulmonary embolus	Rabbit	Release of 1 or 2 blood clots produced in vitro into the lungs via the jugular vein	Determination of the weight of embolus	Streptase (Behringwerke AG, Marburg/Lahn)	10 min after release of the 1st embolus and 5 min before release of the 2nd embolus, 500, 1000, 10000, or 50000 units/h infused over 2 h via the ear vein	Significant reduction of clot weight in each group	NOWAK and GUREWICH, 1974
Coronary thrombus	Dog	Electrical provocation (1 mA, 60 min)	Coronarography	Awelysin (VEB Arzneimittelwerk Dresden)	1, 4 or 24 h after thrombus induction, injection of 96000 units/kg i.v. and infusion of 1200 units/kg/min over 180 min	Recanalization of the right coronary artery if streptokinase was given not later than 4 h after thrombus induction	MARKWARDT et al., 1977
Coronary thrombus	Cat	Electrical provocation (3 mA, 30 sec)	Histological examination	Streptokinase	2, 12 or 24 h after thrombus induction, streptokinase infusion over 5 h	Reduction of the infarcted area by about 60% if streptokinase was given not later than 2 h after thrombus induction	HIEMEYER, 1970

Table 2 (continued)

Type of thrombus	Localization	Animal	Induction of thrombus	Monitoring of thrombus formation and of lysis	Streptokinase preparation	Dosage	Result	References
Micro-thrombi	Liver, lungs, spleen, kidneys	Rabbit	Administration of endotoxin twice within 24 h	Histological examination	Varidase (Lederle Laboratories, Pearl River, New York)	30 min after the 2nd endotoxin dose, 50000 units i.v. every 30 min up to clot lysis time of less than 30 min. Most animals required 100000 units of streptokinase	Bilateral renal cortical necrosis completely prevented, no evidence of reduced extent of thrombosis in the lungs, kidneys, liver and spleen	KLIMAN and McKAY, 1958
Micro-thrombi	Liver, spleen, lungs, kidneys	Dog	Acidosis produced by infusion of lactic acid	Histological examination	Streptase (Hoechst Pharmaceutical Co., Cincinnati, Ohio)	Initial dose 90000–250000 units i.v., infusion of two-thirds the initial dose for 3–4 h, additionally 1 ml/kg/h of human euglobulin fraction	Almost complete reduction of the number of microthrombi	BROERSMA et al., 1970; BROERSMA and MAMMEN, 1971

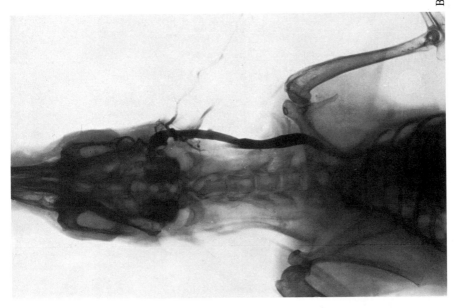

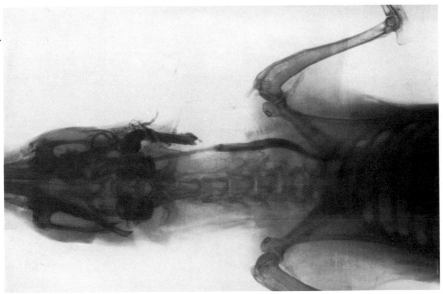

Fig. 9 A and B. Lysis of a venous clotting thrombus in rabbits. Angiography of the jugular vein (A) after thrombus induction, (B) 80 min after the beginning of streptokinase treatment (initial dose 30000 IU/kg i.v., and infusion of 400 IU/kg/min) (MARKWARDT et al., 1976)

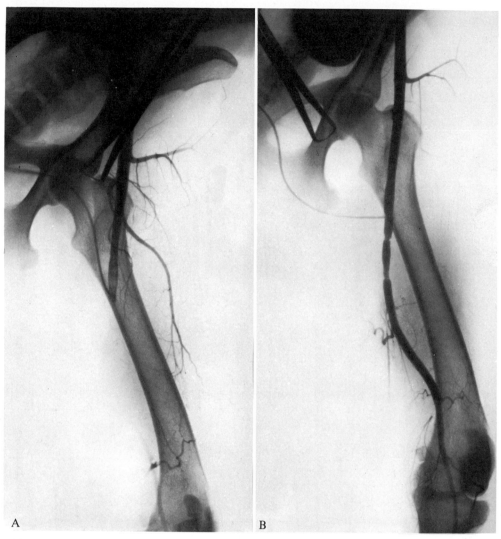

A   B

Fig. 10 A and B. Lysis of an arterial deposition thrombus in dogs. Angiography of the femoral artery (A) after thrombus induction, (B) 180 min after the beginning of streptokinase treatment (initial dose 96 000 IU/kg i.v., and infusion of 1200 IU/kg/min) (MARKWARDT et al., 1976)

observation, angiography and rheography, or the decrease in radioactivity of labeled thrombi was measured. Thrombolysis in animal experiments required high doses of streptokinase, far exceeding the clinico-therapeutic amounts. The dosages employed in animals cannot easily be applied to man, as is evident from the different activation characteristics of the fibrinolytic systems of man and animals (see Section A. 1).

In animal experiments, venous and arterial thrombi up to two days old were in general successfully dissolved by intravenous as well as by local administration of streptokinase (for example see Figs. 9 and 10). There are differences of opinion as to whether higher concentrations are necessarily required for the lysis of arterial as opposed to venous occlusions (SHERRY et al., 1954; GROSSI and CLIFFTON, 1955; FREIMANN et al., 1960).

Induced pulmonary emboli in dogs and rabbits were dissolved with streptokinase (Table 2). In spite of demonstrable clot lysis, however, pulmonary vascular resistance was not reduced in the streptokinase-treated animals (GUREWICH and THOMAS, 1970). These experimental observations serve to emphasize the importance of considering overall response rather than thrombolysis alone in the treatment of pulmonary embolism (THOMAS, 1965; MILLER et al., 1969).

Animal experiments were performed to estimate the efficacy of streptokinase in thrombotic occlusions of the coronary artery (HORT et al., 1966; HIEMEYER, 1970; WENDE et al., 1975; MARKWARDT et al., 1977). When streptokinase infusion was started 2 h after clot formation in the coronary artery, the extent of infarction was clearly diminished, and pathological changes in the ECG showed early normalization. The thrombolytic effect was demonstrated by coronarography (Fig. 11). This beneficial effect was no longer observed when fibrinolytic therapy was started 24 h after the production of coronary thrombosis.

In addition, in myocardial infarction induced in dogs by ligature of a coronary artery, the infarcted area was reduced by streptokinase. This effect was attributed primarily to an improvement in myocardial microcirculation as a result of reduced blood viscosity during periods of decreased blood fibrinogen levels (WENDE et al., 1975). However, in myocardial infarction induced in rats by starch granules, no diminution of the infarcted area occurred after simultaneous administration of streptokinase and human plasma (HORT et al., 1966).

Microthrombosis occurring in endotoxin-induced disseminated intravascular coagulation (DIC) was reduced by streptokinase. Infusions of up to 100000 units per animal after the endotoxin injection prevented bilateral renal cortical necrosis. There was no evidence for the reduction in the extent of thrombosis in the lungs, kidneys, liver, and spleen. However, intravenous injections of 100000–150000 units 30 min after the first endotoxin injection led to a reduction in the number of thrombi in these organs (KLIMAN and MCKAY, 1958).

In experimentally produced hemorrhagic shock in dogs and cats, survival was significantly prolonged when streptokinase was given during the shock phase prior to retransfusion of blood (ENCKE et al., 1966; ENCKE, 1969; LASCH and NEUHOF, 1969).

In animal experiments, an accelerated absorption of hyphema produced by autologous blood was demonstrated after administration of streptokinase into the anterior chamber of the eye (LOHSE and KRAUSE, 1972).

DOROBISZ et al. (1969) attempted to answer the important question as to whether and when postoperative fibrinolysis causes secondary hemorrhage through the walls of alloplastic prostheses. Experiments with dogs showed that the mesh of Dacron prostheses was quickly sealed by a developing thrombus, which remained securely in place even after administration of high doses of streptokinase. On the basis of these observations, the authors advocated early fibrinolytic therapy in thrombotic complications of alloplastic prosthesis implantation.

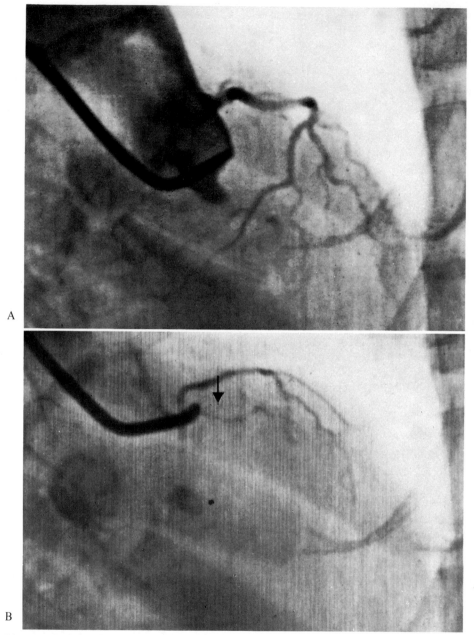

Fig. 11 A–D. Lysis of a coronary thrombus in dogs. Selective angiography of the right coronary artery (A) prior to thrombus induction, (B) 240 min after thrombus induction: (↓) thrombus (compensatory dilatation of the artery leading to the conus pulmonalis), (C) 110 min after the beginning of streptokinase infusion (incomplete recanalization of the right coronary artery, constriction of the peripheral vascular segment): (↓) thrombus, (D) 160 min after the beginning of streptokinase infusion (nearly complete recanalization of the right coronary artery, repatency of the peripheral vasculature, residual thrombotic material (↓), paravascular contrast medium (↑) (MARKWARDT et al., 1977)

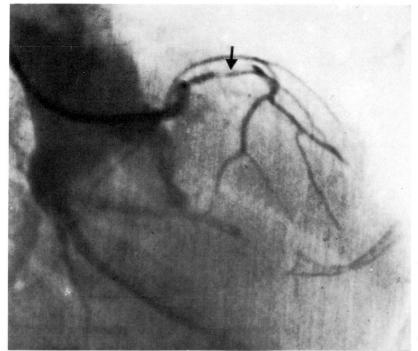

C

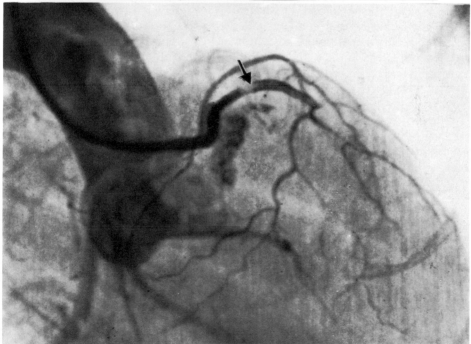

D

F. Clinical Pharmacology

The rational and successful therapeutic use of streptokinase in man requires knowledge of its pharmacokinetics.

As a protein, streptokinase is destroyed in the gastrointestinal tract after oral administration and is, therefore, not absorbed in active form. However, since oral administration of large amounts caused increased proteolytic activity in the urine of man, absorption of at least part of the streptokinase dose must have occurred (INNERFIELD et al., 1966). In practical therapy streptokinase is used only parenterally, mainly as intravenous injections or infusions.

Processes of different kinetics participate in the elimination of streptokinase in man (Fig. 12). Intravenously administered streptokinase is partly inactivated by binding to streptokinase antibodies (TILLET et al., 1934) and is accumulated in the liver (FLETCHER et al., 1958). Because of the high affinity and the rapid reaction between streptokinase and the antibody, small amounts are eliminated from the blood with a half-life of 18 min (FLETCHER et al., 1958). After saturation of antistreptokinase, the main portion of streptokinase interacts with plasminogen to form the activator of fibrinolysis (see p.146). The elimination of streptokinase as a consequence of activator formation occurs with a half-life of 83 min (FLETCHER et al., 1958). Most of the streptokinase is degraded and excreted through the kidneys as amino acids and peptides (SCHWICK, 1964).

After intravenous injection of ^{131}I-streptokinase the radioactivity in blood dropped sharply. After 30 min, 50% of the activity measured at the beginning of lysis was eliminated from the blood. The decrease in ^{131}I-activity in the blood did not run parallel with that of the biological effect of streptokinase (RASCHE et al., 1969). Fifteen to twenty min after administration of ^{131}I-streptokinase, the drug had accumulated in the liver with an activity peak at 20 min, accompanied by a continuous decrease in plasma. Immediately thereafter, the radiolabeled substances entered the extravascular space or were excreted in the urine (6% after 120 min) (PFEIFER et al., 1969a).

The activity measured over the liver was significantly higher than that measured over the heart or spleen, and it decreased gradually (PFEIFER et al., 1969a and b; RASCHE et al., 1969). In the second or third trimester of pregnancy only traces were found to enter the fetal circulation through the intact placenta. They did not suffice to activate the fibrinolytic system of the fetus (PFEIFER, 1965; PFEIFER et al., 1969b;

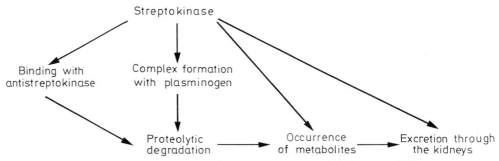

Fig. 12. Scheme of streptokinase elimination (MARKWARDT and KLÖCKING, 1976)

LUDWIG, 1969; PFEIFER, 1970). Treatment with streptokinase of the mother resulted in an increase in antistreptokinase which was transferred to the fetus. The amount of radiolabeled streptokinase entering the mother's milk was extremely low, being about 1/3000 of the amount which crosses the placenta (PFEIFER, 1965).

References

Ablondi, F. B., Hagan, J. J.: Comparison of certain properties of human plasminogen and "proactivator". Proc. Soc. exp. Biol. (N.Y.) **95**, 195 (1957)

Ambrus, J. L., Ambrus, C. M., Back, N., Sokal, J. F., Collins, G. L.: Clinical and experimental studies on fibrinolytic enzymes. Ann. N. Y. Acad. Sci. **68**, 97 (1957)

Astrup, T.: Fibrinolysis in the organism. Blood **11**, 781 (1956).

Back, N., Ambrus, J. L., Mink, J. B.: Distribution and fate of I^{131}-labeled components of the fibrinolysis system. Circulat. Res. **9**, 1208 (1961)

Back, N., Guth, P. S., Munson, A. E.: On the relationship between plasmin and kinin. Ann. N. Y. Acad. Sci. **104**, 53 (1963)

Baillie, A. J., Sim, A. K.: Activation of the fibrinolytic enzyme system in laboratory animals and in man. A comparative study. Thrombos. Diathes. haemorrh. (Stuttg.) **25**, 499 (1971)

Blix, S.: The stability of fibrinolytic inhibitors in human serum and the inhibitor content in animal sera. Scand. J. clin. Lab. Invest. **16**, 614 (1964)

Broersma, R. J., Bullemer, G. D., Mammen, E. F.: Acidosis induced disseminated intravascular microthrombosis and its dissolution by streptokinase. Thrombos. Diathes. haemorrh. (Stuttg.) **24**, 55 (1970)

Broersma, R. J., Mammen, E. F.: Streptokinase in experimental disseminated intravascular coagulation. Thrombos. Diathes. haemorrh. (Stuttg.) Suppl. **47**, 255 (1971)

Brogden, R. N., Speight, T. M., Avery, G. S.: Streptokinase: A review of its clinical pharmacology, mechanism of action and therapeutic uses. Drugs **5**, 353 (1973)

Buluk, K., Malofiejew, M., Czokalo, M.: Activation of fibrinolysis and of plasma-kinin system during venostasis. Thrombos. Diathes. haemorrh. (Stuttg.) **14**, 500 (1965)

Chattopadhyay, D. P., Cliffton, E. E.: Activation of rabbit plasminogen by streptokinase. Amer. J. Physiol. **208**, 190 (1965)

Cliffton, E. E., Cannamela, D. A.: Proteolytic and fibrinolytic activity of serum. Activation by streptokinase and staphylokinase indicating dissimilarities of enzymes. Blood **8**, 554 (1953)

Cliffton, E. E., Downie, G. R.: Variations in proteolytic activity of serum of animals including man. Proc. Soc. exp. Biol. (N. Y.) **73**, 559 (1950)

Cliffton, E. E., Mootse, G.: Species variations in fibrinolytic activity. Thrombos. Diathes. haemorrh. (Stuttg.) **18**, 291 (1967)

Coates, G., DeNardo, S. J., DeNardo, G. L.: Pharmacokinetics of radioiodinated streptokinase. J. nucl. Med. **14**, 623 (1973)

Coates, G., DeNardo, S. J., DeNardo, G. L., Troy, F. A.: Pharmacokinetics of radioiodinated streptokinase. J. nucl. Med. **16**, 136 (1975)

Doleschel, W., Auerswald, W.: Gel filtration studies of the complex forming capacity of streptokinase with human and heterologous plasminogens. Med. Pharm. exp. (Basel) **17**, 248 (1967)

Dorobisz, T., Kaszubkiewicz, C., Osinski, B., Palider, S., Palider-Zaleska, H., Samplawska, B.: Frühe Streptase-Anwendung nach Transplantation von alloplastischen Aortenprothesen bei Hunden. Zbl. Chir. Suppl. **93**, 167 (1969)

Egeblad, K., Bertelsen, S.: Experimental thrombolysis by perfusion. II. Comparative study on the effect of streptokinase, urokinase and plasmin. Acta chir. scand. **135**, 486 (1969)

Eisen, V.: Kinin formation and fibrinolysis in human plasma. J. Physiol. (Lond.) **166**, 514 (1963)

Encke, A.: Untersuchungen zur fibrinolytischen Behandlung des Schocks. Thrombos. Diathes. haemorrh. (Stuttg.) Suppl. **32**, 361 (1969)

Encke, A., Petrich, I., Schmidt, H. D., Schmier, J.: Der Einfluß einer Fibrinolysetherapie auf die Überlebensquote im normotensiven hämorrhagischen Schock. Langenbecks Arch. klin. Chir. **316**, 677 (1966)

Fischer, G.: Untersuchungen über einen Antihistamin-ähnlichen Effekt der Streptokinase am isolierten Meerschweinchen-Ileum. Arzneimittel-Forsch. **19**, 2017 (1969)

Fischer, G., Udermann, H.: Kininfreisetzung aus menschlichem Plasma durch Streptokinase. Arzneimittel-Forsch. **20**, 580 (1970)

Fletcher, A. P., Alkjaersig, N., Sherry, S.: The clearance of heterologous protein from circulation in normal and immunized man. J. clin. Invest. **37**, 1306 (1958)

Freimann, A. H., Bang, N. U., Cliffton, E. E.: Studies on the production of intravascular thrombi and their treatment with fibrinolysin. Circulat. Res. **8**, 409 (1960)

Geiger, W. B.: Involvement of a complement-like factor in the activation of blood protease. J. Immunol. **69**, 597 (1952)

Goodman, L. R., Goodman, C., Greenspan, R. H., Porter, C. D.: Failure to visualize experimentally produced emboli and thrombi using ^{131}I-streptokinase. Investigative Radiology **8**, 377 (1973)

Gottlob, R., Zinner, G.: Treatment of venous thrombosis by continuous local infusions of streptokinase. Experimental investigations. J. internat. Coll. Surg. **28**, 575 (1957)

Gross, R., Hartl, W., Kloss, G., Rahn, B.: Thrombolyse durch Infusion hochgereinigter Streptokinase: Erfahrungen und Untersuchungen an den ersten 50 Kranken. Dtsch. med. Wschr. **85**, 2129 (1960)

Grossi, C. E., Cliffton, E. E.: The lysis of arterial thrombi in rabbits and dogs by use of activated human plasminogen (fibrinolysin) (plasmin). Surgery **37**, 794 (1955)

Guest, M. M., Daly, B. M., Ware, A. G., Seegers, W. H.: A study of antifibrinolysin activity in the plasmas of various animal species. J. clin. Invest. **27**, 785 (1948)

Gurevich, V., Thomas, D. P.: Streptokinase in acute pulmonary embolism. An experimental study. J. thorac. cardiovasc. Surg. **59**, 655 (1970)

Hampton, J. W., Matthews, C.: Similarities between baboon and human blood clotting. J. appl. Physiol. **21**, 1713 (1966)

Haustein, K.-O., Markwardt, F.: Untersuchungen über die Freisetzung gefäßwirksamer Stoffe beim Ablauf der Gerinnungs- und Fibrinolysevorgänge im menschlichen Blut. Acta biol. med. germ. **15**, 386 (1965)

Hawkey, C. M.: Fibrinolysis in animals. Symp. Zool. Soc. **27**, 133 (1970)

Hayashi, T., Maekawa, S.: Studies on the activating factors in fibrinolytic systems. II. Streptococcal and staphylococcal fibrinolysis. Jap. J. Exp. Med. **24**, 287 (1954)

Henry, R. L.: Methods for inducing experimental thrombosis. Angiology **13**, 554 (1962)

Hiemeyer, V.: Die thrombolytische Therapie des Herzinfarktes. Thrombos. Diathes. haemorrh. (Stuttg.) Suppl. **38**, 249 (1970)

Hiemeyer, V., Rasche, H.: Der Mechanismus der streptokinaseinduzierten Thrombolyse und seine Bedeutung für die Therapie akuter Gefäßverschlüsse. Klin. Wschr. **44**, 539 (1966)

Hiemeyer, V., Rasche, H.: Vergleichende Untersuchungen zur Wirkung von Urokinase und Streptokinase im Tierversuch. Thrombos. Diathes. haemorrh. (Stuttg.) **17**, 58 (1967)

Hort, W., Poliwoda, H., DaCanalis, S., Knigge, J.: Untersuchungen über den Einfluß von Antikoagulantien und Fibrinolytika auf die Größe von Mikroinfarkten im Rattenherzen. Klin. Wschr. **44**, 215 (1966)

Hume, M.: Thrombolysis of the experimental radioactive pulmonary embolus. Its demonstration with the use of several agents. New Engl. J. Med. **264**, 471 (1961)

Hume, M.: Lysis of the experimental radioactive pulmonary embolus induced by streptokinase and streptokinase activated plasmin. Thrombos. Diathes. haemorrh. (Stuttg.) **11**, 99 (1964)

Hume, M., Glenn, W. W. L., Grillo, T.: Behavior in circulation of radioactive pulmonary embolus and its application to the study of fibrinolytic enzymes. Ann. Surg. **151**, 507 (1960)

Innerfield, I., Rowley, G., Zweil, P., Siew, C.: Urinary proteolytic activity following oral streptokinase. Enzym. biol. clin. **7**, 149 (1966)

Irfan, M.: Fibrinolytic activity in animals of different species. Quart. J. exp. Physiol. **53**, 374 (1968)

Jestädt, R., Schlüter, G.: Tierexperimentelle Untersuchungen zur percutanen Thrombolyse mit der neuen synthetischen Heparinoid-Salbe. Med. Welt (Stuttg.) **15**, 297 (1964).

Johnson, A. J.: Recent advances in experimental thrombogenesis. Fed. Proc. **24**, 827 (1965)

Johnson, A. J., Tillet, W. S.: Lysis in rabbits of intravascular blood clots by the streptococcal fibrinolytic system (streptokinase). J. exp. Med. **95**, 449 (1952)

Jørgensen, L., Hirsh, J., Glynn, M. F., Buhanan, M. R., Mustard, J. S.: Effect of streptokinase therapy on experimental fibrin-rich arterial thrombi. Amer. J. Path. **62**, 7 (1971)

Kliman, A., McKay, D. G.: The prevention of the generalized Shwartzman reaction by fibrinolytic activity. Arch. Path. **66**, 715 (1958)

Kline, D. L., Fishman, J. B.: Plasmin: The humoral protease. Ann. N. Y. Acad. Sci. **68**, 25 (1957)

Kline, D. L., Fishman, J. B.: Proactivator function of human plasmin as shown by lysine esterase assay. J. biol. Chem. **236**, 2907 (1964)

Klöcking, H.-P.: Zur Pharmakologie des Streptokinasepräparates Awelysin®. Folia haemat. (Lpz.) **103**, 445 (1976a)

Klöcking, H.-P.: Über die Aktivierung von Pferdeplasminogen durch Streptokinase. 1976b (unpublished)

Klöcking, H.-P., Markwardt, F.: Tierexperimentelle Verfahren zur Testung von Fibrinolytika und Antifibrinolytika. Folia haemat. (Lpz.) **92**, 84 (1969)

Klöcking, H.-P., Markwardt, F.: On toxicological examination of streptokinase preparations. III. Symposium on toxicological testing for safety of new drugs. Prague 1976, p. 67

Klöcking, H.-P., Senf, L., Drawert, J., Markwardt, F.: Tierexperimentelle Untersuchungen zur Pharmakokinetik von Streptokinase. Acta biol. med. germ. **34**, 655 (1975)

Lasch, H. G., Neuhof, H.: Die Fibrinolysebehandlung des Schocks. Thrombos. Diathes. haemorrh. (Stuttg.) Suppl. **32**, 355 (1969)

Leger, L., Lande, M., Vergoz, D.: Fibrinolyse au cours de la chirurgie des cirrhoses. J. Chir. (Paris) **80**, 155 (1960)

Levis, G. P.: Formation of plasma kinins by plasmin. J. Physiol. (Lond.) **140**, 285 (1958)

Ling, C., Summaria, L., Robbins, K. C.: Isolation and characterization of bovine plasminogen activator from a human plasminogen-streptokinase mixture. J. biol. Chem. **242**, 1419 (1967)

Lohse, K., Krause, A.: Vergleichende Untersuchungen über die Wirkung und Nebenwirkungen von Varidase und Streptase bei der Behandlung des Hyphaemas am Kaninchenauge. Wiss. Z. Univ. Halle, Reihe M, **21**, 59 (1972)

Ludwig, H.: Experimentelle Untersuchungen zum diaplazentaren Übertritt von Streptokinase. Geburtsh. u. Frauenheilk. **26**, 736 (1966)

Ludwig, H.: Streptokinase während der Gestation. Thrombos. Diathes. haemorrh. (Stuttg.) Suppl. **32**, 307 (1969)

Markwardt, F., Bernstein, K., Drawert, J., Eger, H., Klöcking, H.-P., Sedlarik, K., Vollmar, F., Wilde, J.: Thrombolytische Behandlung einer experimentellen Koronarthrombose mit Streptokinase. Exp. Path. (Jena) **14**, 76 (1977)

Markwardt, F., Klöcking, H.-P.: p-Aminomethylbenzoesäure (PAMBA), ein neues Antifibrinolytikum. Tierexperimentelle Untersuchungen. Münch. med. Wschr. **107**, 2000 (1965)

Markwardt, F., Klöcking, H.-P.: Tierexperimentelle Untersuchungen der Wirkung synthetischer Antifibrinolytika. Acta biol. med. germ. **17**, 746 (1966)

Markwardt, F., Klöcking, H.-P.: Pharmakologie des Streptokinasepräparates Awelysin®. Medicamentum **17**, 197 (1976)

Markwardt, F., Klöcking, H.-P., Sedlarik, K., Perlewitz, J., Drawert, J., Hoffmann, J.: Tierexperimentelle Untersuchungen zur thrombolytischen Wirkung von Streptokinase. Acta biol. med. germ. **35**, 193 (1976)

Markwardt, F., Landmann, H., Klöcking, H.-P.: Fibrinolytika und Antifibrinolytika. Jena: Fischer 1972, p. 46

Martin, M., Hiemeyer, V., Rasche, H.: Zur intravasalen Streptokinase-induzierten Thrombolyse bei der Maus. Vitalmikroskopische und gerinnungsphysiologische Beobachtungen. Thrombos. Diathes. haemorrh. (Stuttg.) **14**, 519 (1965)

McKee, P. A., Lemmon, W. B., Hampton, J. W.: Streptokinase and urokinase activation of human, chimpanzee and baboon plasminogen. Thrombos. Diathes. haemorrh. (Stuttg.) **26**, 512 (1971)

Meyer, W. E.: Proteolytic activity of guinea pig serum activated by streptokinase-human plasminogen preparations. Amer. J. Physiol. **190**, 303 (1957)

Miller, G. A. H., Gibson, R. V., Honey, M., Sulton G. C.: Treatment of pulmonary embolism with streptokinase. A preliminary report. Brit. med. J. **1969 I**, 812

Miller, J. M., Robinson, D. R., Jackson, D. A., Collier, C. S.: Reversal by ipsilon of lytic system in blood stream produced in rabbits by streptokinase. Arch. Surg. **78**, 33 (1959)

Mohler,S.R., Celander,D.R., Guest,M.M.: Distribution of urokinase among the common mammals. Amer. J. Physiol. **192**, 186 (1958)

Mootse,G., Fleming,L.B., Cliffton,E.E.: The mechanism of activation of cat plasma by streptokinase. Thrombos. Diathes. haemorrh. (Stuttg.) **14**, 562 (1965)

Müllertz,S.: Mechanism of activation and effect of plasmin in blood. Acta physiol. scand. Suppl. **38**, 130 (1956)

Niewiarowski,S., Latallo,Z.: Comparative studies of the fibrinolytic system of sera of various vertebrates. Thrombos. Diathes. haemorrh. (Stuttg.) **3**, 404 (1959)

Nowak,A., Gurewich,V.: Thrombolysis with streptokinase in rabbits. Dose response, fibrin-clot specificity and laboratory evaluation of fibrinolytic effect. Thrombos. Diathes. haemorrh. (Stuttg.) **31**, 265 (1974)

Pfeifer,G.W.: Experimentelle Untersuchungen zur Frage eines diaplacentaren Effektes von Streptokinase. Klin. Wschr. **43**, 775 (1965)

Pfeifer,G.W.: Distribution and placental transfer of ^{131}I-streptokinase. Aust. Ann. Med. 1970, Suppl., p. 17

Pfeifer,G.W., Doerr,F., Brod,K.-H.: Zur Pharmakokinetik von ^{131}J-Streptokinase am Menschen. Klin. Wschr. **47**, 482 (1969a)

Pfeifer,G.W., Doerr,F., Brod,K.-H., Berle,P., Dietz,M.: Verteilungsstudien zur Placentapassage von ^{131}J-Streptokinase unter der Geburt. Arch. Gynäk. **207**, 550 (1969b)

Rasche,H., Hiemeyer,V., Heimpel,H.: Verteilungsstudien mit radioaktiv markierter Streptokinase. Thrombos. Diathes. haemorrh. (Stuttg.) Suppl. **32**, 133 (1969)

Reddy,K.N.N., Kline,D.L.: Requirement of human plasmin for streptokinase activation of bovine plasminogen. Thrombos. Res. **6**, 481 (1975)

Ronneberger,H.: Zur gelegentlichen Temperaturerhöhung nach Streptokinase-Infusionen. Tierexperimentelle Befunde. Arzneimittel-Forsch. **25**, 641 (1975)

Sailer,S., Eber,O.: Tierexperimentelle Thrombolyseversuche mit direkt wirkenden Fibrinolytika. Klin. Wschr. **41**, 212 (1963)

Sandritter,W., Schlüter,G., Köppel,G.: Thrombolyse im Tierexperiment. Med. Welt (Stuttg.) 1964, II, 2732

Schick,L.A., Castellino,J.: Interaction of streptokinase and rabbit plasminogen. Biochemistry **12**, 4315 (1973)

Schmalisch,N.: Kollagenolytische Wirkung von Streptokinase. Verh. Dtsch. Ges. inn. Med. **74**, 595 (1968)

Schmidt,H.W.: Zur thrombolytischen Therapie mit Streptokinase. Dtsch. med. Wschr. **88**, 1407 (1963)

Schmutzler,R., Koller,F.: Die Thrombolyse-Therapie. Erg. Inn. Med. Kinderheilk. **22**, 157 (1965)

Schwick,G.: Biochemie der Fibrinolyse. Behringwerk-Mitt. **44**, 128 (1964)

Sherry,S.: The fibrinolytic activity of streptokinase activated human plasmin. J. clin. Invest. **33**, 1054 (1954)

Sherry,S., Alkjaersig,N.: Studies on the fibrinolytic enzyme of human plasma. Thrombos. Diathes. haemorrh. (Stuttg.) **1**, 264 (1957)

Sherry,S., Titchener,A., Gottesman,L., Wassermann,P., Troll,W.: The enzymatic dissolution of experimental arterial thrombi in the dog by trypsin, chymotrypsin and plasminogen activators. J. clin. Invest. **33**, 1303 (1954)

Sodetz,J.M., Brockway,W.J., Castellino,F.J.: Multiplicity of rabbit plasminogen. Physical characterization. Biochemistry **11**, 4451 (1972)

Som,P., Rhodes,B.A., Bell,W.R.: Radiolabeled streptokinase and urokinase and their comparative biodistribution. Thrombos. Res. **6**, 247 (1975)

Spöttl,F., Kaiser,R.: Rapid detection and quantitation of precipitating streptokinase-antibodies. Thrombos. Diathes. haemorrh. (Stuttg.) **32**, 608 (1974)

Tadokoro,S., Kurihara,Y., Shibata,K.: Pharmacological studies on streptokinase-streptodornase (Varidase), especially on its toxicity. Gunma J. med. Sci. **9**, 225 (1960)

Taylor,F.B.,Jr., Singleton,J., Bickford,A.F.,Jr.: In vivo activation of the fibrinolytic enzyme system of dogs. J. appl. Physiol. **18**, 334 (1963)

Thomas,D.P.: Treatment of pulmonary embolic disease: a clinical review of some aspects of current therapy. New Engl. J. Med. **273**, 885 (1965)

Tillet, W. S., Edwards, L. B., Garner, R. L.: Fibrinolytic activity of hemolytic streptococci. The development of resistance to fibrinolysis following acute hemolytic streptococcus infection. J. clin. Invest. **13**, 47 (1934)

Tillet, W. S., Garner, R. L.: The fibrinolytic activity of hemolytic streptococci. J. exp. Med. **68**, 488 (1933)

Tsapogas, M. J.: The role of fibrinolysis in the treatment of arterial thrombosis: experimental and clinical aspects. Ann. roy. Coll. Surg. **34**, 293 (1964)

Tsapogas, M. J., Flute, P. T.: Experimental thrombolysis with streptokinase and urokinase. Brit. med. Bull. **20**, 223 (1964)

Tsapogas, M. J., Flute, P. T., Cotton, L. T., Milroy, S. D.: Lysis of experimental thrombi by streptokinase. Brit. J. Surg. **50**, 334 (1962)

Vogt, W.: Kinin formation by plasmin, an indirect process mediated by activation of kallikrein. J. Physiol. (Lond.) **170**, 153 (1964)

Warren, B. A.: Fibrinolytic activity of vascular endothelium. Brit. med. Bull. **20**, 213 (1964)

Wende, W., Stühlen, H. W., Meyer, J., Bleifeld, W., Holzhüter, H., Wenzel, E.: Die Größe des akuten tierexperimentellen Herzinfarktes unter Streptokinase-induzierter Fibrinolyse. Klin. Wschr. **53**, 755 (1975)

Wulf, R. J., Mertz, E. T.: Studies on plasminogen. VIII. Species specificity of streptokinase. Canad. J. Biochem. **47**, 927 (1969)

Clinical Use of Streptokinase

G. VOGEL

The introduction of classic anticoagulants of the heparin type and of coumarin derivatives into clinical practice has greatly improved the treatment of thromboembolic diseases. These drugs, however, are predominantly suited for prophylaxis. In the case of established thrombosis, anticoagulants are used to prevent it from progressing. It is expected that they will promote the counterregulatory fibrinolysis of the organism. In this way, however, a thrombolytic effect occurs only in exceptional cases. The search for an effective treatment of thrombosis led to the development of thrombolytic agents, of which the most important is streptokinase.

Although spontaneous dissolution of blood clots has been known for centuries, it was not until 1905 that NOLF attempted to induce enhanced fibrinolysis for therapeutic purposes. TILLET and GARNER (1933) discovered that extracts from certain streptococcal strains produce fibrinolytic effects. Such preparations were first used exclusively to dissolve extravascular fibrin deposits (CATHIE and McFARLANE, 1954; CLIFFTON, 1954; TILLET et al., 1955). Intravenous administration of purified streptokinase preparations was first performed by TILLET et al. (1955). These preparations, however, were only partially purified, so that severe side-effects (fever, chills, collapse) frequently occurred. Preparations of higher purity were introduced by FLETCHER and JOHNSON (1957).

Among the various thrombolytic agents tested (plasminogen activated by streptokinase or trypsin, fungal proteases, urokinase), streptokinase in highly purified form is the one most widely used, and the number of patients treated is estimated at 100000.

A. Fundamentals of Clinical Use

I. Thrombolytic Effect

Streptokinase in sufficiently high doses dissolves thrombi. The morphologic alterations of the thrombus undergoing lysis were studied by SANDRITTER (1962), HARMS (1967), BLEYL (1969), and BENEKE (1971). According to these studies, alterations were perceptible at first only by electron microscopy. The transverse striation of the fibrin fiber disappeared, and longitudinal cleavage occurred. Subsequently, alterations appeared that were detectable by light microscopy. First, the structure became homogenous. Following this, the fibrin fibers disintegrated into coarse clumps, and then into small granules.

There are divergent opinions about the molecular biologic details of thrombolysis. SHERRY et al. (1959) believed that streptokinase enters the thrombus and activates the plasminogen contained therein. Plasmin formed in this way is thought to cause endogenous thrombolysis. AMBRUS et al. (1962) started with the assumption that following the administration of streptokinase plasmin is formed in the blood-stream which, however, immediately forms an inactive complex with antiplasmin. Because of the special affinity for fibrin, it was believed that the plasmin-antiplasmin complex is absorbed on the surface of the thrombus, and plasmin is split off. In this way, exogenous thrombolysis would be induced. According to DUDOK DE WIT (1962), streptokinase penetrates into the plasminogen-poor thrombus. Plasminogen from plasma is absorbed on the thrombus, and is activated to plasmin, which also leads to exogenous lysis. OGSTON et al. (1966) believed that plasminogen is not only absorbed, but that it is also capable of diffusing into the thrombus. Thus, in the marginal area of the thrombus, exogenous as well as endogenous lyses occur. GOTTLOB and BLÜMEL (1966) assumed that streptokinase first diffuses into the thrombus and inactivates the plasmin inhibitors. Subsequently, small amounts of plasminogen contained in the thrombus are activated to plasmin, which is especially effective in the inhibitor-free thrombus. Up to now, there is no evidence of the validity of these theories. Thus, depending on one's view of the fibrinolysis mechanism, varying opinions exist about the dosage of streptokinase (see Section B. IV).

II. Effect on Hemostasis

Administration of streptokinase causes changes in the hemostatic system that may become clinically relevant. They are indirectly or directly connected with streptokinase-induced plasminemia. Their extent is, therefore, dependent on the degree and duration of plasminemia which, in turn, depend on the streptokinase dose (see Section B. IV).

During the initial phase of streptokinase therapy, transient hypercoagulability is observed. It appears after administration of 5000–10000 U of streptokinase, and becomes evident by the shortening of the recalcification time in the thrombelastogram and by an increase in factor VIII activity (PRENTICE et al., 1969). Later in the course of therapy, disturbances of hemostasis in the form of hypocoagulability develop. Enhanced vascular permeability, inhibition of platelet functions, as well as impairment of fibrin formation are observed. On the one hand, the disturbances of hemostasis are induced by proteolytic activity of plasmin. Proteolytic degradation of fibrinogen and of clotting factors V and VIII occurs. On the other hand, the products formed during degradation of fibrin and fibrinogen interfere with the thrombin action and also impair the polymerization of fibrin (NIEWIAROWSKI and KOWALSKI, 1957; FLETCHER et al., 1962). Fibrinogen degradation products inhibit the hemostatic platelet functions (KOWALSKI et al., 1964). Furthermore, a decrease in the antithrombin III level and reduction of antiplasmin and α_1-macroglobulin were reported (DEUTSCH and MARSCHNER, 1962; VINAZZER, 1976).

III. Immunologic Reactions

During streptokinase treatment a decrease in γ-globulin fractions and an increase in "acute phase reactants" were observed (RASCHE and HIEMEYER, 1968; LÜBCKE et al., 1972; SPÖTTL et al., 1974). Furthermore, plasmin cleaves certain components of the complement system (JUNG and DUCKERT, 1960; VOGT, 1974). Whether or not the reduced defence against infections can be attributed to this fact (JUNG and DUCK-ERT, 1960) remains unclear.

Because of preceding streptococcal infection, practically all patients possess antibodies against streptokinase, so that administration of the agent leads to an antigen-antibody reaction. Its course depends on the level of the antistreptokinase titer and on the speed of administration. The consequences of this reaction may be prevented by prophylactic administration of a glucocorticoid and/or an antihistaminic agent (DEUTSCH et al., 1960b; DAHLSTRÖM, 1965; AMERY et al., 1970).

On the other hand, administration of streptokinase induces antibody formation. The increase in the titer of antibodies against streptokinase reaches a maximum between the sixth and the twelfth days following administration. The titer persists individually for different time intervals. Three months after administration, the initial values are reached in 92% of the patients (GROSS and HARTL, 1962; AMERY et al., 1963b; BRUHN, 1974). More recent studies showed that antibodies are formed both against the intact molecule of streptokinase and against its individual fragments. There is no evidence for the clinical relevance of these findings (BRUHN, 1974).

IV. Influence on Kinin Formation

The formation of plasma kinins during the initial phase of streptokinase treatment was demonstrated by FISCHER and BLÜMEL (1968). During this phase, reactions of the circulatory system as the consequence of kinin liberation are frequently observed. They may be decreased by simultaneous administration of a protease inhibitor [for example Trasylol or Contrykal (FISCHER and BLÜMEL, 1968)].

B. Therapeutic Use

I. Indications

Treatment with streptokinase is advisable if nonphysiologic fibrin deposits are responsible for the pathologic processes. This is true primarily for thrombosis and embolism of the greater and lesser vessels as well as for hyaline thrombi of the microvasculature occurring during disseminated intravascular coagulation. The dissolution of extravascular fibrin deposits is of minor importance. Streptokinase treatment is justified only as long as fibrous organization of fibrin deposits has not occurred and as long as thrombi did not lead to irreversible damage. Recently, plasma fibrinogen as a substrate of streptokinase treatment has also received growing attention since a decrease in the fibrinogen level improves the rheologic conditions (SANDRITTER, 1962; GROSS, 1963; BOYLES and MEYER, 1964; BENEKE and HEY, 1965; HEY et al., 1966; SCHMIDT, 1966; EHRLY, 1967; HARMS, 1967; HIRSH et al., 1968a, b; SCHWICK and HEIMBURGER, 1969; BLEYL, 1970; BENEKE, 1971; EHRLY and LANGE, 1971).

Based on these considerations, the following indications result for thrombolytic therapy with streptokinase:

    1. Thrombosis of deep veins of the limbs, pelvis, and shoulder area

    2. Thrombosis of veins of organs

   3. Priapism
   4. Thrombosis of retinal veins
   5. Pulmonary embolism
   6. Thrombosis and embolism of arterial vasculature
   7. Myocardial infarction and angina pectoris gravis
   8. Cardiogenic shock
   9. Shock as a consequence of disseminated intravascular coagulation
  10. Arterial occlusion of retinal vessels
  11. Idiopathic perinatal respiratory distress syndrome (hyaline membrane disease)
  12. Extravascular fibrin deposits in burns, peritonitis, bronchitis, pleuritis, and intraocular bleeding

II. Contraindications

Contraindications against streptokinase treatment result, on the one hand, from the defect of hemostasis occurring during therapy, and, on the other hand, from the antigen character of the agent. There are absolute contraindications that do not allow streptokinase therapy, as well as relative ones, which allow streptokinase therapy under strict control, thoroughly considering its risks and its usefulness (THIES, 1967).

Absolute contraindications are:
   1. Hemorrhagic diatheses (with the exception of disseminated intravascular coagulation)
   2. Actual hemorrhage
   3. Sources of hemorrhage in the gastrointestinal tract (ulcus ventriculi et duodeni, colitis, neoplasm)
   4. Postoperative phase (from the fourth to the twelfth day depending on the type of intervention)
   5. Postpartum period (up to the sixth day)
   6. Cerebral stroke (between the sixth hour and the sixth day after its onset)
   7. Malignant hypertension (above 200/110 mm Hg)
   8. Subacute bacterial endocarditis
   9. Severe diabetes mellitus with second degree retinopathy
  10. Pregnancy during the first trimester

Relative contraindications are:
   1. Previous streptokinase therapy (the antibody titer is decisive)
   2. Preceding streptococcal infection (the antibody titer is decisive)
   3. Defect of anticoagulant-induced hemostasis
   4. Severe damage of the liver
   5. Renal insufficiency
   6. Primary tuberculosis
   7. Arteriography

III. Administration

Streptokinase is usually administered as intravenous or intraarterial infusion. The required amount (see Section B. IV. 2.) is dissolved in a basic solvent. The following solvents are utilized: sodium chloride solution, glucose solution, levulose solution, Michaelis buffer, dextran solution, gelatine solution, or albumin solution.

The stability of the streptokinase solution depends on the type of the solvent, on the streptokinase concentration, and on temperature. When gelatine or albumin solutions are used, solutions with a streptokinase concentration of 5 U/ml are stable for about 60 min; with the use of other media, the solutions are stable for only a few minutes (MARTIN, 1975b). At a concentration of 100 U/ml, streptokinase is stable for 8 h in sodium chloride solution, glucose solution, and levulose solution. In gelatine solution however, it is stable for 24 h (ZEKORN, 1967). At a streptokinase concentration of 1500 U/ml, the solutions are stable for 48 h independent of the type of solvent.

The streptokinase dose is usually administered continuously as an infusion or injection by means of an infusion pump. Several authors recommend discontinued administration. In both cases the reactions of the hemostatic system are practically identical (GROSS, 1962; MARX, 1962; DEUTSCH and STACHERL, 1963; VERSTRAETE et al., 1964; LASCH and KRAUSE, 1968; RASCHE and HIEMEYER, 1970; AIACH et al., 1975).

There are varying opinions as to whether or not streptokinase should be administered as close as possible to the thrombus, or whether it should be infused into the site of choice independent of the location of the thrombus (BOYLES et al., 1960; BENZER et al., 1963). In animal experiments, GOTTLOB and ZINNER (1957) found that after infusion of streptokinase near the thrombus, thrombolysis occurred more rapidly than after systemic administration. Based on clinical observations, LUDWIG (1968), HIRSH (1970), and POLIWODA (1970a) recommended administration near the thrombus, whereas FISCHER (1976) and VINAZZER (1976a) did not admit the advantages of this route of administration.

In order to diminish the risk of hemorrhage in special situations, e.g. during the immediate postoperative phase, several authors proposed administration of streptokinase near the thrombus in combination with systemic administration of an antifibrinolytic agent (GOTTLOB and ZINNER, 1957; TOPALOW, 1974).

Local administration of streptokinase given as injection into the thrombus, or by means of through drainage is performed for some indications, i.e., thrombosis in arteriovenous shunts in renal dialysis patients, peritonitis, ulcus cruris, and burns. Furthermore, in chronic bronchitis, inhalation therapy with streptokinase was reported. Although oral absorption of streptokinase is not expected because of its chemical properties, oral administration was attempted (FISCHBACHER, 1967). The results obtained are not convincing.

The duration of streptokinase treatment depends primarily on the therapeutic effect. On the sixth day, a significant increase in the antistreptokinase titer has been observed, so that marked anaphylactic reactions are to be expected. Therefore, the duration of treatment should not exceed 6 days. However, in individual cases, duration of 12–18 days was reported (HAAF, 1976). As a rule, anticoagulant therapy with heparin or coumarin derivatives is performed immediately after the termination of streptokinase treatment (OHLER, 1966; MARX, 1969; MARTIN, 1975a).

IV. Dosage

During the initial phase of streptokinase therapy (see Section B. IV. 1.) an antigen-antibody reaction occurs accompanied by the corresponding clinical symptoms. Its consequences may be diminished or prevented by administration of 20–50 mg prednisolone i.v. and/or an antihistaminic agent prior to treatment.

The guidelines for the dosage of streptokinase were determined empirically, or they were deduced from the mechanism of the fibrinolytic-thrombolytic action. According to the varying opinions about these questions (see Section A.I.) different dosage schemes were proposed. There is agreement that two phases of treatment are to be distinguished. During the initial phase, a high streptokinase dose is given in order to neutralize the streptokinase antibodies and to initiate activation of the fibrinolytic system. During the following phase, an adequate dose is given in order to maintain the desired fibrinolytic activity (DEUTSCH et al., 1960a, b; DAHLSTRÖM, 1965; DONNER, 1965; VERSTRAETE et al., 1966; VERMYLEN et al., 1968; LEUBE, 1968; HIRSH, 1970; HIRSH et al., 1970b).

1. Initial Dose

The initial dose to be administered within 15–30 min can be determined individually, taking into account the antistreptokinase titer of the patient. By means of the streptokinase tolerance test (DEUTSCH et al., 1960b) the streptokinase dose is estimated in vitro which is able to dissolve completely a defined clot from the patient's blood within 10 min at 37° C. The individual initial dose is calculated by multiplication of the detected value of streptokinase tolerance with the approximate blood volume. In children, the following initial doses were proposed (SCHREINERT, 1973):

Initial dose = streptokinase tolerance

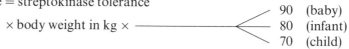

$$\times \text{ body weight in kg} \times \underline{\hspace{4cm}} \begin{cases} 90 & \text{(baby)} \\ 80 & \text{(infant)} \\ 70 & \text{(child)} \end{cases}$$

The distribution of streptokinase tolerance in the normal population of central Europe has been repeatedly investigated (GROSS and HARTL, 1962; SCHMUTZLER and KOLLER, 1969). More than two-thirds of the calculated values were found to be between 40 and 160 U, so that determination of a standard dose became possible. According to SCHMUTZLER and KOLLER (1969), sufficient activation of the fibrinolytic system is expected in 82% at an initial dose of 250000 U, in 93% at 450000 U, and in 98% at 600000 units.

2. Maintenance Dose

The short half-life of streptokinase requires a maintenance dose high enough to maintain the degree of activation reached. Its amount is particularly determined by the conception of the desirable fibrinolysis mechanism. Such dosages are most widely used which cause formation of the greatest possible amount of activator and which prevent plasmin formation. A maintenance dose of 20 U/ml blood volume/h is considered to be sufficient. In adults, in most cases a standard dose of 100000 U/h is chosen. The level of activation of fibrinolysis is controlled by adequate clotting tests (see Section B. V.). If necessary, the dose has to be adjusted. In case of undesired plasminemia, the dose has to be doubled for 2–3 h.

3. Special Dosage Schemes

Several authors used other dosage schemes. BREDDIN et al. (1973) reported a "short-term fibrinolysis" in myocardial infarction with an initial dose of 250 000 U, followed by a maintenance dose of 500 000 U within 2.5 h. KOPEĆ (1976) reported "low-dose streptokinase therapy" in venous thrombosis with an initial dose of 600 000 for 60 min, and for the next 3 days a single dose of 250 000 U each is infused for 30 min.

V. Control of Therapy

Determination of thrombin time is considered the most important laboratory test for the control of streptokinase therapy. Prolongation of up to three to six times the initial value, i.e., in principle, up to 60–120 s is desirable. Longer thrombin times indicate hyperplasminemia, involving the risk of hemorrhage. On the other hand, shorter thrombin times indicate insufficient protection from new thrombus formation. Several authors ascribe special importance to the determination of the fibrinogen level, which should not decrease below 80 mg/100 ml. It has to be taken into consideration that the determination of fibrinogen is interfered with by the fibrin-(ogen) degradation products formed during the treatment. In this case, the coagulation tests reveal values that are too low. Heat-precipitate determination of fibrinogen, which also includes high-molecular-weight degradation products, reveals values that are too high. The most precise values during thrombolytic therapy are obtained by the time-consuming chemical estimation of fibrinogen (for methods see RATNOFF and MENZIE, 1951). The streptokinase-induced coagulation defect can also be demonstrated by other tests such as reptilase time, thrombin coagulase time, or partial thromboplastin time (AMBRUS and MARCUS, 1960, OLOW, 1963; DE VREKER, 1965; POLIWODA, 1967; BLIX, 1969; BOYLES and MEYER, 1971; MINN and MANDEL, 1972; BRUNSWIG, 1974).

VI. Side-Effects

During streptokinase therapy in several patients side-effects were observed, some attributed to the antigen character of the preparation, some to the induced fibrinolytic activity (SCHMUTZLER, 1965; PEZOLD, 1969b).

General reactions: During the initial phase of streptokinase therapy general reactions (chills, nausea, vomiting, backache) occur, which may be considered harmless. The frequency of such reactions depends on individual factors, on the premedication, on the dosage, and on the type of preparation (Table 1).

Fever was also observed later in the course of streptokinase treatment. These instances, however, are not necessarily side-effects in the literal sense. Such reactions are rather assumed to be caused by an inflow of proteolytically degraded thrombus constituents. Moreover, during long-term lysis, fever was observed and considered to be equivalent to serum sickness.

Bleeding: Treatment with streptokinase leads in all cases to a more or less pronounced defect of hemostasis. Bleeding is, therefore, a frequent side-effect of this therapy, which in the majority of the cases, appears as slight oozing from the puncture sites of previous injections and from skin and mucous membranes. Different frequencies of such hemorrhages, which in most cases are clinically irrelevant, were

Table 1. Early reactions under thrombolytic therapy with streptokinase in 708 patients with chronic arterial occlusions

	Slight		Severe	
	No. of patients	%	No. of patients	%
General early reaction[a]	180	25.4	—	—
Allergic reaction	14	2	2	0.3
Joint pains	33	4.7	1	0.1
Decrease in blood pressure[b]	64	43.5	28	19

[a] Excitation, nausea, sweating, tachycardia, flush.
[b] Related to 147 patients.
Summarized data according to the results of TILSNER (1975).

Table 2. Side-effects of streptokinase therapy in 458 patients with arterial (252 embolic, 206 thrombotic) occlusions

	Total		Fatal	
	No. of patients	%	No. of patients	%
Embolism	25	5.6	11	2.3
Cerebral	15	3.2	8	1.7
Pulmonary	4	0.9	2	0.4
In other organs	5	1.1	1	0.2
during lysis	1	0.4	—	—
Hemorrhage	42	8.6	23	4.9
From puncture sites	8	1.8	4	0.9
Parenchymatous	13	2.8	7	1.5
Subdural and cerebral	9	1.9	7	1.5
Gastrointestinal	3	0.6	2	0.4
From surgical wounds	7	1.5	1	0.2
From aneurysm	2	0.4	2	0.4

Summarized data according to the results of HESS (1967).

Table 3. Side-effects of streptokinase therapy in 708 patients with chronic arterial occlusions

	Total		Fatal	
	No. of patients	%	No. of patients	%
Embolism in limbs	15	2.1	—	—
Hemorrhages				
Intestinal	8	1.1	—	—
Urologic	57	8.0	—	—
Intracranial	10	1.4	5	0.7
Other	134	18.9	—	—

Summarized data according to the results of TILSNER (1975).

Table 4. Side-effects of streptokinase therapy in 175 patients with deep vein thrombosis

	Total		Fatal	
	No. of patients	%	No. of patients	%
Pulmonary embolism	7	4	2	1.1
Hemorrhage	7	4	1	0.5

Summarized data according to the results of HESS (1967).

reported. More detailed reports were given on severe hemorrhages that, because of the marked loss of blood or of their location, led to the withdrawal of treatment or even to the death of the patient (Tables 2, 3, 4).

Embolism: Since thrombi are commonly formed inhomogenously, it can be presumed that during thrombolysis segments disintegrate and embolize. A distinction between an embolism induced in this way and a spontaneously occurring one is hardly possible. The data available on this problem must be evaluated with some reservation (Tables 2, 3, 4).

C. Results of Therapy

I. Venous Thrombosis

1. Thrombosis of Deep Veins

Since the introduction of streptokinase treatment, deep vein thromboses (DVT) of the limbs and pelvis are considered to be the most important indications of thrombolytic therapy. There are many reports of successful treatment of DVT with streptokinase. The majority of them are based on experiences obtained in the treatment of patients who were not compared with a control group. In these patients, the therapeutic effects were evaluated only clinically. Reviews on these uncontrolled trials were given by GROSS and KLOSS (1962), HAAN and TILSNER (1965), SCHMUTZLER and KOLLER (1965), HESS (1967), BIGGS (1970), and KAKKAR (1974). The objections to the evaluations of these results, which are based on uncontrolled trials, are justified (KAKKAR, 1974; VAN DE LOO, 1975). In 30% of DVT recanalization was attained without specific treatment and, although the occlusion continued, clinical signs subsided with the development of collateral circulation. Therefore, the effect of thrombolytic therapy in DVT is demonstrable only by controlled comparative studies, and the reliability of the diagnosis and of the therapeutic effect has to be performed by objective methods, such as phlebography, isotope phlebography, and Doppler ultrasound technique. Such comparative studies are represented in Table 5. The results obtained in the group treated with streptokinase are much better than in the control group treated with heparin or Arvin. Further evidence for the therapeutic effect was provided by STORM et al. (1971), who treated patients suffering from DVT with streptokinase-activated or with nonactivated pig plasminogen. In the group treated with activated plasminogen, the phlebograms showed improvement in 60% of the cases, whereas the controls showed improvement in only 10%.

Table 5. Results of noncomparative, phlebographically controlled trials
of streptokinase therapy in deep vein thrombosis

Study	No. of patients	Lysis	No lysis
Hiemeyer, 1967	18	14	4
Kakkar et al., 1969 b, c	10	8	2
Mavor et al., 1969	10	9	1
Robertson et al., 1970	11	11	—
Olow et al., 1970	10	8	2
Kakkar and Flute, 1972	30	26	4
Madar et al., 1972	100	70	30

The effect of streptokinase treatment is not solely expressed by the repatency of the vessel, but also by a reduction of the complications. After streptokinase treatment of DVT, the frequency of pulmonary embolism decreases. In uncontrolled trials, Schmutzler (1969) found in patients treated with streptokinase 4% nonfatal embolism and 1.1% fatal pulmonary embolism. The cumulative statistical analysis of Hess (1967) revealed nonfatal pulmonary embolism of 2.9% and fatal pulmonary embolism of 1.1% in 175 patients with DVT. In a controlled trial (Kakkar, 1974), among 39 heparin-treated patients, two were found with nonfatal and one with fatal pulmonary embolism, whereas in a group of 42 patients treated with streptokinase, pulmonary embolism did not occur.

Studies on the influence of streptokinase treatment in DVT on the functioning of the venous valves were made by Kakkar (1974). Phlebograms were taken 6 and 12 months, respectively, after termination of streptokinase treatment. Four out of seven streptokinase-treated patients showed normal valvular function, and one patient showed disturbed valvular function, whereas in two patients the vascular valves were unable to function. In the control group, consisting of eight heparin-treated patients, in one case the valvular function was normal, and in another case it was impaired. In six cases a loss of valvular function was seen. Analogous results were obtained by Robertson et al. (1968) and Olow et al. (1970). However, the number of patients treated under controlled conditions is relatively small, so that the results obtained need further confirmation (for details see Table 6).

The effects of streptokinase treatment in DVT are influenced by numerous factors. The cumulative statistical analysis of Hess (1967) showed that the longer thrombosis existed prior to treatment, the less effective the lysis (Table 7). The conclusions drawn from these findings, that streptokinase therapy of DVT is reasonable only within the first 6 days after the appearance of clinical symptoms (Back et al., 1958) proved to be wrong. In more than 50% of venous thromboses older than 6 days, Gottlob et al. (1973) found no signs of fibrous organization. He concluded that in these cases thrombolytic therapy is indicated. Alexander et al. (1971) and Tilsner et al. (1972) reported successful streptokinase treatment in occlusions older than 6 days. The rate of success was about 20%. At present, no criteria for favorable streptokinase treatment in thromboses older than 6 days are known. Streptokinase treatment of deep vein thrombosis can also be performed during pregnancy, beyond the first trimester (Ludwig, 1964, 1970a; Pfeifer, 1965, 1967; Walter and Köstering, 1969; Skiftis, 1971). Thrombosis of the axillary veins as in Paget-van Schroet-

Table 6. Results of comparative, phlebographically controlled trials of streptokinase and heparin therapy in deep vein thrombosis

Study	No. of patients	Lysis achieved		
		Complete	Partial	None
GORMSEN and LAURSEN, 1967	11 Streptokinase	4	4	3
	10 Heparin	1	2	7
BROWSE et al., 1968	5 Streptokinase	—	4	1
	5 Heparin	—	—	5
ROBERTSON et al., 1968	8 Streptokinase	5	2	1
	8 Heparin	1	2	5
KAKKAR et al., 1969a	9 Streptokinase	6	1	2
	9 Heparin	2	4	3
ROBERTSON et al., 1970	9 Streptokinase	5	1	3
	7 Heparin	1	1	5
TSAPOGAS et al., 1973	19 Streptokinase	10	—	9
	15 Heparin	1	—	14
DUCKERT et al., 1975	93 Streptokinase	39	23	31
	42 Heparin	—	4	38
BIEGER et al., 1976	5 Streptokinase	4	1	—
	5 Heparin	3	1	1
	5 Phenprocoumon	—	1	4

Table 7. Results of streptokinase therapy of phlebothromboses depending on age of thrombosis at the start of treatment

Age of thrombosis	Total Nr. of cases	Thrombolytic therapy	
		Success	No success
Up to 1 h	4	3 (75%)	1 (25%)
1 day	69	47 (68%)	22 (32%)
2–3 days	50	35 (70%)	15 (30%)
4–5 days	24	13 (54%)	11 (46%)
6–9 days	18	6 (33%)	12 (67%)
10 days-3 weeks	10	0 (0%)	10 (100%)
Total	175	104 (60%)	71 (40%)

Results of HESS (1967).

ter's syndrome is an absolute indication for thrombolytic therapy with streptokinase (for review see VOGEL et al., 1972). Even old thromboses of the axillary veins responded to streptokinase treatment (KRIESSMANN et al., 1971; TILSNER et al., 1972).

2. Thrombosis of Veins of Organs

Effective streptokinase treatment of thrombosis of renal veins was reported by FRIOLET et al. (1964) and by HONKOMP (1966). MIES et al. (1974) reviewed seven successfully treated patients. Thrombolytic therapy may also be performed in cases of renal insufficiency, if necessary, even during peritoneal dialysis (VOGEL and HUYKE, 1976).

KÖSTERING et al. (1971) reported recanalization in a case of Budd-Chiari's syndrome after streptokinase treatment for 13 days. Case reports on streptokinase treatment of thrombosis of mesenteric veins were given by MAYER and MATIS (1962), PEZOLD (1969a), VUJADINOVIC (1969) and ZSCHENKER (1971).

3. Priapism

Patients with priapism were successfully treated with streptokinase. The advantage over the conventional surgical treatment is that in most cases the potentia coeundi is maintained. Streptokinase may be injected topically into the corpora cavernosa (MARX et al., 1967); systemic administration, however, is preferred (VOGEL and SCHLOSSER, 1971). The indication for streptokinase treatment is given only when evidence for thrombosis of the corpora cavernosa was provided. Neurofunctional forms of this disease do not respond to thrombolytic therapy.

4. Special Forms of Venous Thrombosis

Phlegmasia cerulea dolens: Phlegmasia cerulea dolens is an indication for thrombolytic therapy with streptokinase. Reports exist mainly on individual patients. PAQUET et al. (1970), however, observed complete recovery in nine out of ten patients. The number of reports does not suffice to draw parallels to surgical treatment. In those cases of phlegmasia cerulea dolens in which severe shock had already developed, thrombolytic therapy seems to be superior to surgical treatment (SCHMUTZLER, 1970). SENN (1976) recommended combination of thrombectomy with local streptokinase treatment.

In several cases streptokinase was used in thrombosis of intracranial veins and sinuses. The results allow the conclusion that streptokinase treatment is justified only in isolated noninfected thrombosis of sinuses (for review see FRIEDMANN, 1971).

In renal dialysis patients, thromboses in arteriovenous shunts were successfully treated with streptokinase. Local administration seemed to be superior to the systemic one (Table 8).

Table 8. Results of streptokinase therapy in thromboses of arteriovenous shunts in renal dialysis patients

Author	Streptokinase administration	Number of treated thromboses	Results	
			Shunt reopened	No success
ANDERSON et al., 1967	6000– 10000 U[a] (rinsing)	54	48	6
VERMYLEN et al., 1968	20000– 50000 U[a] (rinsing)	9	6	3
LUNDBERG and ERLANDSSON, 1968	1000 U[a] (rinsing)	73	60	13
EPSTEIN, 1969	90000–110000 U (systemically)	12	8	4
ARISZ, 1970	50000 U (locally)	27	25	2
GONZALES and COCKE, 1971	500000 U (systemically)	18	17	1
POGGLITSCH and STÖCKL, 1972	250000 U (locally)	19	12	7

[a] per ml.

Septic thrombosis: Thrombolytic therapy with streptokinase is contraindicated in cases of septic processes. In an individual case, KOPP and HOLZKNECHT (1966) demonstrated effective treatment of septic thrombosis of the leg-pelvic veins. Septic thromboses of intracranial veins and sinuses werc frequently treated with streptokinase (for review see FRIEDMANN, 1971). In the majority of cases, however, severe complications were observed, so that the indications for treatment are given only in exceptional cases.

II. Pulmonary Embolism

Clots occluding the pulmonary vasculature in pulmonary embolism consist mainly of dissoluble material (BENEKE, 1969). As demonstrated in animal experiments, therapeutic effects were obtained in pulmonary embolism by thrombolytic agents (BROWSE and JAMES, 1964; HUME, 1964). Lysis was used even on thrombi 7–14 days old (GENTON and WOLF, 1967; GENTON, 1974). BROWSE and JAMES (1964) reported the first successful thrombolytic therapy of pulmonary embolism in man. For diagnosis and evaluation of the therapeutic effect, however, they used only clinical criteria. Further clinical trials confirmed these first observations (HUME, 1964; FRIEDMANN, 1965; EMANUEL et al., 1966; FRED et al., 1966; HIRSH et al., 1968c; DALEN et al., 1969; MILLER, 1969; TILSNER, 1969; McDONALD et al., 1970; MOTIN et al., 1973; SCHWARTZ et al., 1963; STICKLAND et al., 1973). In 1967, using two patients, HIRSH et al. performed pulmonary angiography, pulmonary scintigraphy, and pulmonary function tests prior to and following streptokinase treatment. They observed rapid normalization of the findings. In a further study, HIRSH et al. (1971) found clinical improvement in 14, and angiographically detectable lysis in 12 out of 16 streptokinase-treated patients. The results were significantly better than in patients treated with heparin alone (HIRSH et al., 1970a).

TIBBUTT et al. (1974) treated patients suffering from pulmonary embolism with streptokinase or with heparin. Angiography was performed aftcr streptokinase treatment of 72 h. In the streptokinase group the results were significantly better than in the group treated with heparin. The decrease in pulmonary pressure was more pronounced in the streptokinase group compared with the heparin group. In a recent study (BELL, 1976), heparin, urokinase, and streptokinase treatments were compared in regard to their therapeutic value in pulmonary embolism. The angiographic, scintigraphic, and hemodynamic findings improved more rapidly and more completely in the urokinase and streptokinase groups than in the heparin group. With regard to the improvement of angiographic findings, there were no differences among the groups.

III. Arterial Thrombosis and Embolism

1. Acute Occlusion

Acute occlusions of arterial vessels by thrombi or emboli were found to respond to streptokinase treatment (COTTON et al., 1962; LINKE, 1962; MÜLLER et al., 1962; AMERY et al., 1963a; McNICOL et al., 1963; VERSTRAETE et al., 1963; McNICOL and DOUGLAS, 1964; HIEMEYER et al., 1965; HESS and GOOSSENS, 1966; HIEMEYER and RASCHE, 1966; SACK, 1968; SAILER et al., 1968a; HIEMEYER, 1969; MARTIN et al.,

Table 9. Global result of streptokinase therapy in 458 patients with arterial (252 = 55% embolic, 206 = 45% thrombotic) occlusions

	Total	Complete lysis		Partial lysis		No lysis	
		No. of patients	%	No. of patients	%	No. of patients	%
Embolism	252	129	51	34	14	89	35
Thrombosis	206	69	34	40	19	97	47
Total	458	198	43	74	16	186	41

Results from Hess (1967).

1969; POLIWODA et al., 1969; CHESTERMANN and BIGGS, 1970; MARTIN, 1970; HUME et al., 1971; SCHMITT et al., 1971).

In the cumulative statistical analysis of Hess (1967) 458 patients were reported on (Table 9). The earlier streptokinase therapy was started, the better were the results. Beyond the fifth day after the appearance of the occlusion, incomplete resolution was seen in some cases. Randomized studies comparing thrombolytic therapy with surgical treatment have not yet been made. Since surgical treatment leads more rapidly to repatency, streptokinase treatment of acute arterial occlusion is justified only when surgical intervention cannot be carried out, i. e., primarily in occlusions distal to the knee joint and to the cubital joint (MUSSGNUG and ALEMANY, 1967).

In some cases, acute occlusions of cerebral vessels were successfully treated (STRICKER and SCHMUTZLER, 1964; SCHMUTZLER, 1969); they involve, however, an extremely high complication rate (SCHMEISSER et al., 1975), so that streptokinase treatment is justified only in exceptional cases.

2. Chronic Occlusion

Attempts at streptokinase treatment for chronic arterial occlusions were stimulated by experimental findings on the dissolubility of arterial thrombi. ROSOLLECK (1961) and GOTTLOB and BLÜMEL (1968) demonstrated that thrombi about 6 days old were partially or completely lysed by streptokinase. An explanation of these unexpected findings was given by BENEKE (1969) and GOTTLOB and BLÜMEL (1970). They found that under certain conditions, fibrous organization and epithelization of arterial thrombi did not necessarily occur after months or even after years. SCHOOP et al. (1968) performed streptokinase therapy in patients with chronic arterial occlusions. Depending on the location of the pathologic process, therapeutic effects were seen in 20–60% of arterial stenoses and in 4.2–33% of arterial occlusions. Similar findings were reported by ALEXANDER et al. (1968), POLIWODA (1970b), and EHRINGER et al. (1974). In 1975, HEINRICH published the results of a multicenter study: 708 patients suffering from arterial stenosis or occlusion were treated with streptokinase. The therapy was not performed under the same conditions, so that the results obtained are hardly comparable. Therapeutic effects were seen in 50.5% of stenoses and in 26.1% of occlusions. In arterial occlusions, correlations were found between the duration of occlusion and the effect of treatment. In 15-day-old occlusions, the rate

Table 10. Indication for an attempt of thrombolytic therapy in chronic arterial occlusions

	Occlusion		Stenosis	
	Preocclusive lumen of the vessel	Age of occlusion	Structure of stenosis	Age of stenosis
Aorta	>15 mm	<2 years		Many years
Common iliac artery External iliac artery	> 8 mm	<1 year	„Crumbly"	<2 years
Femoral artery Popliteal artery	?	<6–8 weeks		

Results from SCHULTE (1975).

of success was 52.6%, in 6-month-old occlusions 37.9%, and in occlusions 35 months old the rate was 10.6%. In stenoses of the aorta, of the common iliac artery, of the external iliac artery, and of the common femoral artery, the therapeutic effect was more significant than in stenoses of the femoral artery, of the popliteal artery, and of the vessels of the lower legs.

In arterial occlusions, no correlations were found between location and therapeutic effect. However, correlations existed between the therapeutic effect and the risk factors. In case of diabetes mellitus, of hypertriglyceridemia, or of severe hypercholesterinemia, the occlusion was influenced less frequently than in the absence of these risk factors. Based on their findings, HEINRICH (1965) considered thrombolysis as justified when the criteria listed in Table 10 were met. In general, streptokinase treatment of chronic arterial occlusion is reasonable solely when surgical intervention is not possible. The risk involved in streptokinase treatment is higher in the group with preexisting vascular injury than in other groups. However, studies of HEINRICH et al. (1975) revealed that severe side effects are to be expected in less than 1% of the cases (for details see Table 3).

IV. Ischemic Heart Disease

The theoretic basis of streptokinase treatment of myocardial infarction is that the following thromboembolic processes are relevant to the occurrence of myocardial infarction and its complications:

1. Primary thrombi (formed prior to infarction) or secondary thrombi (formed after the occurrence of infarction) in the extramural branches of coronary arteries

2. Microthrombi in arterioles, capillaries, and venules in the marginal infarcted area

3. Microthrombi in the terminal vasculature of the whole organism, and

4. Macrothrombi in peripheral vessels

The question of the relevance of these substrates to the pathogenesis of infarction or its complications has yielded various answers. A critical review of the different points of view was given by BENEKE (1971). More recently, the decrease in the fibrinogen level was considered an important mechanism in the streptokinase treat-

Table 11. Results of controlled trials on streptokinase therapy of acute myocardial infarction

Author	Number of patients		Age of in- farction (h)	Duration of treat- ment (h)	Mortality		Signif- icance (p)
	Control group	Strepto- kinase			Control group (%)	Strepto- kinase (%)	
SCHMUTZLER et al., 1966	261	297	< 12	18	21.7	16.1	0.03
AMERY et al., 1969	83	84	< 72	72	24.1	17.9	0.5
GORMSEN, 1972	68	67	< 24	20	29.4	23.8	n.s.
VERSTRAETE et al., 1971	339	357	< 24	24	27.4	19.0	0.01
DIOGUARDI et al., 1971	157	164	< 12	12	11.4	11.5	n.s.
HEIKINHEIMO et al., 1971	207	219	< 72	1–48	9.2	9.0	n.s.
SCHMUTZLER et al., 1971	131	138	< 12	18	26.0	14.5	0.01
BETT et al., 1973	227	230	< 24	18	12.8	10.9	n.s.
BREDDIN et al., 1973 I	95	134	< 12	3	21.0	18.0	n.s.
II	104	102	< 12	3	27.9	12.7	0.01

ment of myocardial infarction. The decrease in blood viscosity caused by the lowered fibrinogen level was thought to lead to considerable improvement of hemodynamics (EHRLY, 1970).

In animal experiments, contradictory results were obtained on the influence of streptokinase on myocardial infarction. In experiments on dogs RUEGSEGGER et al. (1959) observed a diminution of the infarcted area after streptokinase administration, whereas HORT et al. (1966) did not find any differences between the animals treated with streptokinase, and the controls. HIEMEYER et al. (1965, 1969) and HIEMEYER and RASCHE (1974) demonstrated in cats with experimental infarction a diminution of the infarcted area from 20–60%, depending on the start of treatment.

FLETCHER et al. (1959) performed the first streptokinase treatment in patients with myocardial infarction, and obtained positive results. Many case reports confirmed these first experiences (for review see SCHNEIDER, 1974). A decreased mortality, a reduction in the number of penetrating infarction in favor of rudimentary infarction, a more rapid course of enzyme reactions, and more rapid electrocardiographic changes typical of infarction were reported (DEWAR et al., 1963; SINAPIUS, 1965, 1969; POLIWODA et al., 1966; HENNING and LOOK, 1967; SAILER et al., 1968b; HESS, 1969; VAN DE LOO, 1969; LÜBCKE, 1969; HALE, 1970; GOLDEN et al., 1971; HIEMEYER, 1971a, b; VERSTRAETE, 1971; VÖLCKER, 1971; GILLMANN et al., 1973; PRÄTORIUS et al., 1973; SCHREIBER and EULITZ, 1973; SHERRY, 1974).

However, definite statistical proof for the usefulness of streptokinase treatment in myocardial infarction is still lacking. Therefore, attempts have been made to obtain a clear idea about this therapeutic method by prospective, randomized comparative studies. At present, ten such studies have been published (Table 11). These trials, however, did not solve the problem under study, especially because of inappropriate methods, such as inadequacy of randomization and differences in doses. Moreover, in most studies the number of cases did not suffice to obtain statistical reliability. Starting from the present knowledge of epidemiology, the American Heart and Lung Institute has calculated that 4142 patients would be required (SHAW et al., 1974).

At present, attempts are in progress to solve this question by multicenter studies that meet all requirements (VAN DE LOO, 1974). Particular problems arise from the observations of a specific complication possibly caused by streptokinase; this is the so-called hemorrhagic myocardial infarction. SCHACHENMEYER and HAFERKAMP (1972) and BERRY (1975) observed that patients treated with streptokinase showed changes in the morphologic picture of myocardial infarction expressed by diffuse hemorrhages. It is not yet known whether these changes represent a complication or whether they are part of the therapeutic effect. A relationship to ruptures of the cardiac wall was not suspected, because their frequency in streptokinase-treated patients did not differ from that in the control group (VAN DE LOO, 1974). BENDA et al. (1971) and BENDA (1974) reported streptokinase treatment in patients with angina pectoris gravis, in whom frequency and duration of attacks decreased.

V. Thrombosis and Embolism of Retinal Vessels

Acute occlusions of retinal arteries were reported to respond to streptokinase therapy (for review see BÖCK et al., 1963; ROSSMANN, 1967, 1974; MÜLLER and HIEMEYER, 1970; DEJACO and HAMMER, 1972; LOHSE and WELLER, 1976). The therapeutic effect depends both on the extent of the occlusion and on the time of the start of the treatment. In contrast to earlier assumptions that thrombolytic therapy is indicated only up to the second hour after the occurrence of occlusion, DEJACO and HAMMER (1972) believed that treatment should be attempted up to 24 h after the appearance of clinical symptoms, if relative or absolute contraindications are not given.

VI. Thrombosis of the Microvasculature

There are close relationships between the regulatory mechanisms of hemostasis (synthesis, activation, inactivation, and clearance of specific components of the coagulation and fibrinolytic systems) and circulation. Therefore, disturbances of hemostasis often cause impairment of the circulation, especially of the microcirculation; on the other hand, these disturbances occur as a consequence of impaired hemodynamics.

In all forms of shock, the coagulation system becomes activated which leads to thrombus formation in the microvasculature. The course of shock depends particularly on the extent of microthrombosis. In several cases, microthrombi can be dissolved by streptokinase treatment, thus reducing disturbances of the circulation. In contrast to the controls, the survival time of experimental animals treated with streptokinase was enhanced. The number of fibrin thrombi in the glomeruli decreased. The pathologically reduced oxygen consumption normalized (LASCH et al., 1962; HARDAWAY and BURNS, 1963; ENCKE et al., 1966; BROERSMA et al., 1969; HEY et al., 1969; NEUHOF, 1970; NEUHOF and LASCH, 1974).

Several case reports showed that shock conditions in man can also be improved by streptokinase (SCHIMPF, 1969; LUDWIG, 1970b; NEUHOF et al., 1970; BREDDIN, 1971; EHRLY and LANGE, 1971; LUCAS, 1971; SCHMUTZLER et al., 1971; VOGEL and FIEHRING, 1972; MITTERSTIELER et al., 1973; PRESTON and EDWARDS, 1973; SCHREINERT, 1973; WEINMANN et al., 1976). In some cases of Waterhouse-Friderichsen's syndrome death was prevented by streptokinase (KÜNZER et al., 1972; SCHREINERT,

1973). In case of hemolytic uremic syndrome mortality was decreased (MONNENS et al., 1972; HEIMSOTH et al., 1973; POWELL and EKERT, 1974).

DEYSINE and co-workers (1965) reported accelerated demarcation of burns in streptokinase-treated rabbits. After experimental burns under streptokinase, the necrotic area was diminished (HETTICH, 1974). WEBER et al. (1969) used streptokinase for treatment of burns in man. No shift from stage II to stage III was observed. STETTER (1974) reported the results obtained in 90 patients with burns. Necrosis was restricted to primarily irreversibly damaged areas. Wound healing was accelerated and scar formation was improved with regard to cosmetic appearance and function.

VII. Other Fields of Application

Several authors have used streptokinase for the dissolution of extravascular fibrin deposits. Local administration into the anterior chamber of the eye caused accelerated absorption of hyphema and prevented secondary glaucoma (for review see LOHSE and WELLER, 1976). MÜHE (1974) reported prevention of peritonitis by rinsing with streptokinase.

BOTTKE (1965) used streptokinase for inhalation therapy of the bronchitis syndrome. On three successive days, 50 000 u each were administered. After treatment, the viscosity of the bronchial secretion was reduced to 40% of the initial value. The authors observed an increase in the antistreptokinase titer, and concluded absorption of streptokinase by the bronchial mucosa.

In respiratory distress, streptokinase treatment did not lead to satisfactory results (for review see AMBRUS et al., 1971; WEINMANN et al., 1976). Failures of therapy often observed in this disease are thought to be caused by plasminogen deficiency. The problem of whether or not therapeutic effects may be obtained by simultaneous administration of plasminogen being studied (VERSTRAETE, 1976).

References

Aiach, M., Fiessinger, J.-N., Devanley, M., Lagneau, P., Housset, E., Leclerc, M.: Traitement thrombolytique discontinu: premiers résultats biologiques. Sem. Hôp. Paris **51**, 1285 (1975)

Alexander, K., Buhl, V., Holsten, D., Poliwoda, H., Wagner, H. H.: Fibrinolytische Therapie des chronischen Arterienverschlusses. Med. Klin. **63**, 2067 (1968)

Alexander, K., Jester, H. G., Poliwoda, H., Wuppermann, T., Bargon, G., Dowidat, H., Lange, M., Wagner, H. H.: Fibrinolytische Therapie chronischer Phlebothrombosen. Dtsch. med. Wschr. **96**, 1873 (1971)

Ambrus, C. M., Ambrus, J. L., Weintraub, D. H., Foote, R. J., Courey, N. G., Niswander, K. R.: Thrombolytic therapy in hyaline membrane disease. Thrombos. Diathes. haemorrh. (Stuttg.) Suppl. **47**, 269 (1971)

Ambrus, C. M., Back, N., Ambrus, J. L.: On the mechanism of thrombolysis by plasmin. Circulat. Res. **5**, 161 (1962)

Ambrus, C. M., Marcus, G.: Plasmin-antiplasmin complex as a reservoir of fibrinolytic enzyme. Amer. J. Physiol. **199**, 491 (1960)

Amery, A., Donati, M. B., Vermylen, J., Verstraete, M.: Comparison between the changes in the plasma fibrinogen and plasminogen levels induced by a moderate or high initial dose of streptokinase. Thrombos. Diathes. haemorrh. (Stuttg.) **23**, 504 (1970)

Amery, A., Roeber, G., Vermeulen, H. J., Verstraete, M.: Single-blind randomised multicentre trial comparing heparin and streptokinase treatment in recent myocardial infarction. Acta med. scand. Suppl. **505**, 35 (1969)

Amery, M., Vermylen, J., Verstraete, M.: Feasibility of adequate thrombolytic therapy with streptokinase in peripheral arterial occlusions. II. Changes in the peripheral blood and thrombolysis in vivo. Brit. med. J. **1**, 1505 (1963a)

Amery, M., Verstraete, M., Vermylen, J., Maes, A.: The streptokinase reactivity test (SKRT). I. Standardization. Thrombos. Diathes. haemorrh. (Stuttg.) **9**, 175 (1963b)

Anderson, D. D., Martini, A. M., Clunie, G. J. A., Stewart, W. K., Robson, J. S.: Eight months experience in the use of streptokinase locally for declotting arteriovenous cannulas. Proc. Europ. Dial. Transpl. Ass. (Amst.) **4**, 55 (1967)

Arisz, L.: Fibrinolytic agents in the treatment of the thrombosed arteriovenous shunt. Ned. T. Geneesk. **114**, 1484 (1970)

Back, N., Ambrus, J. L., Simpson, C. L., Shulman, S.: Study on the effect of streptokinase-activated plasmin (fibrinolysin) on clots in various stages of organization. J. clin. Invest. **37**, 864 (1958)

Bang, N. U., Fletcher, A. P., Alkjaersig, N., Sherry, S.: Pathogenesis of the coagulation defect developing during pathological plasma proteolytic ("fibrinolytic") states. III. Demonstration of abnormal clot structure by electron microscopy. J. clin. Invest. **41**, 935 (1962)

Bell, W. R.: Streptokinase and urokinase in the treatment of pulmonary thromboemboli. Thrombos. Haemostas. (Stuttg.) **35**, 57 (1976)

Benda, L.: Die fibrinolytische Therapie des Herzinfarktes: Fibrinolyse bei Angina pectoris. In: Schneider, W. (Ed.): Fibrinolytische Therapie, p. 175. Marburg: Medizinische Verlagsges. 1974

Benda, L., Redtenbacher, L., Spiess, A., Steinbach, T.: Fibrinolytische Behandlung bei schwerer Angina pectoris. Dtsch. med. Wschr. **96**, 771 (1971)

Beneke, G.: Der Thrombus als pathologisch-anatomisches Substrat. Thrombos. Diathes. haemorrh. (Stuttg.) Suppl. **32**, 217 (1969)

Beneke, G.: Das Substrat für die Fibrinolyse beim Herzinfarkt. In: Hiemeyer, V. (Ed.): Die thrombolytische Behandlung des Myokardinfarktes, p. 3. Stuttgart: Schattauer 1971

Beneke, G., Hey, D.: Modelluntersuchungen zur fermentativen Löslichkeit von Fibrin im histologischen Schnitt. Histochemie **5**, 366 (1965)

Benzer, H., Blümel, G., Gottlob, R., Piza, F.: Die Behandlung von Thrombosen durch lokale Infusion fibrinolytischer Fermente. Langenbecks Arch. Klin. Chir. **304**, 775 (1963)

Berry, C. L.: Thrombolytic therapy and myocardial infarction. J. clin. Path. **28**, 352 (1975)

Bett, J. H. N., Biggs, J. C., Castaldi, P. A., Chestermann, C. N., Hale, G. S., Hirsh, J., Isbister, J. P., McDonald, I. G., McLean, K. H., Morgan, J. J., O'Sullivan, E. F., Rosenbaum, M.: Australian multicentre trial of streptokinase in acute myocardial infarction. Lancet **1973 I**, 57

Bieger, R., Boekhut-Mussert, R. I., Hohmann, F., Loeliger, E. A.: Is streptokinase useful in the treatment of deep vein thrombosis? Acta med. scand. **199**, 81 (1976)

Biggs, J. C.: Thrombolytic therapy in arterial and venous thrombosis. Aust. Ann. Med. **19**, Suppl. 1, 19 (1970)

Bleyl, U.: Fibrinolyse durch Leukozyten. Thrombos. Diathes. haemorrh. (Stuttg.) Suppl. **32**, 59 (1969)

Bleyl, U.: Pathologie des endotoxischen Schocks. In: Intensivtherapie beim septischen Schock, p. 15 (Ahnefeld, F. W., Halmagyi, M., Eds.). Berlin-Heidelberg-New York: Springer 1970

Blix, S.: The control of plasminogen and plasmin during thrombolytic therapy. Acta med. scand. **186**, 479 (1969)

Böck, J., Bornschein, H., Hommer, K.: Die Überlebens- und Wiederbelebungszeit der menschlichen Netzhaut. Wien. med. Wschr. **113**, 855 (1963)

Bottke, H.: Behandlung des bronchitischen Syndroms mit Streptokinase. Experimentelle und klinische Ergebnisse. Med. Klin. **60**, 1398 (1965)

Boyles, P. W., Meyer, W. H.: A quantitative method for the study of thrombolysis. Angiology **15**, 326 (1964)

Boyles, P. W., Meyer, W. H.: Blood changes following thrombolysin therapy. Thrombos. Diathes. haemorrh. (Stuttg.) Suppl. **47**, 301 (1971)

Boyles, P. W., Meyer, W. H., Graf, J., Ashley, C. C., Ripic, R. G.: Comparative effectiveness of intravenous and intra-arterial fibrinolysin therapy. Amer. J. Cardiol. **6**, 439 (1960)

Breddin, K.: Die Wirkung der Fibrinolyse im kardiogenen Schock. Med. Welt (Stuttg.) **22**, 1206 (1971)

Breddin, K., Ehrly, A. M., Fechler, L., Frick, D., König, H., Kraft, H., Krause, H., Krzywanek, H. J., Kutschera, J., Lösch, H. W., Ludwig, O., Mikat, B., Rausch, F., Rosenthal, P., Sartory, S., Voigt, G., Wylicil, P.: Die Kurzzeitfibrinolyse beim akuten Myokardinfarkt. Dtsch. med. Wschr. **98**, 861 (1973)

Broersma, R. J., Bullemer, G. D., Mammen, E. F.: Blood coagulation changes in hemorrhagic shock and acidosis. Thrombos. Diathes. haemorrh. (Stuttg.) Suppl. **36**, 171 (1969)

Browse, N. L., James, D. C.: Streptokinase and pulmonary embolism. Lancet **1964 II**, 1039

Browse, N. L., Thoma, M. L., Pim, H. P.: Streptokinase and deep vein thrombosis. Brit. med. J. **3**, 717 (1968)

Bruhn, H. D.: Neue Befunde zur Bedeutung des Anti-Streptokinase-Titers für die Streptokinase-induzierte Thrombolysetherapie. Dtsch. med. Wschr. **99**, 1410 (1974)

Brunswig, D.: Dosierung und Überwachung der fibrinolytischen Therapie. In: Schneider, K, W. (Ed.): Fibrinolytische Therapie, p. 11. Marburg: Medizinische Verlagsges. 1974

Cathie, I. A. B., MacFarlane, I. C. W.: Adjuvants to streptomycin in treating tuberculous meningitis in children. Lancet **1954 II**, 784

Chestermann, C. N., Biggs, J. C.: Thrombolytic therapy with streptokinase. Med. J. Aust. **2**, 839 (1970)

Cliffton, E. E.: The present status of therapeutic use of enzymes. Amer. J. med. Sci. **228**, 568 (1954)

Cotton, L. T., Flute, P. T., Tsapogas, M. J. C.: Popliteal artery thrombosis treated with streptokinase. Lancet **1962 II**, 1081

Dahlström, H.: Theorie und Praxis der Streptokinasebehandlung. Z. inn. Med. **20**, 709 (1965)

Dalen, J. E., Banas, J. S., Brooks, H. L., Evans, C. L., Paraskos, J. A., Dexter, L.: Resolution rate of acute pulmonary embolism in man. New Engl. J. Med. **280**, 1194 (1969)

Dejaco, R. M., Hammer, G.: Fibrinolyse-Therapie der Netzhautgefäßverschlüsse. In: Sailer, S. (Ed.): Aktuelle Probleme der Fibrinolyse-Behandlung, p. 57. Wien: Brüder Hollinek 1972

Deutsch, E., Elsner, P., Fischer, N.: Medikamentös induzierte Fibrinolyse. Wien. Z. inn. Med. **41**, 457 (1960a)

Deutsch, E., Fischer, M., Marschner, J., Kock, M.: Die Wirkung intravenös applizierter Streptokinase auf Fibrinolyse und Blutgerinnung. Thrombos. Diathes. haemorrh. (Stuttg.) **4**, 482 (1960b)

Deutsch, E., Marschner, I.: Verhalten der Antiplasmine während der thrombolytischen Therapie. Thrombos. Diathes. haemorrh. (Stuttg.) Suppl. **3**, 59 (1962)

Deutsch, E., Stacherl, A.: Vergleichende Untersuchungen über die Wirkung von Streptokinase und streptokinaseaktiviertem Plasminogen bei der thrombolytischen Therapie. Wien. klin. Wschr. **75**, 667 (1963)

Dewar, H., Stephenson, P., Horler, A., Cassells-Smith, A., Ellis, P.: Fibrinolytic therapy of coronary thrombosis. Brit. med. J. **1963 I**, 915

Deysine, M., Clarke, R. L., Clifton, E. E.: Treatment of experimental burns with systemic human fibrinolysin. Arch. Surg. **91**, 526 (1965)

Dioguardi, N., Mannucci, P. M., Lotto, A., Rossi, P., Levi, G. F., Lomanto, B., Rota, M., Mattei, G., Proto, C., Fiorelli, G., Agostoni, A.: Controlled trial of streptokinase and heparin in acute myocardial infarction. Lancet **1971 II**, 891

Donner, L.: Klinische Erfahrung mit Plasmin und Streptokinase. Z. inn. Med. **20**, 721 (1965)

Duckert, F., Müller, G., Nyman, D., Benz, A., Prisender, S., Madar, G., DaSilva, M. A., Widmer, L. K., Schmitt, M. E.: Treatment of deep vein thrombosis with streptokinase. Brit. med. J. **1975 I**, 479

Dudok de Wit, C.: The role of plasminogen in fibrinolysis. Vox Sang. **7**, 526 (1962)

Ehringer, H., Dudczak, R., Lechner, K., Widhalm, F.: Streptokinasetherapie bei Gliedmaßenarterienverschlüssen. In: Schneider, K. W. (Ed.): Fibrinolytische Therapie, p. 19. Marburg: Medizinische Verlagsges. 1974

Ehrly, A. M.: Hämorrheologische Probleme bei Venenerkrankungen. Zbl. Phlebol. **6**, 338 (1967)

Ehrly, A. M.: Zur Wirkung von Streptokinase beim Herzinfarkt: Rheologische Untersuchungen. Med. Tribune **24**, 973 (1970)

Ehrly, A. M., Lange, B.: Reduction in blood viscosity and disaggregation of erythrocyte aggregate by streptokinase. In: Hartert, H. H., Copley, A. L. (Eds.): Theoretical and Clinical Hemorrheology, p. 366. Berlin-Göttingen-Heidelberg: Springer 1971

Emanuel, D. A., Sautter, R. D., Wenzel, F. J.: Conservative treatment of massive pulmonary embolism. J. Amer. med. Ass. **197**, 924 (1966)

Encke, A., Lutz, H., Lasch, H.-G., Scheele, K.: Der Einfluß der Fibrinolyse auf die Verbrauchskoagulopathie im hämorrhagischen Schock. Réanim. Org. artif. **2**, 77 (1965)

Encke, A., Peterich, I., Schmidt, H. D., Schmier, J.: Der Einfluß einer Fibrinolysetherapie auf die Überlebensquote im normotensiven hämorrhagischen Schock. Langenbecks Arch. klin. Chir. **316**, 677 (1966)

Epstein, I.: Treatment of clotting in external arterio-venous shunts with a fibrinolytic enzyme. Med. J. Aust. **2**, 137 (1969)

Fischbacher, W.: Streptokinase wird peroral nicht resorbiert. Schweiz. med. Wschr. **97**, 211 (1967)

Fischer, M.: Personal communication, 1976

Fischer, M., Blümel, G.: Veränderungen des Plasmakininogenspiegels während der thrombolytischen Therapie mit Streptokinase und Urokinase. Med. Welt **44**, 1044 (1968)

Fletcher, A. P., Alkjaersig, N., Sherry, S.: The maintenance of a sustained thrombolytic state in man. I. Induction and effects. J. clin. Invest. **38**, 1096 (1959)

Fletcher, A. P., Alkjaersig, M., Sherry, S.: Fibrinolytic mechanism and the development of thrombolytic therapy. Amer. J. Med. **33**, 738 (1962)

Fletcher, A. P., Johnson, A. I.: Methods employed for purification of streptokinase. Proc. Soc. exp. Biol. (N.Y.) **94**, 233 (1957)

Fred, H. L., Axelrad, M. A., Lewis, J. M., Alexander, K.: Rapid resolution of pulmonary thromboemboli in man. An angiographic study. J. Amer. med. Ass. **196**, 1137 (1966)

Friedmann, D. G.: Pathologic observations on experimental and human pulmonary thromboembolism. In: Sasahara, A. A., Stein, M. (Eds.): Pulmonary Embolic Disease, New York-London: Grune and Stratton 1965

Friedmann, D. G.: Problematik der Antikoagulantien- und Thrombolysetherapie bei Sinus- und Hirnvenenthrombose. Radiologe **11**, 424 (1971)

Friolet, B., Gugler, E., Bettex, M., Gautier, E., Muralt, G. de: Über 6 Fälle von Nierenvenenthrombose im Kindesalter. Helv. paediat. Acta **19**, 243 (1964)

Genton, E.: Fibrinolytic treatment of pulmonary thromboembolism. Thrombos. Diathes. haemorrh. (Stuttg.) Suppl. **59**, 213 (1974)

Genton, E., Wolf, P. S.: Experimental pulmonary embolism: effects of urokinase therapy on organizing thrombi. J. Lab. clin. Med. **70**, 311 (1967)

Gillmann, H., Colberg, H. K., Keller, H. P., Orth, H. F., Börner, W., Fritze, E., Gebauer, D., Grosser, K. D., Heckner, F., Körtge, P., Loo, J. van de, Pezold, F. A., Poliwoda, H., Prätorius, F., Schmutzler, R., Schneider, B., Zekorn, D.: Zur fibrinolytischen Behandlung des akuten Herzinfarktes. II. Deutsch-Schweizerische Gemeinschaftsuntersuchung: Ergebnisse der elektrokardiographischen Untersuchungen. Z. Kreisl.-Forsch. **62**, 193 (1973)

Golden, L. H., Schultz, R. W., Ambrus, C. M., Dean, D. C., Lippschütz, E. J., Sanne, M., Ambrus, J. L.: Streptokinase and urokinase activated plasmin therapy in myocardial infarction. Thrombos. Diathes. haemorrh. (Stuttg.) Suppl. **47**, 217 (1971)

Gonzales, F. M., Cocke, T. B.: Use of streptokinase in occluded arteriovenous shunts. Thrombos. Diathes. haemorrh. (Stuttg.) Suppl. **47**, 201 (1971)

Gormsen, J.: Thrombolytic therapy of acute phlebothrombosis. Thrombos. Diathes. haemorrh. (Stuttg.) Suppl. **32**, 267 (1969)

Gormsen, J.: Biochemical evaluation of standard treatment with streptokinase in acute myocardial infarction. Acta med. scand. **191**, 77 (1972)

Gormsen, J., Laursen, B.: Treatment of acute phlebothrombosis with streptase. Acta med. scand. **181**, 373 (1967)

Gottlob, R., Blümel, G.: Über den Nachweis der Plasminogenverarmung in retrahierten Vollblutgerinnseln und über deren Bedeutung für die Lysierbarkeit mit Streptokinase. Thrombos. Diathes. haemorrh. (Stuttg.) **15**, 570 (1966)

Gottlob, R., Blümel, G.: Der Einfluß der vier Thrombenalter auf die Lysierbarkeit mit Streptokinase. Med. Welt **19**, 2627 (1968)

Gottlob, R., Blümel, G.: Altersveränderungen im Thrombus und ihre Bedeutung für die Fibrinolyse. Haematologia hung. Suppl. **1**, 1970

Gottlob, R., Donas, P., El Nashef, B.: Experimentelle Thrombolyse mit besonderer Berücksichtigung chronischer venöser Verschlüsse. Folia angiol. Suppl. **1**, 29 (1973)

Gottlob, R., Zinner, G.: Treatment of venous thrombosis by continuous local infusion of strepto-kinase. Experimental investigations. J. Int. Coll. Surg. **28**, 575 (1957)

Gross, R.: Einige klinische Aspekte von Fibrinolyse und Thrombolyse. Behringwerk-Mitteilun-gen **41**, 68 (1962)

Gross, R.: Findings with labelled streptokinase in vitro and in vivo. Proc. 9th Congr. Europ. Soc. Haemat. Lisbon. Basel-New York: Karger 1963

Gross, R., Hartl, W.: Antistreptokinase und Streptokinaseresistenz. Klin. Wschr. **40**, 813 (1962)

Gross, R., Kloss, G.: Klinischer Bericht über die Anwendung von Streptase®. Behringwerk-Mitteilungen **41**, 123 (1962)

Haaf, E.: Personal communication, 1976

Haan, D., Tilsner, V.: Fibrinolyse-Therapie von Thrombosen und Embolien. Münch. med. Wschr. **13**, 638 (1965)

Hale, G. S.: Streptokinase in acute myocardial infarction: Rational and preliminary results of a combined therapeutic trial. Aust. Ann. Med. **19** (Suppl. 1), 63 (1970)

Hardaway, R. M., Burns, J. W.: Mechanism of action of fibrinolysin in the prevention of irrevers-ible hemorrhagic shock. Ann. Surg. **157**, 305 (1963)

Harms, D.: Beitrag zur Morphologie des Fibrinabbaus. Behringwerk-Mitteilungen **48**, 22 (1967)

Heikinheimo, R., Ahrenberg, P., Honkapohja, H., Iisalo, E., Kallio, V., Konttinen, Y., Leskinen, O., Mustaniemi, H., Reinikainen, M., Siitonen, I.: Fibrinolytic treatment in acute myocardial in-farction. Acta med. scand. **189**, 7 (1971)

Heimsoth, V. M., Blümcke, S., Bohlmann, H. G., Haupt, H., Küster, F.: Erfolgreiche thrombolyti-sche Therapie bei bilateraler Nierenrindennekrose. Dtsch. med. Wschr. **98**, 1895 (1973)

Heinrich, F.: Ziel und Aufbau der Studie. In: Heinrich, F. (Ed.): Streptokinase-Therapie bei chronischer arterieller Verschlußkrankheit. Marburg: Medizinische Verlagsges. 1975, p. 1

Henning, H., Look, D.: Elektrokardiographische Beobachtungen bei fibrinolytischer Frühbe-handlung des Herzinfarktes. Med. Klin. **62**, 1799 (1967)

Hess, H. (Ed.): Thrombolytische Therapie. Stuttgart: Schattenauer 1967

Hess, H.: Zur Streptokinasetherapie akuter Verschlüsse von Gliedmaßengefäßen. Thrombos. Diathes. haemorrh. (Stuttg.) Suppl. **32**, 275 (1969)

Hess, H., Goossens, N.: Behandlung rezidivierender Embolien in Extremitätenarterien mit Strep-tokinase und Urokinase. Fortschr. Med. **84**, 296 (1966)

Hettich, R.: Spezielle Indikationen für die fibrinolytische Therapie: Tierexperimentelle Untersu-chungen mit der fibrinolytischen Therapie bei Verbrennungen. In: Schneider, W. (Ed.): Fibri-nolytische Therapie, p. 117. Marburg: Medizinische Verlagsges. 1974

Hey, D., Beneke, G., Sandritter, W.: Die fermentative Löslichkeit von Fibrin in Thromben und bei fibrinösen Entzündungen. Klin. Wschr. **44**, 70 (1966)

Hey, D., Budinger, U., Lasch, H. G.: Verbrauchskoagulopathie im Verbrennungsschock. Verh. Dtsch. Ges. inn. Med. **75**, 481 (1969)

Hiemeyer, V.: Thrombolytische Therapie bei akuten Gefäßverschlüssen. Dtsch. med. Wschr. **92**, 955 (1967)

Hiemeyer, V.: Streptokinasetherapie bei akuten Verschlüssen von Gliedmaßenarterien. Throm-bos. Diathes. haemorrh. (Stuttg.) Suppl. **32**, 261 (1969)

Hiemeyer, V. (Ed.): Die thrombolytische Behandlung des Myokardinfarktes. Stuttgart: Schat-tauer 1971 a

Hiemeyer, V.: Grundlagen und Durchführung der fibrinolytischen Therapie. In: Hiemeyer, V. (Ed.): Die thrombolytische Behandlung des Myokardinfarktes, p. 13. Stuttgart: Schattauer 1971 b

Hiemeyer, V., Rasche, H.: Der Mechanismus der Streptokinase-induzierten Thrombolyse und seine Bedeutung für die Therapie akuter Gefäßverschlüsse. Klin. Wschr. **44**, 539 (1966)

Hiemeyer, V., Rasche, H.: Die fibrinolytische Therapie des Herzinfarktes: Klinische und experi-mentelle Ergebnisse. In: Schneider, W. (Ed.): Fibrinolytische Therapie, p. 161. Marburg: Me-dizinische Verlagsges. 1974

Hiemeyer, V., Rasche, H., Diehl, K.: Der Einfluß von Antikoagulantien und Streptokinase auf den Verlauf des akuten Herzinfarktes. Klin. Wschr. **47**, 371 (1969)

Hiemeyer, V., Schoop, W., Winckelmann, G.: Erfahrungen mit der thrombolytischen Behandlung akuter Verschlüsse von Extremitätenarterien. Med. Klin. **60**, 583 (1965)

Hirsh, J.: Dosage regimens for streptokinase treatment: evaluation of a standard dosage schedule. Aust. Ann. Med. **19**, (Suppl. 1), 12 (1970)

Hirsh, H., Buchanan, M., Glynn, M. F., Mustard, J. F.: Effect of streptokinase on haemostasis. Blood **32**, 726 (1968a)

Hirsh, J., Buchanan, M., Glynn, M. F., Mustard, J. F.: Effect of activation of the fibrinolytic mechanism on experimental platelet-rich thrombi in rabbits. J. Lab. clin. Med. **72**, 245 (1968b)

Hirsh, J., Hale, G. S., McDonald, I. G., McCarthy, R. A., Cade, J. F.: Resolution of acute massive pulmonary embolism after a pulmonary arterial infusion of streptokinase. Lancet **1967 II**, 593

Hirsh, J., Hale, G. S., McDonald, I. G., McCarthy, R. A., Pitt, A.: Streptokinase therapy in acute major pulmonary embolism: effectiveness and problems. Brit. med. J. **1968 c IV**, 729

Hirsh, J., McDonald, I. G., Hale, G.: Streptokinase in the treatment of major pulmonary embolism. Experience with twenty-five patients. Aust. Ann. Med. **19**, (Suppl. 1), 54 (1970a)

Hirsh, J., McDonald, I. G., Hale, G., O'Sullivan, E. F., Jelinek, V. M.: Comparison of the effects of streptokinase and heparin on the early rate of resolution of major pulmonary embolism. Canad. med. Ass. J. **104**, 488 (1971)

Hirsh, J., O'Sullivan, E. F., Gallus, A. S., Gilford, E. J.: Arterial thrombosis in a patient with chronic thrombocytopenia. Successful treatment with intra-arterial infusion of streptokinase. J. med. Aust. **2**, 1304 (1969)

Hirsh, J., O'Sullivan, E. F., Martin, M.: Evaluation of a standard dosage schedule with streptokinase. Blood **35**, 341 (1970b)

Honkomp, J.: Thrombolyse bei Nierenvenenthrombose. Med. Klin. **61**, 1205 (1966)

Hort, W., Poliwoda, H., Canalis, S. da, Knigge, J.: Untersuchungen über den Einfluß von Antikoagulantien und Fibrinolytica auf die Größe von Mikroinfarkten im Rattenherzen. Klin. Wschr. **44**, 215 (1966)

Hume, M.: Lysis of experimental radioactive pulmonary embolus induced by streptokinase and streptokinase-activated plasmin. Thrombos. Diathes. haemorrh. (Stuttg.) **11**, 99 (1964)

Hume, M., Gurewich, V., Dealy, J. B., Gajewski, J. Jr.: Streptokinase for chronic arterial disease — effective lysis and thromboembolic complications. Thrombos. Diathes. haemorrh. (Stuttg.) Suppl. **47**, 229 (1971)

Jung, E. G., Duckert, F.: Der Einfluß von Plasmin (Fibrinolysin) auf die Blutgerinnungsfaktoren. Schweiz. med. Wschr. **90**, 1239 (1960)

Kakkar, V. V.: Fibrinolytic treatment of venous thrombosis. Thrombos. Diathes. haemorrh. (Stuttg.) Suppl. **59**, 227 (1974)

Kakkar, V. V., Flanc, C., Howe, C. T., O'Shea, M., Flute, P. T.: Treatment of deep vein thrombosis. A trial of heparin, streptokinase and Arvin. Brit. med. J. **1969 a I**, 806

Kakkar, V. V., Flanc, C., O'Shea, M. J., Flute, P. T., Howe, C. T., Clarke, M. B.: Treatment of deep vein thrombosis with streptokinase. Brit. J. Surg. **56**, 178 (1969b)

Kakkar, V. V., Flute, P. T.: Treatment of deep vein thrombosis with streptokinase. In: Kakkar, V. V., Jouhar, A. J. (Eds.): Thromboembolism: Diagnosis and Treatment, p. 169. London: Livingstone 1972

Kakkar, V. V., Howe, C. T., Laws, J. W., Flanc, C.: Late results of treatment of deep vein thrombosis. Brit. med. J. **1969 c I**, 810

Körtge, P., Prätorius, F., Schneider, B., Heckner, F., Loo, J. van de, Pezold, F. A., Poliwoda, H., Schmutzler, R., Zekorn, D.: Zur thrombolytischen Therapie des frischen Herzinfarktes. III. Zusammenfassende Beurteilung unter Einschluß der Enzymauswertung. Dtsch. med. Wschr. **92**, 1546 (1967)

Köstering, H., Brunner, G., Heimburg, P., Creutzfeldt, W.: Thrombolyse beim Budd-Chiari-Syndrom infolge partieller Thrombose der Vena cava inferior und Lebervenen. Dtsch. med. Wschr. **96**, 1532 (1971)

Kopeć, M.: Personal communication, 1976

Kopp, P. H., Holzknecht, F.: Fibrinolytische Therapie bei septischer Phlebothrombose. Wien. klin. Wschr. **78**, 927 (1966)

Kowalski, E., Kopeć, M., Wegrzynowicz, A.: Influence of fibrinogen degradation products (FDP) on platelet aggregation, adhesiveness and viscous metamorphosis. Thrombos. Diathes. haemorrh. (Stuttg.) **10**, 406 (1964)

Kriessmann, A., Wirtzfeld, A., Weiss, G.: Erfolgreiche Langzeit-Fibrinolyse bei subchronischer Thrombose der Vena axillaris. Med. Klin. **66**, 1198 (1971)

Künzer, W., Schindera, F., Schenk, W., Schumacher, H.: Waterhouse-Friderichsen-Syndrom. Dtsch. med. Wschr. **97**, 270 (1972)

Lasch, H. G., Krause, W.: Grundlagen und Indikation fibrinolytischer Therapie. Ärztl. Fortbild. **16**, 343 (1968)

Lasch, H. G., Mechelke, K., Nusser, E., Sessner, H. H.: Fibrinolysetherapie im Schock. Experimentelle und klinische Ergebnisse. Thrombos. Diathes. haemorrh. (Stuttg.) **7**, 237 (1962)

Lechner, K., Ehringer, H., Ludwig, E., Niessner, H., Stych, H., Thaler, E.: Das fibrinolytische System unter Streptokinase- und Arvin-Therapie. In: Sailer, S. (Ed.): Aktuelle Probleme der Fibrinolyse-Behandlung, p. 99. Wien: Brüder Hollinek 1972

Leube, G.: Vereinfachtes Verfahren der Fibrinolyse beim Herzinfarkt. Ärztl. Prax. **20**, 2568 (1968)

Leube, G., Kuehn, J.: Schnelltest zur Bestimmung der Streptokinase-Initialdosis. Med. Welt **40**, 2181 (1969)

Linke, H.: Kritischer Beitrag zur Antikoagulantien- und Fibrinolysetherapie bei arteriellen Durchblutungsstörungen im Gliedmaßenbereich. Therapiewoche **12**, 905 (1962)

Lohse, K., Weller, P.: Zur Anwendung von Fibrinolytika in der Augenheilkunde. Folia haemat. (Lpz.) **103**, 483 (1976)

Loo, J. van de: Kritische Überlegungen zur Thrombolysetherapie des frischen Herzinfarktes. In: Müller-Wieland, K. (Ed.): Fibrinolyse-Therapie, p. 22. Stuttgart: Schattauer 1969

Loo, J. van de: Möglichkeiten und Grenzen kontrollierter klinischer Therapiestudien zum Wirkungsnachweis antithrombotischer Therapie. Folia haemat. (Lpz.) **102**, 172 (1975)

Loo, J. van de, Verstraete, M.: Fibrinolytic treatment of acute myocardial infarction: a question still open. Thrombos. Diathes. haemorrh. (Stuttg.) Suppl. **59**, 203 (1974)

Lucas, D.: Neuere Erkenntnisse in der Schocktherapie und deren Anwendung bei Kindern. Pädiat. Fortbild.-Prax. **10**, 625 (1971)

Ludwig, H.: Erfahrungen mit der thrombolytischen Behandlung durch Infusion hochgereinigter Streptokinase in der Frauenklinik. Behringwerk-Mitteilungen **44**, 173 (1964)

Ludwig, H.: Therapeutische Fibrinolyse in der Gravidität. Gynaecologia (Basel) **166**, 20 (1968)

Ludwig, H.: Thrombolytische Therapie in der Frauenheilkunde. Die gelben Hefte **19**, 988 (1970a)

Ludwig, H.: Der Endotoxinschock in der Gynäkologie. In: Ahnefeld, F. W., Halmagyi, M. (Eds.): Intensivtherapie beim septischen Schock, p. 49. Berlin-Heidelberg-New York: Springer 1970b

Lübcke, P.: Klinische Erfahrungen mit der Fibrinolysetherapie beim akuten Herzinfarkt. In: Müller-Wieland, K. (Ed.): Fibrinolyse-Therapie, p. 25. Stuttgart: Schattauer 1969

Lübcke, P., Hauschildt, K., Thürmer, J.: Theoretische und klinische Aspekte bei der Streptokinase-Therapie. Med. Welt **23**, 1747 (1972)

Lundberg, M., Erlandsson, P.: Streptokinase treatment in clotting in arterio-venous shunt. Nord. Med. **80**, 1338 (1968)

Madar, G., Widmer, L. K., Schmitt, H. E., Müller, G.: Zur Therapie der akuten tiefen Thrombophlebitis. Phlebographische Beobachtungen bei 100 Patienten. Ergebn. Angiol. **5**, 47 (1972)

Martin, M.: Indikation und Ergebnis der Streptokinasebehandlung bei arteriellen Verschlüssen. Med. Welt **21**, 1861 (1970)

Martin, M.: Antikoagulatorische und sonstige Zusatz-Therapie. In: Heinrich, F. (Ed.): Streptokinase-Therapie bei chronischer arterieller Verschlußkrankheit, p. 23. Marburg: Medizinische Verlagsges. 1975a

Martin, M.: Streptokinase stability pattern during storage in various solvents and at different temperatures. Thrombos. Diathes. haemorrh. (Stuttg.) **33**, 586 (1975b)

Martin, M., Schoop, W., Zeitler, E.: Erfolgreiche Streptokinasebehandlung bei chronisch-arterieller Verschlußkrankheit. Herz Kreislauf **1**, 31 (1969)

Marx, R.: Bemerkungen zur klinischen Anwendung der gereinigten Streptokinase (Streptase®). Behringwerk-Mitteilungen **41**, 103 (1962)

Marx, R.: Grundlagen der Fibrinolysetherapie. In: Müller-Wieland, K. (Ed.): Fibrinolyse-Therapie, p. 1. Stuttgart: Schattauer 1969

Marx, R., Schmiedt, E., Avenhaus, H., Marx, F., Kolle, P.: Zur antithrombotischen-thrombolytischen Differentialtherapie des Priapismus. Urologe **6**, 347 (1967)

Mavor, G. E., Bennett, B., Galloway, J. M. D., Karmody, A. M.: Streptokinase in ilio-femoral venous thrombosis. Brit. J. Surg. **56**, 564 (1969)

Mayer, W., Matis, P.: Beitrag zur Streptase® -Behandlung thromboembolischer Zustände. Behringwerk-Mitteilungen **41**, 148 (1962)

McDonald, I. G., Hirsh, J., Hale, G. S.: The rate of resolution of pulmonary embolism and its effect on early survival. Aust. Ann. Med. **19** (Suppl. 46), 53 (1970)

McNicol, G. P., Douglas, A. S.: Treatment of peripheral vascular occlusion by streptokinase perfusion. Scand. J. clin. Lab. Invest. **16** (Suppl. 78), 23 (1964)

McNicol, G. P., Read, W., Bain, W. H., Douglas, A. S.: Treatment of peripheral arterial occlusion by streptokinase perfusion. Brit. med. J. **1963 I**, 1508

Mies, R., Asbeck, F., Kux-Greve, I., Wehrle, H. J.: Spätthrombolyse der Nierenvenenthrombose. Med. Welt **25**, 146 (1974)

Miller, G. A. H.: Haemodynamic and angiographic findings in patients with pulmonary embolism treated with streptokinase. J. clin. Path. **22**, 367 (1969)

Minn, S. K., Mandel, E. E.: The use of laboratory determinations in the control of streptokinase therapy. J. clin. Path. **58**, 415 (1972)

Mitterstieler, S., Kurz, R., Waltl, H., Berger, H.: Zur fibrinolytischen Therapie des septischen Schocks im Kindesalter. Pädiat. Pädol. **8**, 225 (1973)

Monnens, L., Kleynen, F., Munster, P. von, Schretlen, E., Bonnerman, A.: Coagulation studies and streptokinase therapy in the haemolytic-uraemic syndrom. Helv. paediat. Acta **27**, 45 (1972)

Motin, J., Bouletreau, P., Petit, P., Latarjet, J.: Le traitement de l'embolie pulmonaire grave par la streptokinase (à propos de 8 observations). Lyon méd. **229**, 753 (1973)

Mühe, E.: Spezielle Indikationen für die fibrinolytische Therapie: Peritonitisprophylaxe durch Saug-Spül-Drainage mit Streptokinase. In: Schneider, W. (Ed.): Fibrinolytische Therapie, S. 125. Marburg: Medizinische Verlagsges. 1974

Müller, G., Hiemeyer, V.: Netzhautgefäßverschlüsse unter thrombolytischer Therapie. Die gelben Hefte **19**, 1011 (1970)

Müller, K. H., Herfarth, C., Hupe, K.: Für und Wider einer Antikoagulantienbehandlung nach Embolektomie mit besonderer Berücksichtigung der Thrombolyse durch Streptokinase. Langenbecks Arch. klin. Chir. **300**, 271 (1962)

Mussgnug, G., Alemany, J.: Fibrinolytische Therapie nach Gefäßoperationen im Iliaca-femoralis-poplitea-Bereich. Symposium über thrombolytische Therapie mit Streptokinase. Kopenhagen, März 1967 (abstr.)

Neuhof, H.: Die Sauerstoffaufnahme des Organismus im hämorrhagischen Schock in Beziehung zu Veränderungen der Hämodynamik und Hämostase. Habilitationsschrift Med. Fakultät Gießen, 1970

Neuhof, H., Glaser, E., Hey, D., Lasch, H. G.: Pathophysiologic mechanism in endotoxin shock and its therapeutic approaches. Adv. exp. med. Biol. **9**, 159 (1970)

Neuhof, H., Lasch, H. G.: Spezielle Indikationen für die fibrinolytische Therapie: Verbrauchskoagulopathie und Schock. In: Schneider, W. (Ed.): Fibrinolytische Therapie, S. 95. Marburg: Medizinische Verlagsges. 1974

Niewiarowski, S., Kowalski, E.: Formation of an antithrombin-like anticoagulant during proteolysis of fibrinogen. Bull. Acad. pol. Sci. **5**, 169 (1957)

Nolf, P.: Contribution à l'étude de la coagulation du sang. (5ième mémoire) La fibrinolyse. Arch. int. Physiol. **6**, 306 (1905)

Ogston, D., Ogston, C. M., Fullerton, H. W.: The plasminogen content of thrombi. Thrombos. Diathes. haemorrh. (Stuttg.) **15**, 220 (1966)

Ohler, W. G. A.: Antikoagulantienbehandlung nach thrombolytischer Therapie. Med. Klin. **61**, 140 (1966)

Olow, B.: Effect of streptokinase on postoperative changes in some coagulation factors and the fibrinolytic system. Acta chir. scand. **126**, 197 (1963)

Olow, B., Johanson, C., Andersson, I., Eklöf, B.: Deep venous thrombosis treated with a standard dosage of streptokinase. Acta chir. scand. **136**, 181 (1970)

Paquet, K. J., Popov, S., Egli, H.: Richtlinien und Ergebnisse der konsequenten fibrinolytischen Therapie der Phlegmasia coerulea dolens. Dtsch. med. Wschr. **95**, 903 (1970)

Pezold, F. A.: Einige außergewöhnliche Fälle von fibrinolytischer Therapie. Thrombos. Diathes. haemorrh. (Stuttg.) Suppl. **32**, 311 (1969a)

Pezold, F. A.: Analyse der Todesursachen im Zusammenhang mit fibrinolytischer Therapie. Thrombos. Diathes. haemorrh. (Stuttg.) Suppl. **32**, 315 (1969 b)

Pfeifer, G. W.: Experimentelle Untersuchungen zur Frage eines diaplazentaren Effektes von Streptokinase. Klin. Wschr. **43**, 775 (1965)

Pfeifer, G. W.: Thromboembolische Komplikationen bei Schwangeren und die thrombolytische Therapie. Therapiewoche **17**, 49, 2021 (1967)

Pogglitsch, H., Stöckl, G.: Die Streptokinasebehandlung von Shunt-Thrombosen. In: Sailer, S. (Ed.): Aktuelle Probleme der Fibrinolyse-Behandlung, p. 67. Wien: Brüder Hollinek 1972

Poliwoda, H.: Technik und Überwachung der thrombolytischen Therapie. Behringwerk-Mitteilungen **48**, 32 (1967)

Poliwoda, H.: Grundlagen der thrombolytischen Therapie. Die gelben Hefte **19**, 1003 (1970 a)

Poliwoda, H.: Treatment of acute and chronic arterial occlusions with streptokinase. Aust. Ann. Med. **19** (Suppl. 1), 25 (1970 b)

Poliwoda, H., Alexander, K., Buhl, V., Holsten, D., Wagner, H. H.: Treatment of chronic arterial occlusions with streptokinase. New Engl. J. Med. **280**, 689 (1969)

Poliwoda, H., Diederich, K. W., Schneider, B., Rodenburg, R., Heckner, F., Körtge, P., Loo, J. van de, Pezold, F. A., Praetorius, F., Schmutzler, R., Zekorn, D.: Zur thrombolytischen Therapie des frischen Herzinfarktes. II. Ergebnisse der elektrokardiographischen Untersuchungen. Dtsch. med. Wschr. **91**, 978 (1966)

Powell, H. R., Ekert, H.: Streptokinase and anti-thrombotic therapy in the hemolytic-uremic syndrome. J. Pediat. **84**, 345 (1974)

Prätorius, F., Körtge, P., Schneider, B., Leonhardt, H., Börner, W., Fritze, E., Gebauer, D., Gillmann, H., Grosser, K. D., Heckner, F., Loo, J. van de, Pezold, F. A., Poliwoda, H., Schmutzler, R., Zekorn, D.: Kinetik der Serumenzyme bei Behandlung des Herzinfarktes mit Streptokinase. Ergebnisse der II. Deutsch-Schweizerischen Gemeinschaftsstudie. Klin. Wschr. **51**, 397 (1973)

Prentice, C. R. M., McNicol, G. P., Douglas, A. S.: Plasminogen activation and the coagulation process. J. clin. Path. **22**, 367 (1969)

Preston, F. E., Edwards, I. R.: Postpartum purpura fulminans: successful management with streptokinase. Brit. med. J. **1973 III**, 329

Rasche, H., Hiemeyer, V.: Über die Beeinflussung verschiedener Plasmaeiweißkörper durch eine fibrinolytische Behandlung. Verh. dtsch. Ges. inn. Med. **74**, 154 (1968)

Rasche, H., Hiemeyer, V.: Theoretische und experimentelle Gesichtspunkte zur thrombolytischen Therapie mit Streptokinase. In: Pezold, F. A. (Ed.): Fibrinolyse-Therapie heute, p. 3. Stuttgart: Schattauer 1970

Ratnoff, O. D., Menzie, C.: A new method for the determination of fibrinogen in small samples of plasma. J. Lab. clin. Med. **37**, 316 (1951)

Robertson, B. R., Nilsson, I. M., Nylander, G.: Value of streptokinase and heparin in treatment of acute deep venous thrombosis. Acta chir. scand. **134**, 203 (1968)

Robertson, B. R., Nilsson, I. M., Nylander, G.: Thrombolytic effect of streptokinase as evaluated by phlebography of deep venous thrombi of the leg. Acta chir. scand. **136**, 173 (1970)

Rosolleck, H.: Lyse von humanen Blutgerinnseln im Reagenzglas. Klin. Wschr. **39**, 440 (1961)

Rossmann, H.: Thrombolyse in der Augenheilkunde. Behringwerk-Mitteilungen **48**, 64 (1967)

Rossmann, H.: Spezielle Indikationen für die fibrinolytische Therapie: Zur Behandlung von Gefäßverschlüssen der Netzhaut durch Fibrinolyse. In: Schneider, W. (Ed.): Fibrinolytische Therapie, p. 89. Marburg: Medizinische Verlagsges. 1974

Ruegsegger, P., Nydick, J., Hutter, R., Freimann, A. H., Bang, N. U., Cliffton, E., Ladue, J. S.: Fibrinolytic (plasmin) therapy of experimental coronary thrombi with alteration of the evolution of myocardial infarction. Circulation **19**, 7 (1959)

Sack, K.: Thrombolytische Therapie bei Thrombangiitis obliterans. Internist. prax. **8**, 529 (1968)

Sailer, S. von, Wehrschütz, E., Tilz, G. P.: Die thrombolytische Behandlung peripherer Gefäßverschlüsse mit Streptokinase. Wien. med. Wschr. **118**, 1 (1968 a)

Sailer, S. von, Wehrschütz, E., Tilz, G. P.: Die thrombolytische Behandlung des frischen Herzinfarktes. Wien. med. Wschr. **118**, 283 (1968 b)

Sandritter, W.: Die pathologische Anatomie der Thrombose und Lungenembolie. Behringwerk-Mitteilungen **41**, 37 (1962)

Schachenmayr, W., Haferkamp, O.: Der hämorrhagische Herzinfarkt. Dtsch. med. Wschr. 97, 1172 (1972)

Schimpf, K.: Thrombolysetherapie. Dtsch. med. Wschr. 94, 2292 (1969)

Schmeisser, G., Vogel, G., Vollmar, F., Heidrich, R.: Subarachnoidalblutung unter Streptokinase-Therapie bei Karotisthrombose. Dtsch. Gesundh.-Wes. 30, 1941 (1975)

Schmidt, H. W.: Zur Thrombolyse mit verschiedenen Fibrinolytica. I. Mitteilung. Untersuchungen an experimentellen menschlichen Nativblutthromben. Klin. Wschr. 44, 618 (1966)

Schmitt, W., Wack, H.-O., Beneke, G.: Das Substrat chronischer arterieller Stenosen und Okklusionen. Dtsch. med. Wschr. 39, 1522 (1971)

Schmutzler, R.: Nebenwirkungen der Fibrinolytika. Thrombos. Diathes. haemorrh. (Stuttg.) Suppl. 15, 99 (1965)

Schmutzler, R.: Klinik der thrombolytischen Behandlung. Internist (Berl.) 10, 21 (1969)

Schmutzler, R.: Fibrinolyse peripherer venöser Thromben. Die gelben Hefte 19, 979 (1970)

Schmutzler, R.: Die fibrinolytische Therapie des Herzinfarktes: Ergebnisse der bisherigen Herzinfarktstudien. In: Schneider, W. (Ed.): Fibrinolytische Therapie, p. 169. Marburg: Medizinische Verlagsges. 1974

Schmutzler, R., Fritze, E., Gebauer, D., Gillmann, H., Heckner, F., Körtge, P., Loo, J. van de, Pezold, F. A., Poliwoda, H., Prätorius, F., Schneider, B., Zekorn, D.: Die fibrinolytische Behandlung des frischen Herzinfarktes. In: Hiemeyer, V. (Ed.): Die thrombolytische Behandlung des Myokardinfarktes, p. 23. Stuttgart: Schattauer 1971

Schmutzler, R., Heckner, F., Körtge, P., Loo, J. van de, Pezold, F. A., Poliwoda, H., Prätorius, F., Zekorn, D.: Zur thrombolytischen Therapie des frischen Herzinfarktes. I. Einführung, Behandlungspläne, allgemeine klinische Ergebnisse. Dtsch. med. Wschr. 91, 581 (1966)

Schmutzler, R., Koller, F.: Die Thrombolyse-Therapie. Ergebn. inn. Med. Kinderheilk. 22, 157 (1965)

Schmutzler, R., Koller, F.: Thrombolytic therapy. In: Poller, L. (Ed.): Recent Advances in Blood Coagulation. London: Churchill 1969

Schneider, K. W.: Die fibrinolytische Therapie des Herzinfarktes: Übersichtsreferat über die fibrinolytische Therapie beim Myokardinfarkt. In: Schneider, W. (Ed.): Fibrinolytische Therapie, p. 145. Marburg: Medizinische Verlagsges. 1974

Schoop, W., Levy, H., Zeitler, E.: Spätergebnisse der thrombolytischen Therapie chronischer Arterienverschlüsse. Dtsch. med. Wschr. 95, 1827 (1970)

Schoop, W., Martin, M., Zeitler, E.: Beseitigung alter Arterienverschlüsse durch intravenöse Streptokinase-Infusion. Dtsch. med. Wschr. 93, 2321 (1968)

Schreiber, F., Eulitz, H.-J.: Streptokinasebehandlung des frischen Herzinfarktes. Med. Klin. 68, 592 (1973)

Schreinert, A.: Thrombolytische Therapie im Kindesalter. Mschr. Kinderheilk. 121, 394 (1973)

Schulte, M.: Nachuntersuchungen. In: Heinrich, F. (Ed.): Streptokinase-Therapie bei chronisch arterieller Verschlußkrankheit, p. 65. Marburg: Medizinische Verlagsges. 1975

Schwartz, J. M., Friedman, S. A., Schreiber, Z. A., Tsao, L. L., Richter, I. H.: Problems with streptokinase therapy in acute pulmonary embolism. Surgery 74, 727 (1973)

Schwick, G., Heimburger, N.: Biochemie der Fibrinolyse. Thrombos. Diathes. haemorrh. (Stuttg.) Suppl. 32, 9 (1969)

Senn, A.: Besonderheiten der Phlegmasia coerulea dolens. Dtsch. med. Wschr. 101, 1005 (1976)

Shaw, L. W., Cornfield, J., Cole, C. M.: Statistical problems in the design of clinical trials and interpretation of results. Thrombos. Diathes. haemorrh. (Stuttg.) Suppl. 59, 191 (1974)

Sherry, S.: Trial and error, questions and answers. Thrombos. Diathes. haemorrh. (Stuttg.) Suppl. 59, 263 (1974)

Sherry, S., Fletcher, A. P., Alkjaersig, N.: The mechanism of clot dissolution by plasmin. J. clin. Invest. 38, 1086 (1959)

Sinapius, D.: Häufigkeit und Morphologie der Coronarthrombose und ihre Beziehungen zur antithrombotischen und fibrinolytischen Behandlung. Klin. Wschr. 43, 37 (1965)

Sinapius, D.: Das pathologisch-anatomische Substrat des Herzinfarktes. Thrombos. Diathes. haemorrh. (Stuttg.) Suppl. 32, 327 (1969)

Skiftis, T.: Therapeutische Fibrinolyse in der Schwangerschaft. Geburtsh. u. Frauenheilk. 31, 568 (1971)

Spöttl, F., Kaiser, R., Mosuni, M. S.: Acute phase reaction following intravenous administration of streptokinase. Thrombos. Diathes. haemorrh. (Stuttg.) **31**, 429 (1974)

Stetter, H.: Spezielle Indikationen für die fibrinolytische Therapie: Fibrinolytische Therapie bei Verbrennungen. In: Schneider, W. (Ed.): Fibrinolytische Therapie, p. 105. Marburg: Medizinische Verlagsges. 1974

Stickland, J., McDonald, I. G., O'Sullivan, E. F.: Response of massive pulmonary embolism with protracted circulatory failure to thrombolytic therapy. Med. J. Aust. **2**, 125 (1973)

Storm, O., Ollendorf, E., Drewsen, E., Tang, P.: Deep venous thrombosis treated with plasmin. Results of a double-blind trial (preliminary report). II. Congr. Int. Soc. Thrombos. Haemostas. Oslo, 1971, p. 136

Stricker, E., Schmutzler, R.: Erfolgreiche Behandlung eines arteriellen zerebralen Gefäßverschlusses. Schweiz. med. Wschr. **18**, 615 (1964)

Thies, H. A.: Kontraindikationen und Nebenwirkungen der Thrombolytika. Behringwerk-Mitteilungen **48**, 28 (1967)

Tibbutt, D. A., Davies, I. A., Anderson, I. A., Fletcher, E. W. L., Hamill, I., Holt, I. M., Thomas, M. L., Lee, G. de J., Miller, G. A. M., Sharp, A. A., Sutton, G. C.: Comparison by controlled clinical trial of streptokinase and heparin in treatment of life-threatening pulmonary embolism. Brit. med. J. **1974 I**, 343

Tillet, W. S., Garner, R. L.: Fibrinolytic activity of haemolytic streptococci. J. exp. Med. **58**, 485 (1933)

Tillet, W. S., Johnson, A. J., McCarthy, W. R.: The intravenous infusion of the streptococcal fibrinolytic principle (streptokinase) into patients. J. clin. Invest. **34**, 169 (1955)

Tilsner, V.: Streptokinasetherapie bei Lungenembolien und die Beurteilung ihres therapeutischen Effektes. Thrombos. Diathes. haemorrh. (Stuttg.) Suppl. **32**, 279 (1969)

Tilsner, V.: Nebenwirkungen. In: Heinrich, F. (Ed.): Streptokinase-Therapie bei chronisch arterieller Verschlußkrankheit, p. 55. Marburg: Medizinische Verlagsges. 1975

Tilsner, V., Johannes, E., Kalmar, P., Westermann, K. W., Marcsek, M.: Thrombolytische Therapie bei älteren venösen Gefäßverschlüssen. Med. Klin. **67**, 16 (1972)

Topalow, B.: Kombinierte chirurgisch-thrombolytische Behandlung der tiefen Venenthrombose. X. Intern. Angiol. Congr., Florenz, 1974 (abstr.)

Tsapogas, M. I., Peabody, R. A., Wu, K. T., Karmody, A. M., Devaray, K. T., Eckert, C.: Controlled study of thrombolytic therapy in deep vein thrombosis. Surgery **74**, 973 (1973)

Vermylen, I., Amery, A., Dirix, P., Verstraete, M.: Keeping arteriovenous shunts patent. Lancet **1967 II**, 1968

Verstraete, M.: The difficulty of appraisal of streptokinase therapy of myocardial infarction. Angiologica **8**, 43 (1971)

Verstraete, M.: Registry of prospective clinical trials. Second report. Thrombos. Haemostas. (Stuttg.) **36**, 239 (1976)

Verstraete, M., Amery, A., Vermylen, J.: Feasibility of adequate thrombolytic therapy with streptokinase in peripheral arterial occlusions. 1. Clinical and arteriographic results. Brit. med. J. **1963 I**, 1499

Verstraete, M., Amery, A., Vermylen, J.: Streptokinase in recent myocardial infarction. A controlled multicentre trial. Brit. med. J. **1971 III**, 325

Verstraete, M., Vermylen, J., Amery, A., Vermylen, C.: Thrombolytic therapy with streptokinase using a standard dosage scheme. Brit. med. J. **1966 I**, 454

Verstraete, M., Vermylen, J., Vreker, R. de, Amery, A., Vermylen, C.: Efficacy of thrombolytic therapy with streptokinase using a new administration scheme. Scand. J. clin. Lab. Invest. **16** (Suppl. 78), 15 (1964)

Vinazzer, H.: Gerinnungsphysiologische Erscheinungen und klinische Nebenwirkungen bei Streptokinasetherapie. Folia haemat. (Lpz.) **103**, 468 (1976 b)

Vinazzer, M.: Personal communication, 1976 a

Völcker, A.: Thrombolytische Behandlung des Myokardinfarktes. Med. Welt **22**, 290 (1971)

Vogel, G., Eger, H., Zuber, W., Fuchs, R., Huyke, R., Raith, S., Warzok, H.: Beitrag zum klinischen Bild des Paget-von-Schroetter-Syndroms unter besonderer Berücksichtigung der thrombolytischen Therapie. Dtsch. Gesundh.-Wes. **27**, 2020 (1972)

Vogel, G., Fiehring, H.: Klinische Erfahrungen mit der Streptokinase-Behandlung beim kardiogenen Schock. Folia haemat. (Lpz.) **97**, 44 (1972)

Vogel, G., Huyke, R.: Klinik der thrombolytischen Therapie mit Streptokinase. Folia haemat. (Lpz.) **103**, 456 (1976)

Vogel, G., Schlosser, R.: Über einen Fall von Priapismus bei aufsteigender Beinvenenthrombose. Erfolgreiche Therapie mit Streptokinase. Z. gcs. inn. Med. **26**, 667 (1971)

Vogt, W.: Activation, activities and pharmacologically active products of complement. Pharmacol. Rev. **26**, 125 (1974)

Vreker, R. A. de: A technique for routine evaluation of plasminogen in humans during streptokinase therapy. Acta haemat. (Basel) **34**, 305 (1965)

Vujadinovic, B.: Nos expériences dans le traitement des affections thromboemboliques avec streptase. Arch. Serb. Med. Gen. (Beograd) **98**, 435 (1969)

Walther, C., Koestering, H.: Therapeutische Thrombolyse in der neunten Schwangerschaftswoche. Dtsch. med. Wschr. **94**, 32 (1969)

Weber, G., Stetter, H., Sessner, H. H.: Zur intravasalen Fibrinolyse-Therapie bei drittgradigen Verbrennungen. Dtsch. med. Wschr. **94**, 899 (1969)

Weinmann, G., Giertler, U., Schwela, S.: Thrombolytische Therapie in der Pädiatrie. Folia haemat. (Lpz.) **103**, 472 (1976)

Zekorn, D.: Biochemische Grundlagen der Thrombolysetherapie mit Streptokinase. Behringwerk-Mitteilungen **48**, 8 (1967)

Zschenker, H.: Über die Behandlung eines Mesenterialverschlusses durch Thrombektomie, ausgedehnte Dünndarmresektion und nachfolgende Streptasebehandlung. Chirurg **42**, 332 (1971)

Urokinase

F. DUCKERT

Introduction

The wide distribution in human body fluids and tissues of fibrinolysis activators most probably reflects their outstanding physiologic importance. The proteolytic activity of urine was discovered in 1861 by VON BRÜCKE, its ability to dissolve fibrin clots by SAHLI in 1885. The existence of several proteolytic enzymes, some with pH optimum in the weak alkaline range, was soon recognized (GEHRIG, 1886; GRÜTZ-NER, 1891).

In 1947 MACFARLANE and PILLING established on the one hand, the fibrinolytic activity of urine at very high dilution, and, on the other, the fast disappearance of blood fibrinolytic activity after an activation stimulus, i.e., trauma, adrenaline injection, or other stimuli. They demonstrated that the blood and urine activities or enzymes attack the same substrates and are impaired by similar inhibitors. They assumed that the blood activity could simply be excreted through the kidney. They failed, however, to show a relationship between the variations of activity in blood and those in urine.

WILLIAMS (1951) attributed the fibrinolytic activity of urine to a kinase able to activate the plasminogen present as impurity in fibrinogen preparations and in fibrin clots. SOBEL et al. (1952) named the potent urine activator of plasminogen, urokinase.

A. Origin of Urokinase

I. Urokinase as Excreted Blood Activator

A quantitative relationship between blood and urine activity has never been consistently established and, in addition, is not automatically a good proof since the production and/or release of two different activators could very well be due to a single stimulus. In most instances even an absence of relationship has been observed after stimulation of the fibrinolysis system by exercise, trauma, adrenaline injection (MACFARLANE and PILLING, 1947), or nicotinic acid treatment (HOLEMANS et al., 1966). The lack of a quantitative relationship between plasma and urine activity is also insufficient to establish their nonidentity. The differences may be due to a variable stability and to the presence of specific inhibitors of plasma and urine. A study of the biochemical and immunologic properties will offer better arguments for or against this hypothesis (see below).

II. Urokinase Produced in the Ureters and Bladder

This possibility can be eliminated. Kidney urine and bladder urine are equally active (BJERREHUUS, 1952). The bladder epithelium is inactive. An activator activity, strongly bound to the cell in contrast to urokinase, is confined to the deeper layers of the bladder wall (HISAZUMI et al., 1973). This information confirms previous results of ALBRECHTSEN (1957a, b) and ROBERTS and ASTRUP (1957) who extracted no or very little activity out of these tissues. However, these findings did not remain unchallenged. LADEHOFF (1960) found more activity in the ureter and mucous membrane of the bladder than in the kidney parenchyma.

III. Urokinase Produced in the Kidneys

Here also the results differ greatly. Three methods have been used to demonstrate the presence of fibrinolytic activators in kidney tissues: the extraction method (ASTRUP and STAGE, 1952), the fibrin slide method of TODD (1958, 1964) which allows the localization of the fibrinolytic activity, and finally the measurement of a difference of activator activity between arterial and venous renal blood. None of these methods is able to distinguish between urokinase and other activators. Variable results have been reported partly due to species differences. Investigating human and rabbit organs, ASTRUP and STERNDORFF (1956) found in the citrate suspension of disintegrated whole kidney or kidney cortex, an activator activity in both the sediment and the supernatant. In contrast no activity was found in the supernatants of lungs and adrenals. An identity between the soluble activator and urokinase is possible but not established. ALBRECHTSEN (1957a, b) found no or moderate activity in the kidneys of several animals and a moderate activity in human kidneys. The experiments of the localization of activity in the kidneys gave the following results:

In man, pig, rabbit, rat, and guinea pig the activator was found in the endothelial cells of the blood vessels. The activity decreases in the following order: (1) peritubular capillary network in the pyramid; (2) interlobal arcuate vessels, perilobular and periureteric capillary bed; (3) interlobular vessels, and (4) glomerular capillaries (KWAAN and FISCHER, 1965). In dogs the kidneys are very active and the activity is localized in the walls of the vasa recta and the tip of the papilla (HOLEMANS et al., 1965; McCONNEL et al., 1966b). The walls of the large renal vessels contain also the activator. In contrast, the tubular and peritubular capillaries are inactive. The activator of the tip of the papilla localized in the distal portion of the collecting channels can be considered as the source of urokinase (McCONNEL et al., 1966b). Some discrepancies may be explained by the existence of a preurokinase which is activated on secretion (ÅSTEDT, 1975), as shown by the primary inactivity of fetal and mature kidney glomeruli followed by the development of activity in the culture of glomeruli.

The measure of fibrinolytic activity in renal blood, both arterial and venous, under normal and experimental conditions underlines the important role of the kidneys. The activity is slightly higher in venous blood than in arterial blood.

This normally low activity increases after venous stasis and even more after ligation of the ureters (BULUK and FURMAN, 1962). The exclusion of the kidney circulation causes a decrease of blood activity (JANUSZKO et al., 1966). The fibrinolytic activity also diminishes after intoxication with mercury chloride and necrosis of the tubular cells (WOROWSKI et al., 1964; NIEWIAROWSKI et al., 1964) as shown by an increase of fibrinogen factor VIII and plasminogen (NIEWIAROWSKI et al., 1964) and the disappearance of activity in the juxtaglomerular cells, the macula densa, and the Goormaghtigh cells after intoxication with a simultaneous decrease in the endothelial cells.

According to BULUK and MALOFIEJEW (see WOROWSKI et al., 1964) as much as 94% of the "urokinase" activity from isolated rabbit kidney goes to the general circulation whereas the remaining 6% is excreted into the urine. In dogs, the activity appears in the perfusates of blood-free kidneys only after stimulation by a histamine injection in the renal artery. A second injection is inefficient because of the depletion of plasminogen activator from the vasa recta (HOLEMANS et al., 1965). The activator release is specific and not associated with a general rise of the protein concentration in the perfusate. The perfusate of veins, even after histamine stimulation, is inactive. HOLEMANS et al. (1965) assume that the release depends on the wall surface, which is relatively much larger in the capillary bed of the kidneys than in the larger veins. The difference, however, may simply reflect the higher solubility and easier release of the kidney activator. All these accumulated data characterize the importance of the kidneys as a source of fibrinolytic activator. They allow no conclusions on the identity or lack of identity of this activator with urokinase.

IV. Comparison of Urokinase with Other Activators

These investigations are based mainly on the comparison of the biochemical and immunologic properties of urokinase and other activators. They can at the same time throw some additional light on the urokinase origin.

KUCINSKI et al. (1966, 1968) obtained a specific antiurokinase antiserum by immunization of guinea pig with purified urokinase. The antiserum inhibits the activity of purified urokinase and urine, also that of primate urokinase. It has no or practically no effect on the urokinase of other animals and on the activity of other activators (KUCINSKI and FLETCHER, 1976; KUCINSKI et al., 1968). Inhibition is limited to the caseinolytic and fibrinolytic assay, whereas esterolysis is not modified. Apparently the antibody cannot block the access of the esters to the active center of urokinase. Using the same antibody, KUCINSKI et al. (1968) were unable to detect urokinase in the renal veins of volunteers. The result excludes the possibility of a distribution of urokinase between blood and urine as postulated by BULUK and MALOFIEJEW (see WOROWSKI et al., 1964). The importance of these results has been weakened by BERNIK et al. (1974) who report that a specific antiserum against urokinase, prepared in rabbits, is able to neutralize 80% of the activity of native tissue activator and of the blood vessel activator obtained from perfusates of peripheral veins. Double diffusion and immunoelectrophoresis showed the same pattern of identity. The discrepancy between the data of KUCINSKI et al. (1968) and of BERNIK et al. (1974) may be tentatively explained by qualitative differences of the antisera. The action of the guinea pig antiserum is limited to urokinase-specific determinant(s) whereas the rabbit antibodies are directed against other parts of the molecules immunologically similar in the different activators detecting only a partial identity. This is possible if the rabbit antisera are directed against the active part of urokinase which may be very similar to the active portion of other fibrinolytic activators.

The interpretation of the biochemical data is even more difficult since the experiments have been performed on urokinase and activators of different animal species and on preparations of variable purity.

For example, ALI and EVANS (1968) assume a similarity, even identity, of urokinase and other activators extracted from lysosomes and microsomes; the molecular weights are similar (50000). Both are competitively inhibited by EACA and AMCA, inhibited by cysteine and arginine, and not altered by iodoacetamide or p-chloromercuribenzoate. In these experiments human urokinase has been compared to activators extracted form different animal organs. THORSEN (1973) came to the same conclusion when testing urokinase and tissue activator against a series of natural inhibitors, the trypsin inhibitors of pancreas, urine, soybeans, peanuts, mingin, and the inhibitor of normal plasma.

Other experimental data prove the lack of identity between urokinase and the tissue activator of the hog ovaries (KOK and ASTRUP, 1969). The inhibition of tissue activator increases with increasing EACA and AMCA concentrations whereas the inhibition of urokinase is biphasic (THORSEN and ASTRUP, 1969). The placenta inhibitor is less potent against tissue activator extracted from the human femoral arteries and veins than against urokinase. Their K_M for the esterolysis of acetyllysine methylester are different and the molecular weight of the tissue activator is higher than that of urokinase (AOKI and VON KAULLA, 1971). LIPINSKI et al. (1975) find a very crucial difference which is reflected by the absence of fibrinogenolysis with the vascular activator in contrast to urokinase. The vascular activator is specifically bound to a plasma inhibitor; the complex is dissociated only in presence of fibrin which explains the lack of fibrinogenolysis. The plasma inhibitor in opposition does not alter the action of urokinase.

The wide disparity of the reported results makes any definitive conclusion impossible. Urokinase is most probably synthetized in the kidney. The identity or partial identity of urokinase with one tissue activator is possible but not established, a total nonidentity of urokinase with all other activators remains also possible. Further qualitative comparisons are required before origin and identity of urokinase with other activators of the plasminogen-plasmin conversion can be considered as definitely acquired.

V. Urokinase from Tissue Cultures

BARNETT and BARON (1958, 1959) detected the presence of a plasminogen activator in kidney cell cultures. PAINTER and CHARLES (1962) confirmed the presence of a soluble activator in the fluid of cultures of kidney cells of both rhesus monkey and dog. Not sedimented with the cells, the activator was thought to be identical to urokinase.

In cultures of primary human kidney explants (BERNIK and KWAAN, 1967) the plasminogen activator activity was found in the outgrowth of small vessels, the cells were predominantly endothelial cells, and the release of activator a function of the living cells. BERNIK and KWAAN (1967) using the antiserum prepared by KUCINSKI and FLETCHER (1966) demonstrated the immunologic identity of this activator with urokinase. Interestingly enough BERNIK and KWAAN (1969) found that even though kidney cells contain an activator immunologically different from urokinase, the same cells, when they survive and grow after implantation, release in the supernatant an activator activity able to neutralize an antiurokinase antiserum. According to the same authors the synthesis of a urokinase-like activator is not limited to the kidney cells. Such an activator accumulates in the supernates of fetal lung and ureter cultures. Serially propagated cells continue to produce a urokinase-like activator. This property is confined to the diploid cell lines. On a quantitative base the antiurokinase antiserum neutralizes 70–95% of the activity produced by the kidney cells and only 30–90% in ureter cultures. Therefore the synthesis of a second activator beside urokinase seems possible.

This tissue activator could be released after the death of the cells. The interpretation of these results is complicated by the simultaneous synthesis of urokinase inhibitors in the cultures of other tissues, i.e., bladder or lung.

The urokinase-like activity found in tissue culture is enhanced by plasmin and thrombin which may activate a urokinase precursor particularly sensitive to their action (BERNIK, 1973). According to MACIAG et al. (1977), a precursor of the plasminogen activator found in the cell of adult pig kidney is increasingly released in the presence of Hageman factor. The zymogen is also activated by proteolytic enzymes such as thrombin, plasmin, trypsin, and Hageman factor protease. The production on a larger scale of this urokinase-like activator seems possible. In addition to the primary culture of embryonic kidney cells the subcultures without karyologic alterations at least up to the 30th generation, preserve their ability to synthetise the urokinase-like activator (BARLOW et al., 1976, 1977). The productivity of the subcultures depends on several yet incompletely defined factors such as amino acids and small peptides which may favor the synthesis and also the release of a precursor in the medium. The precursor is converted by traces of proteolytic enzymes or autocatalytically in urokinase-like activator. The molecular weight, first 54000 is slowly converted to the 31500 moiety. The proportion of the two different molecules evolves toward the 31500 sort upon incubation time.

Several properties of the cell culture activator are similar or identical to those of urokinase. They are immunologically identical. Both enzymes have the same pH optimum at 7.8 for the hydrolysis of the acetyl-glycyl-lysine methyl ester (AGLME). The correlation between the esterolytic activity and the plasminogen activation is identical. Their electrophoretic mobility is the same between pH 5 and pH 9. The elution pattern from Sephadex is similar for the single activators and their mixtures. These still incomplete results make their identity quite probable (BARLOW and LAZER, 1972).

B. Physiology and Pathophysiology

Urokinase is probably present in the urine of all mammals (MOHLER et al., 1958). In humans the urokinase activity in urine is inversely proportional to the urine volume (BJERREHUUS, 1952). The daily production varies from individual to individual between 300 and 900 units (GUEST and CELANDER, 1961). It amounts in average to 6000 CTA units per day, it is independent of age and sex and varies little in time-of-day function (ALKJAERSIG, 1975). However, GUEST and CELANDER (1961) found an important daily variation in a single individual and demonstrated that the urokinase excretion is influenced by the salt-intake. At high salt-intake urokinase activity tends to diminish to low values and increases to the highest normal values at low salt intake. This behavior is the reverse of that of renin. One may postulate a certain correlation between both mechanisms (LARAGH et al., 1972). Apparently no special studies have been undertaken on this particular point.

On the contrary, BOOMGARD et al. (1966) found a constant daily production with a constant production rate over the 24 h. The excretion reaches 6800 ± 1350 Ploug units/day. An enhanced blood fibrinolytic activity was not associated with a concomitant rise of urokinase activity.

As already demonstrated above, it is not at all certain that urokinase is a normal component of the plasma. However if it were, its half-life time, as judged from the experimental data collected after urokinase injection, must be very short. According to BACHMANN (1966) the activity appears in the bile already 5 min after injection and reaches a peak activity 2–3 times higher than in plasma 35–60 min later. The bile activity is neutralized by an antiurokinase antiserum prepared in guinea pig. Only 2% of the activity could be recovered in urine. The liver has probably an active transport system for urokinase, possibly for other plasminogen activators, which would explain a rise of fibrinolytic activity in liver disease. The urokinase is removed from the blood very rapidly with a T 1/2 of 16 ± 7 min. SOM et al. (1975) described a two-phase clearance with a very fast clearance followed by a slower disappearance rate of 3.0 ± 0.8 h for ^{99m}Tc-labeled urokinase and 4.8 ± 0.9 h for ^{131}I-labeled urokinase in dogs. The excretion of bound radioactivity in urine is very small. It is higher in the bile: 0.5–3%. SOM et al. (1975) found labeled urokinase in liver, kidneys, and in the gastrointestinal tract. Similar results had already been reported by BACK et al. (1961) and TAJIMA et al. (1974). The exact value of these data is difficult to appreciate in real physiologic terms since the distinction between free radioactivity and unaltered, labeled urokinase is hardly possible and due to the fact that the injected urokinase is far from the native urokinase. In addition, the experiments in animals were conducted with heterologous urokinase.

Under pathologic conditions urokinase activity in urine is reduced in the postoperative phase of cardiac surgery (VON KAULLA et al., 1958), in recurrent thrombophlebitis and carcinoma (VON KAULLA and RIGGENBACH, 1960), in neoplasms, cardiac disease, muscular dystrophy, and severe burns (GUEST and CELANDER, 1961), in uremia, in carcinomatosis, independent of the tumor site, in congestive cardiac failure, slightly reduced in essential hypertension, chronic glomerulonephritis, and hepatitis (SMYRNIOTIS et al., 1959). Short-term disseminated intravascular coagulation (DIC) results in a transient decrease of urokinase excretion and impairment of renal function. After cessation of DIC there is a reverse reaction which helps lyse the fibrin deposits (THEISS et al., 1970). Urokinase activity is significantly elevated after myocardial infarction, coronary insufficiency, slightly elevated in thrombophlebitis and pneumonia (SMYRNIOTIS et al., 1959).

VREEKEN et al. (1966) find a correlation between renal function expressed by the creatinin clearance and the urokinase excretion. However, the activity detected by the slide technique was present in the diseased kidneys of patients with various nephrologic affections (BERGSTEIN and MICHAEL, 1972) except in renal homograft rejection where the activator activity was absent (BERGSTEIN and MICHAEL, 1974).

The reason for the altered "urokinase" activity in these patients can be due to the following: consumption because of abnormal fibrin deposition, increase of inhibitors, or defective production as in renal homograft rejection. Unfortunately the urine activity was not determined in these patients.

Urokinase activity can be impaired by several natural inhibitors. Their activity is difficult to determine but at least 10 Ploug U/ml are required to get a good lytic activity (DUDOK DE WIT, 1964). The inhibitor level against urokinase varied in several diseases together with the antiplasmin which seems to exclude the existence of a specific urokinase inhibitor.

The inhibitor of urokinase is increased in pregnancy (BRAKMAN and ASTRUP, 1963). This inhibition is most probably due to the liberation of a placenta inhibitor (ÅSTEDT et al., 1972) extracted in large amounts by KAWANO et al. (1968). The abrupt return to normal activity is explained by the removal of the placenta (Shaper et al., 1966). This inhibitor has no effect on plasmin. DEN OTTOLANDER et al. (1967) found two different antiurokinases, one partially soluble and bound to platelet structures, and the other one in plasma.

Platelet antiurokinase is more stable than antiplasmin and other antiactivators and behaves differently in patients (DEN OTTOLANDER et al., 1969a). The antiurokinase is not altered in patients with cirrhosis or fresh thrombosis (DEN OTTOLANDER et al., 1969b).

It is difficult to determine how far the inhibitors are specific for urokinase. According to KWAAN (1973) the platelet inhibitor is mainly directed at urokinase as also in pregnancy (BRAKMAN and ASTRUP, 1963) and in cancer (SOONG and MILLER, 1970; KWAAN, 1973).

C. Purification and Isolation of Urokinase

The main efforts have been aimed at the isolation of human urokinase and its production for clinical purposes. The classical precipitation methods gave products of poor solubility (ASTRUP and STERNDORFF, 1952; SOBEL et al., 1952). The first urokinase pure enough to be injected in animals was obtained by the foaming process (CELANDER et al., 1955). The urokinase is enriched in the foam phase of urine and the isolation is completed by adsorption on silicic acid and precipitation of urokinase in the eluate (GUEST and CELANDER, 1961). Since urokinase has a marked affinity for several adsorbents the purification of urokinase generally begins with a concentration by adsorption, sometimes quantitative on $BaSO_4$ (VON KAULLA, 1954, 1956; SGOURIS et al., 1960), silica gel (PLOUG and KJELDGAARD, 1956), $Ca_3 (PO_4)_2$, $Al (OH)_3$, $Zn (OH)_2$, bentonite, norite (DOLESCHEL and AUERSWALD, 1960), cellulose phosphate (SGOURIS et al., 1960, 1962), or on diatomaceous earth or hyflosupercel (BERGSTRÖM, 1963). Kaolin has been often preferred to the other adsorbents for the preparation of clinical urokinase. The elution is achieved with ammonia at high pH or with rivanol solution. $BaSO_4$ adsorbs both the thromboplastic activity which is eluted with distilled water and urokinase with a citrate solution (VON KAULLA, 1956).

Urokinase in the eluate is precipitated by either sodium chloride, alcohol, or ammonium sulfate (PLOUG and KJELDGAARD, 1956; WHITE et al., 1966). Further purification is obtained by column chromatography on ion exchangers (KICKHÖFEN et al., 1958; CELANDER et al., 1959; SGOURIS et al., 1962; WHITE et al., 1966), and hydroxylapatite (WHITE et al., 1966). With a chromatography on DEAE-cellulose, CELANDER et al. (1959) obtained a highly purified urokinase with a specific activity of about 6000 Ploug U per mg protein. WHITE et al. (1966) purified the eluate by means of repeated gel filtration on Sephadex G-100. The purification of urokinase for therapeutic purposes is based on these procedures. Recently OGAWA et al. (1975) obtained a highly purified urokinase by adsorption from urine on polyacrylonitrile fibers followed by chromatography on ion exchangers. The specific activity was 224000 CTA U/mg protein.

The new technique of affinity chromatography has been applied to the purification of urokinase. The ligands are directly linked to the insoluble matrix or through a long pendant arm to facilitate the binding of the protein to be purified. PYE et al. (1977) used as ligand a competitive inhibitor of urokinase α-benzylsulfonyl-p-aminophenylalanine (BAPA), bound to Sepharose by the carboxyl groups. Chemical modification of the adsorbent can considerably increase the specificity of the adsorption. The elution is best with the inhibitor itself. The degree of purity is higher. However, the separation of urokinase from the inhibitor is often associated with difficulties and a low yield with a specific activity of 156000 CTA U per mg. With concentrated NaCl (8%) the yield reaches 100% but unfortunately the specific activity decreases to 13000 CTA U. JOHNSON et al. (1977) isolated urokinase from concentrates by affinity chromatography on agmatine affinity columns.

The affinity chromatography procedure lends itself to a cyclic use where adsorption is followed by washing, elution, washing, and again adsorption. This system may in the future greatly facilitate the obtaining of highly purified urokinase, completely devoid of thromboplastic activity, pyrogens, and hepatitis virus.

D. Biochemical Properties of Urokinase

I. Characterization

Urokinase is an enzyme of mammalian urine with a definite species specificity. Experiments made in animals or with animal urokinase cannot be extrapolated to humans. Cat urokinase is able to activate several plasminogens: cat, human, cow, dog, rat, rabbit, and hamster. Hamster urokinase is unable to activate cat, rat, and cow plasminogen. Guinea pig urokinase is a weak activator of human plasminogen whereas human urokinase easily activates the guinea pig plasminogen (MOHLER et al., 1958; RAAB, 1964; MOOTSE et al., 1967; HILGARD, 1972). However, there is no species specificity for the activation of human, chimpanzee, and baboon plasminogen by human urokinase (MCKEE et al., 1971).

Urokinase is stable at 50° C between pH 1 and pH 10. However, it is sensitive of the action of proteolytic enzymes, especially uropepsin in acid urine (PLOUG and KJELDGAARD, 1957). After electrophoretic separation the activator activity is found either in one single band (PLOUG and KJELDGAARD, 1957) or in several fractions with different mobilities (KICKHÖFEN et al., 1958). GUEST and CELANDER (1961) isolated, by chromatography on DEAE-cellulose, two different active components and concluded that urokinase is heterogeneous. These data could actually be explained by the existence in urine of two unrelated activators of the plasminogen-plasmin conversion. Later, LESUK et al. (1965) succeeded in crystallizing urokinase from a purified preparation with a specific activity of at least 40000 CTA U/mg protein. Crystallization was obtained between pII 5.0 and 5.3 in an almost saturated solution of sodium chloride. The specific activity increased after each of three successive crystallizations to reach a maximum of 104000 CTA U/mg protein. The activity loss was minimal and the final urokinase was homogeneous in the polyacrylamide gel electrophoresis. The molecular weight varied very little from 52000 at pH 2.1 to 53000 at pH 10.5, a value confirmed by gel filtration (LESUK et al., 1966). Using different experimental methods and urokinase preparations, several groups of investigators reported on the existence of several forms of urokinase. BURGES et al. (1965) measured by gel electrophoresis on Sephadex G-75 or G-100, a molecular weight of 34500 ± 2000, constant at different pH's and in concentrated protamin chloride solution to prevent aggregation. DOLESCHEL and AUERSWALD (1967) found, beside the 54000 type, a 104000 component, probably a dimer, and a 27000 inactive subunit able to reform the active molecule. The relationship between two forms of urokinase was better demonstrated by WHITE et al. (1966). The two active moieties, isolated by chromatography on hydroxylapatite, with molecular weights of 31500 and 54700, showed with an antiurokinase antiserum, a partial immunologic identity in double diffusion. In addition, the specific activity of the two urokinases was inversely proportional to the molecular weight, 31500 and 218000 CTA U/mg protein compared to 54700 and 93500 CTA U/mg protein, suggesting that the affinity for plasminogen remained very similar. WHITE et al. (1966) assumed that the smaller urokinase was the result of a proteolytic degradation of native urokinase by uropepsin either in urine or during purification. The enzymatic degradation of native urokinase was demonstrated experimentally by LESUK et al. (1967, 1968). They obtained, by limited proteolysis of the 54000 urokinase with either trypsin or subtilisin, a second urokinase with a molecular weight of 36000 and a specific activity of 175000 CTA U/mg protein without alterations of the active center. The smaller urokinase has lysine as N-terminal amino acid (WHITE et al., 1966), the "native" urokinase an isoleucine. Urokinase is constituted by a single polypeptide chain.

The existence of active intermediate forms of urokinase has been established. These intermediates, more sensitive to proteolysis, are rapidly converted into the smaller and more stable species. CELANDER and GUEST (1955) suspected the presence of a prokinase (prourokinase) in urine because of an activity increase during the foaming process. This observation was never confirmed and probably is due to separation of inhibitors. However, BERNIK (1973), BARLOW et al. (1977), and MACIAG et al. (1977), demonstrated that in tissue cultures the appearance of urokinase is preceded by an inactive precursor converted into urokinase by thrombin, plasmin, insolubilized trypsin, trypsin, and Hageman factor protease. Using affinity chromatography on agmatine chromatography colums, JOHNSON et al. (1977) found two different urokinases with apparent molecular weights of 47000 and 33500. These two molecules are homogeneous in polyacrylamide gel electrophoresis and are equally inhibited by ^{3}H-DFP. JOHNSON et al. (1977) report the separation of two different polypeptide chains after reduction of disulfide bridges of the larger urokinase species. The heavy chain is similar to the 33500 urokinase form and has the active site serine labeled by ^{3}H-DFP. The specific activity is also a function of the molecular weight,

104 000 CTA U/mg for the 47 000 form and 226 000 CTA U/mg for the lighter 33 500 urokinase. Each urokinase form shows subforms with slightly different isoelectric points. The 47 000 moiety has a major subform at 8.6 and a minor at 8.9. The highly purified urokinase of OGAWA et al. (1975) is electrophoretically homogeneous but shows five active fractions by electrofocusing or electrophoresis at alkaline pH 9.4.

The 33 500 moiety has three major subforms with isoelectric points of 8.35, 8.60, and 8.70. In opposition PYE et al. (1977) found only two different isoelectric points of 8.3 and 4.7 for 53 000–55 000 urokinase without evidence for a urokinase of lower molecular weight. VUKOVICH et al. (1975) found a series of definite pI's between 6.3 and 10.2 for the 31 000 urokinase and below 5.2 for the active material over 100 000. On storage they obtained a still smaller yet active molecule with a molecular weight of 10 000 and a pI lower than 4.0. ANDRASSY et al. (1975) found in the Leo urokinase two isoenzymes with pI of 6.8 and 8.7 and also high molecular weight complexes with serum protein, albumin, or α_2-macroglobulin.

Data on the structure of urokinase(s) are still limited. The amino acid composition has been reported by WHITE et al. (1966) for both the 54 700 and the 31 500 urokinase and by STUDER et al. (1977) for the 33 100 species. The results compare well. STUDER et al. (1977) isolated, by free-flow electrophoresis, a main component, the 53 000 moiety, and two minor components also with urokinase activity and molecular weights of 47 000 and 43 000. ZUBAIROV et al. (1974) isolated a homogeneous urokinase, devoid of thromboplastic activity, and found a molecular weight of $29\,950 \pm 3000$ determined by thin-layer gel filtration. This urokinase is a glycoprotein with the following carbohydrate residues: 1.67% galactose, 1.38% mannose, or 0.74% glucosamine, 0.24 galactosamine, and 1.67 sialic acid. Its stability in 6 M urea indicates a low grade of helicity of the molecule and implies the absence of a hydrophobic nucleus confirmed by the preliminary analysis of the amino acid composition which shows, in urokinase, a very small number of amino acids with hydrophobic radicals (ZUBAIROW et al., 1974).

Table 1. N-terminal sequence of human urokinase (M. W. 31 500) according to Studer et al. (1977)

Ile-Ile-Gly-Gly-Glu-Phe-Ser/Thr(?)-Thr-Ile -Glu-Asn-Gln-Pro-Trp-Phe-Ala-Ala-Ile-Tyr-
1	2	3	4	5	6	7		8	9	10	11	12	13	14	15	16	17	18	19

STUDER et al. (1977) investigated also the N-terminal amino acid sequence of the urokinase with the 33 100 molecular weight. The separation of a minor band, also possessing a urokinase activity was very difficult and both components were analyzed together. They appear to be different, since some steps gave two different amino acids in the same ratio as the major to the minor component. These data suggest the existence of two urokinase isoenzymes. A practically pure major component obtained by chromatography on Sephadex CM-C25 was found to have an N-terminal amino sequence presenting some similarities with other protease, especially the β-chain of bovine thrombin (Table 1).

Insolubilized Urokinase

Urokinase, like other trypsin-like enzymes, can be fixed to an insolubilized matrix without losing its ability to activate plasminogen. AMBRUS et al. (1972a, b) coupled urokinase to carboxymethylcellulose which remained stable for months at 4° C and was able to activate plasminogen 16 times without loss of activity. However the insolubilized urokinase required 50–100-fold the amount of free urokinase for the same effect. Urokinase can be coupled to other matrices: Sepharose-4B (DEUTSCH and MERTZ, 1972; WIMAN and WALLÉN, 1973), and substituted agarose (DEUTSCH and MERTZ, 1972), on acrylamide derivatives or polyanionic copolymer of maleic anhydride and ethylene (CAPET-ANTONINI et al., 1973). In plasma the activation of plasminogen is limited, probably due to the fixation of inhibitors; otherwise the insolubilized urokinase can be reused and is stable. For a clinical purpose (KUSSEROW and LARROW, 1972) urokinase was adsorbed on graphite-coated polycarbonate or polyvinyl chloride tubings and covalently cross-linked. The activator activity of the fixed urokinase was demonstrated by the appearance of fibrinogen split products during incubation with plasma.

II. Urokinase and Plasminogen Activation

Urokinase was related early to proteolysis and fibrinolysis. That it was an enzyme was first assumed by CELANDER and GUEST (1955) and confirmed by SGOURIS et al. (1956) and SHERRY and ALKJAERSIG (1956). The activation of plasminogen by urokinase is a first-order reaction (KJELDGAARD and PLOUG, 1957) associated with the loss of peptidic material (ALKJAERSIG et al., 1958). This reaction becomes a second-order reaction at higher plasminogen concentrations. The temperature optimum is at 42° C (BERG, 1968a, b). The polypeptide is split at a lysine or arginine bond and constitutes about one-fourth of the plasminogen molecule (BERGSTRÖM, 1963). This reaction is potentiated by the venom of *Echis carinata*, which modifies the tertiary structure of plasminogen, making the susceptible bonds more available to urokinase. Urokinase itself is inactivated by prolonged incubation with the venom (FORBES et al., 1966).

ROBBINS et al. (1967), using a degradated plasminogen, were unable to confirm the loss of peptidic material but demonstrated the hydrolysis of an arginine-valine bond leading to the formation of active plasmin with two polypeptide chains held together with a disulfide bridge. RICKLI and OTAVSKY (1973), WIMAN (1973), and WALTHER et al. (1974), with a non-degradated or a less degradated plasminogen, confirmed the loss of 10–20% of the peptidic material upon activation. Using the insoluble Sepharose-4B urokinase, WIMAN and WALLÉN (1973) detected the two-step activation reaction of plasminogen (mol wt 94000) with the separation from the N-terminal end of an 8000 peptide. The remaining fragment is activated as described by ROBBINS et al. (1967). There is general agreement on the second and more important activation step, whereas results about the first differ slightly. The NH_2-terminal amino acid, after loss of activation, is a valine (RICKLI and OTAVSKY, 1973), a methionine (WIMAN and WALLÉN, 1973), a lysine, or valine (WALTHER et al., 1974). The possibility exists that both a large (63 residues) and a small (5 residues) peptide are released successively (WIMAN, 1973).

MÜLLERTZ (1974) describes a still more complicated pathway system depending on the bond first lysed by urokinase. SODETZ and CASTELLINO (1975) report on two possible pathways.

III. Esterolytic and Amidolytic Activity of Urokinase

The enzymatic nature of urokinase can also be demonstrated by its esterolytic action on different esters. Tosylarginine methyl ester and the lysine ethylester (PLOUG and KJELDGAARD, 1956) were first used. Both are competitive inhibitors of the plasminogen-plasmin conversion. The hydrolysis of the N-carbobenzoxy-L-tyrosine-p-nitrophenylester (LORAND and MOZEN, 1964) is not inhibited by the soybean trypsin inhibitor and the urinary inhibitor while TAME and EACA are competitive inhibitors (LORAND and CONDIT, 1965). The affinity and specificity of the N-acetyl-glycyl-L-lysine methyl ester (AGLME) for urokinase is higher (WALTON, 1967) than that of other esters. Its esterolysis with urokinase is not impaired by aprotinin, ε-aminocaproic acid, tranexamic acid, while the esterolytic action of plasmin is totally blocked. This property allows the quantitative assay of urokinase in patients' plasma after inhibition of the plasmin (DUCKERT and BRUHN, 1967).

The amides of basic amino acids are better models of the plasminogen active center. NISHI et al. (1970) demonstrated that optically active α-N-benzoyl-L-arginine-p-nitroanilide is hydrolyzed to 99% by urokinase. The affinity is 6 times higher than that of AGLME ($K_m = 3.3 \ 10^{-3}$ M and $5.9 \ 10^{-4}$ M respectively) and the V_{max} of the reaction 8 times higher than that of the most sensitive substrate (PETKOV et al., 1973). Even more specific substrates can be found in the p-nitroanilides of tri or tetrapeptides (SVENDSEN et al., 1975). The advantage of these substrates is their specificity and the fact that the p-nitroaniline can be easily detected by colorimetry.

IV. Inhibition of Urokinase

According to DUDOK DE WIT (1964), the antiurokinase content of plasma is difficult to determine. Ten Ploug U/Ml are necessary to obtain a lytic activity. At low urokinase concentrations, lower than 9.5 U/ml, 590 U are blocked for every unit of free urokinase (NANNINGA and GUEST, 1971). The fibrinolytic activity and also the esterolytic activity tested on N-acetyl-L-lysine methyl ester, are not impaired by α_1-antitrypsin (CRAWFORD and OGSTON, 1974). DEN OTTOLANDER et al. (1967) found two different antiurokinases, one in the thrombocytes that was partly soluble and partly bound to the platelet structure, and the other in plasma. Their biochemical properties differ and the platelet antiurokinase is more stable than antiplasmin and other antiactivators. According to KWAAN (1973), the platelet antiactivator is mainly directed at urokinase. This inhibitor is found in a fraction of low molecular weight and the activity of one unit urokinase is totally inhibited by 10^7 platelets; however, the effect on plasmin is similar (KOCH et al., 1975). The platelets have besides this inhibitor, two high molecular weight activators whose action is maximal at 200000 platelets for one urokinase unit. The action of the platelet inhibitor is different from α_2-macroglobulin, α_1-antitrypsin, antithrombin III, and the C_1 inactivator (MURRAY et al., 1974). The stability at 20° C is low in opposition to the results reported by DEN OTTOLANDER et al. (1967). The rise of urokinase inhibition in the blood during pregnancy (BRAKMAN and ASTRUP, 1963) may be due to the placenta inhibitor extracted by KAWANO and UEMURA (1971) and found to be a stronger inhibitor of urokinase—20 U are inhibited by 100–200 Ploug U inhibitor whereas 1000 Ploug U of inhibitor are just able to inactivate 25–50% of only 6 Ploug U of tissue activator.

The sensitivity of urokinase to synthetic inhibitors can vary widely in function of the test system. As serine protease urokinase is irreversibly inhibited by diisopropyl-fluorophosphate and by 4′-nitrobenzyl-4-guanidinobenzoate but not by L-lysine and the chloromethylketone (LANDMANN and MARKWARDT, 1970). The inhibitors, EACA, AMCA, and PAMBA competitively inhibit urokinase (ALKJAERSIG et al., 1959; ALI and EVANS, 1968) possibly in a biphasic manner (THORSEN and ASTRUP, 1969). Urokinase is slightly activated by EACA between 10^{-1} mM and 1 mM and by AMCA between 10^{-2} mM and 5 mM. Both inhibit urokinase above and below these concentration limits. This biphasic effect depends on the fibrinogen and urokinase concentration and the adequate conditions for such a phenomenon to occur can be realized in vivo (THORSEN and ASTRUP, 1974).

EACA, AMCA, and PAMBA are weak inhibitors of urokinase in comparison to the strong inhibition produced by the benzamidines (LANDMANN, 1973; GERATZ and CHENG, 1975).

Whereas the respective inhibition of urokinase and other plasminogen activators can be well characterized in vitro and in more or less purified systems, the action of some therapeutic inhibitors is much more difficult to establish in vivo, and it is even more difficult to establish in vivo, which activator is the physiologic target of a particular inhibitor. It must be emphasized that the use of urokinase to measure changes in the inhibiting capacity of blood, however practical it might be, could just as well be a mistake from the physiologic point of view. Solid data are not yet available to make a definitive judgement on the validity of urokinase inhibitor tests.

V. Determination of Urokinase Activity and Units

The activity can be determined by fibrinolytic, caseinolytic, and esterolytic assays. The first unit was described by PLOUG and KJELDGAARD (1957) and is still in use. This Ploug unit corresponds to 1/10 of the GUEST and CELANDER unit (1961) and to 1/100 of the VON KAULLA (1959a, b), whereas the Smyrniotis unit is only 1/8 of the Ploug unit. This information is given to facilitate the comparison of physiologic and pathophysiologic data expressed with these various units. BALL and DAY (1970) report on a microassay able to detect 2.5 to 50 CTA U urokinase. It is doubtful if the test, based on the separation of the fibrin split products on a sucrose gradient, is sensitive enough to assay the circulating urokinase, even at a high therapeutic dose.

Under the auspices of the NIH, JOHNSON et al. (1969) proposed a set of assays, a fibrinolytic, a caseinolytic, and an esterolytic method, and defined in the three systems a CTA urokinase unit (Committee on Thrombolytic Agents). A CTA unit is equivalent to 0.74 Ploug unit, both units are in use. The equivalence of the CTA unit in the three test methods presents some difficulties. It is complicated by the diversity of the urokinase molecules, at least two major forms—or more as shown by DAY et al. (1969) by means of an immunologic assay—and possibly several isoenzymes, which react differently in the different tests and in presence of various inhibitors. The differences are particularly evident between the esterolytic assay on one side and the fibrinolytic and caseinolytic methods on the other. The same difficulties are encountered for the international unit which should replace all other units. The international unit is defined by the International Reference Preparation established by the WHO in 1969. The reference is a vial of lyophilized urokinase whose total activity has been arbitrarily fixed at 4800 IU. This unit is not very different from the CTA unit. This standard urokinase is unfortunately not entirely characterized and is mainly constituted by the 31 500 component.

The use of the fibrinolytic assay for urokinase is complicated by the fact that it involves a multienzyme system as pointed out by BERG (1968 b) and BERG et al. (1968). In this assay system the concentration, relative and absolute, of urokinase and plasminogen is very important and that of fibrinogen and thrombin slightly less critical.

E. Experimental Pharmacology

I. Urokinase Preparation for Thrombolysis

The more refined isolation methods, such as affinity chromatography, will facilitate the preparation of high quality urokinase. However, some minimal requirements must be fulfilled and controlled, especially the absence of thromboplastic activity, pyrogens, and hepatitis virus. ALKJAERSIG et al. (1965) have proposed an assay system to quantify the residual thromboplastic activity by measuring the shortening of the recalcification time of normal plasma in the presence of different urokinase concentrations. An extrapolation to the zero value (no shortening of the clotting time) allows one to find out the maximal urokinase concentration which will not influence the recalcification time. The zero value should be reached for urokinase concentrations over 200 CTA U per ml plasma. The clinical preparations must satisfy the minimal requirements for pyrogens and toxicity. Pyrogens can be reduced or eliminated by 4 days incubation at 37° C (SGOURIS et al., 1962), the hepatitis risk reduced by 10 h heating at 60° C. Urokinase can be sterile-filtrated with minimal loss of activity. The minimal specific activity has been fixed at 35000 CTA U per mg protein. This degree of purity, even much higher purity, is not a guarantee that all urine component sources of side-effects have been eliminated. The residual impurities depend specifically on the purification procedure. Other tests have been performed, e.g., the effect of a bolus injection of 20000 CTA U/kg body weight on the blood pressure of the dog. The best preparations have practically no effect.

Indeed, the best urokinase preparations have only exceptionally been the origin of the side-effects, except, naturally, the bleeding tendency.

II. Experimental Thrombolysis

It is always difficult and sometimes dangerous to predict, from results obtained in animals, the response of human beings. The experimental results, however, are of value when correctly interpreted. The data accumulated on the dog seem to correlate well with the more recent applications in humans. The activator activity in vivo was first demonstrated by GUEST and CELANDER (1961). As evidence for the lytic activity they reported a drop of the plasminogen and fibrinogen level in dogs with a concomitant rise in fibrinolytic activity after an i.v. injection of urokinase. Even adsorbed on tanned red cells, the urokinase retained its activity when infused to the animals. TSAPOGAS and FLUTE (1964) demonstrated the thrombolytic effect of urokinase on experimental thrombi. Thrombolysis was achieved locally in the infused limbs, whereas the thrombi were not altered in the contralateral limb. The short duration of the treatment, they administered, 200000–500000 Ploug U over 3 h, may explain the failure of a systemic application and simultaneously make evident the importance of the local urokinase concentration. The infusions were well tolerated at doses sufficient to make the blood incoagulable. The side-effects were the usual hemorrhages in thrombolytic treatment, including hematuria (HIEMEYER and RASCHE, 1967). Clots in the femoral artery of cats are easily lysed by an intraarterial infusion of 800000–950000 units in 2 or 3 h. This very high dosage, despite the formation of a strong plasmin activity, caused neither a lowering of the fibrinogen concentration nor bleeding.

GENTON and WOLF (1967), during the preparation phase of the American pulmonary embolism trial, examined the thrombolytic effect of urokinase on freshly embolyzed thrombi of different ages in dogs.

The in vivo preformed clots were embolized in the pulmonary circulation of the dog and the animals were treated for 8–12 h with a continuous urokinase infusion of 4000–6000 CTA U per kg body weight an hour. Angiography and autopsy examination showed that urokinase is able to lyse rapidly 2 week-old freshly embolized thrombi.

F. Clinical Use of Urokinase

I. General Aspects

Urokinase now available in a highly purified form, presents as a fibrinolytic activator and thrombolytic agent several advantages in comparison with the widely used streptokinase. Isolated from human urine, urokinase should be nonantigenic. However, the clinical urokinase preparations contain urokinase molecules different from the native ones, and impurities. The alteration of the structure may simultaneously modify their antigenic properties. Several investigations with different urokinase preparations have shown that these preparations do not contain antigens. Repeated infusions of urokinase, followed or not by skin tests, never revealed the formation of antibodies, nor was the fibrinolytic action of urokinase diminished (MCNICOL et al., 1963; DUCKERT, 1967; FISCHER and PILGERSTORFER, 1969; GENTON and CLAMAN, 1970). In opposition to streptokinase the fibrinolytic action of urokinase can be more easily predicted and the relationship between the applied dose and response is more constant (FLETCHER et al., 1965; DUCKERT et al., 1971). This is partly due to the absence of antibodies against urokinase in human plasma, partly due to the direct activation of the plasminogen by urokinase in opposition to the complex reaction with streptokinase. These advantages are clear-cut and well established. HEDNER and NILSSON (1971) found, in opposition, a wide variation in urokinase inhibitors of patients with various diseases. According to these authors the response of the patients to a urokinase infusion also showed wide variation. However, our experience has demonstrated that most of the patients tested in this series will hardly receive a thrombolytic treatment because of other contraindications.

The adsorption of urokinase to the fibrin or thrombus has been discussed often and the results are quite divergent. Some see in urokinase an activator which activates the fibrinolytic system in direct connection with fibrin resulting in a more pronounced fibrinolysis than fibrinogenolysis (SAWYER et al., 1961). On the contrary, BLIX (1962) demonstrated that urokinase is not or only insignificantly adsorbed onto the clot after fibrin formation in opposition to spontaneous activator and the SK-pro-activator complex. The adsorption of urokinase onto the thrombus is illusory and the lytic action can only be obtained by diffusion. As could be foreseen, the fibrin and plasminogen content of a plasma clot are responsible in vitro for the extent of the lytic effect caused by a given concentration of urokinase. Increasing urokinase concentrations enhance the lysis of the clot, except very high concentrations which are inhibitory (OGSTON et al., 1968). One may assume similar conditions in vivo where circulating urokinase diffuses into the thrombus or embolus and activates the plasminogen in situ.

These results are confirmed by CAMIOLO et al. (1971). THORSEN et al. (1972) demonstrated also that the tissue activator (porcine) is more evenly distributed and adsorbed on plasminogen-free fibrin than urokinase (human) which is not present everywhere on the fibrin network and in much smaller amounts. However labeled urokinase in vivo is partly bound to fibrin and able to detect thromboembolic occlusions in patients (NEIDHART et al., 1974; MILLAR and SMITH, 1974).

Besides well-established and some still problematic advantages, urokinase preparations have adverse properties. Residual urine thromboplastic activity remains even in highly purified preparations (ALKJAERSIG et al., 1965; FLETCHER et al., 1965) and provokes a sort of transient stage of hypercoagulability, characterized by an elevation of the factor VIII at the beginning of the infusion, and a shortening of partial thromboplastin time; cryofibrinogen increased but the ethanol gelation test never became positive during the urokinase infusion. The simultaneous administration of EACA did not have a clear-cut effect (DUCKERT et al., 1971; PRENTICE et al., 1972). However, a comparison with streptokinase treatment shows that part of the activation of the coagulation may be directly due to the fibrinolytic activity itself (DUCKERT et al., 1971). An enhancement of platelet aggregation has been observed in vitro and in vivo with urokinase and also streptokinase (DUBBER et al., 1967). GRIGUER (1973) attributes the mentioned effect to secondary reactions which are normalized in vivo by dipyridamole, but not by heparin.

A further disadvantage is the short duration of the in vivo activator effect of urokinase.

Despite their potential activation effect on the coagulation system, the best clinical urokinase preparations have never been the cause of side-effects due to hypercoagulability.

II. Thrombolysis with Urokinase

1. Preliminary Investigations

The first investigations have in common a rather low dosage of urokinase and a treatment of short duration. First, HANSEN et al. (1961) observed in 22 patients a decrease of the urokinase inhibitors, McNICOL et al. (1963) a decrease of plasminogen to half the normal value with only a slight change of the fibrinogen. JOHNSON et al. (1963a, b) obtained with larger urokinase doses (230000 to 7142000 CTA U per patient) an intense fibrinolytic effect associated with a reduction of plasminogen and fibrinogen. Under this urokinase regimen, lysis of experimental venous thrombi of the arm veins of volunteers was successfully demonstrated in eight of nine veins and partial lysis in the ninth. A urokinase dose, calculated with a tolerance assay (DUCK-ERT, 1967) is able to produce a sustained state of hypofibrinogenemia and strong lytic activity absolutely similar to that caused by streptokinase.

2. Urokinase in Pulmonary Embolism

Two consecutive trials were organized under the auspices of the National Heart and Lung Institute since 1967 and preceded by limited feasibility studies (SAUTTER et al., 1967; TOW et al., 1967; SASAHARA et al., 1967; GENTON and WOLF, 1968). The ability of urokinase to accelerate the fibrinolysis of pulmonary emboli was demonstrated. The results of the larger trial confirmed the previous findings (Editorial Committee, 1973, 1974). Eighty-two randomized patients received an initial urokinase dose of 2000 CTA U/lb body weight in 10 min, followed by 2000 CTA U/lb/h during 12 h and were compared to 78 heparinized patients. Evaluation showed a significant difference toward normalization for the following parameters: pulmonary artery and right arterial mean pressures, right ventricular systolic and right end-diastolic pressures, total pulmonary resistance, and lung angiograms. However, the clinical changes were less impressive. Bleeding occurred more frequently in the urokinase groups (45%) than in the heparinized group (23%). Recurrent pulmonary embolism is inversely less frequent after urokinase (17%) than after heparin (23%). The rate of mortality was low and not significantly different between the two groups. The second trial compared three treatments: 12-h urokinase, 24-h urokinase, and 24-h streptoki-nase under the same general conditions as previously. The streptokinase patients received an initial dose of 250000 CTA U and a maintenance dose of 100000 CTA U/h. The fibrinolytic activity of streptokinase was more pronounced than that of urokinase as shown by the low plasminogen and fibrinogen values. There was no significant difference for the lung angiograms and the hemodynamic parameters in the three groups. Lung scans were almost significantly better in the 24-h urokinase treatment as compared to the 24-h streptokinase group. This difference became significant in favor of urokinase for the lung scans and the pulmonary artery pressure in patients with massive embolism. Recurrent embolism was present and its fre-quency similar in the three groups: 7% in UK 24 h, 4% in SK 24 h, and 1% in UK 12 h.

The rather high rate of recurrent embolism is manifestly due to the short period of treatment, absolutely inadequate to remove the venous occlusions, sources of further emboli (DUCKERT and MÜLLER, 1970).

DICKIE et al. (1967), COOLEY et al. (1969), and DICKIE et al. (1974) reported good results controlled by pulmonary angiograms and hemodynamic measurements after a bolus infusion in the pulmonary artery of 15000 CTA U/kg in 10 min.

EDWARDS et al. (1973) in a similar approach judged the effectiveness of urokinase on clinical data alone and without control patients, a non-informative study. BRO-CHIER et al. (1973) and BROCHIER and GRIGUER (1974) chose a low dose (112500 CTA

U/h) administered over 24h and obtained very rapid improvement of lung scans in 15 out of 18 patients with massive lung embolism.

In conclusion, thrombolytic treatment, preferably with urokinase is beneficial in massive life-threatening pulmonary embolism, not in well-tolerated embolism. A treatment of short duration (24 h) does not protect against recurrent embolism and may, in this respect, be dangerous.

3. Urokinase in Myocardial Infarction

Thrombolytic treatment in myocardial infarction is very controversial. A European Collaborative Study (1975) was started in 1969 in six European centers and terminated in 1973. It included for all patients a 1-year follow-up. The urokinase regimen consisted of an initial dose of 7200 CTA U/kg in 10 min followed by i.v. infusion of 3600 CTA U/kg/h over 18 h. It produced a regular and pronounced decrease of plasminogen and fibrinogen—341 patients with established acute myocardial infarction were randomized in a urokinase group of 172 patients and a heparin group of 169 patients. A statistically significant improvement in favor of urokinase was shown for the normalization of the ST segment of the electrocardiogram on days 4, 5, and 7, and for the regression of necrosis on days 4, 5, 7, and 14 after the start of therapy. These improvements were not reflected in the mortality rate which remained similar in both groups. However the enzymatic values indicate a better irrigation of the infarcted area. The peak of enzyme activity in the serum appears after a much shorter interval in the urokinase group. The difference is significant for LDH and HBDH $(P < 0.01)$ and for CPK and PHI $(P < 0.05)$.

For example the average delay for the LDH peak activity was shortened from 37.7 h in the control group to 25.7 h in the urokinase-treated patients (WITTEWEEN et al., 1975). The higher rise of α_1-antitrypsin in the urokinase group is further evidence for a better irrigation of the infarcted area, whereas the significant decrease of α_2-macroglobulin indicates that plasmin was formed in large amounts and preferentially inhibited by α_2-macroglobulin (ARNESEN and FAGERHOL, 1972). Another study conducted by BROCHIER et al. (1975) includes 120 patients with either pending infarction or myocardial infarction who were randomized into a urokinase-heparin group receiving 112500 CTA U/h over 24 h and 24000 IU heparin, and a heparin group treated with 30000 IU over 24 h. The statistically significant normalization of the ECG parameter, characterized by a faster regression of necrosis and cardiac insufficiency, corresponds to a significantly reduced mortality.

A feasibility study by LITMAN et al. (1971) failed to show any positive effects but was accompanied by rather frequent bleeding complications not seen in other trials. GORMSEN et al. (1973) compared a placebo with a low-dose urokinase regimen. The patients received 74500 CTA U initially and 37250 CTA U/h over 22 h as maintenance dose. The dosage was too low to show more than a discrete fall of plasminogen and practically no change of the α_2-macroglobulin. ECG parameters and enzyme levels were unchanged. HASHIDA et al. (1972) assumed a very high penetration rate of urokinase into the thrombus and justified the administration of as little as 20000–30000 CTA U daily during 3–14 days. Despite the absence of control patients, HASHIDA et al. (1972) claim that treatment was efficient in accelerating the normalization of the elevated enzyme values and of the electrocardiographic ST segments.

The collected data allow no definitive conclusion on the value of urokinase therapy in acute myocardial infarction. However, the odds are not very favorable.

4. Urokinase in Cerebral Vascular Disease

The treatment of cerebrovascular disease with urokinase is based on the presence in the patient's blood of fibrinogen-fibrin monomer complexes or of fibrinogen-fibrin-proteolysis product complexes. These complexes are regarded as a sign of blood hypercoagulability characteristic of thromboembolic disorders (FLETCHER and ALKJAERSIG, 1971).

BROOKS et al. (1970) and FLETCHER and ALKJAERSIG (1977) showed a complete disappearance of the signs of hypercoagulability as soon as 1 h after urokinase treatment. The clinical improvement judged on 13 treated patients was excellent in 3 patients with partial hemiplegia and impressive, without neurologic sequellae, in 5 patients with massive cerebral venous thrombosis despite the fact that in at least 4 patients, angiography failed to show any improvement. The control of hypercoagulability alone with urokinase seems to have a therapeutic value.

5. Urokinase in Peripheral Thrombosis

The use of urokinase in the treatment of peripheral occlusions has been impaired by both the high costs and the limited availability of urokinase. SILVER (1968) obtained an efficient thrombolysis, demonstrated by angiography with very variable urokinase doses administered to patients with either arterial or venous occlusions. Taking advantage of the lack of antigenicity, GREUL and TILSNER (1977) have treated their patients for as long as 32 days with 50% success in 59 patients with arterial occlusions. Apparently when the treatment can be pursued over 10–14 days a daily dose of 500000 CTA U is effective. BOUCHER et al. (1973) applied urokinase locally for arterial occlusions.

6. Urokinase in Ophthalmology

Good results have been reported with a local application of urokinase in traumatic hyphema with secondary glaucoma by PIERSE and LE GRICE (1963, 1964). They obtained a clearance of the clots and a normalization of the intravascular tension without side-effects. Comparable and favorable results have been published by BRODRICK and HALL (1971), RAKUSIN (1971), DUGMORE and RAICHAND (1972), WILLIAMSON and FORRESTER (1972, 1973), and FORRESTER and WILLIAMSON (1973). KWAAN et al. (1977) found the combination of urokinase and heparin superior to streptokinase and heparin or to heparin alone.

Thrombolytic treatment with urokinase or streptokinase in central retinal vein occlusions has been attempted. The results were not very convincing. However, KWAAN et al. (1977) found in a small group that occlusions of the central retinal vein are more frequently improved by a systemic urokinase treatment (80% improvement, 20% failure) than by streptokinase (60% improvement, 30% no change, and 10% deterioration), whereas all untreated patients deteriorated.

7. Local Use of Urokinase

ROBINSON et al. (1970) and DUCKERT et al. (1970) found urokinase to be an efficient fibrinolytic agent in deblocking arteriovenous shunts of patients on regular dialysis. The treatment may greatly prolong the life of these shunts as long as the occlusions are not caused by purely mechanical disturbance of the blood flow.

STURROCK et al. (1974) applied urokinase intraarticularly in knees of patients with rheumatic arthritis. The effect was not better than that of water alone.

III. Urokinase as Diagnostic Tool

It has been repeatedly advanced that urokinase has a more pronounced fibrinolytic action and a less marked fibrinogenolytic effect than streptokinase (SAWYER et al., 1961; DUDOK DE WIT et al., 1962). The assumption has also been repeatedly contradicted (BLIX, 1962; CAMIOLO et al., 1971) or weakened (THORSEN et al., 1972).

The diagnostic use of urokinase is based on its possible binding to venous or arterial thrombi still in formation or older ones. In this case urokinase would be superior to fibrinogen which binds very slowly or not at all on already formed thrombi. It has been demonstrated that labeled ^{131}I-streptokinase and ^{99m}Tc-urokinase are able to locate thrombi in the dog (SIEGEL et al., 1972; DUGAN et al., 1973). Urokinase can be labeled with either ^{125}I, ^{131}I, or ^{99m}Tc without loss of activity. Experimental thrombi in the femoral artery or femoral veins of the dog were labeled $1\frac{1}{2}$ h after their formation by an i.v. infusion of radioactive ^{99m}Tc-urokinase (RHODES et al., 1972). The arterial thrombi were on an average 8.2 times more radioactive than the same volume of circulating blood. The venous thrombi were, however, less intensively labeled. Urokinase has potentially another advantage over labeled fibrinogen. It cannot only detect older thrombi which no longer accumulate any fibrin but also detects them more rapidly and disappears faster than fibrinogen from the circulation due to the very short survival time of urokinase itself.

Both ^{131}I- and ^{99m}Tc-labeled urokinase have been experimentally tested in humans (NEIDHART et al., 1974; MILLAR and SMITH, 1974). NEIDHART et al. (1974) injected 100000 CTA U urokinase, labeled with ^{131}I corresponding to 0.45–0.75 mCi in an arm vein. The first measure was made 60–80 min after the injection with a rectolinear scanner. The thrombi were simultaneously documented by phlebography and the ^{125}I-fibrinogen test. From 12 cases of deep vein thrombosis detected by phlebography, 9 were well identified by ^{131}I-urokinase with 3 false negative, and only 7 with ^{125}I-fibrinogen, with 2 uncertain diagnoses. In pulmonary embolism, the diagnosis of both positive and negative, was exact in the two controlled cases. Despite the good agreement between phlebography and ^{131}I-urokinase scans (evaluated without knowledge of the phlebographic information), the difference of radioactivity between the thrombus or embolus and its immediate neighborhood is in general too small to be easily and routinely interpreted. Excretion of radioactive material in the bladder made an evaluation of the pelvic region impossible.

MILLAR and SMITH (1974) tested the ^{99m}Tc-urokinase and injected 5000 Ploug U labeled with 3 mCi. They started the scanning 20 min after the injection. They report quite good results in agreement with phlebography in 17 of 18 patients.

These results may be encouraging, but the replacement of phlebography with this less demanding technique does not seem possible. Its superiority over the fibrinogen test as a screening method remains to be demonstrated, as also the relative value of ^{131}I- and ^{99m}Tc-urokinase.

At this time a more precise evaluation of both ^{131}I- and ^{99m}Tc-urokinase is complicated by the fact that the clinical preparations still contain about 50% impurities.

G. Conclusion

Urokinase is a natural proteolytic enzyme of mammalian urine with a rather specific function as an activator of plasminogen. It originates almost certainly in the kidneys and in their urine-collecting system. The presence of urokinase in the plasma is improbable. Its identity or nonidentity with other activators, especially with the tissue activator of plasminogen conversion, has been discussed and they appear to be different. A urokinase-like activator is synthetized by tissue culture and released in the culture medium. It is found not only in kidney tissue culture but also in the culture of other tissues even though the primary tissue has no activator immunologically identical to urokinase. Proteolytic enzymes favor the excretion of urokinase into the medium and allow the activation of preurokinase to urokinase. Urokinase exists under severeal different forms due to proteolytic degradation of the native molecule without loss of activity. The molecular weights of the main components are 54700 and 33500. The existence of isoenzymes has been suggested. Besides its proteolytic functions, urokinase has esterolytic and amidolytic properties. Urokinase is a powerful thrombolytic agent in patients and can be administered on repeated occasions without allergic or immunologic complications and without side-effects besides hemorrhage.

References

Åstedt, B.: Release of plasminogen activators from isolated human glomeruli. Thrombos. Diathes. haemorrh. (Stuttg.) **34**, 339 (1975)

Åstedt, B., Pandolfi, M., Nilsson, I. M.: Inhibitory effect of placenta on plasminogen activation in human organ culture. Proc. Soc. exp. Biol. (N.Y.) **139**, 1421—1424 (1972)

Albrechtsen, O. K.: The fibrinolytic activity of animal tissues. Acta physiol. scand. **39**, 284—290 (1957a)

Albrechtsen, O. K.: The fibrinolytic activity of human tissues. Brit. J. Haemat. **3**, 284—291 (1957b)

Ali, S. Y., Evans, L.: Purification of rabbit kidney cytokinase and a comparison of its properties with human urokinase. Biochem. J. **107**, 293—303 (1968)

Alkjaersig, N., Fletcher, A. P.: Metabolism of urokinase. In: Paoletti, R., Sherry, S. (Eds.): Thrombosis and Urokinase pp. 129—141 London: Academic Press. Proceedings of the Serono Symposia vol. 9, 1977

Alkjaersig, N., Fletcher, A. P., Sherry, S.: The activation of human plasminogen II. A kinetic study of activation with trypsin, urokinase and streptokinase. J. biol. Chem. **233**, 86—90 (1958)

Alkjaersig, N., Fletcher, A. P., Sherry, S.: ε-Aminocaproic acid: an inhibitor of plasminogen activation. J. biol. Chem. **234**, 832—837 (1959)

Alkjaersig, N., Fletcher, A. P., Sherry, S.: The assay of urokinase preparations for contamination with thromboplastic moieties. J. Lab. clin. Med. **65**, 732—738 (1965)

Ambrus, C. M., Ambrus, J. L., Roholt, B. K., Shields, R. R.: Insolubilized activators of the fibrinolytic system: in vitro studies. J. Med. exp. clin. **3**, 270—281 (1972b)

Ambrus, C. M., Roholt, O. A., Meyer, B. K.: Enzymatic activity of insolubilized streptokinase (I-SK) and urokinase (I-UK). Fed. Proc. **31**, 267 (1972a)

Andrassy, K., Ritz, E., Bleyl, U., Egbring, R.: Purification of human urokinase and its topographical localisation in renal parenchyma. Thrombos. Diathes. haemorrh. (Stuttg.) **34**, 338 (1975)

Aoki, N., Kaulla, K. N. von: Dissimilarity of human vascular plasminogen activator and human urokinase. J. Lab. clin. Med. **78**, 354—362 (1971)

Arnesen, H., Fagerhol, M. K.: α_2-Macroglobulin, α_1-antitrypsin and antithrombin III in plasma and serum during fibrinolytic therapy with urokinase Scand. J. clin. Lab. Invest. **29**, 259—263 (1972)

Astrup, T., Stage, A.: Isolation of a soluble fibrinolytic activator from animal tissue. Nature (Lond.) **170**, 929 (1952)

Astrup, T., Sterndorff, I.: An activator of plasminogen in normal urine. Proc. Soc. exp. Biol. (N.Y.) **81** 675—678 (1952)

Astrup, T., Sterndorff, I.: Fibrinolysokinase activity in animal and human tissue. Acta physiol. scand. **37**, 40—47 (1956)

Bachmann, F.: The role of the human liver in the regulation of thrombolytic activity. J. Lab. clin. Med. **68**, 854—855 (1966)

Back, N., Ambrus, J. L., Muik, I. B.: Distribution and fate of I^{131}-labeled compounds of the fibrinolysin system. Circulat. Res. **9**, 1208—1216 (1961)

Ball, A. P., Day, E. D.: Urokinase-induced fibrinolysis of ^{125}I-fibrin. Thrombos. Diathes. haemorrh. (Stuttg.) **24**, 463—474 (1970)

Barlow, G. H., Lazer, L.: Characterization of the plasminogen activator isolated from human embryo kidney cells. comparison with urokinase. Thrombos. Res. **1**, 201—208 (1972)

Barlow, G. H., Lazer, L., Rueter, A., Tribby, I.: Production of plasminogen activator by tissue culture techniques. In: Paoletti, R., Sherry, S. (Eds.): Thrombosis and Urokinase pp. 75—81 London: Academic Press. Proceedings of the Serono Symposia vol. 9, 1977

Barlow, G. H., Rueter, A., Tribby, I.: Production of plasminogen activator by tissue culture technique. In: Proteases and Biological Control, pp. 325—331. Cold Spring Habor Laboratory 1975

Barnett, E. V., Baron, S.: Cell culture produced activator for serum proteolytic proenzyme and its presence in poliomyelitis vaccine. Fed. Proc. **17**, 503 (1958)

Barnett, E. V., Baron, S.: An activator of plasminogen produced by cell cultures. Proc. Soc. exp. Biol. (N.Y.) **102**, 308—311 (1959)

Berg, W.: Activation of plasminogen and spontaneous inactivation of the plasmin formed. A kinetic study. Thrombos. Diathes. haemorrh. (Stuttg.) **19**, 145—160 (1968a)

Berg, W.: A method to correct for the continuing activation during the second stage in a two-stage assay. Thrombos. Diathes. haemorrh. (Stuttg.) **19**, 161—168 (1968b)

Berg, W., Korsan-Bengsten, K., Ygge, J.: Theoretical basis and standardization of the one-stage lysis time method for determination of urokinase. Thrombos. Diathes. haemorrh. (Stuttg.) **19**, 169—177 (1968)

Bergstein, J. M., Michael, Jr., A. F.: Cortical fibrinolytic activity in normal and diseased human kidneys. J. Lab. clin. Med. **709**, 701 (1972)

Bergstein, J. M., Michael, Jr. A. F.: Glomerular plasminogen activator activity in renal homograft rejection. Transplantation **17**, 443—446 (1974)

Bergström, K.: A preparative method for the partial purification of human urokinase. Ark. Kemi **21**, 535—546 (1963)

Bergström, K.: Purified bovine plasminogen preparation. N-terminal amino acid sequence, isoelectric point, and activation with urokinase. Ark. Kemi **21**, 547—554 (1963)

Bernik, M. B.: Increased plasminogen activator (urokinase) in tissue cultures after fibrin deposition. J. clin. Invest. **52**, 823—834 (1973)

Bernik, M. B., Kwaan, H. C.: Origin of fibrinolytic activity in cultures of the human kidney. J. Lab. clin. Med. **70**, 650—661 (1967)

Bernik, M. B., Kwaan, H. C.: Plasminogen activator activity in cultures from human tissues. An immunological and histochemical study. J. clin. Invest. **48**, 1740—1753 (1969)

Bernik, M. B., White, W. F., Oller, E. P., Kwaan, H. C.: Immunologic identity of plasminogen activator in human urine, heart, blood vessels and tissue culture. J. Lab. clin. Med. **84**, 546—558 (1974)

Bjerrehuus, I.: Fibrinolytic activity in urine. Scand. J. clin. Invest. **4**, 179—182 (1952)

Blix, S.: The effectiveness of activators in clot lysis with special reference to fibrinolytic therapy. Acta med. scand. Suppl. **386**, 1—24 (1962)

Boomgard, J., Vreeken, J., Bleyenberg, A., Deggeller, K.: Studies on urokinase. Some physiological considerations concerning normal urokinase excretion. Clin. chim. Acta **13**, 484—490 (1966)

Boucher, B. J., Connolly, E. M., Farrow, S. C.: The use of intraarterial urokinase in a case of recurrent arterial occlusion. Postgrad. med. J. **49**, 365—367 (1973)

Brakman, P., Astrup, T.: Selective inhibition in human pregnancy blood of urokinase induced fibrinolysis. Scand. J. clin. Lab. Invest. **15**, 603—609 (1963)

Brochier, M., Griguer, P.: L'emploi de l'urokinase à doses modérées dans le traitement des embolies pulmonaires de haute gravité. Journées angéiologiques de langue française. Expansion scientifique. 82—86 (1974)

Brochier, M., Raynaud, R., Griguer, P., Fauchier, J.-P., Morand, Ph., Archamband, D., Ginies, G., Bienvenu, P.: Traitement thrombolytique par urokinase des embolies pulmonaires de haute gravité. Sem. Hôp. (Paris) **49**, 1825—1836 (1973)

Brochier, M., Raynaud, R., Planiel, T., Fauchier, J. P., Griguer, P., Archamband, D., Pellois, A., Clisson, M.: Le traitment par l'urokinase des infarctus du myocarde et des syndromes de menace. Arch. Mal. Coeur **68**, 563—569 (1975)

Brodrick, J. D., Hall, R. D.: Management and prognosis of secondary hyphaema. Proc. roy. Soc. Med. **64**, 931—934 (1971)

Brooks, J., Davis, D., Devivo, G.: Blood hypercoagulability in acute cerebrovascular syndroms: its control with urokinase therapy. J. Lab. clin. Med. **76**, 879—880 (1970)

Brücke, E. von: Die verdauende Substanz im Urin. S-B Akad. Wiss. (Wien) math.-nat. Kl. **43**, 601 (1861)

Buluk, K., Furman, M.: On the controlling function of kidneys in fibrinolysis. Experientia (Basel) **18**, 146—147 (1962)

Burges, R. A., Brammer, K. W., Coombes, J. D.: Molecular weight of urokinase. Nature (Lond.) **208**, 894 (1965)

Camiolo, S. M., Thorsen, S., Astrup, T.: Fibrinogenolysis and fibrinolysis with tissue plasminogen activator, urokinase, streptokinase-activated human globulin and plasmin. Proc. Soc. exp. Biol. (N.Y.) **138**, 277—280 (1971)

Capet-Antonini, F. C., Grimard, M., Tamenasse, J.: Properties of two types of solid-phase urokinase preparations. Thrombos. Res. **2**, 479—486 (1973)

Celander, D. R., Guest, M. M.: Purification and properties of a urinary activation of plasma profibrinolysin. Fed. Proc. **14**, 27 (1955)

Celander, D. R., Langlinais, P., Guest, M. M.: The application of foam technique to the partial purification of urine activator of plasma profibrinolysin. Arch. Biochem. **55**, 286—287 (1955)

Celander, D. R., Schlagenhauf, G. K. Jr., Guest, M. M.: Purification of urokinase and some characteristics of the product. Thrombos. Diathes. haemorrh. (Stuttg.) **3**, 359 (1959)

Cooley, R. N., Howard, M. D., De Groot, W. J., Dickie, K. J., Guest, M. M.: Angiographic observations on the treatment of pulmonary thromboembolism with urokinase. Amer. J. Roentgenol. **106**, 576—590 (1969)

Crawford, G. P. M., Ogston, D.: The influence of α-1-antitrypsin on plasmin, urokinase and Hageman factor cofactor. Biochim. biophys. Acta (Amst.) **354**, 107—113 (1974)

Day, E. D., Ball, A. P., Jeffords, D., Woodard, W. T., Jr., Silver, D.: The immunoassay of human urokinase. Thrombos. Diathes. haemorrh. (Stuttg.) **21**, 273—286 (1969)

Deutsch, D. G., Mertz, E. T.: Activation of plasminogen with insoluble derivation of urokinase. J. Med. exp. clin. **3**, 224—230 (1972)

Dickie, K. J., DeGroot, W. J., Cooley, R. N., Bond, T. P., Guest, M. M.: Hemodynamic effect of bolus infusion of urokinase in pulmonary embolism. Amer. Rev. resp. Dis. **109**, 48—56 (1974)

Dickie, K. J., DeGroot, W. J., Cooley, R. N., Guest, M. M., Bond, T.: Urokinase in pulmonary thromboembolic disease: preliminary report. Tex. Rep. Biol. Med. **25**, 613—624 (1967)

Doleschel, W., Auerswald, W.: Physiko-chemische Untersuchungen an humaner Urokinase mit besonderer Berücksichtigung ihres Verhaltens gegen Adsorbentien. Wien. Z. inn. Med. **41**, 49—58 (1960)

Doleschel, W., Auerswald, W.: Determination of the molecular weights of uroprotein fractions with urokinase activity by means of molecular sieving. Med. Pharm. Exp. **16**, 225—231 (1967)

Dubber, A. H. C., McNicol, G. P., Wilson, P. A., Douglas, A. S.: Studies with a preparation of urokinase. Thrombos. Diathes. haemorrh. (Stuttg.) **18**, 133—149 (1967)

Duckert, F.: Lack of antigenicity of human urokinase. Unpublished data (1967)

Duckert, F., Bruhn, H. D.: Urokinase and plasmin assay. Unpublished data (1967)

Duckert, F., Gurland, H. J., Bounameaux, Y.: Urokinase in shunts. Unpublished data (1970)

Duckert, F., McNicol, G. P., Godal, H. C., Herold, R.: Influence of various initial doses of urokinase on coagulation parameters. Thrombos. Diathes. haemorrh. (Stuttg.) Suppl. **45**, 23—36 (1971)

Duckert, F. Müller, G.: Thrombolysis and pulmonary embolism. Unpublished observations (1970)

Dudok de Wit, C.: Investigations on the inhibition of the fibrinolytic system. Thrombos. Diathes. haemorrh. (Stuttg.) **12**, 105—118 (1964)

Dudok de Wit, C., Den Ottolander, G. J. H., Krijnen, H. W.: The measurement of fibrinolytic activity with I^{131}-labeled clots. II. Application. Thrombos. Diathes. haemorrh. (Stuttg.) **8**, 322—332 (1962)

Dugan, M. A., Kozar, J. J., Ganse, G., Charkes, N. D.: Localization of deep vein thrombosis using radioactive streptokinase. J. nucl. Med. **14**, 233—234 (1973)

Dugmore, W. N., Raichand, M.: Intravitreal urokinase in treatment of vitreous haemorrhage. Lancet **1972/II**, 660

Editorial Committee: The urokinase pulmonary embolism trial. A national cooperative study. Circulation **47**, Suppl. 2, 1—108 (1973)

Editorial Committee: Urokinase-streptokinase embolism trial. A cooperative study. J. Amer. med. Ass. **229**, 1606—1613 (1974)

Edwards, I. R., MacLean, K. S., Dow, J. D.: Low-dose urokinase in major pulmonary embolism. Lancet **1973/II**, 409—413

European Collaborative Study: Controlled trial of urokinase in myocardial infarction. Lancet **1975/II**, 624—626

Fischer, M., Pilgerstorfer, H. W.: Urokinase "Green Cross", eine neue Urokinasepräparation. II In-vivo Untersuchungen. Int. J. clin. Pharmacol. **2**, 142—149 (1969)

Fletcher, A. P., Alkjaersig, N.: Blood hypercoagulability, intravascular coagulation and thrombosis. New diagnostic concepts. Thrombos. Diathes. haemorrh. (Stuttg.) Suppl. **45**, 389—394 (1971)

Fletcher, A. P., Alkjaersig, N.: Use of urokinase therapy in cerebrovascular disease. In: Paoletti, R., Sherry, S. (Eds.): Thrombosis and Urokinase pp. 203—215 London: Academic Press. Proceedings of the Serono Symposia vol. 9, 1977

Fletcher, A. P., Alkjaersig, N., Sherry, S., Genton, E., Hirsh, J., Bachmann, F.: The development of urokinase as a thrombolytic agent. Maintenance of a sustained thrombolytic state in man by its intravenous infusion. J. Lab. clin. Med. **65**, 713—731 (1965)

Forbes, C. D., Turpie, A. G., McNicol, G. P.: Enhancement of the activity of optimum concentration of urokinase by the venom of *Echis carinata*. Nature (Lond.) **211**, 989—990 (1966)

Forrester, J. V., Williamson, J.: Resolution of intravitreal clots by urokinase Lancet **1973 II**, 179—181

Gehrig, F.: Über Fermente im Harn. Pflügers Arch. ges. Physiol. **38**, 35—93 (1886)

Genton, E., Claman, H. N.: Urokinase: Antigenic studies in patients following thrombolytic therapy. J. Lab. clin. Med. **75**, 619—621 (1970)

Genton, E., Wolf, P. S.: Experimental pulmonary embolism: effects of urokinase therapy on organizing thrombi. J. Lab. clin. Med. **70**, 311—325 (1967)

Genton, E., Wolf, P. S.: Urokinase therapy in pulmonary thromboembolism. Amer. Heart. J. **76**, 628—637 (1968)

Geratz, J. D., Cheng, M. C.-F.: The inhibition of urokinase by aromatic diamidines. Thrombos. Diathes. haemorrh. (Stuttg.) **33**, 230—243 (1975)

Gormsen, J., Tidstrøm, B., Feddersen, C., Ploug, J.: Biochemical evaluation of low dose of urokinase in acute myocardial infarction. Acta med. scand. **194**, 191—198 (1973)

Greul, W., Tilsner, V.: Thrombolysis with urokinase in arterial and venous thrombosis. In: Paoletti, R., Sherry, S. (Eds.): Thrombosis and Urokinase pp. 235—242 London: Academic Press. Proceedings of the Serono Symposia vol. 9, 1977

Griguer, P.: L'augmentation de l'agréagation plaquettaire. Effet inattendu de la thérapeutique fibrinolytique. Ann. Cardiol. Angéiol. **22**, 223—230 (1973)

Grützner, P.: Über Fermente im Harn. Dtsch. med. Wschr. **17**, 10—13 (1891)

Guest, M. M., Celander, D. R.: Urokinase. Physiologic activator of profibrinolysin. Tex. Rep. Biol. Med. **19**, 89—105 (1961)

Hansen, P. F., Jørgensen, M., Kjeldgaard, N. O., Ploug, J.: Urokinase an activator of plasminogen from human urine. Eperiences with intravenous application on twenty-two patients. Angiology **12**, 367—371 (1961)

Hashida, E., Maekawa, F., Mori, Y., Rin, K., Yamada, T.: Feasibility of urokinase in the treatment of acute myocardial infarction. Jap. Circulat. J. **36**, 941—944 (1972)

Hedner, U., Nilsson, I. M.: Urokinase inhibitors in serum in a clinical series. Acta med. scand. **189**, 185—189 (1971)

Hiemeyer, V., Rasche, H.: Vergleichende Untersuchungen zur Wirkung von Urokinase und Streptokinase im Tierversuch. Thrombos. Diathes. haemorrh. (Stuttg.) **17**, 58—64 (1967)

Hilgard, O.: Comparative studies of the fibrinolytic system in rats and humans. Haemostasis **1**, 101—107 (1972)

Hisazumi, H., Naito, K., Misaki, T.: Fibrinolytic activity in normal and cancerous tissues of the bladder. Invest. Urol. **11**, 28—34 (1973)

Holemans, R., Johnston, J. G., Reddick, R. L.: Release of plasminogen activator by the isolated perfused dog kidney. Nature (Lond.) **208**, 291—292 (1965)

Holemans, R., McConnell, D., Johnston, J. G.: Urokinase levels in urine after nicotinic acid injection. Thrombos. Diathes. haemorrh. (Stuttg.) **15**, 192—204 (1966)

Januszko, T., Furman, M., Buluk, K.: The kidneys and the liver as the organs regulating the fibrinolytic system of the circulating blood. Thrombos. Diathes. haemorrh. (Stuttg.) **15**, 554—560 (1966)

Johnson, A. J., Kline, D. L., Alkjaersig, N.: Assay methods and standard preparations for plasmin, plasminogen and urokinase in purified systems, 1967—1968. Thrombos. Diathes. haemorrh. (Stuttg.) **21**, 259—272 (1969)

Johnson, A. J., McCarty, W. R., Newman, J.: Thrombolysis in man with urokinase (UK). Proc. IXth Congr. Europ. Soc. Haemat. (Lissabon) p. 1389. Basel: Karger 1963 b

Johnson, A. J., McCarty, W. R., Newman, J., Lackner, H.: Thrombolysis in man with urokinase. Blood **22**, 829 (1963 a)

Johnson, A. J., Soberano, M. E., Ong, E. B., Levy, M., Schoellmann, G.: Urinary urokinase, two molecules or one? In: Paoletti, R., Sherry, S. (Eds.): Thrombosis and Urokinase pp. 59—67 London: Academic Press. Proceedings of the Serono Symposia vol. 9, 1977

Kaulla, K. N. von: Urin adsorbate with fibrinolytic and thromboplastic properties. J. Lab. clin. Med. **44**, 944 (1954)

Kaulla, K. N. von: Methods for preparation of purified human thromboplastin and fibrinolysokinase from urine. Acta haemat. (Basel) **16**, 315—321 (1956)

Kaulla, K. N. von: Components of the human fibrinolytic system in blood and urine and their relationship to therapeutic and spontaneous fibrinolysis. In: Page, I. H. (Ed.): Connective Tissue, Thrombosis and Atherosclerosis, pp. 259—279. New York: Academic Press 1959 a

Kaulla, K. N. von: Urokinase studies. Thrombos. Diathes. haemorrh. (Stuttg.) **3**, 358—359 (1959 b)

Kaulla, K. N. von, Riggenbach, N.: Urokinase excretion in man: A method of determination and consideration of its significance. Thrombos. Diathes. haemorrh. (Stuttg.) **5**, 162—178 (1960)

Kaulla, K. N. von, Schneeberger, E., Curry, M.: Quantitative determination of urokinase. Fed. Proc. **17**, 167 (1958)

Kawano, T., Morimoto, K., Uemura, Y.: Urokinase inhibitor in human placenta. Nature (Lond.) **217**, 253—254 (1968)

Kawano, T., Uemura, Y.: Inhibition of tissue activator by urokinase inhibitor. Thrombos. Diathes. haemorrh. (Stuttg.) **25**, 129—133 (1971)

Kickhöfen, B., Struwe, F. E., Bramesfeld, B., Westphal, O.: Über einige Beobachtungen am Uropepsinogen und Plasminogen-Aktivator des menschlichen Urins. Biochem. Z. **330**, 467—482 (1958)

Kjeldgaard, N. O., Ploug, J.: Urokinase. An activator of plasminogen from human urine. I. Mechanism of plasminogen activation. Biochim. biophys. Acta. (Amst.) **24**, 283—289 (1957)

Koch, M., Binder, B., Auerswald, W.: Release of fibrinolytically active compounds during plate-let-UK interactions. Thrombos. Diathes. haemorrh. (Stuttg.) **34**, 318 (1975)

Kok, P., Astrup, T.: Isolation and purification of a tissue plasminogen activator and its comparison with urokinase. Biochemistry **8**, 79—86 (1969)

Kucinski, C., Fletcher, A. P.: Immunologic distinction between human plasma plasminogen activator and human urokinase. Fed. Proc. **25**, 194 (1966)

Kucinski, C., Fletcher, A. P.: Immunological studies with urokinase. Fed. Proc. **26**, 647 (1967)

Kucinski, C., Fletcher, A. P., Sherry, S.: Effect of urokinase antiserum on plasminogen activators: Demonstration of immunologic dissimilarity between plasma plasminogen activator and urokinase. J. clin. Invest. **47**, 1238—1253 (1968)

Kusserow, B. K., Larrow, R.: Use of surface bonded, covalently crosslinked urokinase as an approach to the creation of a thromboresistant synthetic surface with fibrinolytic capability. Circulation **46**, Suppl. 2, II—54 (1972)

Kwaan, H. C.: Inhibitors of fibrinolysis. Thrombos. Res. **2**, 31—40 (1973)

Kwaan, H. C., Dobbie, J. G., Fetkenhour, C. L.: The use of anticoagulants and thrombolytic agents in occlusive retinal vascular disease. In: Paoletti, R., Sherry, S. (Eds.): Thrombosis and Urokinase pp. 191—198 London: Academic Press. Proceedings of the Serono Symposia vol. 9, 1977

Kwaan, H. C., Fischer, S.: Localization of fibrinolytic activity in kidney tissues. Fed. Proc. **24**, 387 (1965)

Ladehoff, A. A.: The content of plasminogen activator in the human urinary tract. Scand. J. clin. Invest. **12**, 136—139 (1960)

Landmann, H.: Studies on the mechanism of action of synthetic antifibrinolytics. Thrombos. Diathes. haemorrh. (Stuttg.) **29**, 253—275 (1973)

Landmann, H., Markwardt, F.: Irreversible synthetische Inhibitoren der Urokinase. Experientia (Basel) **26**, 145—147 (1970)

Laragh, J. H., Bär, L., Brunner, H. R., Bühler, F. R., Sealey, J. E., Darracott Vaughan, Jr., E.: Renin, angiotensin and aldosterone system in pathogenesis and management of hypertensive vascular disease. Amer. J. Med. **52**, 633—652 (1972)

Lesuk, A., Terminiello, L., Traver, J. H.: Crystalline human urokinase: some properties. Science **147**, 880—882 (1965)

Lesuk, A., Terminiello, L., Traver, J. H.: Sephadex gel-filtration of human urokinase preparations. Fed. Proc. **25**, 194 (1966)

Lesuk, A., Terminiello, L., Traver, J. H., Le Groff, J. L.: Proteolytic degradation of urokinase to active fragments. Fed. Proc. **26**, 647 (1967)

Lesuk, A., Terminiello, L., Traver, J. H., Le Groff, J. L.: Biochemical and biophysical studies of human urokinase. Thrombos. Diathes. haemorrh. (Stuttg.) **18**, 293—294 (1968)

Lipinski, B., Gurewich, V., Hyde, E.: Fibrinolysis versus fibrinogenolysis: the specificity of human vascular activator (VA) as compared to urokinase (UK) and streptokinase (SK). Thrombos. Diathes. haemorrh. (Stuttg.) **34**, 351 (1975)

Litman, G. I., Smiley, R. B., Wenger, N. K.: The feasibility of urokinase therapy in acute myocardial infarction. Amer. J. Cardiol. **27**, 636—640 (1971)

Lorand, L., Condit, E. V.: Ester hydrolysis by urokinase. Biochemistry **4**, 265—270 (1965)

Lorand, L., Mozen, M. M.: Ester hydrolyzing activity of urokinase preparations. Nature (Lond.) **201**, 392—393 (1964)

MacFarlane, R. G., Pilling, J.: Fibrinolytic activity of normal urine. Nature (Lond.) **159**, 779 (1947)

Maciag, T., Mochan, B., Pye, E. K., Iyengar, M. R.: Plasminogen activator stimulation by plasma components in tissue culture. In: Paoletti, R., Sherry, S. (Eds.): Thrombosis and Urokinase, pp. 103—118. London: Academic Press. Proceedings of the Serono Symposia, vol. 9, 1977

McConnell, D., Johnston, D. G., Holemans, R., Cohen, L. A.: Blood plasminogen activator: mechanism of its release and lack of identity with urokinase. Fed. Proc. **25**, 194 (1966a)

McConnell, D., Johnston, J. G., Young, I., Holemans, R.: Localization of plasminogen activator in kidney tissue. Lab. Invest. **15**, 980—986 (1966b)

McKee, P. A., Lemmon, W. B., Hampton, J. W.: Streptokinase and urokinase activation of human, chimpanzee and baboon plasminogen. Thrombos. Diathes. haemorrh. (Stuttg.) **26**, 512—522 (1971)

McNicol, G. P., Gale, S. B., Douglas, A. S.: In vitro and in vivo studies of a preparation of urokinase. Brit. med. J. **1963** I, 909—915

Millar, W. T., Smith, J. F. B.: Localization of deep venous thrombosis using technetium-99 m-labelled urokinase. Lancet **1974** II, 695—696

Mohler, S. R., Celander, D. R., Guest, M. M.: Distribution of urokinase among mammals. Amer. J. Physiol. **192**, 186—190 (1958)

Mootse, G., Marley, C., Cliffton, E. E.: Species-specific activation of plasminogen: comparison of human urokinase and cat urine. Amer. J. Physiol. **212**, 657—661 (1967)

Müllertz, S.: Different molecular forms of plasminogen and plasmin produced by urokinase in human plasma and their relation to protease inhibitors and lysis of fibrinogen and fibrin. Biochem. J. **143**, 273—283 (1974)

Murray, J., Crawford, G. P. M., Ogston, D., Douglas, A. S.: Studies on an inhibitor of plasminogen activators in human platelets. Brit. J. Haemat. **26** 661—668 (1974)

Nanninga, L. B., Guest, M. M.: Antiactivation (antikinase) activity of human plasma and its blocking by parachloromercuribenzoate and salicylate. Thrombos. Diathes. haemorrh. (Stuttg.) **26**, 541—556 (1971)

Neidhart, P., Hofer, B., Duckert, F., Fridrich, R.: Die diagnostische Verwendung von ^{131}I-Urokinase. Schweiz. med. Wschr. **104**, 141—142 (1974)

Niewiarowski, S., Prokopowicz, J., Poplavski, A., Worowski, K.: Inhibition of dog fibrinolytic system in experimental tubular necrosis of kidney. Experientia (Basel) **20**, 101—103 (1964)

Nishi, N., Tokura, S., Noguchi, J.: The synthesis of benzoyl-L arginine p-nitroanilide. Bull. chem. Soc. Jap. **43**, 2900 (1970)

Ogawa, N., Yamamoto, H., Katamine, T., Tajima, H.: Purification and some properties of urokinase. Thrombos. Diathes. haemorrh. (Stuttg.) **34**, 194—209 (1975)

Ogston, C. M., Ogston, D., Fullerton, H. W.: Observations on the lysis of artificial thrombi by urokinase. Thrombos. Diathes. haemorrh. (Stuttg.) **19**, 107—116 (1968)

Ottolander, G. J. H., den, Leijnse, B., Cremer-Elfrink, H. M. J.: Plasmatic and platelet antiplasmins and anti-activators. Thrombos. Diathes. haemorrh. (Stuttg.) **18**, 404—415 (1967)

Ottolander, G. J. H., den, Leijnse, B., Cremer-Elfrink, H. M. J.: Plasmatic and thrombotic antiplasmins and anti-activators II. Thrombos. Diathes. haemorrh. (Stuttg.) **21**, 26—34 (1969 a)

Ottolander, G. J. H., den, Leijnse, B., Cremer-Elfrink, H. M. J.: Plasmatic and platelet anti-plasmins and anti-activators III. Thrombos. Diathes. haemorrh. (Stuttg.) **21**, 35—41 (1969 b)

Painter, R. H., Charles, A. F.: Characterization of a soluble plasminogen activator from kidney cell cultures. Amer. J. Physiol. **202**, 1125—1130 (1962)

Petkov, D., Christova, E., Karadjova, M.: Amidase activity of urokinase I. Hydrolysis of α-N-acetyl-L-lysine p-nitroanilide. Thrombos. Diathes. haemorrh. (Stuttg.) **29**, 276—285 (1973)

Pierse, D., Legrice, H.: Urokinase in ophtalmology. Lancet **1963** II, 1143—1144

Pierse, D., Legrice, H.: The use of urokinase in the anterior chamber of the eye. J. clin. Path. **17**, 362 (1964)

Ploug, J., Kjeldgaard, N. O.: Isolation of a plasminogen activator (urokinase) from urine. Arch. Biochem. **62**, 500 (1956)

Ploug, J., Kjeldgaard, N. O.: Urokinase. An activator of plasminogen from human urine. 1. Isolation and properties. Biochem. biophys. Acta (Amst.) **24**, 278—282 (1957)

Prentice, C. R. M., Turpie, A. G. G., McNicol, G. P., Douglas, A. S.: Urokinase therapy: Dosage schedules and coagulant side effects. Brit. J. Haemat. **22**, 567—577 (1972)

Pye, E. K., Maciag, T., Kelly, P., Iyengar, M. R.: Purification of urokinase by affinity chromatography. In: Paoletti, R., Sherry, S. (Eds.): Thrombosis and Urokinase pp. 43—58 London: Academic Press. Proceedings of the Serono Symposia vol. 9, 1977

Raab, W.: Die Urokinase des Meerschweinchens. Experientia (Basel) **20**, 546—547 (1964)

Rakusin, W.: Urokinase in the management of traumatic hyphaema. Brit. J. Ophthal. **55**, 826—832 (1971)

Rhodes, B. A., Turhisi, K. S., Bell, W. R., Wagner, H. N., Jr.: Radioactive urokinase for blood clot scanning. J. Nucl. Med. **13**, 646—648 (1972)

Rickli, E. E., Otavsky, W. I.: Release of an N-terminal peptide from human plasminogen during activation with urokinase. Biochim. biophys. Acta. (Amst.) **295**, 381—384 (1973)

Robbins, K. C., Summaria, L., Hsieh, B., Shak, R. J.: The peptide chains of human plasmin mechanism of activation of human plasminogen to plasmin. J. biol. Chem. **242**, 2333—2342 (1967)

Roberts, H. R., Astrup, T.: Content of tissue activator of plasminogen in monkey tissues. Thrombos. Diathes. haemorrh. (Stuttg.) **1**, 376—379 (1957)

Robinson, B. J., Glanville, J. N., Smith, P. H., Rosen, S. M.: Management of clotting in arteriovenous cannulae in patients on regular dialysis therapy. Brit. J. Urol. **42**, 590—597 (1970)

Sahli, W.: Über das Vorkommen von Pepsin und Trypsin im normalen menschlichen Harn. Pflügers Arch. ges. Physiol. **36**, 209—229 (1885)

Sasahara, A. A., Cannilla, J. E., Belko, J. S., Morse, R. L., Criss, A. J.: Urokinase therapy in clinical pulmonary embolism. New Engl. J. Med. **277**, 1168—1173 (1967)

Sautter, R. D., Emanuel, D. A., Fletcher, F. W., Wenzel, F. J., Matson, J. I.: Urokinase for the treatment of acute pulmonary thromboembolism. J. Amer. med. Ass. **202**, 215—218 (1967)

Sawyer, W. D., Alkjaersig, N., Fletcher, A. P., Sherry, S.: A comparison of the fibrinolytic and fibrinogenolytic effects of plasminogen activators and proteolytic enzymes in plasma. Thrombos. Diathes. haemorrh. (Stuttg.) **5**, 149—161 (1961)

Sgouris, J. T., Inman, J. K., McCall, K. B.: The preparation of human urokinase. Amer. J. Cardiol. **6**, 406—408 (1960)

Sgouris, J. T., Storey, M. W., McCall, K. B., Anderson, H. D.: The purification, assay, sterilization and removal of pyrogenicity of human urokinase. Vox Sang. (Basel) **7**, 739—749 (1962)

Sgouris, J. T., Taylor, H. L., McCall, K. B.: Urokinase activation of human plasminogen. National Meet. Amer. chem. Soc. **129**, Abstr. 13 (1956)

Shaper, A. G., MacIntosh, D. M., Kyobe, J.: Fibrinolytic activity in pregnancy during parturition and in the puerperium. Lancet **1966 II**, 874—876

Sherry, S., Alkjaersig, N.: Studies on the activation of plasminogen (profibrinolysin). J. clin. Invest. **35**, 735 (1956)

Siegel, M. E., Malmud, L. S., Rhodes, B. A., Bell, W. S., Wagner, H. N., Jr.: Scanning of thromboemboli with ^{131}I-streptokinase. Radiology **103**, 695—696 (1972)

Silver, D.: Urokinase in the management of acute arterial and venous thrombosis. Arch. Surg. (Chic.) **97**, 910—916 (1968)

Smyrniotis, F. E., Fletcher, A. P., Alkjaersig, N., Sherry, S.: Urokinase excretion in health and its alteration in certain disease states. Thrombos. Diathes. haemorrh. (Stuttg.) **3**, 257—270 (1959)

Sobel, G. W., Mohler, S. R., Jones, N. W., Dowdy, A. B. C., Guest, M. M.: Urokinase: an activator of plasma profibrinolysin extracted from urine. Amer. J. Physiol. **171**, 768—769 (1952)

Sodetz, J., M., Castellino, F. J.: Mechanism of activation of rabbit plasminogen by urokinase. J. biol. Chem. **250**, 3041 (1975)

Som, P., Rhodes, B. A., Bell, W. R.: Radiolabeled streptokinase and urokinase and their comparative biodistribution. Thrombos. Res. **6**, 247—253 (1975)

Soong, B. C. F., Miller, S. P.: Coagulation disorders in cancer. III. Fibrinolysis and inhibitors. Cancer (Philad.) **25**, 867—874 (1970)

Studer, R. O., Roncari, G., Lergier, W.: Characterization of urokinase from human urine. In: Paoletti, R., Sherry, S. (Eds.): Thrombosis and Urokinase pp. 89—90 London: Academic Press. Proceedings of the Serono Symposia vol. 9, 1977

Sturrock, R. D., Watkin, C., Williamson, T., Dick, W. C.: Intra-articular urokinase in rheumatical arthritis. Ann. rheum. Dis. **33**, 124—125 (1974)

Svendsen, L., Senn, H. P., Amundsen, E.: Determination of urokinase and urinkallikrein by means of new chromogenic amide substrates, chromozym UK and chromozym GK. Int. Symp. on Vasopeptides (Fiesole) (1975)

Tajima, H., Ishiguro, J., Nonaka, R., Kurita, M., Tanaka, S., Ogawa, N.: Metabolic fate of urokinase. Chem. pharm. Bull. **22**, 727—735 (1974)

Theiss, W., Gräff, H., Bleyl, U., Immich, H., Kuhn, W.: Reversible Stadien intravaskulärer Gerinnung und ihre Auswirkungen auf Nierenfunktion und Urokinaseausscheidung. Thrombos. Diathes. haemorrh. (Stuttg.) **23**, 369—385 (1970)

Thorsen, S.: The inhibition of tissue plasminogen activator and urokinase induced fibrinolysis by some natural proteinase inhibitors and by plasma and serum from normal and pregnant subjects. Scand. J. clin. Lab. Invest. **31**, 51—59 (1973)

Thorsen, S., Astrup, T.: Biphasic inhibition of urokinase-induced fibrinolysis by ε-aminocaproic acid; distinction from plasminogen tissue activator. Proc. Soc. exp. Biol. (N.Y.) **130**, 811—814 (1969)

Thorsen, S., Astrup, T.: Substrate composition and the effect of ε-aminocaproic acid on tissue plasminogen activator and urokinase induced fibrinolysis. Thrombos. Diathes. haemorrh. (Stuttg.) **32**, 306—324 (1974)

Thorsen, S., Glas-Greenwalt, P., Astrup, T.: Differences in the binding to fibrin of urokinase and tissue plasminogen activator. Thrombos. Diathes. haemorrh. (Stuttg.) **28**, 65—74 (1972)

Todd, A. S.: Fibrinolysis autographs. Nature (Lond.) **181**, 495—496 (1958)

Todd, A. S.: Localization of fibrinolytic activity in tissues. Brit. med. Bull. **20**, 210—212 (1964)

Tow, D. E., Wagner, H. N., Holmes, R. A.: Urokinase in pulmonary embolism. New Engl. J. Med. **277**, 1161—1167 (1967)

Tsapogas, M. J., Flute, P. T.: Experimental thrombolysis with streptokinase and urokinase. Brit. med. Bull. **20**, 223—227 (1964)

Vreeken, J., Boomgard, J., Deggeler, K.: Urokinase excretion in patients with renal diseases. Acta med. scand. **180**, 153—157 (1966)

Vukovich, T., Binder, B., Auerswald, W.: "Different" forms of urokinase. Thrombos. Diathes. haemorrh. (Stuttg.) **34**, 338 (1975)

Walther, P. J., Steinman, H. M., Hill, R. L., McKee, P. A.: Activation of human plasminogen by urokinase. Partial characterization of a pre-activation peptide. J. biol. Chem. **249**, 1173—1181 (1974)

Walton, P. L.: The hydrolysis of N-acetyl-glycyl-L-lysine methyl ester by urokinase. Biochim. biophys. Acta (Amst.) **132**, 104—114 (1967)

White, W. F., Barlow, G. H., Mozen, M. M.: The isolation and characterization of plasminogen activators (urokinase) from human urine. Biochemistry **5**, 2160—2169 (1966)

Williams, J. R. B.: The fibrinolytic activity of urine. Brit. J. exp. Path. **32**, 530—537 (1951)

Williamson, J., Forrester, J. V.: Urokinase in the treatment of vitreous haemorrhage. Lancet **1972 II**, 488

Williamson, J., Forrester, J. V.: Treatment of vitreous haemorrhage with urokinase. Lancet **1973 II**, 888

Wiman, B.: Primary structure of peptides released during activation of human plasminogen by urokinase. Europ. J. Biochem. **39**, 1—9 (1973)

Wiman, B., Wallén, P.: Activation of human plasminogen by an insoluble derivative of urokinase. Europ. J. Biochem. **36**, 25—31 (1973)

Witteween, S. A. G. J., Hemker, H. C., Hollaar, L., Hermens, W. T.: Quantitation of infarct size in man by means of plasma enzyme levels. Brit. Heart J. **37**, 795—805 (1975)

Worowski, K., Niewiarowski, S., Prokopowicz, J.: Fibrinolysis and fibrinogen breakdown products (antithrombin VI) in renal venous blood (RVB) in dogs. Thrombos. Diathes. haemorrh. (Stuttg.) **12**, 87—104 (1964)

Zubairov, D. M., Asadullin, M. G., Zinkevich, O. D., Chenborisova, G. S., Timerbaev, V. N.: The isolation and some properties of human urokinase. Biokhimiya **39**, 378—383 (1974)

Synthetic Fibrinolytic Agents
Induction of Fibrinolytic Activity In Vitro

K. N. VON KAULLA

Introduction

Various asymmetric organic anions have been shown to possess the important capacity to enhance the endogenous fibrinolytic activity in human plasma in vitro. Their further development may well permit induction with them of the thrombolytic activity in human blood in vivo resulting in intravascular clot (thrombi, emboli) dissolution (thrombolysis) by the body's own fibrinolytic system alone, without the necessity for use of extensive enzyme preparations, which have various drawbacks. The reasons for this statement are as follows:

Streptokinase, a plasminogen activator produced by alpha-hemolytic streptococci, which is being used therapeutically as a thrombolytic agent, is a protein that is foreign to the body. Among other disadvantages, its application is restricted because it induces the appearance of antibodies, thus limiting its use in the individual patient. Urokinase as a human plasminogen activator is also currently being used clinically for thrombolytic therapy, although the cost of this treatment is exceedingly high. Urokinase, however, and this is the decisive point, is not identical with the plasminogen activator occurring in the human blood, namely the vascular activator. The differences between these two plasminogen activators have been clearly demonstrated by various investigators; the molecular weights of the two activators are different (AOKI and VON KAULLA, 1971; AOKI, 1974). Antisera against urokinase do not react with vascular activator (KUCINSKI et al., 1968; AOKI and VON KAULLA, 1971). These two plasminogen activators hydrolyze acetylglycine lysine methyl ester with different kinetics and have a different stability in salt solution.

Most important, when incubated in plasma, streptokinase and urokinase induce not only fibrinolytic activity, but also destruction of the clottable proteins, and they produce fibrin degradation products whereas the vascular activator has none of these effects, but induces clot lysis at much lower concentrations (as measured in CTA units) than do streptokinase and urokinase under the same conditions (GUREWICH et al., 1975). The destruction of the clottable proteins creates a bleeding potential which, at least theoretically, could be avoided by using the vascular activator as the thrombolytic agent. The vascular activator has a very high affinity to fibrin, which is higher than that of urokinase or streptokinase (GUREWICH et al., 1975). This essential point is very relevant to natural thrombolysis and its relation to the fibrinolysis-inducing effect of the synthetic compounds. Since in all likelihood the human vascular activator is the body's own thrombolytic agent, it would be highly desirable to enable this activator to obtain full activity and to induce uninhibited dissolution of thrombi and emboli. The synthetic fibrinolytic agents have the important potential to induce or to enhance this process, thus permitting the human blood to develop its own fibrinolytic activity without the need to resort to exogenous fibrinolytic enzymatic activators such as streptokinase and urokinase. The basic mechanism for this approach is as follows:

A. Plasminogen is adsorbed onto the fibrin strands of the clot and thrombi. The actual amount of adsorption is presently under discussion (Hedner et al., 1966; Ogston et al., 1966; Gottlob, 1975).

B. The vascular activator is also adsorbed onto fibrin, much more specifically and to a much greater extent than streptokinase and urokinase are (Gurewich et al., 1975). Obviously this feature would permit the vascular activator to induce fibrinolysis by activating the adsorbed plasminogen. However, this process might be completely prevented or proceeds only to a very limited extent because,

C. inhibitors of fibrinolytic activity are also adsorbed onto fibrin, as has been, for instance, clearly demonstrated by immunological methods (Gottlob, 1975), thus interfering with the fibrinolytic process. It is at this point that synthetic compounds exert the desirable fibrinolysis-inducing action by an indirect pathway. This involves several interrelated mechanisms.

D. The compounds exert very marked antiactivator (Aoki and Von Kaulla, 1969a) and antiplasmin activity (von Kaulla, 1963b, 1975a), thus permitting plasminogen to be activated to plasmin in the presence of these inhibitors and the plasmin thus formed to dissolve fibrin.

E. The compounds diffuse very quickly and deeply into the clot, as shown with fluorescent compounds (von Kaulla et al., 1975a), and

F. the compounds are strongly adsorbed onto the fibrin strands from which they cannot be removed any more. These facts were also distinctly demonstrated with fluorescent compounds (von Kaulla et al., 1975b). Obviously, the compounds inhibit or destroy the antiactivator and the antiplasmin adsorbed to the fibrin strands, thus permitting the vascular activator to induce plasminogen activation. These fibrinolysis-enhancing effects of the synthetic compounds are best demonstrated by the fact that maximally retracted human clots, which contain no serum at all, are no longer lysed when exposed to streptokinase and urokinase. They are, however, lysed when exposed to the synthetic compounds (von Kaulla, 1970), because their small molecules diffuse into the clot and are adsorbed onto fibrin, inactivating the adsorbed inhibitors and thus permitting the equally adsorbed vascular activator to activate the adsorbed plasminogen to plasmin, which subsequently induced fibrinolysis.

It has been shown briefly above that induction of endogenous fibrinolysis by vascular activator is the only pathway by which natural thrombolysis can be obtained under optimal conditions and it is highly likely that this pathway can be opened and/or enhanced by synthetic fibrinolytic compounds. Descriptive details will be discussed in the following sections. At this point, it should be added that drugs are known which induce the release of vascular activator into the circulation. These compounds had no effect on the fibrinolytic activity in the test tube, quite in contrast to the compounds referred to above, which themselves—with a few exceptions—do not induce activator release. However, many of the compounds inducing activator release also have some additional properties such as induction of hypercoagulability (for literature see Mishenko et al., 1972) which would make their potential

Table 1. Vascular activator-induced fibrinolytic activity. Mechanism of its inhibition and enhancement

Steps for development of fibrinolytic activity induced by vascular activator	Vascular activator-induced fibrinolytic activity	
	Inhibition	Enhancement
1. Vascular activator is released from vascular wall into circulation	Liver removes activator from circulation	a) Vascular activator release enhanced by certain drugs b) Liver bypass prevents removal by liver
2. Vascular activator converts plasminogen into plasmin	Antiactivator blocks vascular activator activity	Antiactivator activity suppressed by many asymmetric organic anions
3. Plasmin breaks fibrin strands of thrombus (thrombolysis)	Antiplasmin blocks plasmin activity	Antiplasmin activity suppressed by many asymmetric organic anions

Table 2. Potential pathway for drug-induced fibrinolytic activity

1. Inhibition of antiactivator and antiplasmin activity
2. Enhancement of activator release from vascular wall
3. Blockage of activator removal by liver
4. Combination of 1 and 2 (optimal)

usefulness questionable. Others induce activator release in a protracted way but may not exhibit these undesirable properties. The properties and functions of compounds which enhance the vascular activator activity in vitro will be discussed in the following sections. This includes also a problem to be solved. It should be added that we have found one synthetic compound which induces fibrinolytic activity in animals in vivo and in animal plasma in vitro, in other words by both pathways (VON KAULLA, 1974). This will be included in the compound descriptions.

Table 1 summarizes the basic steps in the development of endogenous thrombolytic activity, the endogenous inhibition of these pathways and of the potential pathways for their enhancement. The enhancement of fibrinolytic activity by liver-bypass has no clinical potential but it is an excellent arrangement for experimental creation of high fibrinolytic activity in vivo without resorting to exogenous enzymes, thus enabling the study of the synergism of synthetic fibrinolytic compounds with endogenous fibrinolytic activity (VON KAULLA et al., 1975c). The enhancement of fibrinolytic activity by liver-bypass, however, indicates, at least theoretically, that a drug-induced blockage of the plasminogen activator removal by the liver would also markedly enhance endogenous fibrinolytic activity. No experiments relating to this approach have been reported so far.

Table 2 summarizes the potential pathways for drug-induced fibrinolytic activity. The mechanism involved, the properties of the active compounds, their structure-function relationship and experiences relating to the points of Table 2, primarily point one, will be described below.

Historical Remarks

Chemical induction of fibrinolysis is not a new discovery; it actually dates back to 1889 when two French scientists, Denys and De Marbaix, observed that proteolytic activity could be generated in human serum by treatment with chloroform (Denys and De Marbaix, 1889). In 1903, Delezenne and Pozerski demonstrated that chloroform-treated serum developed the ability to digest gelatine and casein; this activity was inhibited by addition of untreated serum. Nolf (1921) showed that proteolytic activity accompanied by fibrinolysis could be generated in mammalian and avian plasma by chloroform. Later, it was suggested that chloroform destroys an inhibitor of fibrinolytic activity in the euglobulin fraction (Christensen, 1946).

Treatment of the euglobulins obtained from pig plasma with acetone was also found to increase their fibrinolytic activity thus permitting to obtain fibrinolytic preparations from plasma without the use of enzymatic activator. These fibrinolytic preparations were used for the first reported induction of fibrinolytic activity in vivo in animals (von Kaulla, 1949). In 1938, Juehling and Wöhlisch demonstrated the induction of fibrinolytic activity in equine and porcine plasma with urea (15 percent), and this plasma retained its fibrinolytic activity after the urea had been removed by dialysis. Identical treatment of an equine or porcine fibrinogen solution with urea did not produce the same phenomenon, so that the authors specified the requirement of a plasma factor for this particular ability of urea. These observations indicated that the induction of fibrinolytic activity in plasma by synthetic compounds is basically possible. When we started the search for such compounds, the first preparation tried, Cibalgin, as it was obtainable in the USA, was found to contain three chemical compounds; each of them, however, induced fibrinolytic activity in human plasma at a high concentration only. One of the compounds was urethan (the other two were aminopyrine and ethylurea), which induced us to try ethylurethan, and this proved to be more effective than urethan. With this compound, the observation of Juehling and Wöhlisch that a plasmatic factor is re-

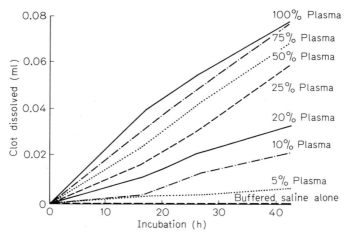

Fig. 1. Dissolution of a preformed bovine standard fibrin clot (see A in the following section of Methodology) by 4% ethylurethan in presence of increasing amounts of human defibrinated plasma. Note the ineffectiveness of ethylurethan in absence of human plasma and increasing activity with increasing plasma concentrations (von Kaulla and Smith, 1961)

quired for fibrinolysis induction was confirmed and extended. This is illustrated in Figure 1. The rotating preformed standard clot (see Section A.I.) was used. This figure shows that application of ethylurethan dissolved in buffered saline on a clot made from bovine fibrinogen does not induce lysis. However, the clot was lysed when the buffered saline in which the ethylurethan was dissolved contained human plasma and the progress of fibrinolysis was enhanced in direct proportion to the amount of human plasma that was present (VON KAULLA and SMITH, 1961). This can be clearly recognized from Figure 1. We found that several urea and urethan derivatives induced marked fibrinolytic activity in human plasma. It was thought that their common denominator might be hydrotropic or solubilizing properties of the compounds. JUEHLING and WÖHLISCH suggested as early as 1938 that hydrotropism and ability to induce fibrinolysis might be related phenomena. This suggestion caused us to attempt fibrinolysis induction in human plasma with a compound that had a quite different structure but well known hydrotropic properties. This compound, 2,4-dimethylbenzene sulfonic acid, did prove to be quite active, thus "opening the door" for the search of synthetic fibrinolysis inducers active in vitro by using various structures primarily with hydrotropic properties (VON KAULLA, 1962). The underlying mechanism was investigated in subsequent years (see Section D). It might be added that, as already mentioned, compounds have recently been found which induce fibrinolysis both in vivo and in vitro (VON KAULLA, 1974).

A. Methods for the In Vitro Assessment of the Fibrinolysis-Inducing Capacity of Synthetic Organic Compounds

The assessment of a potential fibrinolysis-inducing capacity of synthetic compounds is primarily carried out in human plasma as substrate, because obviously dissolution of human thrombi is the final goal for the development of synthetic fibrinolytic agents. Several testing methods were developed, selection for use depending on the type of information needed (VON KAULLA, 1961 and 1965). These methods are described below:

I. Rotating Standard Clot

This clot is designed to imitate a vessel completely occluded by a thrombus which can be attacked fibrinolytically from one small side only. This type of clot allows reading of the progress of clot lysis at any time, thus permitting the progress of fibrinolysis to be plotted as a curve rather than recorded as a single value. The tube used is shown in Figure 2. It is a so-called protein tube, with a graduated hollow stem. In this stem a clot of human plasma is formed by recalcification. The compound to be tested, usually dissolved in human plasma, is placed in the enlarged upper part of the tube, above the plasma clot in its stem. A glass bead and an air space in the enlarged part permit the plasma containing the compound to fluctuate slowly, thus avoiding its dilution close to the clot surface by the serum from the lysed clot. The tube is slowly rotated in an oblique position in an incubator.

Figure 1 (see section on historical remarks) gives an example of progressive clot lysis. In this case, a bovine fibrin clot was formed in the stem of the tube which was not dissolved by the synthetic compounds but which was lysed when human plasma is added to the compound solution. This method proved to be very useful for the testing of synthetic fibrinolytic agents alone or in combination with enzymatic acti-

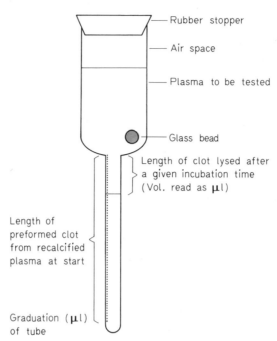

Fig. 2. Tube used for rotating standard clot imitating a human vessel completely occluded by a thrombus. The plasma containing the compounds to be tested is placed on top of the plasma clot formed in the stem of a tube. The tube is rotated at 4 r.p.m. in an incubator at 37° C in an oblique position

vators and plasma obtained from "fibrinolytic" animals in combination with compounds (see Section B on Mechanism of Action), or any fibrinolytic arrangement using primarily human plasma clots as substrate where the dynamics of dissolution were to be studied. The method requires technical skill and is therefore little used for serial testing of compounds. The relatively simple hanging clot method was developed for serial testing.

II. Hanging Clot

A cylinder-shaped clot (0.5 ml) is formed from citrated human plasma (usually obtained from outdated blood-bank plasma) by recalcification in a cylinder-shaped siliconized small glass tube with a flat bottom. Immediately after recalcification a glass rod is suspended in the plasma reaching to the bottom of the tube. Approximately 30 min after the plasma has been clotted, the glass rod with the cylinder-shaped clot attached to it is removed from the tube and suspended in 2.5 ml buffered saline solution of the compound to be tested at 37° C; the solution is adjusted to pH 7.42. The lowest molarity of the compound to induce complete lysis of the clot within 24 h is determined. This method has proved to be well adapted for serial testing. It is, very importantly, not much influenced by the binding of the synthetic fibrinolytic compounds to the albumin contained in the clot, because the volume of the compound solution is five times greater than that of the clot to be dissolved. Binding to albumin of the compound diffusing into the clot thus has little effect on the concentration of the free compound in the solution in which the clot is submerged.

A characteristic example of test results with the hanging clot method is shown in Table 3. The results indicate several important items. They show that fibrinolytic activity can be induced by an active compound not only in human plasma, but also in rat plasma. It should be added that dog, guinea pig and mouse plasmas respond just as well as the human plasma does, whereas plasmas from cat, pig and pigeons respond to a lesser degree, and plasma from rabbit, goat, ox and horse and rhesus monkey respond very poorly or not at all (VON KAULLA, 1966). The upper line represents the results of the normal routine testing with the hanging clot method when the clot is suspended in buffered saline containing the compound. In the example given in Table 3, complete lysis is obtained at 3 mM with flufenamic acid; no lysis is obtained at concentrations higher than 7 mM. This absence of lysis induction at higher concentrations has been observed with all compounds tested (see Section B: Mechanism of Action). The second line shows similar results obtained with a micro-hanging clot method which requires only 0.05 ml of rat plasma. Lines 3 and 4 indicate results obtained with the hanging clot suspended in compound-containing human plasma instead of the buffered saline solution used for the routine testing. With plasma much higher concentrations are required to dissolve the hanging clot. The main reason for this is the binding of the compound to the albumin in the plasma used, thus reducing the concentration available for fibrinolysis induction (see Section E). This variation of the hanging clot method is therefore not used for serial testing.

III. Plasma Clot

The simplest method of testing asymmetric organic anions for their potential for induction of fibrinolysis is to dissolve the compound directly in citrated plasma or to add it to the plasma in highly concentrated (in order to avoid dilution of the plasma) solution. The pH of the plasma after compound addition should be kept at 7.42. The plasma is subsequently clotted by recalcification. Again, the lowest concentration is determined at which the clot will dissolve within 24 h.

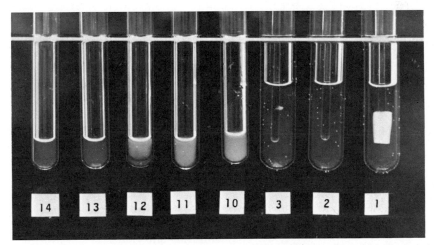

Fig. 3. Assessment of fibrinolysis-inducing capacity of 3-cinnamyl salicylic acid with the plasma clot (left) and the hanging clot (right) methods. Note the difference between the results of the two methods in regard to the lowest active compound concentration.

Table 3. Fibrinolysis induction in vitro. Results with the hanging clot method, including a micro-method, using clots made from human and rat plasma. Clots were suspended in compound-containing buffered saline or in compound-containing plasma of the same species

Plasma	Compound	H.C. or M.H.C.	B.S. or Plasma	mM															
				16	15	14	13	12	11	10	9	8	7	6	5	4	3	2	1
Human	Flufenamic acid	H.C.	B.S.									(+)	(+)	(+)	+	+	+	(+)	−
Rat	Flufenamic acid	M.H.C.	B.S.									−	(+)	(+)	+	+	(+)	−	−
Human	Flufenamic acid	H.C.	Plasma	−	(+)	(+)	(+)	+	+	+	(+)								
Rat	Flufenamic acid	M.H.C.	Plasma	−	(+)	(+)	(+)	+	+	+	+								

H.C. = Hanging clot (0.5 ml); M.H.C. = Micro-hanging clot (0.05 ml); + clot completely dissolved within 24 h; (+) clot partially dissolved; − clot not dissolved.

An (at least theoretical) objection to this simple method is that the compounds could influence the structure of the clot being formed in their presence in the sense of a reduction of the fibrin network, resulting in incorrect information regarding their fibrinolysis-inducing capacity. On the other hand, testing of compounds with both hanging clot and plasma clot appears to suggest binding of the compound to plasma proteins other than those involved in fibrinolysis induction. The nonspecific binding seems to diminish in direct proportion to the difference in required concentration between the hanging clot and the plasma clot (see Section E). Figure 3 shows a test run with 3-cinnamyl salicylic acid with both the plasma clot (left) and the hanging clot methods (right). The picture was taken after 24 h incubation.

B. Mechanism of Action

The mechanism of in-vitro induction of fibrinolytic activity by synthetic compounds has been briefly described in the introduction. Table 4 indicates the basic mechanism by which the compounds act inducing fibrinolytic activity in vivo or in vitro. Table 4 also indicates that there are synthetic compounds—one example is given—which induce fibrinolytic activity by both pathways, i.e., in vitro and in vivo (see Section G). The clot-dissolving activity induced by the synthetic organic anions in vitro is based on the following properties of the compounds: 1. They diffuse rather quickly and deeply into preformed clots. This diffusion endows them with a good "thrombolytic" potential. 2. They are adsorbed onto fibrin. 3. They reduce or eliminate antiplasmin and antiactivator activity. By this reduction or elimination of the inhibitor activity, they actually induce fibrinolytic activity.

I. Diffusion into Clots

This diffusion of the compounds is proved in two ways, namely lysis of flat clots and

Table 4. Synthetic fibrinolytic agents. Basic mechanism of action

A. Release of plasminogen activator from vascular wall	in vivo	Vascular active drugs
B. Reduction or elimination of antiplasmin and antiactivator activity	in vitro	Asymmetric organic anions
C. Combination of A and B	in vivo in vitro	Niflumic acid

photographic evidence of diffusion of fluorescent synthetic fibrinolytic compounds into plasma clots. Flat clots are obtained from recalcified clotted citrated human plasma which is centrifuged serum-free by high-speed centrifugation resulting in flat clots; they are washed several times with buffered saline. These flat clots suspended and incubated in buffered compound solution will lyse completely within 24 h. Suspension of the flat clots in solutions of urokinase or streptokinase has no lytic effect whatsoever because the large molecules of these plasminogen activators cannot diffuse into the maximally retracted clots (VON KAULLA, 1970). Table 5 compares the concentrations of four fibrinolytic compounds needed to induce fibrinolytic dissolution of flat clots, hanging clots, and plasma clots. The molarity required for the dissolution of flat clots is the lowest, most probably, because the flat clot does not contain proteins, in particular albumin, that are not required for the fibrinolytic process; these would bind the compounds, thus making them available for fibrinolysis induction. The mechanism by which the compounds induce lysis of the flat clot (and other types of clots) is as follows: the fibrin strands have plasminogen, adsorbed plasminogen activator, antiactivators and antiplasmin. The compounds are also adsorbed onto fibrin (see "B") therein inactive antiactivator and antiplasmin (see "C"), thus permitting the plasminogen activator to activate plasminogen to plasmin, which subsequently induces lysis of the fibrin strands. The compounds diffuse also concentration-dependently into preformed clots obtained from recalcified plasma. This is clearly demonstrated when niflumic acid is used as fibrinolytic compound (VON KAULLA, 1976). Its ability to diffuse is particularly important because the compound diffuses from the plasma (not from buffered saline solution) in which it is dissolved into the preformed cylinder-shaped clots which expose only one small side.

Table 5. Concentrations in mM of synthetic organic anions required for inducing fibrinolytic dissolution of the 3 types of test clots prepared from human plasma

Compound	Flat	Hanging	Plasma
N-(m-trifluoromethylphenyl)anthranilic acid	0.8	3	10
N-(4-isopropylphenyl)anthranilic acid	0.7	8	13
5-cyclohexyl-γ-resorcylic acid	0.6	3	9
3-(2-chlorobenzyl)salicylic acid	0.5	2	10

Table 6. Evidence of the adsorption onto fibrin of synthetic fibrinolytic agents

1. Hanging clot incubated for a few hours in B.S. which contains the fibrinolytic compounds, is transferred into compound-free B.S. and incubated: Clot dissolves

2. Compound is dissolved in human plasma, plasma is clotted, centrifuged at 36000 g, the clot washed 3 times with B.S., then incubated compound-free in B.S.: Clot dissolves

3. Fluorescent fibrinolytic compound is added to plasma previously clotted on a slide, following this the clot is washed 3 times with B.S. The fibrin strands remain highly fluorescent (see Fig. 5) due to the firmly adsorbed compound

This indicates an important potential, at least theoretically, namely that an appropriate compound would diffuse in vivo from the bloodstream in which it is kept at a certain level into thrombi or emboli and there induce their fibrinolytic dissolution.

II. Adsorption onto Fibrin

The adsorption of synthetic fibrinolytic agents onto fibrin is clearly proved by the procedures listed in Table 6 and by photographs of the fibrin network of human plasma clots following exposure to fluorescent synthetic compounds. Figure 4 gives an example of the adsorption of the fluorescent fibrinolytic compound pamoic acid onto the fibrin strands. The adsorption of the compounds onto the fibrin strands is an essential step in the induction of fibrinolysis, because antiactivator and antiplasmin are also adsorbed onto fibrin. As already mentioned, it is by inactivation of these two inhibitors that the synthetic fibrinolytic compounds induce fibrinolytic activity.

III. Suppression of Antiplasmin and Antiactivator Activity

The fibrinolytic compounds also suppress antiplasmin activity of the human serum. This effect develops within one hour of incubation and reaches its maximum after several hours. The substrate used was bovine fibrinogen clots, which were exposed to bovine or human plasmin, together with human serum which had been preincubated (except for the control) with the compounds. The compounds reduce or eliminate antiplasmin activity of the serum with a concentration-dependent time reaction. Minor structural changes which abolish the fibrinolysis-inducing capacity of the compounds also eliminate their ability to reduce antiplasmin activity (von Kaulla, 1963a and 1970). Alpha-2-macroglobulin also inhibits fibrinolytic activity; thus an immunologically pure preparation inhibits the dissolution of bovine fibrin clots by chloroform-activated plasmin. In pilot studies it was found that this inhibition was completely abolished by preincubation of the alpha-2-macroglobulins with various synthetic fibrinolysis-inducing compounds (von Kaulla, 1970). The antiurokinase activity of human plasma is also suppressed by the fibrinolytic compounds. This has been demonstrated for all of the seven compounds tested for this effect (von Kaulla, 1970). It was further shown that the amount of urokinase required to

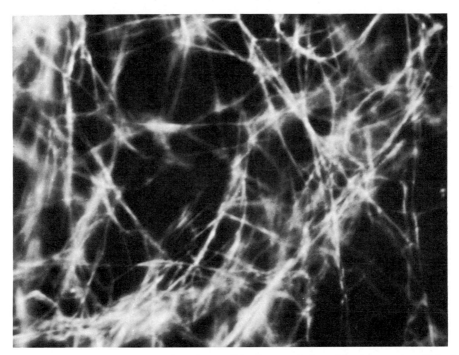

Fig. 4. Human citrated plasma was clotted on a slide, then a solution of 3 mM pamoic acid in B.S. was added; 15 min later the clot was very well rinsed 3 times with B.S. free of compound. Following this the fibrin network was photographed in the darkroom using ultraviolet light. The adsorption of the fluorescent pamoic acid onto the fibrin strands is obvious and makes the strands clearly visible. (VON KAULLA, 1976)

dissolve the human plasma clot rapidly within 15 minutes is reduced from 200 CTA units to 20 CTA units in the presence of 5 mM of the fibrinolytic 3,5-diiodo salicylic acid by blocking the binding of the urokinase to the inhibitor (NANNINGA, 1975). It was also shown that substituted benzoates block the inhibition of urokinase by plasma fibrinolytic antiactivators (NANNINGA, 1974). These findings point to probably the most important effect of the synthetic fibrinolytic compounds: suppression of antiactivator activity in human plasma or serum. This suppression has been proved with various compounds, including flufenamic acid, for the antiactivator which inhibits the vascular activator, the body's own plasminogen activator. The inactivation of antiactivator by the compounds is irreversible (AOKI and VON KAULLA, 1969a). Minor structural changes that abolish the fibrinolysis-inducing capacity also abolish their effect on the serum or plasma antiactivator activity. A suppression of antiactivator activity with regard to vascular activator could also be demonstrated for dog plasma with ortho-thymotic acid. With this plasma it was also observed that high compound concentrations which do not induce fibrinolysis (an effect observed with all compounds tested) do not reduce but potentiate the activity of antiactivator (DAVER and DESNOYERS, 1974). This effect may explain the inhibitory effect of the high compound concentration.

It has also been claimed that the fibrinolysis-inducing flufenamic acid liberates a plasminogen activator from a latent activator. This latent activator is distributed between euglobulin precipitate and euglobulin supernatant of serum in the ratio 3:7. This effect of the compound is thought to be different from its suppression of antiactivator and antiplasmin activity (Tomikawa and Abiko, 1973).

It should be added that the fibrinolytic compounds reduce also on incubation the C'-complement activity of human plasma at concentrations which are practically identical to those that would induce fibrinolytic activity in the plasma. Minor modifications of the molecule, such as shifting of the substituent from the para- to the ortho-position or introduction of a second carboxylic group into the molecule, which would abolish the fibrinolytic activity of a given compound abolish also its ability to inactivate complement C' and to suppress antiplasmin activity. Further studies revealed that the compounds actually inactivate β_1C-globulin in the serum without interaction with other components of the complement system. Whether or not this inactivation is related to fibrinolysis induction is an open question. Blocking of the fibrinolytic activity induced by the compounds with Epsilon-aminocaproic acid does not inhibit their effect on β_1C-globulin (Aoki and von Kaulla, 1969b).

C. Synergism of Action Between Synthetic Fibrinolytic Compounds, the Natural Plasminogen Activators and Proteolytic Enzymes

I. Synergism with Urokinase

Rather early in our investigations with the synthetic fibrinolytic compounds it was observed that the compounds act synergistically with the plasminogen activator urokinase. This effect is very clear-cut: a marked fibrinolytic activity results when a plasminogen activator such as urokinase is used at concentrations which induce little or no fibrinolytic effect together with the synthetic fibrinolytic compounds also at concentrations that induce little or no fibrinolytic effect. This synergistic effect is well demonstrated with the rotating human plasma standard clot, as shown in Figures 5 and 6. Figure 5 shows results obtained 15 years ago with urokinase prepared in our laboratories. The synergistic effect of ethylurethan dissolved in human plasma at a

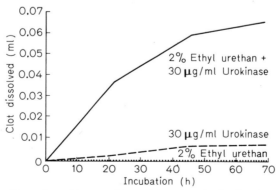

Fig. 5. Synergistic effect of urokinase with etyhlurethan both dissolved in the same human plasma. Both agents were used combined with the rotating standard clot at concentrations which alone have little or no fibrinolytic effect on this clot. (von Kaulla and Smith, 1961)

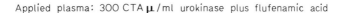

Applied plasma: 300 CTA μ/ml urokinase plus flufenamic acid

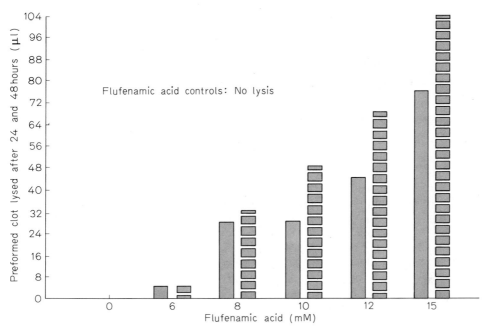

Fig. 6. Synergistic effect of urokinase and flufenamic acid both dissolved in the same human plasma. The two agents were used together with the rotating standard clot, at concentrations which individually had no fibrinolytic effect on this clot. Note the increasing volume of dissolved clot with increasing amounts of flufenamic acid. Black columns: 24 h incubation; striped columns: 48 hours' incubation. (VON KAULLA et al.: New York: 1975b)

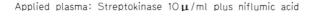

Applied plasma: Streptokinase 10 μ/ml plus niflumic acid

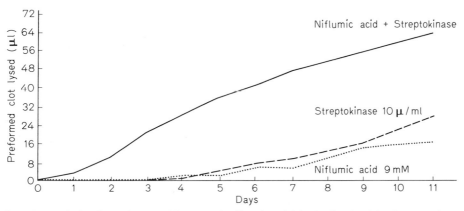

Fig. 7. Synergistic effect of streptokinase and niflumic acid both dissolved in the same human plasma. The two agents were used together with the rotating standard clot, at concentrations which individually had only a weak fibrinolytic effect on this clot

concentration which has no fibrinolytic effect on the rotating standard clot together with urokinase at a concentration which exerts only a very weak effect is very pronounced. A similar synergistic effect is observed when other fibrinolytic compounds are used. This is shown with flufenamic acid as an example in Figure 6: Urokinase and flufenamic acid are used, dissolved in the same human plasma at concentrations at which each agent when used alone produced no fibrinolytic activity whatsoever with the rotating standard clot.

II. Synergism with Streptokinase

A synergistic effect can also be observed with streptokinase. An example with streptokinase, using niflumic acid as synthetic fibrinolytic agent and the rotating standard clot as substrate, is shown in Figure 7. Niflumic acid, at a concentration which is nearly ineffective, speeds up and enhances the poor and delayed fibrinolytic activity induced by streptokinase. A similar synergism with streptokinase using the hanging clot method was observed for thymotic acid (DESNOYERS et al., 1971).

III. Synergism with the Endogenous Plasminogen Activator

Actual proof of the potential usefulness of the enhancing fibrinolytic effect of a combination of enzymatic activators with synthetic fibrinolytic agents requires a demonstration of this effect with the body's own activator. For this purpose plasma obtained from blood in which the fibrinolytic activity had been increased in vivo with no use of external stimulation (such as treatment with certain vasoactive drugs) was applied. The best method for induction of the required endogenous fibrinolytic activity is the liver bypass. This bypass prevents the liver from removing vascular activator from the circulation (TYTGAT et al., 1968), thus inducing a marked and increasing fibrinolytic activity in the circulation. When plasma from pigs with liver bypass was used, the synergistic effect of the synthetic compounds with endogenous activator was distinctly demonstrated. Figure 8 indicates that plasma clots made from pig plasma before the bypass do not dissolve within 24 h. No lysis occurs when these clots contain flufenamic acid (tested up to 8 mM) (column on the left). After a liver bypass of thirty minutes duration, the compound-free clotted plasma lyses in approximately four hours. This lysis time is progressively shortened with increasing concentrations of flufenamic acid (column in the center). After 90 min bypass, the fibrinolytic activity has further increased in the control and is markedly enhanced by the compound, to the point where with the two highest concentrations (7 and 8 mM) no clot can be obtained, because it dissolves as fast as it is being formed. A marked synergistic effect is also obtained, as has been shown for urokinase and streptokinase, when the preformed rotating clot is used as substrate. Example: Pig plasma obtained before bypass containing 9 mM flufenamic acid did not induce any lysis of the rotating standard clot after 24 and 48 h incubation. Nor does the fibrinolytic plasma (without compound) obtained after 30 min bypass have an effect on this type of preformed clot. However, the addition of 9 mM flufenamic acid to this bypass plasma very markedly enhances its fibrinolytic activity, to the point where it dissolves the preformed clot: 40 µl are lysed within 24 h and 60 µl within 48 h, which actually indicates a shortening of 4 mm and 6 mm, respectively, of this cylinder-

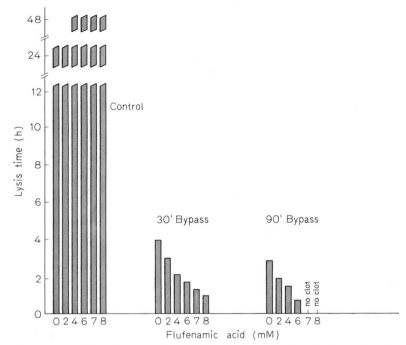

Fig. 8. Enhancement of liver bypass-induced fibrinolytic activity in pig plasma by the synthetic fibrinolytic compound flufenamic acid at concentrations which do not themselves induce fibrinolysis. Control values before bypass on the left. Lysis times of plasma clots obtained after 30 min bypass are shown in the center and those obtained after 90 min on the right. Note the marked enhancing effect of flufenamic acid. (VON KAULLA et al., 1975b)

shaped preformed clot which can be fibrinolytically attacked from one small side only. In this connection it should be stated that compounds tested for a thrombolytic potential should always be tested with preformed clots obtained from human plasma, such as the one described herein (the rotating standard clot). Use of the lysis time only can give very misleading results. This is shown in Table 7, which illustrates use of fibrinolytic pig bypass plasma with or without fibrinolytic compounds. After 30 min liver bypass, an average plasma clot dissolution time is reduced from more

Table 7. Enhancement of endogenously increased (liver bypass in the pig for 30 min) fibrinolytic activity upon addition of flufenamic acid (FFA) to the bypass plasma. Average of 7 runs. Fibrinolytic (A) vs. "Thrombolytic" activity (B)

mM FFA added	A Plasma clot lysis (min)	B µl of preformed rotating standard clot lysed
0	204 (100–325)	4 (0–8)
8	60 (30–85)	44 (20–84)

than 48 h in the pre-bypass control to 204 min. When, however, this fibrinolytic bypass plasma is applied to the small side of the cylinder-shaped preformed clot, practically no lysis of the exposed side of this clot occurs, indicating clearly that this increased fibrinolytic activity does not exert or reflect any "thrombolytic" activity. Only further marked enhancement of this fibrinolytic activity to an average lysis time of about 60 min upon addition of the synthetic compound at a concentration that applied alone does not induce fibrinolytic activity, endows the liver-bypass plasma with "thrombolytic" activity, as indicated by the induced shortening of the preformed clot.

From these observations of the enhancing effect of synthetic fibrinolytic compounds with urokinase, streptokinase and, in particular, with endogenously induced fibrinolytic activity, one may conclude that for clinical use an intermediate step for the development of synthetic fibrinolytic compounds may well be their enhancement on the fibrinolytic activity induced by enzymatic plasminogen activators. This potential is of practical interest, because it has been shown above that the synergism can be obtained with activator and compound concentrations which alone are too low to induce fibrinolytic activity. It should be pointed out that only testing of these combinations on preformed clots such as the rotating standard clot would reflect a potential clinical effectiveness.

IV. Synergismen with Proteolytic Enzymes

The synthetic fibrinolytic compounds also enhance the activity of proteolytic enzymes. An example of this enhancement is shown in Figure 9: pronase, brinase, and trypsin dissolved in buffered saline have been applied to the rotating standard clot at concentrations which do not induce any clot dissolution. The addition of flufenamic acid to these solutions induces a concentration-dependent proteolytic activity. Whereas the enhancement of pronase and brinase activities is concentration-dependent, the activity of trypsin is first enhanced and then, with further increases in compound concentrations, inhibited. No further studies of this particular synergism have been carried out.

V. Synergism Among Synthetic Fibrinolytic Compounds

It has been reported that an increased fibrinolysis-inducing effect can be obtained when two synthetic fibrinolytic compounds are simultaneously applied at half their optimal concentrations (BAUMGARTEN et al., 1970).

D. Structure-Activity Relationship of Synthetic Fibrinolytic Compounds

As previously stated, the first compounds found to induce in vitro fibrinolytic activity in human plasma were urea and urethan derivatives. Alterations of the urea and urethan molecules increased the activity in the following order: urea (inactive)→ thiourea→ethylthiourea→allyl-2-thiourea; urethan (poorly acitve)→methylurethan→ethylurethan. It was hypothesized that the common denominator of the active compounds might be hydrotropic properties. Indeed, a well known hydrotropic compound, 2,4-dimethylbenzene sulfonic acid, was found to induce fibrino-

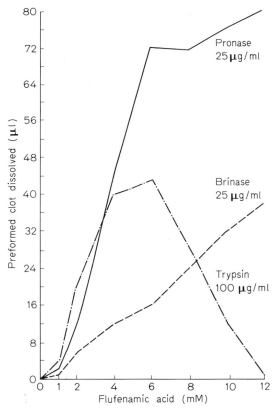

Fig. 9. Enhancing effect of a synthetic fibrinolytic compound (flufenamic acid) on ineffective concentrations of proteolytic enzymes dissolved in buffered saline pH 7.42. Substrate: Rotating human plasma standard clot

lysis at a much lower concentration than the urea and urethan derivatives did (VON KAULLA, 1962a and b). Subsequently, various organic anions were found to be active, and the first observations of the relation of the type and position of substitutions with the extent of the induced fibrinolytic activity were made. Thus, ortho-toluic acid was inactive, meta-toluic acid induced a weak activity, and para-toluic acid was the most active one of these three compounds (VON KAULLA, 1962b). The same relationship of the position of the substitution applied to bromo-benzoic acid and to chlorophenoxy acetic acid. Substitutions with methyl groups in 2,4-position resulted in a compound with higher activity than substitution in the 2,5-position, as shown for dimethylbenzene sulfonic acid; with naphthalene sulfonic acid, substitution of the hydrophilic group in the alpha-position produced compounds with higher activity than substitution in the beta-position, to give a few examples (VON KAULLA, 1962b, 1963). Ethylalcohol was one of the active compounds only when used at high concentrations, however.

Derivatives of salicylic acid were next observed to induce fibrinolysis of human plasma clots; 2-methyl-5-sec-butyl salicylic acid was the most active of these (at 5 mM) (RADER and WULF, 1966). Derivatives of anthranilic acid, the N-arylanthrani-

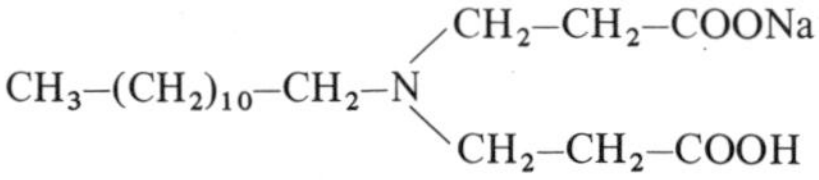

$$CH_3-(CH_2)_{10}-CH_2-N\begin{cases}CH_2-CH_2-COONa\\CH_2-CH_2-COOH\end{cases}$$

N–lauryl–β–iminodipropionic
acid (monosodium)
— 10 mM —

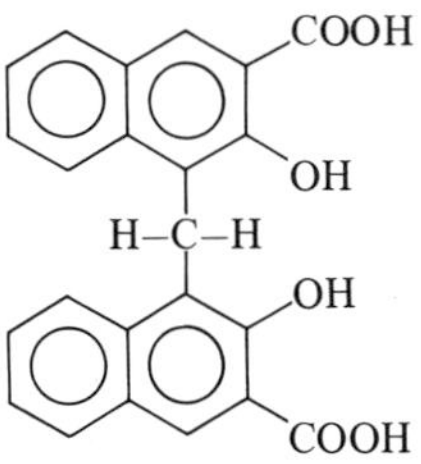

methylene–di–(β–hydroxy
naphthoic acid)
— 2 mM —

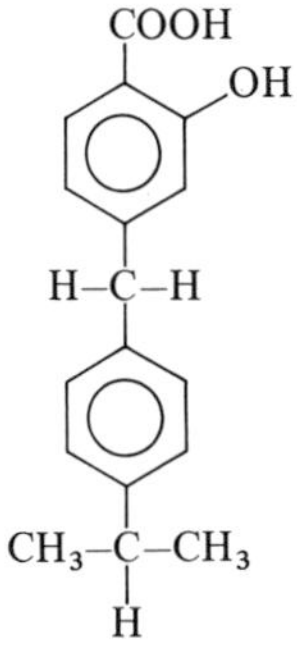

3–(4′–isopropylbenzyl)
salicylic acid
— 2 mM —

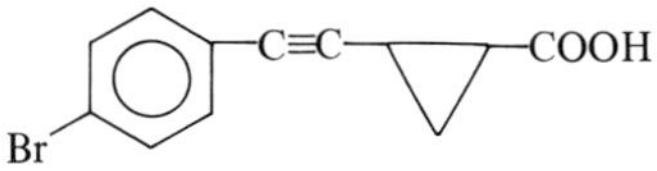

trans–4–bromophenethynyl–
cyclopropane carboxylic acid
— 15 mM —

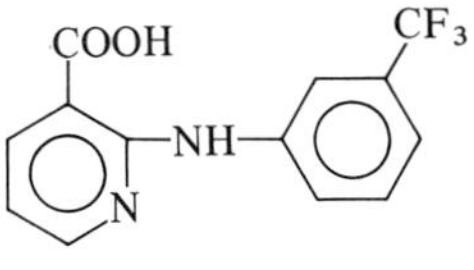

niflumic acid
— 8 mM —

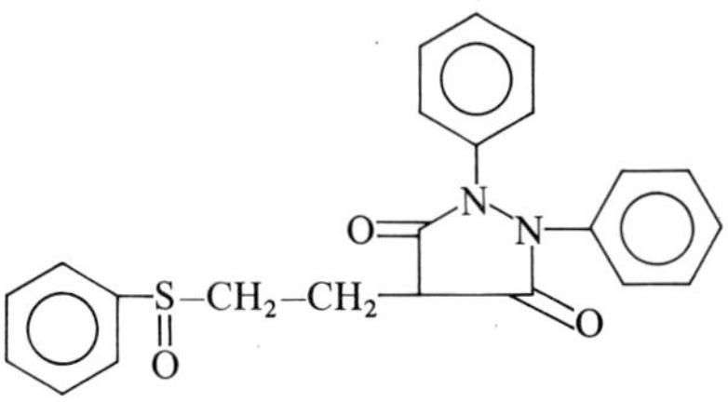

4–phenylsulfonylethyl–1,2–diphenyl–
3,5–pyrazolidinedione
— 10 mM —

lates, were found to induce fibrinolytic activity at rather low concentrations. (N-(3-trifluoromethyl-phenyl)-anthranilate was the compound with highest activity of the compounds checked in this series [activity at 38 mg/100 ml] [Gryglewski and Gryglewska, 1966]). A number of derivatives of diarylcarboxylic acids were noted to induce marked fibrinolytic activity in vitro. Simple diphenylcarboxylic acid was inactive but when the carboxyl group is attached to the ring through an alkyl or

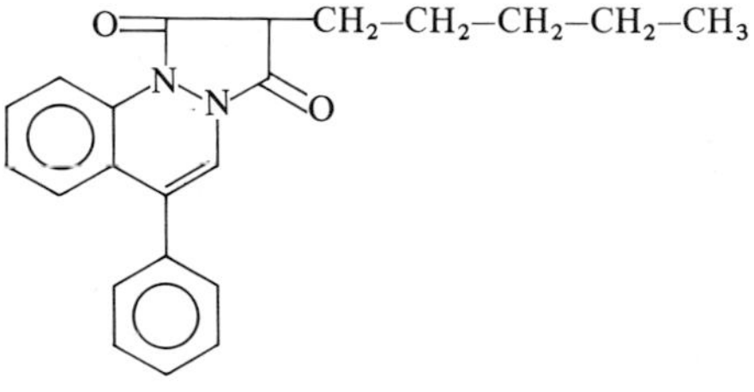

O=⟨ring⟩—CH₂–CH₂–CH₂–CH₂–CH₃   1,2–(pentylmalonyl)–
                                 1,2–dihydro– 4–phenylcinnoline

                                 – 0,7 mM –
                                 (with (NH₂)₂)

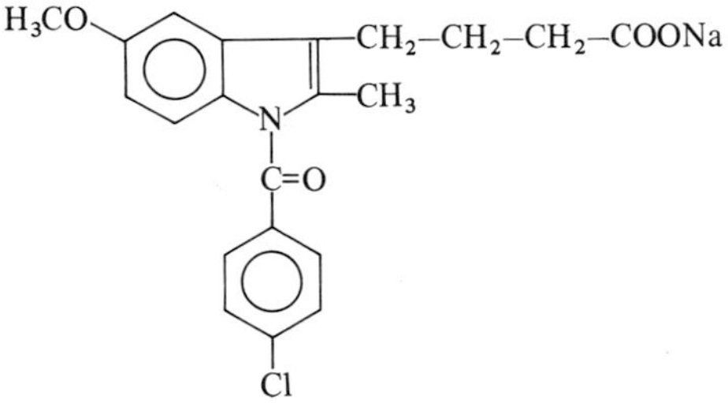

H₃CO—⟨indole⟩—CH₂–CH₂–CH₂–COONa
                —CH₃   1–(p–chlorobenzoyl)–2–
          N   methyl–5–methoxy–3–
          C=O   indole–γ–butyric acid
                                     –4 mM– 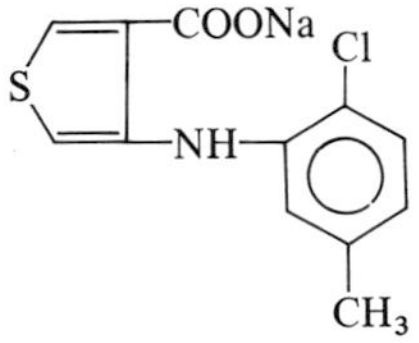
          Cl

⟨thiophene⟩—COONa Cl
   S   N–(2′–chloro–5′–
         —NH—⟨ring⟩   methylphenyl)–
                                  4–aminothiophene–3–
                                  carboxylic acid
              CH₃   – 3 mM –

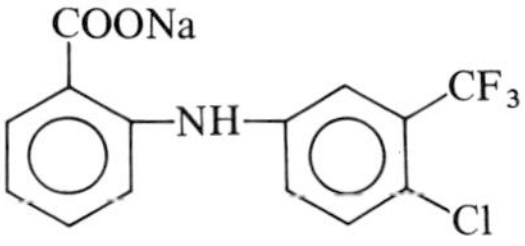

COONa
⟨ring⟩—NH—⟨ring⟩—CF₃   N–(3–trifluoromethyl–4–
                    Cl   chlorophenyl) anthranilic acid
                                     – 2 mM –

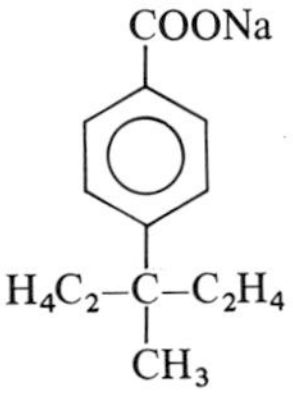

COONa
⟨ring⟩   4–(1′,1′–diethyl)–
                                  ethylbenzoic acid
H₄C₂–C–C₂H₄   – 6 mM –
      CH₃

Fig. 10. Various structures of organic anions which induce fibrinolytic activity in human plasma. Lowest effective concentration in mM. Hanging clot method

alkylene chain but not through an alkoxy chain, there is a rather high fibrinolysis-inducing capacity (GRYGLEWSKI and ECKSTEIN, 1967). It was further observed that a number of anti-inflammatory compounds (and many of their derivatives) including benzopyrazone, phenylbutazone, ketophenylbutyzone and indomethacin, induced marked fibrinolytic activity in the test tube (ROUBAL and NEMECEK, 1966; VON KAULLA, 1968), and that with some diphenyldioxy pyrazolidine derivatives, there is a parallel between their anti-inflammatory effectiveness and their fibrinolysis-inducing capacity (ROUBAL and NEMECEK, 1966).

Numerous other groups of organic anions were subsequently found to induce fibrinolytic activity in the test tube, for instance, thiophene-3-carboxylic acid derivatives. N-(2-chloro-3-methylphenyl)-4-amino-thiophene-3 carboxylic acid, with activity at 3 mM, was the most active of these compounds, though only over a narrow range (von KAULLA, 1970).

For studies of structure-activity relationship, alkylated 3-enol tautomers, for instance, were used to hinder the keto-enol tautomerism. This hindrance did not cause loss of fibrinolytic activity, suggesting that the keto-enol tautomerism is not a major factor in rendering compounds fibrinolytically active. With substitution changes of the tri-methazone related compound Kebuzone (1,2-diphenyl-3,5-dioxo-4-(3-oxobutyl)-pyrazolidine), for instance, it could be shown that branching on the carbon atom next to the carboxyl group substantially enhanced the fibrinolytic activity of the compound. The fibrinolytic activity was further enhanced when the terminal methyl group was substituted by phenyl or furyl groups. Substitution of the terminal phenyl group by an alpha-substituted benzyl group resulted in additional enhancement of fibrinolytic activity, although the activity was exerted over a rather narrow range (ROUBAL et al., 1975). In this connection it should be mentioned that compounds active over a narrow concentration range were observed to inhibit only plasmin and trypsin activity in the caseinolytic test. This inhibitory activity increased interestingly enough with the fibrinolytic activity in the hanging clot test (BAILLIE and SIM, 1972). We found that flufenamic acid at low concentrations enhanced activity of trypsin, while at higher concentrations it reduced the activity of trypsin but not of other proteolytic enzymes (see Figure 9).

The number of organic anions which have so far been found to induce fibrinolytic activity is very large, and their structures vary widely. This is documented with examples shown in Figure 10. The lowest activity is indicated in mMols as measured with the hanging clot test. Only structures of compounds with an activity of 15 mM or less are given. Space does not permit discussion of all the many compounds observed so far to be active. However, two of entirely different structures should be mentioned, as the substituted derivative of both exhibited a very marked activity. The one group is made up of derivatives of trans-phenethynylcyclopropane carboxylates: Substitution of the benzene ring increases the fibrinolytic activity in the following order: 4-F; 4-Me; 2-Me; 4-Cl; 3-Me; 3-Cl; 4-Br (YOSHIMOTO et al., 1975). The other group of compounds are derivatives of azopropazon (5-dimethylamino-9-methyl-2-propyl 1 H pyrazolo [1,2a] [1,2,4]benzotriazene-1,3[2 H]-dione). The mother compound itself is inactive, but replacement of the methyl group on the benzene ring by trifluoromethyl induces a marked fibrinolytic activity, which is further enhanced by additional substitutions (WAGNER-JAUREGG et al., 1973). Some other compounds which induce fibrinolytic activity in vitro are tribenoside (ethyl-tri-0-benzyl-D-glucofuranoside) (RUEGG et al., 1972) and bencyclane (N-[3-(1-benzyl cycloheptyl-oxy)propyl]-N,N-dimethyl ammonium hydrogen fumarate). It was claimed that this last-mentioned compound induces fibrinolytic activity in vitro and in vivo (KOVACS et al., 1971). A similar claim was made for a bencyclane derivative (see Section G). Furthermore, it was found that dextrane sulfate increases the fibrinolytic activity of the euglobulin fraction of human plasma and also induces

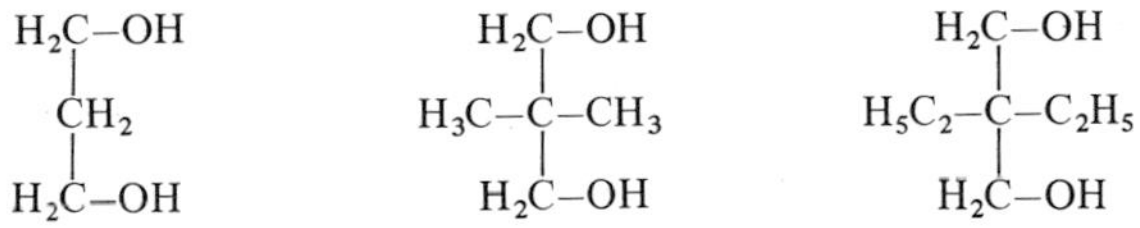

H₂C—OH   H₂C—OH   H₂C—OH

CH₂   H₃C—C—CH₃   H₅C₂—C—C₂H₅

H₂C—OH   H₂C—OH   H₂C—OH

1,3–propanediol   2,2–dimethyl–   2,2–diethyl–
          1,3–propanediol   1,3–propanediol
– 3000 mM –   – 1500 mM –   – 300 mM –

Fig. 11. Induction and enhancement of fibrinolytic activity by substitutions of the inactive 1,3 propanediol. Substitution with ethyl groups is five times more effective than substitution with methyl groups. Hanging clot method

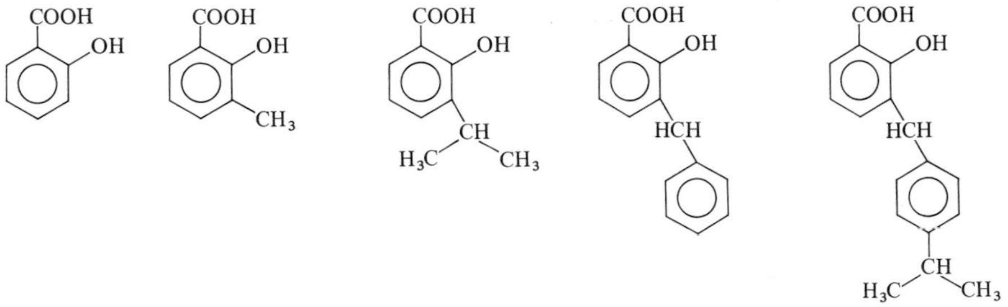

salicylic   3–methylsalicylic   3–isopropylsalicylic   3–benzylsalicylic   3–(4′–isopropylbenzyl)
acid   acid   acid   acid   salicylic acid
– 150 mM –   – 60 mM –   – 8 mM –   – 5 mM –   – 2 mM –

Fig. 12. Induction and marked enhancement of fibrinolytic activity by asymmetric substitutions of the poorly active salicylic acid. Hanging clot method

such activity in the supernatant of the euglobulin fraction. These effects of dextrane sulfate were interpreted as direct production of an activator from a proactivator by the compounds (ASTRUP and ROSA, 1974).

The question arises as to what might be the common denominator for the fibrinolysis-inducing capacity of the compounds of various structures. Generally speaking, the enhancing effect of substitutions on the fibrinolysis-inducing capacity is obvious. Even a symmetrical substitution can induce fibrinolytic activity in an inactive compound, as shown in Figure 11. Appropriate substitutions resulting in an asymmetric molecule, however, are much more effective, as indicated with salicylic acid derivatives as example in Figure 12. A similar effect (as another example for many) is obtained by substitution of the inactive anthranilic acid. As can be seen in Figure 13, in addition to the effect of asymmetry of the compound, the position of a methyl group or the more efficient tri-fluoro methyl group on the substituting benzen ring plays a clear-cut role in the extent of the enhancement of fibrinolytic activity. It seems as though the anionic and, in particular, the lipophilic character of the compounds has a clear-cut relation to their fibrinolytic activity, as shown by mathematical analysis (HANSCH and VON KAULLA, 1970 and 1975). Similar conclusions were reached by ČEPELAK et al. (1976). These authors state that fibrinolytic activity signifi-

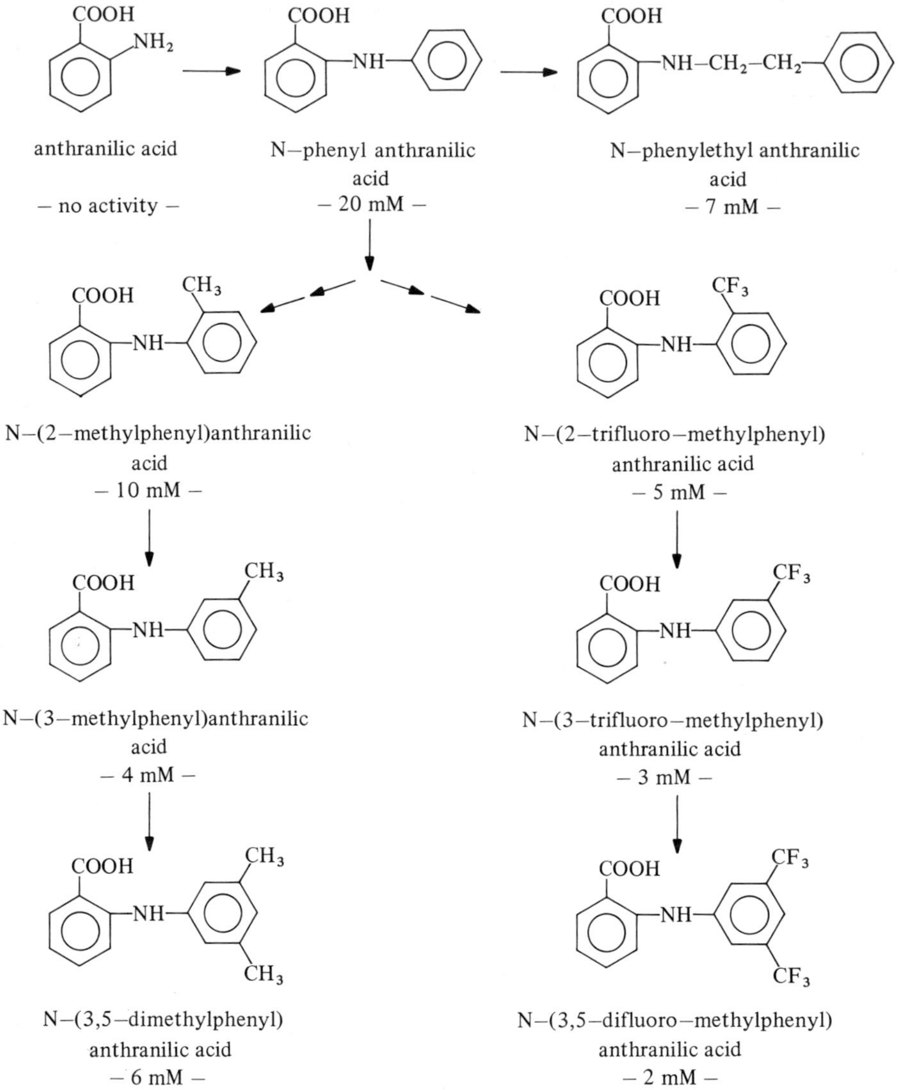

Fig. 13. Induction and marked enhancement by asymmetric substitution of inactive anthranilic acid. Various effects of the position of methyl and trifluoromethyl groups on the substituting benzen ring. (von Kaulla et al., 1975 b)

cantly increases with increasing lipophilia of either aromatic or beta-alkyl substituents, and that the steric effect of beta-alkyls plays merely an accessory role and manifests itself by lowering fibrinolytic activity. The electronic effect of aromatic substituents does not influence the fibrinolytic activity. These findings will assist in the search for more active compounds. One basic problem, however, the binding of the compounds to albumin (see Section E), remains to be solved.

E. Binding of Synthetic Fibrinolytic Compounds to Albumin

The differences of the required molarity to induce dissolution of hanging clots and of plasma clots indicate that a large portion of the compound is adsorbed onto proteins unrelated to fibrinolysis induction. With the hanging clot, the compound is present in excess (dissolved in the 2.5 ml buffered saline solution in which the hanging clot with a volume of 0.5 ml is suspended). This is not the case with the plasma clot. The compounds are dissolved in plasma before clot formation and their adsorption to inert proteins markedly reduces the concentration available for fibrinolysis induction after clotting.

Albumin is primarily the inert compound-binding protein, as can be shown in various ways. Thus, reduction of the albumin content of plasma reduces the compound molarity required for fibrinolysis induction: the concentration of flufenamic acid required for lysis induction of a clot made from plasma with 4.1 g albumin per 100 ml amounts to 10 mM. In plasma with an albumin content reduced to 0.4 g/100 ml only 3 mM is required. Blocking of the binding site of albumin with oxacillin has a similar effect: the concentration of flufenamic acid required to lyse hanging clots is 4 mM; that required to lyse hanging clots made from plasma containing 20 mg/ml oxacillin is 0.9 mM (von KAULLA, 1975b). With flufenamic acid, it has been found that the aromatic portion of the compounds is inserted into a hydrophobic crevice of the albumin while the carboxylate group of the compound interacts with the cationic site of the protein surface (CHIGNELL, 1969). Due to the binding, 3.3 times more flufenamic acid is needed to dissolve a plasma clot than to dissolve a hanging clot. When ^{125}I-labeled 3,5-diiodo salicylic acid was used, it was found that about 85 percent of the compound is bound to albumin (von KAULLA, 1970). With this highly albumin-bound compound, the activity relationship between hanging clot and plasma clot was 1:6 (2 mM vs. 12 mM). For fibrinolysis-inducing bety-aryl aliphatic acids it has been also reported that they prevent the thermal denaturation of serum albumin, and it was suggested that the extent of lipophilia plays a role in the binding of the compound to albumin, as it does for the induction of fibrinolytic activity (ČEPELAK et al., 1976).

Are there any observations indicating a potential solution of the problem of the binding to albumin of synthetic fibrinolysis inducers? Possibly the variation in the different concentrations required for lysis of plasma clots and of hanging clots gives an indication. As mentioned, the hanging clots are not much influenced by the albumin binding of the compounds, because these are present in "excess" so that the albumin binding by the hanging clot reduces their concentration in the solution in which the clots are suspended to a small extent only, whereas the binding to albumin in the plasma clot, with no surrounding compound solution, reduces the concentration available for fibrinolysis induction very markedly. For this reason, higher compound concentrations are required to dissolve plasma clots. It was noticed, however, that the ratio between the concentrations required to lyse the two types of clot varies widely. Example: The following three compounds induce plasma clot lysis at 10 mM. However, lysis of the hanging clot is induced with 2 mM by 3-(4-chlorobenzyl)-salicylic acid, with 3 mM by N-(3-trifluoromethylphenyl)anthranilic acid and by 7 mM with 3-(2,3-xylylanilino)-4-thiophene carboxylic acid, resulting in ratios of 1:5, 1:3.3, and 1:1.4, respectively. Does a relationship close to 1:1 indicate a reduced binding of the compound to albumin? If this were the case, compounds, for instance, of the type of Deriphat 160 C (N-lauryl-beta-imino-dipropionic acid Na) deserve further investigation, because with this compound the relationship was found to be 1:1 (von KAULLA and von KAULLA, 1976). In other words, the same molarities (14 mM) are required to lyse both types of clots.

F. Enhancement by Hydrazine and Cobra Venom Factor of the Fibrinolytic Activity Induced by Synthetic Compounds In Vitro

Hydrazine at 20 mM was reported to reduce the antiplasmin activity of human serum (RATNOFF et al., 1954). Investigations were therefore carried out to find whether or not hydrazine might enhance the activity of synthetic fibrinolysis-inducing compounds. This is indeed the case, with the most effective concentration being only 2.5 mM. Benzylhydrazine and isopropyl-hydrazine were considerably less effective (von KAULLA, 1970). With the use of human serum together with bovine plasmin and bovine fibrin clots, the reduction of antiplasmin activity could be confirmed; the optimal concentration was again 2.5 mM (von KAULLA, 1975a). Hydrazine was also reported to reduce the alpha-2-macroglobulin content of human plasma by 50% (DESNOYERS and SAMAMA, 1976). Whether these two ways of reducing the antiplasmin activity of plasma are the only explanations of the enhancing effect of the synthetic fibrinolytic agents is still an open question. It has also been claimed that there is a relationship between the lipophilic character of the molecules and the enhancement of the fibrinolysis-inducing capacity by hydrazine, the enhancement increasing with the lipophilic properties of the compounds (HANSCH, 1975). Hydrazine did not, however, enhance the fibrinolytic activity of streptokinase or urokinase (von KAULLA, 1976). The enhancing effect of hydrazine on the fibrinolysis-inducing capacity of the synthetic compounds is proven in three ways. 1. Hydrazine reduces the molarity required for the fibrinolytic dissolution of hanging clots. Example: The required molarity of flufenamic acid is reduced from 3 mM to 0.9 mM. The hanging clot was exposed for 4 h to the 2.5 mM hydrazine solution and then transferred into the compound solution. 2. Hydrazine unmasks the potential for fibrinolysis induction of apparently inactive compounds which theoretically—that is to say, according to their structure—should be quite potent. This was shown with the hanging clot and with plasma clots. Example: The inactive 3-n-nonyl salicylic acid was active with hydrazine at 0.4 mM and 7 mM, respectively. 3. Hydrazine shortened the dissolution time of plasma clots. Example: Niflumic acid at 13 mM induced dissolution of the human plasma clot within 24 h and after preincubation with 2.5 mM hydrazine for 60 min of the plasma from which the clot was made within 5 h (von KAULLA, 1975a). Pretreatment with hydrazine was also observed to enhance and prolong in vivo in rats the fibrinolytic reaction induced after intravenous injection of synthetic compounds which are active both in vitro and in vivo (see Section G). Some of the compounds were observed to increase factor VIII activity in hemophilia A plasma, an effect which is enhanced by hydrazine. This enhancement is particularly marked in plasma of patients with a high inhibitor of factor VIII (von KAULLA, E., unpublished data).

Hydrazine is known to reduce the complement activity of human plasma. Therefore, it was of interest to investigate whether or not another agent reducing the complement activity would have an enhancing effect on the fibrinolysis induction by the compounds. This was indeed the case with cobra venom factor used at a concentration that completely abolished the complement activity of the plasma but neither exerts an appreciable reducing effect on the antiplasmin activity of the plasma nor enhances the antiplasmin inhibition by synthetic fibrinolytic compounds. Thus, pretreatment of human plasma with cobra venom factor for 30 min reduces the molarity required for flufenamic acid to lyse the plasma clot within 24 h from 12 mM to 5 mM, for instance. Similar effects could be demonstrated with a number of other compounds. Cobra venom factor also enhances the fibrinolysis-inducing capacity of the synthetic compounds in dog, rat, and pig plasma. Thus, to give two examples: Deriphat 160 C at 3 mM took more than 24 h to induce lysis of dog plasma clots, but only 60 min or less after previous addition of cobra venom factor to this plasma (VON KAULLA, 1975a). Addition of 6 mM flufenamic acid to pig plasma did not induce lysis within 48 h; pretreatment with hydrazine reduced the lysis time to 24 h and pretreatment with cobra venom factor to 17 h (VON KAULLA, 1976). With a number of compounds it was also observed that combined use of cobra venom factor and hydrazine might have an additive effect (VON KAULLA, 1975a). A clear-cut explanation for the enhancing effect of the cobra venom factor on the fibrinolysis induction by synthetic compounds is not available at present. An analysis of this effect and also of that of hydrazine is likely to contribute to the further development of synthetic fibrinolytic agents.

G. Induction of Fibrinolytic Activity In Vitro and In Vivo

Various vasoactive drugs induce a rather short-lasting but marked fibrinolytic activity in vivo after intravenous injection. These drugs are not active in vitro. Nicotinic acid is an example of this type of compound. However, a derivative of nicotinic acid, 3-fluoromethyl-3-phenylamino-2-nicotinic acid, the niflumic acid, is active both in vitro (hanging clot at 8 mM, plasma clot at 12 mM) and in vivo in rats, and is thus able to induce fibrinolytic activity by two different pathways, a "chemical" one and a "pharmacological" one. Niflumic acid represents a prototype of an optimal synthetic fibrinolytic agent. The in vivo fibrinolysis-inducing capacity is demonstrated with rats using a micro-euglobulin lysis time permitting a number of blood specimens to be taken from the same rat from the tail, thus making it possible to follow the trend of fibrinolytic activity in an individual animal for some hours (WASANTAPRUEK and VON KAULLA, 1966). After intravenous injection of 10 mg/kg niflumic acid, the euglobulin lysis time is considerably shortened for one to two hours (VON KAULLA, 1975b). The in vitro enhancement of niflumic acid-induced fibrinolytic activity by blood from rats treated with niflumic acid is demonstrated with the use of the microhanging clot method. Here, plasma clots (from 0.2 ml blood) obtained from rats five minutes after injection of niflumic acid and then suspended in rat plasma containing niflumic acid dissolve at a lower molarity than plasma clots obtained from untreated rats (VON KAULLA et al., 1975b). It is of great interest that hydrazine enhances the fibrinolysis-inducing effect of niflumic acid both in vitro (hanging clot from 8 to 4 mM) and in vivo. Pretreatment of the rats with i.v. injection of 5 mg/kg hydrazine intensifies and prolongs the fibrinolytic activity induced by niflumic acid and abolishes rebound effects which may occur. The enhancing effect of hydrazine both in vivo and in vitro was also shown for a bencyclane derivative (VON KAULLA and VON KAULLA, 1975b): pretreatment of the rat with hydrazine increased and prolonged very considerably the compound-induced fibrinolytic activity. The enhancing effect of hydrazine and its potential are of importance but require further investigation.

The two compound examples described indicate the possibility that drugs which induce fibrinolytic activity both in vitro and in vivo by two different pathways may be developed. It has been claimed that some other compounds, which are active in vitro, induce fibrinolytic activity, although of rather short duration, as measured with the euglobulin lysis time in the rat in vivo after oral administration (100 mg/kg) or after i.v. injection (10% of LD_{50}: approx. 10 mg/kg). The most active compound in this regard was 2-hydroxy-5-(2'-methyl-4-thiazolyl)benzoic acid (DESNOYERS, 1970). It was also observed that regional infusion of trimethazone (in vitro activity at 3 mM) to rabbits with artificial thrombi reduced the size of the thrombi by more than 50% as compared with clots in animals receiving saline only. Systemic infusion had no effect (ČEPELAK et al., 1975).

H. Effect of Synthetic Fibrinolytic Agents on Thrombocytes, Erythrocytes and some Clotting Factors

Collagen-induced aggregation of human platelets left in their plasma was inhibited, at various concentrations, by most of the many synthetic fibrinolytic compounds tested for this particular effect. This observation suggests the possibility of designing drugs with the dual antithrombotic action of prevention of thrombus formation and induction of thrombolysis. There is a rather loose correlation between the structural features which enhance the fibrinolytic action of the compounds and those which enhance their ability to prevent platelet aggregation. Thus, aggregation inhibition was obtained by approximately one-third (e.g. 3-cinnamyl salicylic acid) to one-sixtieth (e.g.: N-(2-chloro-6-methylphenyl)-4-aminothiophene-3 carboxylic acid) of the concentrations required to induce fibrinolysis. The latter compound prevented collagen-induced platelet aggregation at 0.05 mM. The prevention of collagen-induced platelet aggregation was observed, for instance, with fibrinolytic derivatives of anthranilic acid, of salicylic acid and thiophene carboxylic acid (THILO and VON KAULLA, 1970), with fibrinolytic pyrazolidine derivatives (ROUBAL et al., 1972), and with other compounds. The mother compounds had little or no activity, either for prevention of platelet aggregation or for fibrinolysis induction.

Figure 14 reveals, with thiophene derivatives as an example, the rather loose correlation between structural changes which enhance the fibrinolysis-inducing capacity and those which enhance inhibition of platelet aggregation. This figure does not show 3-(2,3-dimethylphenyl)-4-aminothiophene carboxylic acid, which induces fibrinolysis at 7 mM and inhibition of collagen-induced platelet aggregation at 0.2 mM. Combination of the carboxyl group of this compound with an aliphatic chain completely abolishes the fibrinolysis-inducing capacity, but enhances the aggregation inhibition to 0.02 mM. However, substitution of the benzyl ring of the compound with free carboxyl group with C 1 in position 2 together with a methyl group in position 4 endows it with the capacity for both fibrinolysis induction (at 3 mM) and prevention of platelet aggregation (at 0.05 m) (VON KAULLA, 1976). With

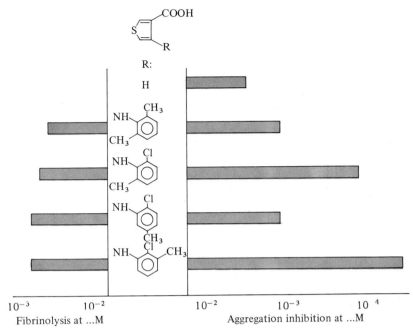

Fig. 14. Thiophene derivatives which induce fibrinolytic activity in vitro as well as prevent platelet aggregation. Loose relationship between the substitutions which at various concentrations endow the compound with ability to exert both activities. Activity assessment: Hanging clot and platelet aggregation by collagen. Human plasma

salicylic acid it has been found, to give another example of the effect of structure modifications, that substitution in the 3- or 5-position with cyclohexyl enhanced fibrinolytic activity but not aggregation inhibition, whereas substitution in position 3 with 2-chlorobenzyl increased the fibrinolysis-inducing activity and reduced by a factor of ten the molarity required for aggregation inhibition (THILO and VON KAULLA, 1970). For pyrazolidine, it was observed that an alpha-substitution in the side chain of 1,2-diphenyl-3,5-dioxopyrazolidine always enhanced the biological activity of the parent compound both for fibrinolysis induction and for platelet aggregation inhibition (ROUBAL et al., 1972). It has been claimed that the lipophilic effect with the fibrinolytic beta-substituted phenylaliphatic acid as an example is equally important for the platelet aggregation inhibition as it is for the fibrinolytic activity, whereas the steric effect plays also yet a less important role with this effect (ROUBAL et al., 1975). Niflumic acid, the fibrinolytic compound which induces fibrinolytic activity both in vitro and in vivo, is also able to reduce collagen-induced platelet aggregation. Actual measurements of this effect with niflumic acid are shown with four different molarities in Figure 15. Although with this compound a higher concentration is required for inhibition of platelet aggregation than with some other compounds, this activity of niflumic acid indicates that it might be possible to develop multi-action antithrombotic drugs inducing fibrinolytic activity by two different pathways and also preventing platelet aggregation. The mechanism involved in the inhibition of colla-

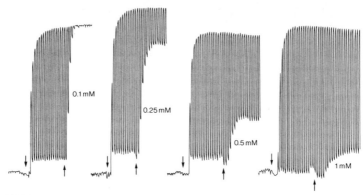

Fig. 15. Inhibition of collagen-induced aggregation of platelets in human plasma by various concentrations of niflumic acid. ↓ Collagen added to compound-free control; ↑ collagen added to plasma containing niflumic acid. Double-aggregometer

gen-induced platelet aggregation by synthetic fibrinolytic compounds has not yet been established.

Two compounds were tested and found to inhibit an entirely different type of platelet aggregation: the aggregation of pig platelets suspended in saline or in pig plasma by dog serum. Dog serum has a powerful preformed humoral antibody against porcine tissue. It is assumed that the antigens on the surface of pig platelets are the same as those in other porcine cells. The dog serum was incubated with 12 mM flufenamic acid or with 7 mM pamoic acid for 30 min and subsequently dialyzed for 15 h at a low temperature to remove the unbound compounds and thus any reduction by them in complement activity of the pig plasma. After this treatment, the dog serum had lost most of its ability to aggregate pig platelets. Within five minutes either compound reduced the complement activity of the dog serum to <5 CH_{50}. Whether or not the elimination of complement activity is the mechanism by which the two synthetic fibrinolytic compounds abolish the ability of dog serum to aggregate pig platelets is not quite clear, because pamoic acid, which in contrast to this compound exhibited the same abolishing effect on the complement as flufenamic acid did, reduces but does not completely prevent the dog serum-induced pig platelet aggregation (GERLOFF and von KAULLA, 1972).

Inhibition of erythrocyte aggregation or increased sedimentation tendency by many synthetic fibrinolytic compounds is an additional mechanism by which they may exert another potential antithrombotic function. On the basis of both clinical observations and experimental evidence, many investigators have suggested that erythrocytes have some role in thromboembolism. The role of erythrocytes in enhancing a thrombosis tendency has been described in two ways: increased aggregability and increased sedimentation rate. The inhibitory function of the compounds on increased sedimentation rate of erythrocytes was shown in two ways: inhibition of increased sedimentation of erythrocytes left in their plasma (citrated blood) and inhibition (measured as sedimentation rate) of aggregation of erythrocytes suspended in buffered saline induced by fibrinogen and also by dextran and gelatine. Figure 16 shows as a characteristic example the inhibiting effect of fibrinolytic com-

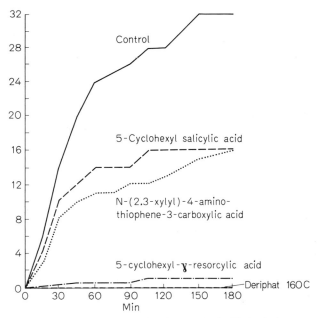

Fig. 16. Inhibition of erythrocyte sedimentation by synthetic fibrinolytic compounds in the citrated blood of a patient with acute myocardial infarction. Compound concentration 0.5 mM

pounds at 0.5 mM concentration on the very markedly enhanced erythrocyte sedimentation rate of a patient with an acute myocardial infarction. Two of the compounds block the sedimentation practically completely. As typical examples, Table 8 lists the extent of inhibition of bovine fibrinogen(final concentration 0.77%)-induced sedimentation of human erythrocytes by five fibrinolytic agents. This inhibition is quite marked for the first three compounds listed. No correlation of the inhibiting

Table 8. Comparison of the inhibiting effects of five fibrinolytic compounds on erythrocyte sedimentation and platelet aggregation

Compound	% Inhibition of fibrinogen-induced erythrocyte sedimentation at 0.1 mM	Lowest molarity (mM) inhibiting by 50% or more collagen-induced platelet aggregation	Lowest molarity (mM) at which a human clot dissolved within 24 hours at 37° C	
			Hanging clot	Plasma clot
Niflumic acid	98	0.5	8	12
3-(2-chlorobenzyl)salicylic acid	83	0.3	2	10
Flufenamic acid	62	0.2	3	10
3-(2-methyl-3-chloro)-anilino-4-thiophene COOH	34	0.05	3	11
3-(2-chloro-3-methyl)-anilino-4-thiophene COOH	0	0.05	3	14

activity of the compounds with the extent of their ability to prevent collagen-induced platelet aggregation could be demonstrated (von Kaulla, 1975c). The mechanism of the compound-induced sedimentation and aggregation inhibition is unknown, although it might have something to do with the interaction of the compound with the erythrocyte membrane. For flufenamic acid, for instance, it has been shown that this compound is adsorbed on the erythrocyte membrane (Tanaka et al., 1973) and it was further shown that the membrane stabilization by synthetic fibrinolytic agents (e.g. with beta-aryl aliphatic acid) prevents the osmotic hemolysis of the erythrocytes (Čepelak et al., 1976). The membrane-stabilizing effect of the compounds was claimed to be correlated primarily with the lipophilic and, in contrast to the fibrino-lysis-inducing capacity, with the electronic effect, and to a lesser degree with the steric effect (Roubal et al., 1975). It should be added that of all 13 compounds tested, niflumic acid exerted the most marked inhibition of fibrinogen-, dextran- and gela-tine-induced erythrocyte sedimentation. At 0.05 mM, only niflumic acid was effective with gelatine.

Besides the described effect on thrombocytes and erythrocytes, some of the com-pounds have another, secondary activity: antihemophilic globulin, i.e. factor VIII activity in hemophilic plasma, is considerably enhanced when the platelet-free plasma is exposed at 4° C to certain synthetic fibrinolytic agents (others are without effect). The induced increase in factor VIII activity is a time reaction with a maxi-mum effect mostly after one to two hours. Thus, to give a few examples: after 90 min exposure flufenamic acid increases factor VIII activity in the plasma of hemophiliacs from 1% to 33%, 3-cinnamyl salicylic acid from 1% to 35%, and N-(2-chloro-6-methylphenyl)-4-aminothiophene-3 carboxylic acid from 2.5% to 48% (von Kaulla and von Kaulla, 1972 and 1975). The thiophene derivative was one of the most active compounds, whereas closely related derivatives such as N-(4-chloro-6-methylphenyl)- and N-(chloro-4-methylphenyl)-4-aminothiophene-3 carboxylic ac-ids induce no activity. Once it has been generated by active compounds, the factor VIII activity is relatively stable when the compound-plasma mixture is stored in a frozen state. It was observed that hydrazine when added to the same hemophilic plasma enhances the factor VIII-increasing effect of the active fibrinolytic com-pounds. The compounds were also able to increase factor VIII activity in plasma of some patients with a high factor VIII inhibitor titer which made blood transfusions useless. Example: Factor VIII activity in plasma of a patient with a factor VIII inhibitor was $\pm 1\%$. After five minutes' incubation with N-(2-chloro-6-methyl-phenyl)-4-amino-thiophene-3 COOH, the activity rose to 16% and with the same compound plus hydrazine to 30%. After 90 min incubation at 4° C the activity rose to 51% and with hydrazine added to over 100%. After 90 min incubation with 3-cinnamyl salicylic acid, factor VIII activity rose to 40% and with hydrazine to 100%; it should be added that in several cases with von Willebrand-disease an increase of factor VIII activity was obtained with the same compounds (von Kaulla, E., un-published data). Space does not permit technical details of the testing procedure. The mechanism by which some of the synthetic compounds improve factor VIII activity in hemophilic plasma is not yet known, but removal of an inhibitor might be the pathway.

The interference of compounds with inhibitors of the coagulation and fibrinolytic system is also demonstrated by their reducing effect on antithrombin III activity.

Thus, exposure of human serum with a pathologically high antithrombin III activity to 8 mM 3-cinnamyl salicylic acid resulted in a progressive reduction of this activity, which almost completely disappeared after 90 min interaction (VON KAULLA, E., VON KAULLA, K. N., 1975). It should be added that some of the compounds reduce in vitro the level of factor XIII. Particularly active in this regard was a bencyclane derivative which at 4 mM suppressed this activity. This compound induced at 7 mM, but only together with hydrazine, fibrinolytic activity in vitro, and 10 mg/kg i.m. in the rat induced a very marked but short-lived fibrinolytic activity. Another active compound at 8 mM was 3-chloro-6-methylphenyl-3-carboxylic acid.

In summary, it should be pointed out that synthetic organic anions inducing fibrinolytic activity in vitro represent the potential for development of multiaction antithrombotic-thrombolytic drugs, a potential which deserves further intensive investigation.

References

Aoki, N.: Preparation of plasminogen activator from vascular trees of human cadavers. Its comparison with urokinase. J. Biochem. (Tokyo) **75**, 731—741 (1974)

Aoki, N., Kaulla, K. N. von: Inactivation of human serum plasminogen antiactivator by synthetic fibrinolysis inducers. Thrombos. Diathes. haemorrh. (Stuttg.) **22**, 251—262 (1969a)

Aoki, N., Kaulla, K. N. von: β_1C-globulin and synthetic fibrinolytic agents. Proc. Soc. exp. Biol. (N.Y.) **130**, 101—106 (1969 b)

Aoki, N., Kaulla, K. N. von: The extraction of plasminogen activator from human cadavers. Some of its properties. Amer. J. clin. Pathol. **55**, 171—179 (1971 a)

Aoki, N., Kaulla, K. N. von: Dissimilarity of human vascular plasminogen activator and human urokinase. J. Lab. clin. Med. **78**, 354—362 (1976)

Astrup, T., Rosa, A. T.: A plasminogen proactivator system in human blood effective in absence of Hageman factor. Thrombos. Res. **4**, 609—613 (1974)

Baillie, A. J., Sim, A. K.: The effects of some synthetic compounds on in vitro fibrinolytic activity measured by different methods and the relevance to activity in vivo. Thrombos. Diathes. haemorrh. (Stuttg.) **28**, 351—358 (1972)

Baumgarten, W., Priester, L. I., Stiller, D. W., Duncan, A. E. W.: Mechanism of action of synthetic fibrinolytic compounds. Thrombos. Diathes. haemorrh. (Stuttg.) **24**, 495—506 (1970)

Čepelak, V., Chudacek, Z., Muratova, J., Roubal, Z., Nemecek, O.: Effect of some non-steroidal antiinflammatory drugs on fibrinolysis activation in vitro and thrombosis in vivo. In: Kaulla, K. N. von, Davidson, J. F. (Eds.): Synthetic Fibrinolytic Thrombolytic Agents. Chemical, Biochemical, Pharmacological and Clinical Aspects, pp. 148—164. Springfield/Ill.: Thomas 1975

Čepelak, V., Roubal, Z., Kuchar, M.: Fibrinolysis induction by synthetic organic acids. Chemical structure and biological activity relationship. Folia haemat. (Leipz.) **103**, 343—350 (1976)

Chignell, C. F.: Optical studies of drug-protein complexes. III. Interaction of flufenamic and other N-arylanthranilates with serum albumin. Molec. Pharmacol. **5**, 955—962 (1969)

Christensen, L. R.: The activation of plasminogen by chloroform. Z. gen. Physiol. **30**, 149—157 (1946)

Daver, J., Desnoyers, P.: Nouvelle hypothèse concernant le mécanisme de la fibrinolyse et de la coagulation. Anesth. Anal. Réan. **31**, 539—549 (1974)

Delezenne, C., Pozerski, E.: Action du sérum sanguin sur la gélatine en présence du chloroforme. C.R. Soc. Biol. **55**, 327—332 (1903)

Denys, J., De Marbaix, M.: Les peptonisations provoquées par le chloroforme. Cellule **5**, 197—251 (1889)

Desnoyers, P. C.: Experimental study of synthetic chemical agents with fibrinolytic activity. In: Schor, J. M. (Ed.): Chemical Control of Fibrinolysis-Thrombolysis. Theory and Clinical Applications, pp. 73—111. New York: Wiley-Interscience 1970

Desnoyers, P. C., Labaume, J., Conard, J., Samama, M.: Essai de contribution au mécanisme d'action thrombolytique de composés chimiques synthétiques. Bibliotheca Haematologica **38**, 2: 776—783 (1971)

Desnoyers, P. C., Samama, M.: Synthetische Verbindungen mit fibrinolytischer und thrombolytischer Aktivität. 2. Teil: Untersuchungen zum Wirkungsmechanismus. Folia haemat. (Leipz.) **103**, 357—361 (1976)

Gerloff, J., Kaulla, K. N. von: Prevention of dog serum-induced aggregation of pig platelets. Proc. Soc. exp. Biol. (N. Y.) **141**, 298—303 (1972)

Gottlob, R.: Plasminogen and plasma plasmin inhibitors in arterial and venous thrombi of various ages. In: Davidson, J. F., Samama, M. M., Desnoyers, P. C. (Eds.): Progress in Chemical Fibrinolysis and Thrombolysis, Vol. 1, pp. 23—35. New York: Raven 1975

Gryglewski, R. J., Eckstein, M.: Fibrinolytic activity of some biarylcarboxylic acids. Nature (Lond.) **214**, 626 (1967)

Gryglewski, R. J., Gryglewska, T. A.: Fibrinolytic activity of N-arylanthranilates. Biochem. Pharmacol. **15**, 117—1175 (1966)

Gurewich, V., Hyde, E., Lipinski, B.: The resistance of fibrinogen and soluble fibrin monomers in blood to degradation by a potent plasminogen activator derived from cadaver limbs. Blood **46**, 555—565 (1975)

Hansch, C.: (1975) Discussion remark: see von Kaulla, 1975a

Hansch, C., Kaulla, K. N. von: Quantitative structure-activity considerations in synthetic fibrinolytics. In: Schor, J. M. (Ed.): Chemical Control of Fibrinolysis-Thrombolysis. Theory and Clinical Applications, pp. 245—257. New York: Wiley-Interscience 1970

Hansch, C., Kaulla, K. N. von: A structure-activity model for certain synthetic fibrinolytics. In: Kaulla, K. N. von, Davidson, J. F. (Eds.): Synthetic Fibrinolytic Thrombolytic Agents. Chemical, Biochemical, Pharmacological and Clinical Aspects, p. 227—239. Springfield/Ill.: Thomas 1975

Hedner, U., Nilsson, I. M., Robertson, B.: Determination of plasminogen in clots and thrombi. Thrombos. Diathes. haemorrh. (Stuttg.) **16**, 38—50 (1966)

Juehling, L., Wöhlisch, E.: Über Fibrinogenolyse unter dem Einfluß hydrotroper Substanzen. Biochem. Z. **298**, 312—319 (1938)

Kaulla, E. von, Kaulla, K. N. von: Factor VIII activity in hemophilic plasma unmasked by synthetic organic anions. Nature (Lond.) New Biology **240**, 144—145 (1972)

Kaulla, E. von, Kaulla, K. N. von: Is inhibitor removal the mechanism for unmasking factor VIII activity in hemophilic plasma by certain synthetic fibrinolytic agents. In: Kaulla, K. N. von, Davidson, J. F. (Eds.): Synthetic Fibrinolytic Thrombolytic Agents. Chemical, Biochemical, Pharmacological and Clinical Aspects, pp. 176—181. Springfield/Ill.: Thomas 1975a

Kaulla, K. N. von: Extraction of fibrinolytic enzyme from blood. Nature (Lond.) **164**, 408 (1949)

Kaulla, K. N. von: The standard clot. Thrombos. Diathes. haemorrh. (Stuttg.) **5**, 489—494 (1961)

Kaulla, K. N. von: Fibrinolysis induction in vitro by aromatic derivatives. Arch. Biochem. Biophys. **96**, 4—12 (1962a)

Kaulla, K. N. von: Chemical structure and fibrinolysis induction. In vitro studies with 126 synthetic compounds. Thrombos. Diathes. haemorrh. (Stuttg.) **7**, 404—420 (1962b)

Kaulla, K. N. von: Chemistry of Thrombolysis: Human Fibrinolytic Enzymes, pp. 261—287. Springfield/Ill.: Thomas 1963a

Kaulla, K. N. von: Inactivation of antiplasmin and complement C' in human plasma rendered fibrinolytic by synthetic organic compounds. Thrombos. Diathes. haemorrh. (Stuttg.) **10**, 151—163 (1963b)

Kaulla, K. N. von: A simple test tube arrangement for screening fibrinolytic activity of synthetic organic compounds. J. med. Chem. **8**, 164—166 (1965)

Kaulla, K. N. von: Animal plasma as substrate for synthetic fibrinolysis inducers. Proc. Soc. exp. Biol. (N. Y.) **121**, 46—69 (1966)

Kaulla, K. N. von: Structure-dependent fibrinolytic (clot-dissolving) activity of antiinflammatory drugs and related compounds. Arzneimittel-Forsch. **18**, 407—412 (1968)

Kaulla, K. N. von: On the in vitro mechanism of synthetic fibrinolytic agents. In: Schor, J. M. (Ed.): Chemical Control of Fibrinolysis-Thrombolysis. Theory and Clinical Applications, pp. 1—41. New York: Wiley-Interscience 1970

Kaulla, K. N. von: Niflumic acid; prototype of a multiaction antithrombotic agent. Experientia (Basel) **30**, 959—960 (1974)

Kaulla, K. N. von: In vitro enhancement by hydrazine and Cobra venom factor of fibrinolytic activity induced by synthetic organic anions. In: Kaulla, K. N. von, Davidson, J. F. (Eds.): Synthetic Fibrinolytic Thrombolytic Agents. Chemical, Biochemical, Pharmacological and Clinical Aspects, pp. 166—174. Springfield/Ill.: C. C. Thomas 1975 a

Kaulla, K. N. von: The synthetic approach to fibrinolysis/thrombolysis. In: Kaulla, K. N. von, Davidson, J. F. (Eds.): Synthetic Fibrinolytic Thrombolytic Agents. Chemical, Biochemical, Pharmacological and Clinical Aspects, pp. 53—76. Springfield/Ill.: C. C. Thomas 1975 b

Kaulla, K. N. von: In vitro inhibition of aggregation of human erythrocytes by synthetic fibrinolytic compounds. Arzneimittel-Forsch. **25**, 152—155 (1975c)

Kaulla, K. N. von: Synthetische Fibrinolytika. Eigene Erfahrungen und Vorschläge. Folia haemat. (Leipz.) **103**, 313—342 (1976)

Kaulla, K. N. von, Fogleman, D., Mueller, H.: Clot penetration and fibrin adsorption of synthetic fibrinolytic compounds. In: Davidson, J. F., Samama, M. M., Desnoyers, P. C. (Eds.): Progress in Chemical Fibrinolysis and Thrombolysis, Vol. 1, pp. 45—54. New York: Raven 1975 a

Kaulla, K. N. von, Kaulla, E. von: Remarks on the euglobulin lysis time. In: Davidson, J. F., Samama, M. M., Desnoyers, P. C. (Eds.): Progress in Chemical Fibrinolysis and Thrombolysis, Vol. I, pp. 131—141. New York: Raven Press 1975 e

Kaulla, K. N. von, Kaulla, E. von: Synthetic fibrinolytic agents active in vitro, the potential optimal approach to induce "natural" thrombolysis and a problem still to be solved. Proceedings of the 3rd International Conference on Synthetic Fibrinolytic Thrombolytic Agents, Glasgow 1976. New York: Raven (in press)

Kaulla, K. N. von, Ostendorf, P., Leppke, L.: In vitro synergism of endogenously increased fibrinolysis with compound-induced fibrinolysis. In: Davidson, J. F., Samama, M. M., Desnoyers, P. C. (Eds.): Progress in Chemical Fibrinolysis and Thrombolysis, Vol. I, pp. 385—394. New York: Raven Press 1975 f

Kaulla, K. N. von, Smith, R. L.: Urea derivatives as fibrinolysis promoting agents. Proc. Soc. exp. Biol. (N.Y.) **106**, 530—533 (1961)

Kovacs, I. B., Csalay, L., Csakavry, G.: Antithrombotic and fibrinolytic effect of bencyclane. Arzneimittel-Forsch. **21**, 1553—1556 (1971)

Kucinski, C. S., Fletcher, A. P., Sherry, S.: Effect of urokinase antiserum on plasminogen activators. Demonstration of immunologic dissimilarity between plasma plasminogen activator and urokinase. J. clin. Invest. **47**, 1238—1253 (1968)

Mishenko, V. P., Kuznik, B. I., Bochkarnikov, V. V.: The mechanism of action of vasoactive agents on the blood clotting and fibrinolysis. Cor vasa **14**, 228—237 (1972)

Nanninga, L. B.: Blocking of urokinase binding to plasma inhibitor by diiodosalicylate. Fed. Proc. **34**, 290 (1975)

Nanninga, L. B., Guest, M.: Blocking of the fibrinolytic antiactivator by substituted benzoates. Life Sci. **14**, 2507—2511 (1974)

Nolf, P.: Action coagulante du chloroforme sur le plasma du chien. Arch. int. de Physiol. **18**, 549—569 (1921)

Ogston, D. C., Ogston, M., Fullerton, H. W.: The plasminogen content of thrombi. Thrombos. Diathes. haemorrh. (Stuttg.) **15**, 220—230 (1966)

Rader, R. W., Wulf, R. J.: Substituted salicylates and chemically induced fibrinolysis. Fed. Proc. **25**, 1734 (1966) (Abstract)

Ratnoff, O. D., Lepow, I. H., Pillemer, L.: The multiplicity of plasmin inhibitors in human serum, demonstrated by the effect of primary amino compounds. Bull. Johns Hopkins Hosp. **94**, 169—179 (1954)

Roubal, Z., Čepelak, V., Nemecek, O.: Newly synthesized pyrazolidine derivatives as potential activators of fibrinolysis and antiaggregating agents. Acta Univ. Carolina, Med. Monogr. **52**, 49—54 (1972)

Roubal, Z., Grimova, J., Kuchar, M., Nemecek, O., Čepelak, V.: An investigation into the interrelationship between structure and fibrinolysis activating capacity of some non-steroidal antiinflammatory drugs in vitro. In: Kaulla, K. N. von, Davidson, J. F. (Eds.): Synthetic Fibrinolytic Thrombolytic Agents. Chemical, Biochemical, Pharmacological and Clinical Aspects, pp. 133—147. Springfield/Ill.: Thomas 1975

Roubal, Z., Nemecek, O.: Antiinflammatory compounds exhibiting fibrinolytic activity. Med. Chem. **9**, 840—842 (1966)

Ruegg, M., Riesterer, L., Jaques, R.: Increase of plasma fibrinolysis by ethyl-tri-benzyl-D-gluco-furanoside. Pharmacology **7**, 51—61 (1972)

Tanaka, K., Kobayashi, K., Kazui, S.: Temperature dependent reaction of flufenamic acid with rat erythrocyte membrane. Biochem. Pharmacol. **22**, 879—886 (1973)

Thilo, D., Kaulla, K. N. von: Structure-dependent inhibition by synthetic fibrinolytic anions of collagen-induced aggregation of human platelets. J. med. Chem. **13**, 503—510 (1970)

Tomikawa, M., Abiko, Y.: The plasminogen-plasmin system. Part VIII. On the mechanism of chemical induction of fibrinolysis. Isolation of a latent plasminogen activator from human plasma. Thrombos. Diathes. haemorrh. (Stuttg.) **29**, 50—62 (1973)

Tytgat, G., Collen, D., Vreker, R. de, Verstraete, M.: Investigations on the fibrinolytic system in liver cirrhosis. Acta haematol. (Basel) **40**, 265—274 (1968)

Wagner-Jauregg, Th., Jahn, U., Bürlimann, W.: Fibrinolytische Antirheumatika. Vergleich von Substanzen der Flufenamsäurereihe mit Trifluormethyl-Analogen des Azapropazons. Arzneimittel-Forsch. **23**, 911—913 (1973)

Wasantapruek, S., Kaulla, K. N. von: A serial microfibrinolysis test and its use in rats with liver bypass. Thrombos. Diathes. haemorrh. (Stuttg.) **15**, 284—293 (1966)

Yoshimoto, M., Kaulla, K. N. von, Hansch, C.: Structure-activity relationship in synthetic fibrinolytics. 2-Phenethynyl-cyclopropanecarboxylates. J. med. Chem. **18**, 950—951 (1975)

Indirect Fibrinolytic Agents

P. C. DESNOYERS

Introduction

The prophylaxis and treatment of thromboembolic disorders have long involved the use of anticoagulants administered either parenterally or via the oral route. However, at the present time, there is no longer unanimity regarding the effectivenes of this medication, due to the difficulties of objective assessment of all of the parameters of thromboembolic disease.

As a new advance, thrombolytic therapy is aimed at obtaining vascular repatency, where anticoagulants can only limit extension of the obliteration. This logical but audacious approach to treatment involves the use of purified factors of human or pig plasma, fractions of human placenta containing plasminogen, urokinase—an important but very costly thrombolytic agent—or finally, streptokinase, which is unfortunately endowed with antigenic properties and whose use requires extremely close surveillance.

In spite of these risks and disadvantages of treatment on an enzyme basis, the development of activation of the endogenous fibrinolytic system appears to be extremely desirable, and in addition seems far more physiological. There exists in the circulating blood a spontaneous but slight fibrinolytic activity due to a labile factor activating circulating plasminogen. This activator, whose existence was demonstrated in 1959 by TODD, following the studies of ASTRUP (1948), is found in the vessel walls, chiefly in the veins. Continual release of this activator into the circulation forms a physiological defense against thrombosis, lysing fibrin deposits at the time of their formation. Numerous clinical studies have shown that patients suffering from arterial thrombosis (CONSTANTINI et al., 1972) or chronic arterial diseases (FEARNLEY, 1964), survivors of myocardial infarction (CHAKRABARTI et al., 1966), patients suffering from type IV hyperlipoproteinemia, from recurrent deep venous thrombosis (ISACSON and NILSSON, 1975), and from cutaneous vasculitis (CUNLIFFE, 1968) show virtually no spontaneous fibrinolytic activity.

Over the last 30 years, numerous agents capable of increasing fibrinolytic activity by various degrees have been described. We are not concerned here with the major thrombolytic agents already mentioned, which act either directly on the conversion of circulating plasminogen to plasmin or by absorption of the clot and subsequent activation of the plasminogen contained within it.

However, VON KAULLA and SMITH (1961) obtained complete lysis of plasma clots in vitro, using synthetic chemical compounds of low molecular weight. This promising discovery led to numerous discoveries and a large number of active compounds have been described. The exact mechanism of action of these compounds is not yet known (VON KAULLA, 1968; DESNOYERS et al., 1971a, 1972a, 1975a) although certain publications have indicated that some of them might act directly on the conversion of plasminogen to plasmin. A general review concerning this type of compound has been given by VON KAULLA in this volume.

We shall thus limit ourselves to a description of those agents that are capable of increasing the liberation of tissue activators of plasminogen.

Some of these agents, which are inactive in tests of thrombolysis in vitro, have been known for a considerable time and numerous publications have been devoted to them. Mention can be made of the work of MacNICOL and DOUGLAS (1964) and STAMM (1964), who in the same year reported an increase in fibrinolytic activity obtained with pyrogenic substances and derivatives of nicotinic acid. VON KAULLA (1963), FEARNLEY (1965, 1966) and KATALIN and JOZSEF (1967), in reviews concerning the pathology and physiology of fibrinolysis, described the best-known indirect fibrinolytic agents. Finally, mention should be made of the reviews of IVLEVA and ZOLOTUKHIN (1973), NILSSON (1974), FEARNLEY (1975), VERSTRAETE (1975), MARKWARDT (1976), and SAMAMA (1976).

These various reviews are concerned essentially with the clinical utilization of these agents. An attempt will be made here to consider in addition their biochemical, pharmacological and toxicological aspects.

We have deliberately abandoned any chronological classification of the discovery of these substances in order to use a more pharmacological classification. For this reason, attention will be paid first to the putative neurotransmitters, then hormones, followed by antidiabetics, anticoagulants and hypolipidemic and diuretic medications, ending with various little studied or abandoned substances such as bacterial pyrogens.

Unfortunately, in this domain, the conclusions drawn from numerous studies contradict each other. This may be due, amongst other things, to the different experimental protocols used, to the different routes of administration and doses, to the type of animal species or the pathological condition of the subjects used in the trials.

A. Neurotransmitters and Autacoids

I. Sympathomimetic Amines

1. Adrenaline

Fibrinolytic properties of adrenaline were first discovered in man and in this area the clinical discovery preceded pharmacological studies.

a) Pharmacological Aspects

SCHOR et al. (1970) showed that in rat the intraperitoneal administration of 50–1000 µg/kg of adrenaline induced a marked degree of fibrinolytic activity. The fibrinolytic response, measured by the dilute blood clot lysis time, is proportional to the dose injected up to 300 µg/kg. At higher doses the activity decreases and at 1000 µg/kg it is essentially identical with that obtained with doses of 150 µg/kg. The activity is maximal towards the 10th minute after injection and lasts for approximately 25 min, except after the dose of 300 µg/kg, when it persists until the 70th minute. The present author's group (DESNOYERS et al., 1975b) obtained a decrease of approximately 40% in the euglobulin lysis time in the rat with an intravenous injection of only 1 µg/kg. The action is maximal from the fifth minute after injection, and does not disappear until after the 30th minute. Administration of a single dose of 1 µg/kg to the rat induces a much more marked fibrinolytic activity than infusion of the same dose of adrenaline over a period of 30 min.

These results are in agreement with previous results obtained in dogs by RAHN and VON KAULLA (1965) and in rats by MOSCHOS et al. (1965).

The intravenous injection of adrenaline into healthy mongrel dogs of either sex produced an increase in the fibrinolytic activity measured by plasma euglobulin lysis time. Usually this fibrinolytic activity is at its maximum five minutes after injection and returns to the initial value within 30 min. This increase was apparently unrelated to the splenic contraction, stimulation of the lymph circulation, or increase in blood glucose, lactic acid or free fatty acids induced by adrenaline. Specific involvement of either alpha- or beta-adrenergic receptors was ruled out (HOLEMANS, 1965). In fact, fibrinolytic activity induced in the rat by adrenaline (1 mg/kg) was inhibited by pretreatment with the α-blockers—phenoxybenzamine, phentolamine and dibenamine—in very low doses of 5, 10, and 100 µg/kg/i.p., respectively. The α-blockers had no inhibitory effect at all if they were injected after the administration of adrenaline. On the other hand, very little effect was observed with the β-blockers pronethanol and practolol, even in doses as high as 10 mg/kg, although propranolol in a dose of 3 mg/kg exerted an inhibitory effect (SASAKI and TAKEYAMA, 1972). Sometimes β-blockers such as practolol, dichloroisoproterenol and pronethalol, given i.p. in rats before adrenaline administration, have a stimulating effect on adrenaline-induced fibrinolysis (SASAKI and TAKEYAMA, 1974).

Adrenaline appears also to be the mediator of the fibrinolytic activity induced by various substances, and in particular by cellulose sulfate. ROSA et al. (1972) showed that the administration of 1 mg/kg of cellulose sulfate i.v. in the rat is associated with fibrinolytic activity that is maximal one minute after the injection, disappearing after 10–20 min.

This fibrinolytic activity is inhibited by adrenalectomy. After adrenalectomy, animals showed an increase in plasma kininogen, which would result from a decrease in the "plasminogen activating mechanism."

A heparin-adrenaline complex obtained from the plasma of rats receiving an intravenous injection of 200–300 units/kg of thrombin at the same time as an injection of 0.2 ml of 0.1% adrenaline solution possesses marked lytic properties on polymerized fibrin clots not stabilized by factor XIII (KUDRYASHOV and LYAPINA, 1971). The heparin-adrenaline complex was studied in vitro and in vivo with i.v. administration in the rat and an increase in the lytic activity of blood was recorded; this was maximal 15 min after injection and disappeared after 45 min. This complex appears to bind with fibrinogen (KUDRYASHOV et al., 1975).

The influence of biogenic amines on the release of plasminogen activator was studied in the isolated perfused pig ear. Of the adrenergic agents, isoproterenol was found to be more effective than noradrenaline and adrenaline. Its effect was suppressed by the β-receptor blocking agent propranolol (MARKWARDT and KLÖCKING, 1976).

b) Clinical Aspects

Adrenaline (Biggs et al., 1947) was the first drug shown to increase the fibrinolytic activity in man. A single dose of 1 or 2 mg, given subcutaneously, produces a transient rise of fibrinolytic activity. When adrenaline is given by the intravenous route, the increase of fibrinolytic activity is achieved within a few minutes. The finding that adrenaline itself stimulated (Sherry et al., 1959) increased fibrinolysis led to the hypothesis that this agent was the common pathway by which the plasminogen activator was released (Genton et al., 1961). It was also noticed that some of the fibrinolysis-inducing drugs lead to significant changes in vessel diameter. These vasoactive changes, whether vasoconstriction or vasodilation, could be the main cause of the alterations in fibrinolysis.

In order to resolve the conflict between these two theories, the correlation between the systemic fibrinolytic and forearm blood flow responses following adrenaline administration (10 µg per 1.95 m^2 surface area per minute) in 10 healthy male volunteers was investigated (Cash et al., 1969). The authors found a significant correlation between the percentage increase in fibrinolytic activity, as assessed by the euglobulin lysis time, and the maximum percentage increase in forearm blood flow following the standard adrenaline infusion. The result suggests that the fibrinolytic response to intravenous adrenaline may be due to the release of plasminogen activator from the skeletal muscle vascular bed. Two years before (Cash and Allan, 1967), the same authors had shown that there was a significant correlation between the fibrinolytic response to adrenaline and moderate exercise in the same individual, but a considerable variation between two individuals, and they suggested the existence of "poor responders." On the other hand, in a recent work Britton et al. (1975) pointed out that the release of plasminogen activator in response to stress in man is not the direct result of changes in plasma adrenaline concentration.

In conclusion, while it is undeniable that the administration of adrenaline is associated with an increase in fibrinolytic potential both in man and in animals, this effect is only transient and would be difficult to exploit on a therapeutic basis. The question of the mechanism of action does not yet seem to be completely clear. The results obtained with α- or β-blockers on the activity of adrenaline appear to be different in man than in animals. In the rat, α-blockers inhibit the fibrinolytic activity of adrenaline, while they appear to have no action in man (Tanser and Smellie, 1964). The β-blockers have a clear influence on the fibrinolytic activity of adrenaline in the animal, while the results obtained in man are highly controversial (Cash et al., 1970).

2. Noradrenaline

Less studied than adrenaline in the domain of fibrinolysis, noradrenaline possesses the same properties. In the rat (Sasaki and Takeyama, 1974), it appears that maximal activity is obtained more rapidly than with adrenaline. The intraperitoneal administration of 0.5 mg/kg/i.p. produces a peak activity at the fifth minute after injection, whilst a similar dose of adrenaline gives the same effect only at the 10th minute. In man, the fibrinolytic activity of noradrenaline was shown by Genton et al. (1961).

3. Phenylephrine

GENTON et al. (1961) also showed in the animal and in man that the fibrinolytic activity of phenylephrine was similar to that of noradrenaline. Repeated injections of this amine do not produce tachyphylaxis (VON KAULLA, 1963). By contrast, on the basis of a study published many years ago by HENRIQUES et al. (1956) it appears that the subcutaneous administration of adrenaline, noradrenaline, and phenylephrine produces a significant increase in blood fibrinogen concentration after 24 h. The results obtained with adrenaline, noradrenaline, or phenylephrine pose the problem of an activation of the α-receptors, but the effects of α-blockers have still to be determined.

4. Dopamine

According to CHO and CHOY (1964), dopamine in the dog increases the level of activator of the fibrinolytic system. This increase is not affected by the depletion in catecholamines produced by reserpine or adrenalectomy. The common denominator of these substances that are capable of producing an increase in activation of the fibrinolytic system seems to be their ability to liberate histamine, since in most instances this action can be blocked by antihistamines. However, in the course of tests of inhibition of thrombosis induced in the marginal ear vein of the wild Burgundy rabbit (induction of platelet thrombi by irritation), BAUMGARTNER et al. (1964) injected to these animals 5 mg/kg of serotonin by the intraperitoneal route in combination with other compounds, and in particular with 4.68 mg/kg of dopamine. These authors were unable to demonstrate any protective action on the part of dopamine. This result could be explained by the well-known platelet-aggregating action of dopamine, which increases the effects of ADP and abolishes the inhibitory effect of adenosine and of ATP on platelet aggregation (ARDLIE et al., 1966).

The increase in fibrinolytic activity induced by dopamine does not seem to be sufficient to outweigh its platelet-aggregation effect in the prevention of experimental thrombosis in the rabbit. The possible participation of a specific dopaminergic receptor has not yet been studied.

5. α- and β-Adrenoceptor Stimulating and Blocking Agents

a) Clinical Aspects

The intravenous administration of adrenaline, noradrenaline and isoprenaline in man suggests that the liberation of plasminogen activator caused by these drugs is mediated via the β-adrenoceptors, and that these receptors could even be classified in the β_2 sub-group (CASH, 1975). YAMAZAKI et al. (1971) showed that the "post-adrenaline plasminogen activator response" in man was abolished by β-adrenergic blockers, such as propranolol or alprenolol, whereas INGRAM and VAUGHAN-JONES (1969) had found contradictory results.

Exercise stress is known to stimulate blood coagulation and fibrinolysis, possibly as a result of sympatho-adrenal stimulation of the β-adrenergic receptor. In order to test this hypothesis five men exercised on four separate occasions with and without previous β-adrenergic blockade with oxprenolol, propranolol and pindolol (BRITTON et al., 1976). The increase in plasma adrenaline and noradrenaline concentration was much greater during exercise under β-blockade but activation of fibrinolysis was also enhanced. These results suggest that the activation of fibrinolysis by exercise is not mediated by the β-adrenergic receptor, which has also been demonstrated by PONARI et al. (1973).

b) Pharmacological Aspects

The present authors sought to determine in the rat (DESNOYERS et al., 1975b) the influence of sympathomimetic agents (catecholamines, α- and β-stimulants) and of "adrenoceptor blocking agents" on fibrinolytic activity measured by plasma euglobulin lysis time according to the method of WASANTAPRUEK and VON KAULLA (1966).

The α-stimulants methoxamine, 50 and 200 μg/kg/i.v., naphazoline 10 μg/kg, and clonidine 50 μg/kg, significantly decrease euglobulin lysis time. The fibrinolytic effect of naphazoline is short-lived while that of clonidine has a certain lag time.

The β-stimulants, isoprenaline and salbutamol may also induce fibrinolytic activity. The acute i.v. administration of high doses of isoprenaline (500 μg/kg) is associated with only a moderate decrease in euglobulin lysis time. By contrast, the infusion of 1 μg/kg/min for 30 min results in a 30–40% decrease in euglobulin lysis time. This was also found with salbutamol. Infusion over 30 min of 50 μg/kg of this agent appears to be much more effective than a single injection of the same dose.

Amongst the β-adrenergic blockers propranolol, practolol, alprenolol, pindolol, and KÖ 1366, only the last two are capable of producing a marked decrease in euglobulin lysis time. It seems reasonable to suppose that the effect observed is due to the β-stimulant action of pindolol and of KÖ 1366. Phentolamine, another α-adrenergic blocker, induces only moderate fibrinolytic activity.

The administration of propranolol or of pindolol decreases, but does not completely eliminate, fibrinolytic effects of the infusion of isoprenaline, while practolol is ineffective. Furthermore, phentolamine does not abolish the effects of methoxamine. The authors therefore suggest that α- and β-adrenergic receptors are involved in the increase of fibrinolytic potential, but the receptors seem to be somewhat different from the classic ones.

II. Cholinomimetics and Cholinolytics

The sympathomimetic agents studied in the preceding chapter appear to induce an acceleration in clotting and an increase in fibrinolytic potential simultaneously, by the liberation of cellular thromboplastic factors and, secondly, by the liberation of plasminogen activators from the endothelial cells of the vascular walls. However, at present there is no precise knowledge of the mechanism by which plasminogen activators are released from these endothelial cells. In a recent article, BRITTON et al. (1975) note that other substances, in particular acetylcholine and kinins, that are capable of activating fibrinolysis, may be liberated by various stimuli, for instance stress.

1. Acetylcholine

SHERRY et al. (1959) have reported that intravenous injection of large amounts of acetylcholine to dogs is followed by a significant rise in fibrinolytic activity of the euglobulin fraction.

As early as 1948, SOULIER and KOUPERNIK had already noted a marked but short-lived increase in lytic activity in man after administration of subtoxic doses of acetylcholine. Later, KWAAN et al. (1958) demonstrated that intravenous or paravenous injection of acetylcholine, like the injection of serotonin, was associated with fibrinolytic activity.

In studies of local fibrinolysis, TESI (1975) used injections of acetylcholine to induce a regional stimulation of fibrinolysis. Both in patients suffering from arterial disease of the lower limbs and in healthy subjects, injection into the femoral artery of 30 mg of acetylcholine was associated with marked lytic activity in femoral venous blood five minutes after this endoarterial injection. The infusion of very high doses of acetylcholine (1 g in 1 h) led to a marked degree of lytic activity. If the infusion was repeated after one hour, no lytic activity was detectable, but if an interval of six hours was allowed before repetition of the infusion, the results were identical to those obtained with the first injection.

2. Atropine

The competitive antagonist of acetylcholine, atropine, seems to be a powerful inducer of lysis. With intravenous injections of massive doses of atropine (10 mg/kg) in dog, RAHN and VON KAULLA (1964, 1965) were able to demonstrate a reduction of 73% in euglobulin lysis time. This marked but transient activation of the fibrinolytic system did not lead to tachyphylactic phenomena with repeated injections. With experimental pulmonary emboli in the rat, DAVID and KENEDI (1971) showed that the administration of atropine permitted survival of the animals during the acute phase of vascular obstruction. The protection endowed by atropine is present even after treatment of the animals with propranolol.

However, atropine seems to possess a procoagulant action (BELIKINA, 1973), and blocks the hypocoagulant action of lipocaïc factor in the rabbit, although SCHIMPF et al. (1958) had found that in healthy human subjects at rest, in contrast to reserpine and dihydroergotoxin, atropine was associated with a decrease in the overall coagulation of peripheral blood.

3. Nicotine

In 1930, HARTMANN and WEISS observed that nicotine, like atropine, possesses an inhibitory action on blood coagulation, this being confirmed by in vitro studies carried out by TUDORANU et al. (1950). By contrast, ZUNZ (1935), followed by WENZEL and SINGH (1962) and SINGH and OESTER (1964a), using human or rabbit plasma or whole blood, observed that the addition of nicotine in vitro or its intravenous administration was followed by a decrease in overall clotting time and in prothrombin time, this effect being partially antagonized by piperoxan. The fibrinolytic activity of nicotine has not yet been studied, either in the animal or in clinical practice. However, given that the administration of this substance may result in the liberation of adrenaline, this being responsible for its procoagulant action in the opinion of SINGH and OESTER (1964b), it seems logical to consider that it may indirectly induce an increase in lytic potential (YOSHIZAKI, 1975).

III. Biogenic Amines

1. Serotonin

In addition to its vasoconstrictor action, serotonin could play a role in the process of blood coagulation (MILNE et al., 1957). In association with intravascular thrombosis, a marked increase in circulating serotonin levels was observed (SULLENBERGER et al., 1959).

In coagulolytic systems in vitro consisting of fibrinogen, plasminogen, buffer and plasmin or urokinase, TSITOURIS et al. (1962) and CORREL and SJOERDSMA (1962) noted that the addition of serotonin to these media inhibited the fibrinolysis generated by plasmin or urokinase, although to a lesser degree than ε-aminocaproic acid. These results were confirmed by HARADA and TAKEUCHI (1964), who showed that serotonin decreased the lytic activity of streptokinase in human, rabbit, and cat plasma. However, when the fibrinolytic activity was determined by thrombelastography, no modification of this activity was observed after the addition of serotonin (BELLI, 1963).

While serotonin behaves in vitro on plasma or artificial coagulolytic systems as an inhibitor of lysis, its action in vivo would be entirely the reverse.

a) Pharmacological Aspects

Although KOKOT (1962) failed to observe any alterations in fibrinolytic activity measured by euglobulin lysis in pigeons fed for seven months with an atherogenic diet under the influence of 0.2 mg/kg/day serotonin administered intramuscularly, numerous authors have demonstrated in experimental animals an activation of lytic processes. BAUMGARTNER et al. (1963) studied the formation of thrombi produced by the lesion of the intima of the marginal ear vein of the rabbit after treatment with serotonin alone or in combination with nialamide, with nialamide alone, or with a serotonin antagonist. The number of thrombi is markedly decreased by serotonin, and totally inhibited by the association of nialamide with serotonin. In contrast, it is markedly increased by serotonin antagonists.

NITYANAND and ZAIDI (1964) produced pulmonary emboli in rabbits by repeated injections of homologous fibrin, adrenaline, or serotonin. At the same time, they observed an increased plasma fibrinolytic activity one hour after administration of the emboligenic agent, this activity returning to normal after the 24th hour. According to these authors, it is the vascular spasm produced by these agents that plays the most important role in the production of these pulmonary lesions, despite the increase in fibrinolytic activity.

Artificial fibrin clots implanted into rats and rabbits were digested by the granulocytes and histiocytes and replaced by connective tissue (HEY et al., 1970). Serotonin stimulates the granulocytic reaction and the generation of fibroblasts, reflecting increased fibrinolytic activity while ε-aminocaproic acid inhibits fibrinolysis, decreasing the number of granulocytes and histiocytes.

The time course of activity generated by three levels of serotonin was determined. Maximum activity occurred at about 45 min after injection of the compound, at two hours some activity was still demonstrable, but at 2.5 h the activity had returned to normal (SCHOR et al., 1970).

The fibrinolytic dose-response curve determined 45 min after intraperitoneal injection of serotonin to rats is linear, and the percentage of clots of diluted blood that undergo lysis varies from approximately 40 for a dose of 0.5 mg/kg to 100 for the dose of 5 mg/kg.

SCHOR et al. (1970) demonstrated that serotonin was also capable of decreasing euglobulin lysis time in the dog, which led them to use the compound as a standard fibrinolytic in studies carried out on synthetic fibrinolytic agents.

b) Clinical Aspects

The intravenous or paravenous administration of serotonin is associated with a fibrinolytic reaction (KWAAN et al., 1958; THOMSON et al., 1964).

The liberation of serotonin by blood platelets results in pulmonary vasoconstriction, which is partially involved in the problems of consumption coagulopathy seen in acute cor pulmonale at the same time as an increase in circulating lytic activity (SCHNEIDER et al., 1960). However, in a study involving 41 cases of venous thrombosis, BOBEK et al. (1961) found blood levels of serotonin that were markedly lower (0.052 µg/ml) than those in a control group (0.125 µg/ml). These levels returned to normal only three to five weeks after the acute phase of thrombosis. The fall in blood serotonin levels could be considered as a reflection of its consumption by fibrinolytic reaction. By contrast, KOKOT (1961) did not find any action of serotonin on euglobulin lysis time or on the clearing factor in man.

2. Histamine

In the various forms of shock or following the injection of endotoxin, the liberation of histamine from the mast cells is largely responsible for the liberation of plasminogen activator and the increase in fibrinolytic potential (HOLEMANS and LANGDELL, 1964; SHERRY, 1961; VON KAULLA, 1958). Fibrinolytic activity may also be increased by administration of substances capable of inducing the liberation of histamine, e.g. compound 48/80, morphine, and tubocurarine (CHO and CHOY, 1964; PATON, 1957). These facts reveal the decisive role played by the liberation of endogenous histamine in the increase in fibrinolytic potential induced via this pathway (RÜEGG, 1975).

a) Biochemical Aspects

The action of histamine on blood coagulation was first demonstrated many years ago. In related studies (1948), CSEFKÓ et al. and GERENDÁS et al. demonstrated that histamine in low concentrations (less than 10 µg/ml of oxalated and recalcified plasma) has no action on coagulation. By contrast, with higher concentrations there is an acceleration of the clotting process, maximum activity being reached with concentrations of 66 µg/ml. Histamine acts by inhibiting the thrombin inactivator system, and in an artificial system containing only purified fibrinogen and thrombin it has no action. With the administration of histamine in the rabbit, the same authors were able to demonstrate an antiheparin action and postulated that coagulolytic balance was controlled by equilibrium between histamine and heparin. Although attractive, this hypothesis would appear to be somewhat oversimplified, the more so since in 1953 Shulman showed that histamine at molar concentrations of between 0.14 and 0.20 and at an ionic strength of 0.51–0.53, behaved as a typical inhibitor of the coagulation of fibrinogen by thrombin.

The in vitro fibrinolytic activity of histamine on human fibrinogen-plasminogen systems activated by urokinase was studied by Correll and Sjoerdsma (1962). They demonstrated, as for serotonin, an inhibitory effect on the lysis induced by urokinase. The same inhibitory action was found by Harada and Takeuchi (1964) on the lysis produced by streptokinase in clots of human plasma or cat or rabbit plasma. The results obtained in this area with histamine are identical with those obtained with serotonin.

b) Pharmacological Aspects

The procoagulant activity of histamine observed in vitro has been confirmed in vivo (Löfgren, 1956; Park and Lee, 1960). This procoagulant activity is manifested in a shortening of overall clotting time and prothrombin time, and appears to be notably greater than that obtained with adrenaline. The administration of histamine in the rabbit is also associated with an increase in thoracic lymph flow. Finally, Mischenko et al. (1972) and Kuznik et al. (1972), working with dogs, were able to demonstrate an increase in clotting, involving a decrease in recalcification time and an increase in plasma heparin tolerance. This action is the result of the liberation of thromboplastin factors and of antiheparin substances from the endothelium of the veins.

Postnov et al. (1964) had found a marked decrease in blood heparin levels following the daily administration of 20 µg/kg of histamine subcutaneously in the rat. These authors had also observed an increase in circulating fibrinogen levels, confirmed by Lazar et al. (1972), and also a concomitant increase in fibrinolytic activity and an increase in the liberation of plasminogen activator, which could result from dystrophy of the cells of the vascular walls. An increase in fibrinolytic potential had already been described by Holemans and Langdell (1964) in the dog, following the intravenous administration of 50–200 µg/kg of histamine. These authors failed to observe any alteration in antiplasmin levels, but did record an increase in glutamo-oxalacetic transaminases, which appeared later than the increase in fibrinolytic activity. However, Holemans (1965), still working with dogs, concluded that repeated injections of this powerful inducer of fibrinolysis could lead to tachyphylactic phenomena.

The results obtained by the group of Holemans were confirmed a few years later by Izhizu and Nobuhara (1970). The only discordant note found in this area involves the studies of Bielski and Owczarek (1970), who observed no action of histamine when administered to the rabbit in a dose of 100 µg/kg subcutaneously, as far as coagulation parameters were concerned. It is possible that with subcutaneous administration the dose of histamine used by these authors would be too low to have any activity upon these parameters.

Studies in the isolated perfused pig ear revealed that histamine causes a release of plasminogen activators. This effect is suppressed by antihistaminic agents (Markwardt and Klöcking, 1976).

c) Clinical Aspects

Although WEINLAND and WEINLAND (1949), using the subcutaneous administration of histamine in man, failed to confirm the decrease in clotting time seen in vitro and in animal experiments, JÜRGENS (1948), followed by WAGNER (1952), BUTLER (1955), and finally STÜTTGEN (1957), observed a procoagulant effect after intravenous, subcutaneous or intramuscular administration of histamine. This effect is demonstrated by an increase in prothrombin time and a decrease in levels of antithrombins and factor V (HENGSTMANN et al., 1960). This procoagulant effect is concomitant with a marked fibrinolytic action, though of short duration (TOYODA and SHIOKAWA, 1950; CASERTANO and PICCININI, 1959; ORLIKOV, 1969).

However, the last-named author found the action of histamine on coagulation to be variable according to the individual patient, and in contrast to most workers he noted an increase in blood heparin levels. Finally, in contrast to serotonin, blood histamine levels are much higher after venous thrombosis than in a control group of healthy individuals (BOBEK et al., 1961).

IV. Biogenic Peptides

1. Hypotensive Polypeptides

The most closely studied of the hypotensive polypeptides is a nonapeptide, bradykinin, which has pharmacological properties fairly close to those of histamine. In vitro, when added to blood in concentrations of 0.1–20 µg/ml, it has no influence on the coagulation process, apart from a slight reduction in recalcification time. Furthermore, it has no action in vitro on fibrinolysis measured by means of euglobulin lysis time or on thrombelastography.

By contrast, in vivo, when administered via the intra-arterial route in patients taking part in venous stasis studies involving use of the "sphygmomanometer cuff technique," bradykinin had no action on coagulation apart from that due to venous stasis, but it activated the fibrinolytic system in 82% of cases. This activation is associated with a slight decrease in plasminogen proactivator and activator levels (NERI et al., 1965).

Bradykinin was found to cause a dose-dependent release of plasminogen activator in the isolated perfused pig ear (MARKWARDT and KLÖCKING, 1976).

2. Hypertensive Polypeptides

Hydrolysis of angiotensinogen, a plasma α_2-globulin, by renin gives a decapeptide, hypertensin I, which is inactive and which is subsequently hydrolyzed in the blood to form an octapeptide, angiotensin II.

While these hypertensive polypeptides have long been the subjects of study with regard to their vascular actions, no consideration seems to have been given to their action on fibrinolytic potential. It is merely known on the basis of the studies of RODIONOV et al. (1971) and RODIONOV (1974) that renin in doses of 0.1–2.0 Goldblatt units and angiotensin II in doses of 0.3–3 µg administered intravenously in dog and rabbit produce an acceleration of blood clotting, an increase in platelet aggregation activity, the liberation of platelet factor 3, and the liberation of platelet serotonin.

B. Hormones

I. Pituitary Hormones

1. Anterior Pituitary Hormones

The injection of pituitary corticotropin (ACTH) results in adrenal hypertrophy and in the secretion of corticosteroids: cortisone, hydrocortisone, and aldosterone.

FEARNLEY and BUNIM (1951) showed that in healthy volunteers a single intramuscular injection of 25–40 mg of ACTH was associated with a fall of plasma fibrinogen. The common occurrence of a slight degree of fibrinolytic activity having been noted in patients suffering from rheumatoid arthritis, and the fact that corticosteroid treatment of patients with rheumatic fever also provoked a decrease in plasma fibrinogen (FEARNLEY, 1951) led the same team (CHAKRABARTI et al., 1964; FEARNLEY, 1965) to treat patients with ACTH in the form of an injectable gel twice daily (60 units/day for 20 days, and 40 units during the subsequent 20 days). These workers observed a marked increase in fibrinolytic activity in all subjects.

Furthermore, given that the secretion of ACTH is increased by stress and adrenaline, it seems reasonable to ask to what extent the fibrinolytic activity induced by adrenaline is in part mediated via ACTH.

2. Posterior Pituitary Hormones

The catecholamines, and in particular adrenaline, increase the level of cyclic AMP in numerous tissues by activating adenylcyclase (ROBINSON et al., 1971). It has been shown by CHASE and AURBACH (1968) and by BECK et al. (1971) that the antidiuretic hormone (ADH) vasopressin also increased the activity of adenylcyclase and the concentration of cyclic AMP. Like adrenaline, ADH is a powerful activator of the fibrinolytic system in man. The first studies published by VON KAULLA (1963) in fact showed that the injection of one unit of vasopressin to each of 17 individuals led to a decrease in euglobulin lysis time by approximately 50%. This action was seen during the first five minutes after injection and lasted for approximately 30 min. Recent studies of MANNUCCI (1975) have demonstrated a marked fibrinolytic activity for ADH, but have also eliminated the hypothesis that cyclic AMP is involved in the physiological regulation of the fibrinolytic system. According to CASH (1975a and b), the fibrinolytic response to ADH is due not to a direct action on the endothelial peripheral receptors, but could depend upon a second humoral factor.

The intravenous administration of ADH is accompanied by undesirable side-effects including pallor, stomach cramps, etc. Research into derivatives with the same action on the liberation of plasminogen activator has been undertaken and has resulted on the one hand in lysine-vasopressin, which has virtually the same side-effects, and secondly in 1-deamino-8-D-arginine-vasopressin (DDAVP), which is free of the unpleasant symptoms associated with its precursors, and in addition is virtually free of the hypertensive actions of this posterior pituitary hormone. Its action is also more prolonged than that of ADH or of lysine-vasopressin (GADER et al., 1973). Similar findings have been confirmed by MANNUCCI (1975) in two anuric patients.

II. Steroid Hormones

1. Nonanabolic Steroids

The fibrinolytic activity of nonanabolic adrenocortical hormones appears to be highly controversial. In a study carried out in rabbit, GRISHIN (1972) showed that a glucocorticoid, dexamethasone, decreased fibrinolytic potential at doses of 1 and 2 mg/kg. Overall coagulability, measured by the amplitude of thrombodynamographic records, estimation of factors II, V, VII and XIII, and resistance to heparin, were increased. By contrast, the administration of 0.125 and 0.25 mg/kg of a mineralocorticoid, aldosterone, decreased coagulation, decreased fibrinogen levels, and increased fibrinolytic activity, in particular when given in subchronic administration, the effect being most marked between days 5 and 10.

However, in a study already mentioned with regard to ACTH, CHAKRABARTI et al. (1964) were able to show that a synthetic glucocorticoid, prednisone, administered *per os* was associated with a marked increase in fibrinolytic potential. Decrease in the lysis time of clots of diluted blood appeared to be less rapid with prednisone than with ACTH, and the type of response also appeared to be different. In these patients, the active dose appears to be 30 mg/day, since reduction of the dose to 20 mg/day is associated with "a swinging escape" of lysis time for a number of days. These results are in disagreement with a more recent study of ISACSON (1971), who noted that the administration of prednisolone to normal subjects was associated with a decrease in fibrinolytic activity. Finally, according to SAMAMA (1976), the effect of cortisone is very slight or virtually nil.

2. Anabolic Steroids

a) Male Sexual Hormones

Steroids with a cyclopentano-perhydrophenanthrenic nucleus (testosterone derivatives) may have androgenic, anti-estrogenic or anabolic properties.

α) Pharmacological Aspects

In this area, while numerous clinical studies have been undertaken, animal experiments remain rare (KUMADA and ABIKO, 1976; ABIKO and KUMADA, 1976). The fibrinolytic activity of an anabolic steroid with very slight androgenic properties, furazabol, was determined in rats (OHTA et al., 1965). This substance was administered for 12 weeks to male rats aged eight weeks at doses varying from 0.04 mg/kg to 0.9 mg/kg. The coagulolytic system of the animals was studied by determination of euglobulin lysis time, fibrinogen levels, and plasma recalcification time. After sacrifice, tissue plasminogen activator was determined in the thoracic and abdominal aorta, the inferior *vena cava*, and the femoral artery and vein after ultrasonication. The capacity for release of this activator was estimated by the technique of venous occlusion used in man by NILSSON and ROBERTSON (1968). The authors also determined plasma plasminogen, antiplasmin, cholesterol, serum albumin, and plasma GOT levels.

The treatment of animals with furazabol is associated with a decrease in euglobulin lysis time that is proportional to the dose ingested and is seen above all from the sixth week of treatment onwards. After the end of treatment, the fibrinolytic index returns to its initial values. Activity of the activator also shows a highly significant correlation with fibrinolytic index, and plasminogen and antiplasmin levels showing no variation during treatment. The authors also observed a marked increase in the content of tissue plasminogen activator in the lungs, also in correlation with the increase in blood activator activity and fibrinolytic index. Administration of furazabol is associated with a slight increase in recalcification time and a decrease in cholesterol levels, while plasma transaminases are unaffected.

The antithrombotic effect at week 12 of treatment, by contrast, was seen only in the group of rats receiving the lowest dose of furazabol. It seems curious despite increased blood fibrinolytic activity, the occurrence rate of experimental pulmonary thromboses did not seem to be altered.

β) Clinical Aspects

A large number of anabolic steroids have been studied in clinical trials since Fearnley and Chakrabarti (1962) observed that the administration of testosterone propionate was associated with an increase in blood fibrinolytic activity. The principal compounds studied have been testosterone, ethylestrenol and stanozolol.

Testosterone: In their study involving testosterone, Fearnley and Chakrabarti also demonstrated that in a case of obliterative vascular disease with mild diabetes, the increase in fibrinolytic activity was parallel with a decrease in fasting blood sugar. The authors proposed the hypothesis that atherosclerosis, carbohydrate metabolism, and fibrinolysis were somehow linked, and found that another anabolic steroid, nandrolone, had a fibrinolytic activity similar to that of testosterone but without its undesirable side-effects.

These results were confirmed by Winther (1965a and b), who treated patients with 250 mg of testosterone propionate by intramuscular injection three times weekly for four weeks.

However, the results were not confirmed by other authors (Heutzer and Cort-Madsen, 1966; Dohn et al., 1968; Genster and Oram, 1971).

It is possible that these failures were due to the use of too-low doses of testosterone or too-infrequent administration. The combination of testosterone with ethinylestradiol and with kallikrein also apparently failed to give satisfactory results (Albrechtsen et al., 1972).

Ethylestrenol: More recently, Allenby et al. (1973) treated female patients aged over 40 years with ethylestrenol, administered in a dose of 8 mg/day for three weeks before a surgical procedure, in a double-blind study. They observed a marked reduction in euglobulin lysis time during the preoperative period. However, after the operation, the authors noted no difference between the two groups in the occurrence of venous thromboses. These observations are in agreement with those of Fearnley (1973), who noted the disappearance of the fibrinolytic effect of ethylestrenol after continuous administration for three to four weeks, despite an increase in dose. Nevertheless it is possible that the duration of preoperative treatment had been too long and had thereby exhausted fibrinolytic capacity at the time of development of postoperative thromboses. At all events, the question as to whether an increase in fibrinolytic potential in an individual can prevent the appearance of postoperative venous thromboses remains open.

In patients with recurrent idiopathic venous thromboses with low fibrinolytic activity of the venous walls, HEDNER et al. (1975) were able to demonstrate a marked decrease in the frequency of thrombotic episodes when the patients were treated with ethylestrenol. The results obtained are in disagreement with those of ALLENBY and of FEARNLEY, inasmuch as the increase in fibrinolytic activity developed after three months and remained constant throughout the period of treatment. It involved both spontaneous fibrinolytic potential and local fibrinolytic activity measured by the venous occlusion test, and the fibrinolytic activity of the vessel walls (HEDNER et al., 1976). Identical results were obtained by WALKER et al. (1975a) in 20 patients who had survived myocardial infarction but were treated, for four weeks only, alternatively with placebo and various anabolic steroids including ethylestrenol, norethandrolone, methylandrostenediol, oxymetholone, and methandienone. These results would support the hypothesis mentioned above concerning the exhaustion of fibrinolysis capacity by excessively prolonged treatment. By contrast, methenolone acetate, unique amongst the steroids studied in having methyl group at position 17α, proved to be inactive. Furthermore, this last-named steroid was not associated with a marked increase in plasma antithrombin III levels during the course of treatment; this was also true of methandienone (WALKER et al., 1975b).

Stanozolol: With a chemical structure differing only slightly from that of ethylestrenol, stanozolol seems to possess more promising fibrinolytic properties. During a double-blind study, DAVIDSON et al. (1972b) demonstrated, in 34 patients suffering from ischemic heart disease, an increase in fibrinolytic activity, measured by plasma euglobulin lysis time.

Stanozolol, unlike another anabolic steroid, ethylestrenol, does not require phenformin to achieve this sustained effect (DAVIDSON et al., 1972a).

The administration of 10 mg/day of stanozolol for 12 months also leads to an increase in plasma plasminogen and to a slight decrease in fibrinogen level, which returns to its basal value at the third month of treatment. The correction by stanozolol of the hypofibrinolysis observed in ischemic heart disease would justify a more thorough study of the activity of this compound in a more extensive controlled trial. In a patient suffering from recurrent deep venous thromboses, SAMAMA (1976) observed that after venous occlusion, fibrinolytic activity that was very slight before treatment was normalized by the administration of stanozolol.

WALKER and DAVIDSON, continuing a study of DAVIDSON et al. (1975) involving the treatment of patients with ischemic heart disease with stanozolol, reported the results of a five-year study of nine subjects (1978). All had suffered a myocardial infarction more than one year previously, and anticoagulant therapy had been stopped for at least six weeks. The patients received 10 mg/day of stanozolol for the first 12 months of the trial, then 5 mg/day for the following 18 months. Treatment was stopped for three months, then restarted and continued for an average of 15 months with various anabolic steroids and finally for the last 12 months with 5 mg/day of stanozolol. Determination of the fibrinolytic activity of each patient was carried out each month by determination of euglobulin lysis time.

Treatment with stanozolol at a dose of 10 mg/day resulted in a marked increase in fibrinolytic activity, without side-effects or tachyphylaxis. By daily administration of 5 mg of stanozolol during the subsequent 15 months the patients were kept within the zone of normality, while the interruption of treatment again put them into a state of hypofibrinolysis. Restarting treatment once again restored them to the zone of normality.

Jarrett et al. (1978a) performed studies in patients suffering from venous lipo-sclerosis of the legs and treated them for three months with 10 mg of stanozolol in two daily doses. These subjects were also seen every month and compared with a group of 48 controls. At the end of treatment, the authors noted a decrease in fibrinogen level, an increase in fibrinolytic potential, a subjective clinical improvement, and healing of a leg ulcer.

In a second study, Jarrett et al. (1978b) used stanozolol in the treatment of patients who had suffered from 4 to 20 episodes of thrombophlebitis over an average of 7.7 years. There was no associated arterial disease. Laboratory studies revealed that before treatment, they all had a significantly increased fibrinogen level and a decrease in fibrinolytic activity (determined by means of Fearnley's test and biopsies of the dorsal veins of the hand). After six months of treatment, the authors observed an increase in fibrinolytic activity, a decrease in fibrinogen levels and a reduction in the number of episodes of phlebitis.

The same authors also used 10 mg of stanozolol divided in two daily doses for three months to treat patients with Raynaud's disease and others with scleroderma. Before treatment, these patients showed a significantly elevated fibrinogen level and a decrease in fibrinolytic activity. At the end of treatment, there was an improvement in circulatory flow, a decrease in fibrinogen levels, and an increase in fibrinolytic activity.

During these various clinical trials with stanozolol, a number of side-effects were observed, in particular water retention requiring diuretic therapy, amenorrhea, digestive complications (constipation or diarrhea) and a few virilizing effects.

In addition, liver function must be monitored, since cases of cholestatic-type jaundice have been described during stanozolol treatment.

b) Female Sexual Hormones

Natural female sexual hormones, in particular 17 β-estradiol, which also possesses anabolic properties, administered for 10 days to 16 women in a dose of 10 mg/day seemed to have no influence on tissue fibrinolytic activity in the superficial veins (Åstedt and Jeppsson, 1974). The synthetic estrogen, ethinylestradiol administered in a dose of 250 μg/day was associated with a marked decrease in the fibrinolytic activity of the venous wall.

III. Thyroid Hormones

In a clinical trial, arteriosclerotic subjects with a reduction in fibrinolytic activity associated with an increase in platelet adhesion and aggregation received 2 mg of D-thyroxine (Cajozzo et al., 1974). Fibrinolytic potential and platelet adhesion and aggregation were measured before and 30 and 60 days after the beginning of treatment.

During D-Thyroxine treatment, fibrinolysis is activated and there is a tendency for platelet aggregation and adhesion to decline, particularly in patients showing definite regression towards normolipemia. The frequent appearance or exacerbation of anginal symptoms or arrhythmias during prolonged treatment is a drawback that must be borne in mind, however. D-Thyroxine may inhibit primary aggregation by acting on the aggregation cofactors or directly on the platelets, or it may inhibit the second phase of aggregation by selectively inhibiting the release of platelet factors.

IV. Insulin

1. Clinical Aspects

In preliminary studies involving the possible fibrinolytic activity of common pharmacological substances, FEARNLEY et al. (1959) showed that insulin reduced this activity. Using the subcutaneous administration of 20 units of soluble insulin in four diabetic patients, the authors demonstrated an initial reduction in fibrinolytic activity, followed, three or four hours after the injection, by an increase, which coincided with the maximum fall in blood sugar levels. This increase in fibrinolytic activity could be due to the liberation of adrenaline induced by hypoglycemia. It does not seem that the hypoglycemia caused by insulin could in itself explain such an increase. As a matter of fact, TSAPOGAS et al. (1962) and TANSER (1966) showed that the fibrinolytic activity was increased after oral administration of glucose in patients suffering from intermittent claudication or in patients in whom fibrinolytic activity was depressed.

2. Pharmacological Aspects

In the rat rendered hyperglycemic by alloxan, LASSMAN et al. (1974) found an increase in fibrinolytic potential. LASSMAN and BACK (1974a and b) subsequently studied alterations in the fibrinolytic system of the rat after induction of a hypoglycemic state. This was achieved by subcutaneous administration of 5 units/kg of insulin and determinations of fibrinolytic potential measured by euglobulin lysis time were carried out four hours, 8 and 24 h after injection. The results obtained show a very marked decrease in fibrinolytic potential at the fourth and eighth hours, the return to normal being seen only after 24 h. The rebound phenomenon with increased lytic potential seen in man by FEARNLEY (1970) was not observed in the rat. In the rat, the administration of insulin is not associated with any alteration in plasminogen or with fast or slow antiplasmin levels.

V. Antidiabetic Drugs

Apart from insulin, the hypoglycemic hormone whose activity has been studied above, two major groups of drugs may be used in the treatment of hyperglycemia: sulfonylureas and biguanides.

1. Sulfonylureas

The increase in fibrinolytic activity seen in diabetics with a lowered blood glucose level following the administration of insulin might have indicated that compounds such as sulfonylureas, tolbutamide or chlorpropamide were capable of increasing fibrinolytic activity in nondiabetic individuals by lowering their blood sugar. In the light of this possibility, FEARNLEY et al. (1960) administered to eight arteriosclerotic patients a dose of 0.5–1.5 g per day of tolbutamide or 250 mg of chlorpropamide. Daily determination of dilute blood clot lysis time and of blood sugar was carried out several days before and during the period of treatment, the treatment being continued for several weeks.

Seven of these patients showed a marked increase in fibrinolytic activity, without any significant fall in blood glucose, leading the authors to conclude that the increase in lytic potential induced by sulfonylureas was not due to their hypoglycemic activity. By contrast, after approximately one month of treatment, the effect of these drugs fell away and the patients became resistant despite an increase in dose.

The fibrinolytic activity of these so-called first generation sulfonylureas was confirmed by TSAPOGAS et al. (1962), using oral administration and by VERSTRAETE et al. (1963), who used the intravenous route for administration. While it is obvious that these sulfonylureas are not satisfactory drugs for the purpose of obtaining a long-lasting increase in fibrinolytic activity in patients with arterial disease (FEARNLEY, 1970b), it is nevertheless true that with oral administration they were the first substances discovered to be capable of increasing fibrinolytic potential over a period of a number of weeks. Within the context of hemobiological studies carried out on second-generation sulfonylureas, DESNOYERS et al. (1970, 1972b) were able to show that a new substance, gliclazide, administered in hypoglycemic doses in the rat and rabbit, possessed both an anti-platelet adhesive action and a fibrinolytic action simultaneously.

This fibrinolytic activity was demonstrated objectively in the circulating blood by a decrease in euglobulin lysis time and by a decrease in fibrin monomer levels. It was also demonstrated in the vessel wall (DESNOYERS et al., 1971b) with the aid of a histochemical technique derived from that of TODD (1959).

An increase in the liberation of plasminogen activator was demonstrated in the inferior *vena cava* of the rat, but also in the eye and the renal glomerulus (DESNOYERS et al., 1973). Other sulfonylureas used in this test proved to be inactive or had only a nonsignificant action. This finding would appear to be extremely important with relation to the angiopathic complications of diabetes, which most frequently involve the eye and the kidney. Long-term double-blind clinical studies are currently under way in order to confirm in man the action of gliclazide on the course of diabetic retinopathy.

2. Biguanides

The results obtained by FEARNLEY et al. (1960) with sulfonylureas naturally led the same author to seek any possible fibrinolytic activity of the biguanides, in particular since he felt that there was a connection between fibrinolysis and carbohydrate metabolism (FEARNLEY, 1970a and b).

a) Phenformin

The first biguanide tested was phenformin. It was administered in a dose of 75–150 mg per day for three months in 16 patients with ischemic disease (FEARNLEY and CHAKRABARTI, 1964). Of these patients, 14 showed a marked decrease in lysis time. An identical result was found by the same authors (FEARNLEY et al., 1965) in patients suffering from rheumatoid arthritis. The increase in fibrinolytic activity appeared in general between days 7 and 28 of treatment. However, beyond the third month of treatment, a tachyphylaxis phenomenon developed. An increase in dose was not possible, firstly because of the poor gastrointestinal tolerance of the drug, and secondly because of the risks of lactic acidosis (ASSAN et al., 1975).

However, in diabetics treated for three months with a daily dose of 115 mg phenformin no intolerance phenomena were observed (FIASCHI et al., 1969). Of these diabetic patients 62% showed a decrease of approximately 50% in euglobulin lysis time. This effect was all the more marked when the initial fibrinolytic potential was lower. In diabetics who had a normal euglobulin lysis time before treatment, phenformin was not associated with any change in fibrinolytic potential.

The fibrinolytic potential of phenformin in the animal was later studied by BACK et al. (1968). In the normal animal (dog, cat, and monkey), the administration of phenformin in a maximal tolerated dose was not associated with any fibrinolytic effect. By contrast, in the dog in which the fibrinolytic system had been previously depressed by insulin, the administration of phenformin was associated with a decrease in euglobulin lysis time. This effect was found again by LASSMAN and BACK (1974a) in the rat receiving 20 mg/kg of phenformin subcutaneously, four hours and 20 hours after the injection of 5 U/kg of insulin subcutaneously. The increase in fibrinolytic potential appears to be due to the activation of plasminogen by an activator that has not yet been identified and appears to be associated with a reduction in the acid-labile inhibitors of plasmin and an increase in fast and slow antiplasmin levels. By contrast, in the normal rat, the acute administration of phenformin produced an overall suppression of the fibrinolysin system due to increased levels of fast antiplasmins and the acid-labile inhibitors of plasmin.

b) Metformin

The discovery of the fibrinolytic properties of phenformin but also its possible side-effects led to studies on another biguanide antidiabetic compound, metformin (CHAKRABARTI et al., 1965). Administered to 27 patients suffering from obliterative vascular disease, in a dose of 1500 mg in three daily doses for four months, metformin induced a marked increase in fibrinolytic activity in 21 of these patients. Fibrinolytic response was given by most cases with initial low or medium fibrinolytic activity. This was indicated by lysis time measurements during treatment, since there was a reduction in euglobulin lysis time caused by elevation of plasminogen activator.

During treatment, serum cholesterol was reduced, as was plasma fibrinogen towards the end of the trial period. Unfortunately, as with phenformin, partial resistance develops during the course of treatment with metformin (HOCKING et al., 1967) which to some extent reduces the hope of activity of this drug in the prophylaxis of arterial obstruction. Such pessimism is reinforced by the results obtained by

Heikinheimo (1969) in a group of 40 patients treated according to a protocol identical with that of the English authors, with 1500 mg per day of metformin for three months. No significant alteration in euglobulin lysis time or in circulating fibrinogen levels was observed.

c) Buformin

More recently, Ghanem et al. (1972) studied the possible fibrinolytic activity of another biguanide, buformin, in patients suffering from rheumatoid arthritis, compared with normal individuals. These patients received 150 mg of buformin in three divided daily doses for one month. The euglobulin lysis time was determined each week and at the end of treatment it showed a decrease of approximately 30%. The authors also observed a fall in fibrinogen levels and in sedimentation rate in the treated group, while blood sugar levels fell only slightly. An increase in fibrinolytic activity following buformin had also been reported by Endo (1970).

The largest study is that of Asbeck et al. (1975), which involved 66 patients suffering from peripheral obliterative atherosclerosis. The patients were divided into three groups, the first receiving a placebo, the second 100 mg/day of phenformin and the third 200 mg/day of buformin. Treatment was continued for four months. Activation of the fibrinolytic system was more pronounced under the influence of buformin, while in the group treated with phenformin there was no significant alteration in fibrinolytic potential. There were no changes in plasminogen concentration during treatment and no free plasmin or activator activities were detected in the euglobulin fractions.

VI. Combination of Biguanides and Anabolic Steroids

After the partial resistance of fibrinolytic effect that developed after treatment with metformin or with phenformin, and the discovery of the fibrinolytic activity of testosterone (Fearnley and Chakrabarti, 1962) had been reported, followed by a similar discovery concerning numerous other anabolic steroids, trials of a combination of biguanides with anabolic steroids were performed (Fearnley et al., 1967).

1. Combination Phenformin-Ethylestrenol

Eighteen patients were treated first with metformin and then with phenformin until a tachyphylactic phenomenon developed. These patients then received 4 mg of ethylestrenol twice daily. Combined use of the two drugs was associated with a decrease in lysis time throughout treatment, which was continued for one year, and then continued with ethylestrenol alone for three months. This resulted in a shortening of blood lysis time, which was restored to its previous level when combined therapy was given for the last three months of the trial.

Twenty out-patients with occlusive vascular disease of the heart, lower limb, or brain were treated for six months with 50 mg of phenformin twice daily together with 4 mg of ethylestrenol twice daily. Response to treatment is often delayed for three months (Chakrabarti and Fearnley, 1967). The influence of this combined therapy on fibrin breakdown product levels was also determined in six patients suffering from rheumatoid arthritis and ten suffering from obliterative vascular disease

(FEARNLEY et al., 1969). In all cases, the authors observed an increase in fibrin breakdown product levels. In healthy volunteers and some arteriosclerotic subjects, increases in fibrin breakdown products were only transient. This was probably due to successful defibrination.

Identical results were obtained by BROWN (1971). Some patients due to be subjected to elective surgery received six weeks' preoperative and ten days' postoperative treatment with phenformin (50 mg twice daily) and ethylestrenol (4 mg twice daily). All patients showed a high level of lytic activity in the immediate postoperative period, but over the next few days lytic activity decreased. Preoperative mean fibrin breakdown product levels were higher in the group that received this treatment, and the postoperative rise was more sustained.

However, when patients surviving myocardial infarction received an identical dose of the combination phenformin-ethylestrenol over three weeks and were compared with normal subjects, in 70% of cases a decrease of approximately 35% in euglobulin lysis time was found but no changes in plasminogen levels or fibrin breakdown product levels were observed (BRUHN et al., 1974).

Similarly, FOSSARD et al. (1974) failed to demonstrate any change in these parameters under the influence of combined therapy in a group of 50 patients in a gynecological surgery department. The treatment had no influence on the development of deep venous thrombosis.

Furthermore, side-effects requiring the interruption of treatment were seen in 10% of the treated patients. According to ROBB et al. (1974), the discordant results obtained by FOSSARD's group could be due to the fact that the patients were treated for only three weeks preoperatively, as against six weeks in the study of BROWN. In addition, the inclusion of a substantial proportion of premenopausal women with wide variations in dilute blood clot lysis time could have affected the results.

In a case of malignant atrophic papulosis reported by DELANEY and BLACK (1975), while treatment with the combination of phenformin-ethylestrenol relieved pruritus and prevented the development of new lesions, it had no influence on euglobulin lysis time, which was normal at the beginning of treatment and remained unchanged.

In addition, it seems that the degree of fibrinolytic response to treatment depends to a certain extent on the status of fibrinolytic potential in the individual before treatment. In a study involving 75 patients suffering from idiopathic recurrent deep venous thrombosis, recurrent superficial thrombophlebitis or, finally, retinal venous thrombosis and being treated with the combination phenformin 100 mg/day and ethylestrenol 8 mg/day for periods varying between three and 48 months, it was shown that of the 34 patients who at the beginning of the trial had an abnormally weak response to the upper limb venous occlusion test, all but three had a normal response after 3 to 12 months of treatment, while no significant increase occurred in any of the 41 patients who had a normal fibrinolytic response to venous occlusion before treatment (NILSSON, 1975).

The mechanism of action of this drug combination has not yet been elucidated. FEARNLEY and CHAKRABARTI (1971) consider it to be due to an increase in blood levels of plasminogen activator. NILSSON and ISACSON (1972) consider it to be due to an increase in activator levels in the venous endothelium. Thus the question as to whether there is an increase in the synthesis of activator or an increase in its liberation at the endothelium persists. It is quite conceivable that these two phenomena could be coexistent. The fact that the increase in release might be greater than the increase in synthesis could possibly explain the tachyphylactic effect seen after several months of treatment.

At all events, while the results obtained with this combination suggest a possible new approach in the long-term prophylaxis of recurrent thromboses, for example, the side-effects seen by certain authors may limit its use. These were in general not serious, however, except for one case of lactic acidosis and one case of megaloblastic anemia due to folic acid deficiency; the phenomena seen most frequently have been anorexia, nausea, vomiting, weight loss, and a few cases of sodium retention that have responded well to the administration of diuretics (CHAKRABARTI and FEARN-LEY, 1972).

2. Combination Phenformin — Stanozolol

An investigation of the influence of a combination of phenformin (50 mg twice daily) and stanozolol (5 mg daily) was carried out by MENON et al (1970); their study was based on blood fibrinolytic activity in two groups, each consisting of 10 patients.

The increased fibrinolytic activity seen in patients who had previously been receiving phenformin-ethylestrenol therapy was maintained when this combination was replaced by phenformin-stanozolol, and no significant difference between the effects of the two combinations could be detected. Blood fibrinolytic activity was significantly higher after phenformin-stanozolol therapy in patients who had previously received anticoagulants, and this increase, which was apparent at the end of 4 weeks' treatment, was still present after 28 weeks. These findings have been confirmed by FEARNLEY (1970) and, more recently, by BIELAWIEC et al. (1978).

3. Combination Metformin — Ethylestrenol

The effects on plasma fibrinogen, platelet stickiness, fibrinolysis and serum cholesterol of combinations of ethylestrenol with phenformin or metformin were studied by FEARNLEY and CHAKRABARTI (1968) in patients with such conditions as ischemic disease of the lower limbs, myocardial infarction. Both drug combinations increased blood fibrinolytic activity by 50%. However, while phenformin plus ethylestrenol decreased platelet stickiness and serum cholesterol levels, metformin plus ethylestrenol raised both.

The combination phenformin-ethylestrenol thus appears to be the most suitable prophylactic agent for use in patients surviving vascular occlusion.

C. Anticoagulants and Related Compounds

I. Heparin

Although according to ADAR and SALZMAN (1975) heparin is the drug of choice in the treatment of deep venous thrombosis of the lower limbs, it cannot be considered as a fibrinolytic agent. Nevertheless, there is no doubt that thrombi in vivo, both in animals and in man, show an increased tendency to spontaneous regression under the influence of heparin therapy (FITZGERALD et al., 1967). However, the question of determining whether anticoagulants, and in particular heparin, increase fibrinolysis, and if so, whether directly or indirectly, remains open. PAYLING WRIGHT et al. (1953) considered the possibility of an indirect influence permitting the continuous action of plasmin, which is normally masked by the continuous deposition of small quantities of fibrin on the surface of the thrombus. FEARNLEY and FERGUSON (1958) found that the inhibition of natural fibrinolytic activity was due either to a naturally occurring process or to a property present in the blood, heparin preventing the normal coagulation process and unmasking the fibrinolytic activity present in total blood. By contrast, SANDRITTER et al. (1954) considered that heparin possessed a direct fibrinolytic action. Thrombi produced in the jugular veins of rabbits sometimes regress rapidly if the animals are treated with heparin 24 h after induction of the thrombus. The same authors (SANDRITTER et al., 1958) obtained identical results using a heparinoid.

However, these in-vivo observations have not been confirmed by studies in vitro. Studies carried out by VON KAULLA and MACDONALD (1958) showed that while heparin in low concentrations could increase the fibrinolytic activity in test tubes, in preformed clots high concentrations of heparin inhibited the fibrinolysis induced by plasma or by human plasminogen activated by urokinase. DESNOYERS et al. (1975a) have shown that the addition of heparin to the incubation medium of standard plasma hanging clots decreased and could even inhibit the lysis induced either by synthetic chemical compounds or by urokinase and streptokinase. This seems to be a specific effect of heparin, although it has proved possible, by mixing heparin and plasma and using fibrin plates, to demonstrate, that commercial heparin preparations all have a slight antiprotease action. This is in agreement with the study of ASTRUP et al. (1966). However, it does not seem that this slight antiprotease action could explain the inhibition observed at a concentration of 0.5 IU/ml.

Studies on the release of plasminogen activator in the isolated perfused pig ear revealed an increase in activator release (MARKWARDT and KLÖCKING, 1977).

The lytic activity of heparin complexes with fibrinogen, and urea was determined after intravenous administration in rat blood (KUDRYASHOV et al., 1970; KUDRYASHOV and LYAPINA, 1975). The complexes showed an increased antithrombin activity compared with its heparin content and lysed fibrin.

The authors feel that these complexes could be formed within the body, as natural anticlotting agents (KUDRYASHOV et al., 1975a and b).

II. Heparinoids

Studies have also been performed on the fibrinolytic and anticoagulant actions of a natural mucopolysaccharide polysulfuric acid ester, eleparon (DE NICOLA et al., 1965a; FRANDOLI et al., 1967). Plasmin- and plasminogen-activating effects of intravenous eleparon were independent of anticoagulant activity and dosage. The duration of activation increased with large and frequent dosage. Depot-eleparon similarly potentiated fibrinolysis, but the effect of a single intramuscular injection lasted more than 12 h.

The principal studies concerning the fibrinolytic activity of ateroid, a complex mucopolysaccharide duodenal extract, were published in 1969 in Italy. Pharmacological studies carried out by PRINO et al. (1969) showed that the administration of ateroid in rat and rabbit was associated with a marked decrease in plasma euglobulin lysis times. Ateroid may also potentialize the thrombolytic action of urokinase and normalize the increase in antiplasmin levels induced in rat by the intravenous injection of triton (PRINO and MANTOVANI, 1969). These pharmacological data have been confirmed in various clinical studies. BIZZI and BUTTI (1969) performed a controlled cross-over trial with arteriosclerotic patients. Similar results were obtained by GUIDI et al. (1969), SPAMPINATO (1969), CENTONZA et al. (1969). Ateroid was compared with a semisynthetic polysaccharide sulfate and proved superior in the long-term prophylaxis of these various disorders (CASCONE and LAMPUGNANI, 1969).

The fibrinolytic and thrombolytic effects of various substances analogous to heparin, and in particular synthetic acid polysaccharides, have been described by OLESEN (1961), KRAFT (1963), SANDRITTER et al. (1964), and above all by HALSE (1962, 1964). The most extensively studied of these synthetic sulfate polyanions is SP 54, whose activity has been compared with that of heparin by RAYNAUD et al. (1965) in vitro and in vivo after intravenous administration. The results obtained show that the fibrinolytic activity of SP 54 is less marked than that of heparin.

More recently, KOESTERING et al. (1973) showed that SP 54, administered orally in a dose of 10 mg/kg to mice, produced a decrease in the size of thrombi induced by electrical lesion in the ear vein. These results are attributed to activation of the fibrinolytic system. This activation of the fibrinolytic system was also found by FRANDOLI et al. (1972) and DE NICOLA (1975). COCCHERI et al. (1978), continuing the studies of RAY and ASTRUP (1974) were also able to demonstrate an activation of the fibrinolytic system by SP 54. This activation appears to be mediated by cyclic AMP.

III. Oral Anticoagulants

Drugs lowering prothrombin activity do not appear to possess any favorable action on fibrinolysis and thrombolysis. According to NIEWIAROWSKA and WEGRZYNO-WICZ (1959), the administration of anti-vitamin K agents, and in particular dicoumarol derivatives, is associated with a prolongation of euglobulin lysis time and an increase in antiplasmin levels. Identical results were obtained by DONNER (1960). After long-term treatment with phenylin dandione, OGSTON (1961) observed no action on fibrinolytic potential measured by plasma clot lysis time. Oral anticoagulants even seem capable of counterbalancing the increase in fibrinolytic activity induced by bacterial pyrogens in man (DONNER et al., 1961). However, in a patient who had suffered three major vascular occlusions of the lower limbs, VERE and FEARNLEY (1968) progressively tailed-off oral anticoagulant treatment and replaced it with the combination phenformin-ethylestrenol. The patient then suffered a severe subcutaneous hemorrhage associated with a superficial venous thrombosis. The problem of the influence of oral anticoagulant therapy on the natural fibrinolytic potential of the blood requires more extensive research.

IV. Clofibrate

According to GOODHART and DEWAR (1966), clofibrate has only a moderate effect on activation of the fibrinolytic system. In a study carried out by CHAKRABARTI and FEARNLEY (1968) in patients suffering from obliterative vascular disease and receiving 1 g of clofibrate twice daily for seven months, the authors noted a decrease of approximately 30% in serum cholesterol levels and a decrease of approximately 20% in fibrinogen levels. Persistent or transient prolongation of blood clot lysis times was seen. Thus CHAKRABARTI and MEADE (1972) concluded that the effects of clofibrate on fibrinolysis may include short-term improvement that fades after about six months and is then even replaced by antifibrinolytic activity.

A combination of diisopropylamine-clofibrate (150 mg) and of 2-dimethylamino-ethanol-clofibrate (100 mg) was studied in arteriosclerotic patients, who received this combination four times per day for 30 days (SPREAFICO et al., 1973). A significant increase in fibrinolytic activity was observed. This was apparent on the 20th day of treatment, and increased as treatment continued.

D. Vasodilators

Activation of the fibrinolytic system following the intravenous administration of nicotinic acid was observed by MENEGHINI and PICCININI (1958) and by WEINER et al. (1958). This action would appear to be independent of the vascular dilation induced by this drug, since other vasodilators, and in particular histamine, are not endowed with similar properties (WEINER et al., 1959; VON KAULLA, 1963). Nevertheless, as mentioned earlier, at least in the animal histamine has a powerful fibrinolytic activity.

According to the majority of experimental workers, the fibrinolytic effect of nicotinic acid is transient and cannot be reproduced with a second administration a short time after the first dose. However, WILSON and FOSTIROPOULOS (1959) demonstrated the presence of a fibrinolytic response after the 7th injection of 100 mg of nicotinic acid given over a 24-h period.

The induction of fibrinolytic activity after oral administration of nicotinic acid has also been demonstrated, but very high doses are necessary. In the animal, studies of thrombolysis using nicotinic acid proved to be negative (RASCHE and HIEMEYER, 1968). In cats with a thrombus in the femoral artery induced by the local injection of thrombin and left *in situ* for eight hours, no repermeabilization was observed. In rat, ANDREENKO and MIGALINA (1971) showed that intravenous administration of small doses of nicotinic acid was associated with a significant increase in fibrinolytic activity but that high doses, in contrast, had an inhibitory effect. In man, oral or parenteral treatment for short periods in arteriosclerotic patients (BIELAWIEC and LUKJAN, 1971; ROBERTSON, 1971) invariably led to a marked activation of the fibrinolytic system, which was sometimes accompanied by an increase in coagulability (KISELEVA and ROMANENKO, 1966). This activation would appear to be even more marked in patients with cirrhosis (FLETCHER, 1966).

The mechanism of action of nicotinic acid has not yet been completely elucidated. It appears to increase the liberation of plasminogen activator, but also that of factor VIII contained in the endothelial cells of the vessel wall (MANNUCCI, 1975).

Using a histochemical technique (sections of thrombosed tissue incubated on plates of human fibrinogen) DENK and FISCHER (1970) were able to demonstrate only a very slight increase in the liberation of plasminogen activator.

BELLER and SELLIN (1960) used a combination of heparin and nicotinic acid, since they had noted that intravenous injection of 2 mg/kg of nicotinic acid induced marked fibrinolytic activity in 70–80% of cases, but at the same time decreased the clotting time as recorded by thrombelastography.

Low doses of heparin do not only eliminate the retardation of clotting time, but appear to potentialize the fibrinolytic activity of nicotinic acid (GOOSSENS, 1967).

The intravenous administration of nicotinic acid in the prophylaxis of thromboembolic disease was rapidly abandoned because activation of fibrinolysis was short and resistance developed rapidly. Oral activation on a long-term basis appeared to be more appropriate for the long-term activation of fibrinolysis. However, in view of the side-effects (liver and metabolic impairment, skin reactions, flush, etc.), derivatives and homologues of nicotinic acid were sought and studied.

GIAROLA et al. (1972) administered pyridylcarbinol in daily doses of 62.5 and 125 mg to rabbits receiving a high-cholesterol diet for 2 months. They noted a marked increase in fibrinolytic activity, associated with a prolongation in recalcification time and a decrease in the maximal amplitude of the thrombodynamographic tracing. These results were more pronounced when the dose administered was higher. The same authors also noted a decrease in cholesterol, total lipid, and triglyceride levels, and concluded that the nicotinyl-alcohol combination had a potential value in thrombophilic states.

The nicotinic derivative that has been most extensively studied is theophylline nicotinate or xanthinol niacinate (Complamin). As early as 1962, AMERY et al. were able to demonstrate the fibrinolytic activity of theophylline nicotinate with various modes of administration, and these results were confirmed by SAMAMA (1963). Both groups also noted the rapid development of a tachyphylactic phenomenon. This resistance effect was confirmed by BOUVIER and BERTHOUD (1978) even with the administration of doses of as much as 18 g per day, though at these doses many of the individuals treated showed manifestations of hypotension. In the 50 patients studied, a shortening of euglobulin lysis time was observed in 34 cases, but activation of the fibrinolytic system was short-lived, being 5 min to 4 h for doses of 150–1000 mg, and with very high doses, activity in general did not persist beyond 6 h. Only a few patients showed continuing signs of activation up to the third day.

Turnover of fibrinogen in elderly patients is greatly increased after one week's intravenous administration of theophylline nicotinate (DE NICOLA et al., 1968; DE NICOLA, 1975).

In a study carried out in rabbit, TURAZZA et al. (1966) showed that daily intravenous administration of theophylline nicotinate for a 28-day period increased plasmin, as measured on fibrin plates. This can be totally inhibited by aprotinin or ε-aminocaproic acid. These results appear to disagree with those obtained by BOUVIER and BERTHOUD (1978) in man.

Aminophylline in a single intravenous injection activated fibrinolysis in patients with low initial activity of the fibrinolytic system, but if fibrinolysis was active initially, aminophylline decreased the activity of the system (BOGOMOLOVA et al., 1975).

An increase in fibrinolytic activity and a decrease in fibrinogen levels were also seen in healthy volunteers treated with three doses per day of 200 mg of pentoxyfylline (Trental) for three months (JARRETT et al., 1978c). In some cases it was necessary to suspend treatment because of nausea and vomiting. Increased fibrinolytic activity in venous blood following bencyclane has been demonstrated in vivo (KOVACS et al., 1971).

E. Diuretic Drugs

The effects of furosemide on fibrinolysis have been studied (BRUHN, 1975; BRUHN et al., 1975). Healthy persons were given a single intravenous injection of 40 mg of furosemide, and its effects on the fibrinolytic system of the blood and urokinase activity in the urine were determined. Patients with terminal uremia and nephrectomized patients were subjected to a similar procedure. In healthy subjects, euglobulin lysis time was shortened by 60% after furosemide, showing a significant activation of the fibrinolytic system. This activation was not found in the uremia/nephrectomy group. This indicates that an intact renal system is necessary for furosemide to exert any fibrinolytic effects. It is suggested that the beneficial effect of large doses of furosemide in acute renal failure with consumption coagulopathy following septic abortion or shock may be in part due to fibrinolysis of glomerular microthrombi.

F. Anti-Inflammatory Drugs

Using standard plasma clots immersed in solutions of the compounds to be studied, VON KAULLA (1965) was able to demonstrate the fibrinolytic properties of derivatives of benzoic acid and of salicylic acid. Subsequently, ROUBAL and NEMECEK (1966) and VON KAULLA (1967) showed that the power of induction of fibrinolysis was a common property of all acid nonsteroid anti-inflammatory agents. A large number of anti-inflammatory substances were then studied GRYGLEWSKI and GRYGLEWSKA, 1966; GRYGLEWSKI and ECKSTEIN, 1967; MURATOVA et al., 1967; WAGNER-JAUREGG et al., 1973; ČEPELAK et al., 1976).

However, given that these agents have a marked lytic action in vitro, their mechanism of action would appear to be very different from that of all the compounds studied in this general review and should therefore be seen rather in the context of the mechanism of action of the direct fibrinolytic agents studied by VON KAULLA (1965).

G. Pyrogens

Pyrogens remain the most powerful known nonenzymatic fibrinolytic agents. MENEGHINI (1949) noted that the intravenous injection of a vaccine was capable of dissolving a clot in the inferior *vena cava*. This fibrinolytic action is not specific and can also be produced by the administration of purified bacterial pyrogens, which give the same favorable results (EICHENBERGER, 1955; MENEGHINI, 1958; VON KAULLA, 1958; DEUTSCH and ELSNER, 1960).

The peak of fibrinolytic activity precedes the hyperthermic peak and seems to be independent of the pyrogenic action itself, since the fibrinolytic action persists if the fever is suppressed by antipyretic agents. However, this fibrinolytic activity is relatively short-lived, not exceeding 6 h. In addition, and in contrast to other compounds administered intravenously that induce fibrinolytic activity in man a few minutes after injection, the fibrinolytic activity provoked by the administration of pyrogenic substances does not appear until about 90 min after injection, unless the pyrogens have been previously incubated in serum prior to injection (HOERDER and WENDT, 1958). Clinical trials involving the use of pyrogenic agents in the treatment of thrombophlebitis have come up against the problem of major side-effects (MENEGHINI and MORANDO, 1961; BATTEZZATI and BELARDI, 1965). In order to eliminate side-effects, instead of the pyrogenic agent, 100 to 200 ml of plasma obtained from presumably healthy individuals who had received 0.25 μg of pyrogenic substances was injected every 8 h for 2–3 days (MENEGHINI, 1961). This plasma from pyrogen-treated donors does not induce fever and is well tolerated. The injection of pyrogenic substances induces a decrease in blood levels of factors V and VII, which is more marked in venous than in arterial blood (HENGSTMANN et al., 1959). Furthermore, it appears that the administration of pyrogenic substances is not capable of inducing fibrinolytic activity in the animal (AMBRUS et al., 1968).

The use of such pyrogenic substances to increase fibrinolytic activity in the prophylaxis or treatment of occlusive vascular diseases seems to have been totally abandoned at present.

H. Miscellaneous Drugs

I. Antibiotics

Fibrinolytic activity following intravenous injection of different antibiotics was studied in rat by IVLEVA (1969). The results showed that the injection of streptomycin was associated with increased blood fibrinolytic activity, with a parallel reduction in fibrinogen level. The period of fibrinolysis activation is complete two hours after injection of the drug. Neomycin, monomycin, and kanamycin caused a persistent inhibition of blood fibrinolytic activity 5–6 h after injection. The fibrinolysis inhibition period after injection of these three drugs precedes an enhanced fibrinolytic activity phase, which is different for each of the drugs tested. More recently, BICK et al. (1976) have shown that daunomycin and adriamycin, extracted from a streptomyces strain and used as cytotoxic agents in the treatment of acute leukemia, are also capable of creating a hyperfibrinolytic state, and that this effect is not due to direct activation of plasminogen.

II. Monoamine Oxidase Inhibitors

A monoamine oxidase inhibitor, nialamide, was administered for periods of up to 60 days, in a daily dose of 200 mg *per os* in man, and a daily dose of 5–10 mg/kg intramuscularly in animals (DE NICOLA et al., 1965b). An increase in fibrinolytic activity was invariably observed, even in animals receiving a high-cholesterol diet, in which there is usually a decrease in fibrinolytic activity. Monoamine oxidase inhibitors inhibit the increase in the fibrinogen level that is always seen when experimental thrombosis is produced (MAGDA and SZEGI, 1970). However, prolonged administration in the prophylaxis of thromboembolic disease does not seem to be possible due to their side-effects, such as acute episodes of hypertension provoked by the ingestion of foods that are rich in serotonin during treatment.

III. Amino Acids and Derivatives

Induced clots in the jugular vein of the dog are lyzed by the local infusion of a mixture containing 100 mg of L-tyrosine and 1 g of sodium gluconate, while a mixture of L-alanine-sodium gluconate or of L-tyrosine-sodium glucuronate is ineffective. The injection of 100 mg of D-gluconyl-L-tyrosine in solution in 1 ml of distilled water into the femoral vein is associated with repermeabilization of the jugular vein over a 15-min period. By contrast, fibrin clots are not lyzed in vitro, implying an indirect fibrinolytic action (KOPPER, 1966).

Administration of a dose of 50 mg/kg per os of taurine increases fibrinolytic activity for several hours. Hyperfibrinolysis can be maintained by repeated administration and there do not appear to be any tachyphylactic phenomena (SICUTERI et al., 1970). When the intravenous route is used, with a dose of 30 mg/kg, hyperfibrinolysis is preceded by a slight decrease in fibrinolytic activity. Similarly, in vitro, taurine reduces spontaneous fibrinolytic activity. FANCIULLACCI et al. (1970) feel that taurine could be a valuable substance in the treatment of arterial disease.

IV. Chemical Emulsifying and Dispersing Substances

A potentiating effect of the lytic action of urokinase by polysorbate 80 (tween 80) was observed in vivo as well as in vitro (KWAAN et al., 1967). Experimental clots produced in the ear vein of rabbits were more rapidly lyzed by urokinase in a 5% solution of tween 80 than by urokinase in solution in isotonic sodium chloride.

V. Vegetable Extracts

The oligosaccharide fraction of florideae extracts administered parenterally has been shown to possess anticoagulant and fibrinolytic actions (KIRSCHNINCK, 1965).

The effect of the ingestion of onions on fibrinolytic activity was studied in patients suffering from gastric ulcer (MENON et al., 1968). After ingestion of 60 g of onions, the patients showed an increase in fibrinolytic activity. AUGUSTI et al. (1975) were able to demonstrate in particular methane-thiol-3-4 dimethylthiophene, propylallyldisulfide, and methyl and propyl cysteine sulfoxides as the active principles leading to an increase in fibrinolytic activity observed following the ingestion of onions.

VI. Animal Extracts

A blood extract administered to the rabbit receiving an atherogenic diet proved capable of provoking an increase in fibrinolytic activity and a decrease in blood coagulability (GIAROLA et al., 1974).

Bile salts, and in particular sodium taurocholate at a dose of 1.5 g per day, are capable of inducing an increase in fibrinolytic activity (Kroll, 1966).

Finally, using plasma and nonheated fibrin plates, Hellmann and Hawkins (1968) were able to demonstrate marked lytic activity of an extract obtained from ticks (*ornithodorus moubata*) or from eggs of *dermacentor andersoni*.

Conclusion

Numerous workers have demonstrated that occlusive vascular diseases are generally related to low spontaneous fibrinolytic activity. Thus, the use of activators of the fibrinolytic system that have a prolonged action and can be administered via the oral route appears to be desirable. This general review has mentioned a large number of substances, physiological or medicinal, that are capable of provoking an increase, varying in degree and duration, in circulating lytic activity. However, it seems that the effectiveness of these agents depends in part on the state of fibrinolytic potential of the individual before treatment, the best results being obtained in patients in whom fibrinolytic activity at the beginning of treatment is substantially decreased. In addition, there seems to be a fairly high proportion of "poor responders," and the increase in fibrinolytic activity, measured by decrease in euglobulin lysis time, dilute blood clot lysis time, or increase in lysis zones on fibrin plates, is often slight.

Described as indirect fibrinolytic agents, these substances do not act directly on the conversion of plasminogen to plasmin, but via an activator theoretically liberated by the endothelial cells of the vascular wall. The mechanism of action has not yet been entirely elucidated, but some of these agents with a very short duration of action, such as nicotinic acid and adrenaline, may act solely on the release of activator from the vessel wall, while others, with an activity lasting for several months or years, may increase both the synthesis and the release of activator. However, if release occurs more rapidly than synthesis, the effect of the substance tails off even if the dose is increased. This appears to be the case, after varying periods, for the compounds described. Furthermore, many of these agents are not free of side-effects, which implies limitation of their use. In addition, the geographical situation and everyday life habits of the patients should also be taken into consideration. Intensive studies of the fibrinolytic activity of anabolic steroids and of biguanides have been carried out almost solely in England or Sweden, whilst Italien workers have turned their attention more to nicotinic acid derivatives and studies in Czechoslovakia have involved nonsteroid anti-inflammatory agents.

At all events, the influence of an increase in fibrinolytic activity on the development or treatment of occlusive vascular disorders has still to be precisely determined, and it seems likely that long and numerous studies will be required.

Acknowledgment. I am very much indebted to Professor H. Schmitt, C.H.U. Broussais — Hôtel Dieu, Medical Faculty of Paris VI for helpful criticism and advices during the writing of the manuscript.

References

Abiko, Y., Kumada, T.: Enhancement of fibrinolytic and thrombolytic potential in the rat by an anabolic steroid Furazabol. Thrombos. Res. **8** (Suppl. II), 107—14 (1976)

Adar, R., Salzman, E. W.: Treatment of thrombosis of veins of the lower extremities. New Engl. J. Med. **292**, 348—50 (1975)

Åstedt, B., Jeppsson, S.: Thromboembolism and oral contraceptives. Brit. med. J. **1974 II**, 333

Albrechtsen, O., Barfod, B., Barfod, E., Laursen, N. P. R., Nordentoft, B., Yde, H.: Hormonal treatment of arterial insufficiency in the lower extremities. Dan. med. Bull. **19**, 157—159 (1972)

Allenby, F., Jeyasingh, K., Calnan, J.: Ethyloestrenol and postoperative venous thrombosis. Lancet **1973 II**, 38—39

Ambrus, J. L., Ambrus, C. M., Stutzman, L., Schimert, G.: Therapeutic studies with fibrinolytic and antifibrinolytic agents. Abstr. Papers, Amer. chem. Soc. **155**, 25 N (1968)

Amery, A., Vermylen, J., Maes, H., Verstraete, M.: Influence d'un dérivé du niacin sur le système fibrinolytique de l'homme. Apparition de l'activité fibrinolytique après différents modes d'administration. Nouv. Rev. franç. Hémat. **2**, 70—78 (1962)

Andreenko, G. V., Migalina, G. A.: Mechanism of action of nicotinic acid in vitro and in vivo. Vopr. Med. Khim. **17**, 423—27 (1971)

Ardlie, N. G., Glew, G., Schwartz, C. J.: Influence of catecholamines on nucleotide-induced platelet aggregation. Nature (Lond.) **212**, 415—17 (1966)

Asbeck, F., Schuchardt, V., Schoop, W., van de Loo, J.: Induction of fibrinolytic activity by buformin and phenformin. A double blind clinical trial. In: Kaulla, K. N. von, Davidson, J. F. (Eds.): Synthetic Fibrinolytic Thrombolytic agents, pp. 338—42. Springfield/Ill.: Thomas 1975

Assan, R., Heuclin, C., Girard, J. R.: Limitations of use of phenformin. In: Davidson, J. F., Samama, M., Desnoyers, P. (Eds.): Progress in Chemical Fibrinolysis and Thrombolysis, Vol. 1, pp. 351—356. New York: Raven 1975

Astrup, T.: Fibrinolytic enzymes. Transactions of 1st Conference on blood clotting and allied problems. New York: Josiah Macy Jr Foundation 1948, p. 28

Astrup, T., Nissen, U., Rasmussen, J.: Effects of preparations of heparin and heparitin sulfate on fibrinolysis. Arch. Biochem. **113**, 634—40 (1966)

Augusti, K. T., Benaim, M. E., Dewar, H. A., Virden, R.: Partial identification of the fibrinolytic activators in onion. Atherosclerosis **21**, 409—16 (1975)

Back, N., Wilkens, H., Barlow, B., Czarnecki, J.: Fibrinolytic studies with biguanide derivatives. Ann. N.Y. Acad. Sci. **148**, 691—713 (1968)

Battezzati, M., Belardi, P.: Terapia fibrinolitica indiretta da pirogeni. La Ricerca scient. No Spécial **27** (1965)

Baumgartner, H. R., Studer, A., Reber, K.: Methods for the production of experimental thrombosis in the rabbit ear, and the significance of 5-hydroxytryptamine for its origination. Thrombos. Diathes. haemorrh. (Stuttg.) **9**, 485—511 (1963)

Baumgartner, H., Studer, A., Reber, K.: Influence of 5-hydroxytryptamine, 5-hydroxytryptophan, dopamine, norepinephrine, and reserpine on thrombotic deposits in the rabbit. Thrombos. Diathes. haemorrh. (Stuttg.) **12**, 169—178 (1964)

Beck, N. P., Kaneko, T., Zor, U., Field, J. B., Davis, B. B.: Effect of vasopressin and prostaglandin E_1 on the adenyl cyclase-cyclic 3'-5' adenosine monophosphate system in the renal medulla of the rat. J. clin. Invest. **50**, 2461—65 (1971)

Belikina, N. V.: Mechanism of lipocain effect on hemocoagulation. In: Anikin, G. D. (Ed.): 6th Mater. Povolzh. Konf. Fiziol. Uchastiem. Biokhim. Farmakol. Morfol. Chuv. Gos. Univ. Cheboksary, URSS **1**, 120—1 (1973)

Beller, F. K., Sellin, D.: Fibrinolyse-Aktivierung durch eine Kombination von Nicotinsäure und Heparin. Arzneimittel-Forsch. **10**, 758—763 (1960)

Belli, C.: In vivo and in vitro analytical studies of the action of some biodynamical substances derived from chromaffin tissue on spontaneous fibrinolysis. Biol. Latina **16**, 771—782 (1963)

Bick, R. L., Murano, G., Fekete, L., Wilson, W. L.: Daunomycin and fibrinolysis. Thrombos. Res. **9**, 201—203 (1976)

Bielawiec, M., Lukjan, H.: Der Einfluß der Fibrinolyse-Aktivierung auf den peripheren Kreislauf bei obliterierenden Gefäßkrankheiten. Med. Mschr. **25**, 312—314 (1971)

Bielawiec, M., Mysliwiec, M., Perzanowski, A.: Combined therapy with phenformin plus stanozolol in patients with occlusive arterial disease and recurrent venous thrombosis. In: Davidson, J. F., Samama, M., Desnoyers, P. (Eds.): Progress in Chemical Fibrinolysis and Thrombolysis, Vol. 3. New York: Raven 1978

Bielski, J., Owczarek, L.: Histamine and blood clotting. Acta haemat. pol. **1**, 47—53 (1970)

Biggs, R., MacFarlane, R. G., Pilling, J.: Observations on fibrinolysis. Experimental activity produced by exercise or adrenalin. Lancet **1947 I**, 402—405

Bizzi, B., Butti, A.: Valutazione clinica di un farmaco fibrinolitico in un disegno sperimentale cross-over. Minerva Med. **60** (Suppl. 99), 5062—5067 (1969)

Bobek, K., Cerhova, M., Čepelak, V., Sidlova, A.: Serotonin and histamine in cases with venous thrombosis. Metab. Parietis Vasorum, Papers Intern. Congr. Angiol. 5th, Prague 921—927 (1961)

Bogomolova, E. K., Sukhanov, A. A., Yastrebova, L. P., Yampolskaya, L. A.: Effect of euphillin on the fibrinolytic system of the blood in patients with atherosclerosis and hypertensive disease. Klin. Med. **53**, 51—53 (1975)

Bouvier, C. A., Berthoud, S.: Effects on the human fibrinolytic system of intravenous infusions of high doses of Complamin, a nicotinic acid derivative. In: Davidson, J. F., Samama, M., Desnoyers, P. (Eds.): Progress in Chemical Fibrinolysis and Thrombolysis, Vol. 3. New York: Raven 1978

Britton, B. J., Wood, W. G., Peele, M., Hawkey, C., Irving, M. H.: The role of sympatho-adrenal stimulation in the release of plasminogen activator. In: Davidson, J. F., Samama, M., Desnoyers, P. (Eds.): Progress in Chemical Fibrinolysis and Thrombolysis, Vol. 1. New York: Raven 1975

Britton, B. J., Wood, W. G., Smith, M., Hawkey, C., Irving, M. H.: The effect of beta adrenergic blockade upon exercise-induced changes in blood coagulation and fibrinolysis. Thrombos. Haemost. **35**, 396—402 (1976)

Brown, I. K.: Pharmacological stimulation of fibrinolytic activity in the surgical patient. Lancet **1971 I**, 774—776

Bruhn, H. D.: Activation of fibrinolysis by furosemide. Thrombos. Diathes. haemorrh. (Stuttg.) **33**, 672—673 (1975)

Bruhn, H. D., Jipp, P., Okoye, S., Oltmann, A.: Hypofibrinolyse beim akuten Myokardinfarkt. Med. Klin. **69**, 1951—1955 (1974)

Bruhn, H. D., Fricke, G., Schmidt, J., Niedermayer, W.: Fibrinolyseaktivierung durch Furosemid. Med. Klin. **70**, 1125—1127 (1975)

Butler, S.: Experiments dealing with the relation of blood histamine to coagulation, hemoconcentration, and arterial blood pressure. Quart. Bull. Northw. Univ. med. Sch. **29**, 100—105 (1955)

Cajozzo, A., Citarrella, P., Abbadessa, V., Di Marco, P.: Effetti della D-tiroxina sulla fibrinolisi e sulla adesivita ed aggregabilita piastrinici in soggetti aterosclerotici. Boll. Soc. ital. Biol. sper. **50**, 984—990 (1974)

Cascone, A., Lampugnani, P.: Studio sperimentale controllato dei rapporti tra attivita fibrinolitica e attivita anticoagulante nella valutazione di attivatori della fibrinolisi. Minerva Med. **60** (Suppl. 99), 5039—5045 (1969)

Casertano, F., Piccinini, F.: Fibrinolytic action in vivo of histamine. Arch. E. Maragliano Pat. Clin. **15**, 267—273 (1959)

Cash, J. D.: Physiological aspects of fibrinolysis. In: Kaulla, K. N. von, Davidson, J. F. (Eds.): Synthetic Fibrinolytic Thrombolytic Agents, pp. 5—19. Springfield: C. Thomas 1975a

Cash, J. D.: Short-term enhancement of plasminogen activator in vivo by drugs. Thrombos. Diathes. haemorrh. (Stuttg.) **34**, 648—651 (1975b)

Cash, J. D., Allan, A. G. E.: The fibrinolytic response to moderate exercise and intravenous adrenaline in the same subjects. Brit. J. Haematol. **13**, 376—383 (1967)

Cash, J. D., Lind, A. R., McNicol, G. W., Woodfield, D. G.: Fibrinolytic and forearm blood flow responses to intravenous adrenaline in healthy subjects. Life Sci. **8**, 207—213 (1969)

Cash, J. D., Woodfield, D. G., Allan, A. G. E.: Adrenergic mechanisms in the systemic plasminogen activator response to adrenaline in man. Brit. J. Haemat. **18**, 487—494 (1970)

Centonza, D., Brina, A., De Cristoforo, A.: Controllo e regolazione della fibrinolisi negli arterio-patici mediante l'impiego di un complesso mucopolisaccaridico estrattivo. Minerva Med. **60** (Suppl. 99), 5023—5033 (1969)

Čepelák, V., Roubal, Z., Kuchař, M.: Fibrinolysis induction by synthetic organic acids. Chemical structure and biological activity relationship. Folia haemat. (Lpz.) **103**, 3: 343—350 (1976)

Chakrabarti, R., Delitheos, A., Clarke, G. M.: Fibrinolytic activity in relation to age in survivors of myocardial infarction. Lancet **1966 I**, 573—574

Chakrabarti, R., Fearnley, G. R.: Phenformin plus ethyloestrenol in survivors of myocardial infarction. Three-year pilot study. Lancet **1972 II**, 556—559

Chakrabarti, R., Fearnley, G. R.: Reduction of platelet stickiness by phenformin plus ethyl-oestrenol. Lancet **1967 II**, 1012—1014

Chakrabarti, R., Fearnley, G. R.: Effects of clofibrate on fibrinolysis, platelet stickiness, plasma-fibrinogen, and serum-cholesterol. Lancet **1968 II**, 1007—1009

Chakrabarti, R., Fearnley, G. R., Hocking, E. D.: Effect of corticosteroid on fibrinolysis in patients with inflammatory and non inflammatory conditions. Brit. med. J. **1964 I**, 534—537

Chakrabarti, R., Hocking, E. D., Fearnley, G. R.: Fibrinolytic effect of metformin in coronary-artery disease. Lancet **1965 II**, 256—259 (1965)

Chakrabarti, R., Meade, T. W.: Trial of clofibrate. Brit. med. J. **1972 I**, 247

Chase, L. R., Aurbach, G. D.: Renal adenylcyclase: anatomically separate sites for parathyroid hormones and vasopressin. Science **159**, 545—547 (1968)

Cho, M. H., Choy, W.: Induction of increased fibrinolytic activator in plasma by various drugs. Thrombos. Diathes. haemorrh. (Stuttg.) **11**, 372—392 (1964)

Coccheri, S., De Rosa, V., Cavallaroni, K., Poggi, M.: Activation of fibrinolysis by means of sul-phated polysaccharides. Present status and perspectives. In: Progress in Chemical Fibrino-lysis and Thrombolysis, Vol. 3 (J. F. Davidson, M. Samama and P. Desnoyers, Eds.). New York: Raven 1978

Constantini, R., Hilbe, G., Spöttl, F., Holzknecht, F.: The plasminogen activator content of the arterial wall in occlusive arterial diseases. Thrombos. Diathes. haemorrh. (Stuttg.) **27**, 649—654 (1972)

Correll, J. T., Sjoerdsma, A.: Inhibition of a human fibrinolytic system by normal and pathologic serums. Proc. Soc. exp. Biol. (N.Y.) **111**, 274—277 (1962)

Csefkó, I., Gerendás, M., Udvardy, M. D. F.: Histamine and the coagulation of blood. Orvosi Hetilap. **89**, 247—250 (1948)

Cunliffe, W. J.: An association between cutaneous vasculitis and decreased blood fibrinolytic activity. Lancet **1968 I**, 1126—1128

David, G., Kenedi, I.: Experimental pulmonary embolism after pharmacological heart denerva-tion in the rat. Acta physiol. **40**, 101—106 (1971)

Davidson, J. F., Conkie, J. A., McDonald, G. A.: Fibrinolytic enhancement with Stanozolol in men with ischaemic heart disease. III th Congress International Society on Thrombosis and Hae-mostasis Washington (August, 1972) Abstract p. 282 (1972 a)

Davidson, J. F., Lochhead, M., McDonald, G. A., McNicol, G. P.: Fibrinolytic enhancement by Stanozolol A double blind trial. Brit. J. Haemat. **22**, 543—559 (1972 b)

Davidson, J. F., McDonald, G. A., Conkie, J. A.: Stanozolol as a fibrinolytic agent in men with ischaemic heart disease. A thirty-month study. In: Kaulla, K. N. von, Davidson, J. F. (Eds.): Synthetic Fibrinolytic Thrombolytic Agents, pp. 328—337. Springfield: C. Thomas 1975

Delaney, T. J., Black, M. M.: Effect of fibrinolytic treatment in malignant atrophic papulosis. Brit. med. J. **1975 III**, 5980: 415

De Nicola, P.: Long-term activation of fibrinolysis in the prophylaxis of thromboembolism. In: Kaulla, K. N. von, Davidson, J. F. (Eds.): Synthetic Fibrinolytic Agents, pp. 343—356. Spring-field/Ill.: Thomas 1975

De Nicola, P., Cultrera, G., Manai, G.: Fibrinogen turnover in the aged subjects following the administration of drugs acting on fibrinolysis. Farmaco, Ed. sci. **23**, 10: 994—998 (1968)

De Nicola, P., Gibelli, A., Frandoli, G.: Recherches cliniques et expérimentales sur le traitement fibrinolytique prolongé. Activation de la fibrinolyse par l'administration prolongée d'un inhibiteur de la mono-amine-oxydase. Hémostase **5**, 11—16 (1965 b)

De Nicola, P., Gibelli, A., Turazza, G., Nadile, L.: Untersuchungen über die fibrinolytische Wir-kung eines Heparinkörpers beim Menschen. Arzneimittel-Forsch. **15**, 1430—1433 (1965 a)

Denk, H., Fischer, M.: Histochemische Untersuchungen der fibrinolytischen Aktivität an experimentell erzeugten Thromben bei Ratten nach Gabe von direkten und indirekten Fibrinolytika. Thrombos. Diathes. haemorrh. (Stuttg.) **24**, 48—54 (1970)

Desnoyers, P., Anstett, M., Labaume, J., Schmitt, H.: Effect of α- and β-adrenoceptor stimulating and blocking agents on fibrinolytic activity in rats. In: Davidson, J. F., Samama, M., Desnoyers, P. (Eds.): Progress in Chemical Fibrinolysis and Thrombolysis, Vol. 1, pp. 367—374. New York: Raven 1975 b

Desnoyers, P., Duhault, J., Beregi, L., Hugon, P.: Effect of new sulfonylureas on different parameters of haemostasis. Diabetologia **6**, 43 (1970)

Desnoyers, P., Labaume, J., Anstett, M., Baudet, M., Cure, R., Herrera, M., Pesquet, J., Sebastien, J., Samama, M.: Pharmacological screening of synthetic fibrinolytic-thrombolytic agents: comparison between synthetic and enzymatic compounds. In: Kaulla, K. N. von, Davidson, J. F. (Eds.): Synthetic Fibrinolytic Thrombolytic Agents, pp. 199—226. Springfield/Ill.: Thomas 1975 a

Desnoyers, P., Labaume, J., Anstett, M., Herrera, M., Pesquet, J., Sebastien, J.: The pharmacology of S 1702, a new highly effectiv oral antidiabetic drug with unusual properties. Part 3: Antistickiness activity, fibrinolytic properties and haemostatic parameters study. Arzneimittel-Forsch. **22**, 1691—1695 (1972 b)

Desnoyers, P., Labaume, J., Baudet, M., Verry, M.: Fibrinolytic activity of vascular endothelium, demonstrated by Todd's method, after administration of a new antidiabetic drug 1702 SE. II th Congress of the Internat. Soc. on Thrombosis and Haemostasis Oslo (12—16 July) Abstract p. 118 (1971 b)

Desnoyers, P., Labaume, J., Brunerie, C.: Diabetic angiopathy: large venous vessels, retinal and kidney vascular endothelium fibrinolytic activity: influence of gliclazide administration on the rat (XII th Congrès International de Thérapeutique, Genève, 1973). Progr. méd. **7**, 274 (1973)

Desnoyers, P., Labaume, J., Conard, J., Samama, M.: Essai de contribution au mécanisme d'action thrombolytique de composés chimiques synthétiques. Bibl. haemat. (Basel) **38**, 776—783 (1971 a)

Desnoyers, P., Labaume, J., Conard, J., Samama, M.: Contribution to the study of mechanism of action of synthetic thrombolytic chemical agents. (III th Symposium on Thrombosis-Pilsen 1970) Acta. Univ. Carol.: Med. Monographia **52**, 33—40 (1972 a)

Deutsch, E., Elsner, P.: Pyrogens as thrombolytic agents. Clinical and experimental studies. Amer. J. Cardiol. **6**, 420—424 (1960)

Dohn, K., Hvidt, V., Nielsen, J., Palm, L.: Testosterone therapy in obliterating arterial lesions in the lower limbs. Angiology **19**, 342—350 (1968)

Donner, L.: Einfluß der Dicumarolpräparate auf die Fibrinolyse. Schweiz. med. Wschr. **90**, 1254—1255 (1960)

Donner, L., Bracová, S., Setkova, O.: The effect of Pelentan (Ethylum dihydroxy-cumarinylaceticum) on fibrinolysis. Blood **18**, 116 (1961)

Eichenberger, E.: Fibrinolyse nach intravenöser Injektion bakterieller Pyrogene. Acta Neuroveget. **11**, 201—209 (1955)

Endo, K.: Blood fibrinolytic activity in diabetics before and after treatment. J. Jap. Soc. int. Med. **59**, 16 (1970)

Fanciullacci, M., Sicuteri, F., Giotti, A., Brunetti, S.: La Taurina come agente fibrinolitico nell' uomo: Prime osservazioni terapeutiche. Clin. Ter. **53**, 3—8 (1970)

Fearnley, G. R.: Proc. 2 nd ACTH Conference, New York, Vol. 2. 1951, p. 561

Fearnley, G. R.: Pharmacological enhancement of fibrinolytic activity of blood. J. clin. Path. **17**, 328—333 (1964)

Fearnley, G. R.: The pharmacology of fibrinolysis. Fibrinolysis. London: Arnold 1965

Fearnley, G. R.: Fibrinolysis and fibrinolytic drugs. Practitioner **196**, 585—592 (1966)

Fearnley, G. R.: Phenformin and Stanozolol in blood fibrinolytic activity. Brit. med. J. **1970 I**, 693 (1970 a)

Fearnley, G. R.: Pharmacological enhancement of fibrinolysis. In: Schor, J. M. (Ed.): Chemical Control of Fibrinolysis-Thrombolysis, pp. 205—243. New York-London-Sydney-Toronto: Wiley-Interscience 1970 b

Fearnley, G. R.: Ethyloestrenol and postoperative venous thrombosis. Lancet **1973 II**, 95

Fearnley, G. R.: Development of oral fibrinolytic therapy. In: Kaulla, K. N. von, Davidson, J. F. (Eds.): Synthetic Fibrinolytic Thrombolytic Agents, pp. 305—311. Springfield/Ill.: Thomas 1975

Fearnley, G. R., Bunim, J. J.: Effect of adrenocorticotropic hormone (ACTH) on the erythrocyte-sedimentation rate and plasma-fibrinogen and serum-protein levels in normal persons. Lancet **1951 II**, 1113—1116

Fearnley, G. R., Chakrabarti, R.: Increase of blood fibrinolytic activity by testosterone. Lancet **1962 II**, 128—132

Fearnley, G. R., Chakrabarti, R.: Effect of ethyloestrenol combined with phenformin or with metformin on platelet stickiness and serum-cholesterol in patients with occlusive vascular disease. Lancet **1968 II**, 1004—1007

Fearnley, G. R., Chakrabarti, R.: Mode of action of phenformin plus éthyloestrenol on fibrinolysis. Lancet **1971 I**, 723—725

Fearnley, G. R., Chakrabarti, R., Evans, J. F.: The pharmacological enhancement of blood fibrinolytic activity with special reference to phenformin. Acta cardiol. (Brux.) **19**, 1—13 (1964)

Fearnley, G. R., Chakrabarti, R., Evans, J. F.: Fibrinolytic and defibrinating effect of phenformin plus ethyloestrenol in vivo. Lancet **1969 I**, 910—914

Fearnley, G. R., Chakrabarti, R., Hocking, E. D.: Phenformin in rheumatoid arthritis. A fibrinolytic approach. Lancet **1965 I**, 9—13

Fearnley, G. R., Chakrabarti, R., Hocking, E. D., Evans, J.: Fibrinolytic effects of biguanides plus ethyloestrenol in occlusive vascular disease. Lancet **1967 II**, 1008—1011

Fearnley, G. R., Chakrabarti, R., Vincent, C. T.: Effect of the sulphonylureas on fibrinolysis. Lancet **1960 II**, 622—625

Fearnley, G. R., Ferguson, J.: Presence of fibrinolytic activity in whole blood, masked by the clotting process. Clin. Sci. **17**, 555—561 (1958)

Fearnley, G. R., Vincent, C. T., Chakrabarti, R.: Reduction of blood fibrinolytic activity in diabetes mellitus by insulin. Lancet **1959 II**, 1067

Fiaschi, E., Barbui, T., Previato, G., Di Luzio, V., Guarnieri, G. F., Todesco, S.: The effects of phenformin on blood fibrinolysis in diabetes mellitus. Arzneimittel-Forsch. **19**, 638—640 (1969)

Fitzgerald, D. E., Szeto, I. L. F., Spero, J., Lewis, J. H.: The thrombolytic effect of heparin and a heparin-like substance, SP 54. Thrombos. Diathes. haemorrh. (Stuttg.) **17**, 418—422 (1967)

Fletcher, A. P.: Pathological fibrinolysis. Fed. Proc. **25**, 84—88 (1966)

Fossard, D. P., Friend, I. R., Field, E. S., Corrigan, T. P., Kakkar, V. V., Flute, P. T.: Fibrinolytic activity and postoperative deep-vein thrombosis. Lancet **1974 I**, 9—11

Frandoli, G., Gibelli, A., Giarola, P. A., De Nicola, P.: Untersuchungen über die prolongierte Aktivierung der Fibrinolyse. Arzneimittel-Forsch. **17**, 1397—1400 (1967)

Frandoli, G., Spreafico, P. L., Lampugnani, P., Tammaro, A. E.: Action on fibrinolysis and platelet aggregation of a synthetic, heparin-like sulfated polyanion (SP 54) given orally and parenterally, as related to lipidic fractions. Arzneimittel-Forsch. **22**, 759—763 (1972)

Gader, A. M. A., Da Costa, J., Cash, J. D.: A new vasopressin analogue and fibrinolysis. Lancet **1973 II**, 1417—1418

Genster, H. G., Oram, V.: Arterial insufficiens i underekstremiteterne behandlet medikamentelt. Ugeskr. Laeg. **6**, 244—246 (1971)

Genton, E., Kern, F., von Kaulla, K. N.: Fibrinolysis induced by pressor amines. Amer. J. Med. **31**, 564—571 (1961)

Gerendás, M., Csefkó, I., Udvardy, M. D. F.: Histamine-heparin-thrombin chain mechanism. Nature (Lond.) **162**, 257—258 (1948)

Ghanem, M. H., Guirgis, F. K., El Sawy, M.: Effect of buformin on fibrinolytic activity in rheumatoid arthritis. Arzneimittel-Forsch. **22**, 1487—1489 (1972)

Giarola, P., Egge, H., Gibelli, A., Mueller, J.: β-Pyridylcarbinol in experimental hypercholesterinemia of the rabbit. Study of lipidic fractions and of the mechanisms of hemostasis. Farmaco, Ed. sci. **27**, 1018—1023 (1972)

Giarola, P., Egge, H., Gibelli, A., Murawski, U.: Die Wirkung eines Blutextraktes auf Plasmalipide, Blutgerinnung, Fibrinolyse und Plättchenaggregation bei der experimentellen Hypercholesterinämie des Kaninchens. Arzneimittel-Forsch. **24**, 925—928 (1974)

Gibelli, A., Turazza, G., Giarola, P., De Nicola, P.: Action of ε-aminocaproic acid and of parotid inhibitor on the fibrinolysis activation due to nicotinic acid derivatives and to heparin-like substances. Farmaco, Ed. sci. **21**, 301—309 (1966)

Goodhart, J. M., Dewar, H. A.: Effect of atromid-S on fibrinolytic activity in patients with ischemic heart disease and normal blood cholesterol levels. Brit. med. J. **1966 I**, 325—327

Goossens, N.: Über Fibrinolyseaktivierung in vitro und in vivo durch Nikotinsäure, Heparin und deren Mischungen. Med. Welt (Stuttg.) **14**, 899—903 (1967)

Grishin, A. I.: Dexametazone and aldosterone action on the blood coagulation system. Farmakol. Toksikol **35**, 90—92 (1972)

Gryglewski, R. J., Eckstein, M.: Fibrinolytic activity of some biarylcarboxylic acids. Nature (Lond.) **214**, 626 (1967)

Gryglewski, R. J., Gryglewska, T. A.: The fibrinolytic activity of N-arylanthranilates. Biochem. Pharmacol. **15**, 1171—1175 (1966)

Guidi, G., Lombardi, V., Torsellini, A.: Azione di un eparinoide estrattivo su alcuni indici della coagulazione del sangue. Minerva Med. **60** (Suppl. 99) 5034—5038 (1969)

Halse, T.: Aktivierung der Fibrinolyse und Thrombolyse durch Polysaccharidschwefelsäureester (Heparinoids). Arzneimittel-Forsch. **12**, 574—582 (1962)

Halse, T.: Polyelectrolytes as activators of fibrinolysis and thrombolysis. Sangre **9**, 149—152 (1964)

Harada, M., Takeuchi, M.: Effect of histamine on clot lysis by streptokinase in vitro. Shionogi Kenhyusho Nempo **14**, 207—209 (1964)

Hartmann, E., Weiss, I.: The effect of alkaloids upon blood coagulation. Klin. Wschr. **9**, 347—349 (1930)

Hedner, U., Nilsson, I. M., Isacson, S.: Effect of ethyloestrenol on fibrinolysis in the vessel wall. Thrombos. Diathes. haemorrh. (Stuttg.) **34** 609 (1975)

Hedner, U., Nilsson, I. M., Isacson, S.: Effect of ethyloestrenol on fibrinolysis in the vessel wall. Brit. med. J. **1976 II**, 729—731

Heikinheimo, R.: Metformin and fibrinolysis. Scand. J. Haematol. **6**, 288—290 (1969)

Hellmann, K., Hawkins, R. I.: The action of tick extracts on blood coagulation and fibrinolysis. Thrombos. Diathes. haemorrh. (Stuttg.) **34**, 609 (1975)

Hengstmann, H., Klien, D., Becker, M.: Behavior of factors V and VII in arterial and venous blood in the pyrogen reaction. Dtsch. Arch. klin. Med. **206**, 30—44 (1959)

Hengstmann, H., Klien, D., Becker, M.: The activity of factor V and factor VII complex in human circulation following administration of histamine. Dtsch. Arch. klin. Med. **206**, 459—467 (1960)

Henriques, S. B., Henriques, O. B., Levy, A.: Slow hyperfibrinogenemic action of adrenaline and related substances. Brit. J. Pharmacol. **11**, 99—103 (1956)

Heutzer, E., Cort-Madsen, P.: Testosterone ved arteriel insufficiens i underekstremiteterne. Nord. Med. **76**, 1307—1312 (1966)

Hey, D., Nazemi, M., Beneke, G.: Experimental approach to lysis of fibrin in vivo. Z. ges. exp. Med. **153**, 169—186 (1970)

Hocking, E. D., Chakrabarti, R., Evans, J.: Effect of biguanides and atromid on fibrinolysis. J. Atheroscler. Res. **7**, 121—130 (1967)

Hoerder, M. H., Wendt, F.: Fibrinolyse und Gerinnungsfaktoren nach Injektion von bakteriellen und endogenen Pyrogenen beim Menschen. (Proc. 7th Congress of the International Society of Hematology, Rome, 1958). New York: Grune and Stratton 1960

Holemans, R.: Enhancement of fibrinolysis in the dog by injection of vasoactive drugs. Amer. J. Physiol. **208**, 511—520 (1965)

Holemans, R., Langdell, R. D.: Histamine-induced increase in fibrinolytic activity. Proc. Soc. exp. Biol. (N.Y.) **115**, 584—587 (1964)

Ingram, G. I. C., Vaughan-Jones, R.: Alterations of fibrinolysis and blood coagulation. Lancet **1969 I**, 310

Isacson, S.: Low fibrinolytic activity of blood and vein walls in venous thrombosis. Scand. J. Haematol. (Suppl. 16) 1—29 (1971)

Isacson, S., Nilsson, I. M.: Antithrombotic effect of a combined phenformin-ethyloestrenol medication. In: Kaulla, K. N. von, Davidson, J. F. (Eds.): Synthetic Fibrinolytic Thrombolytic Agents, pp. 312—316. Springfield: Thomas 1975

Ivleva, A. Y.: Changes in blood fibrinolytic activity following the intravenous injection of aminoglycoside antibiotics. Farmakol. Toksikol. **32**, 321—324 (1969)

Ivleva, A. Y., Zolotukhin, S. I.: Thrombolytic means of non-enzymic character: Review of the literature. Farmakol. Toksikol. **36**, 359—365 (1973)

Izhizu, H., Nobuhara, M.: Fluidity of blood studied on the basis of fibrinolysis. VII: Fibrinolytic activity and blood catecholamine level after the administration of cholinergic stimulants. Nippon Hoigaku Zasshi **24**, 455—461 (1970)

Jarrett, P. E. M., Burnand, K. G., Morland, M., Browse, N. L.: The treatment of venous liposclerosis of the legs by fibrinolytic enhancement. In: Davidson, J. F., Samama, M., Desnoyers, P. (Eds.): Progress in Chemical Fibrinolysis and Thrombolysis, Vol. 3. New York: Raven 1978 a

Jarrett, P. E. M., Morland, M., Browse, N. L.: The fibrinolytic activity and treatment by stanozolol of patients with idiopathic recurrent superficial thrombophlebitis. In: Davidson, J. F., Samama, M., Desnoyers, P. (Eds.): Progress in Chemical Fibrinolysis and Thrombolysis, Vol. 3. New York: Raven 1978 b

Jarrett, P. E. M., Morland, M., Browse, N. L.: The effect of oxpentifylline (Trental) on fibrinolytic activity and plasma fibrinogen levels. In: Davidson, J. F., Samama, M., Desnoyers, P. (Eds.): Progress in Chemical Fibrinolysis and Thrombolysis, Vol. 3. New York: Raven 1978 c

Jürgens, J.: The hemostyptic effect of histamine and its relation to the function of the stomach. Z. ges. inn. Med. **3**, 272—281 (1948)

Katalin, M., Jozsef, S.: A Fibrinolizis es Gyogyszertana. Gyogyszereszet **11**, 97—100 (1967)

Kaulla, K. N. von: Intravenous protein-free pyrogen: a powerful fibrinolytic agent in man. Circulation **17**, 187—198 (1958)

Kaulla, K. N. von: Experimental and clinical approaches toward thrombolysis by mobilizing the body's own fibrinolytic system. In: Chemistry of Thrombolysis: Human fibrinolytic enzymes, pp. 240—260. Springfield, Ill.: Thomas 1963

Kaulla, K. N. von: A simple test tube arrangement for screening fibrinolytic activity of synthetic organic compounds. J. med. Chem. **8**, 164—166 (1965)

Kaulla, K. N. von: Structure-dependent fibrinolytic (clot-dissolving) activity of anti-inflammatory drugs and related compounds. Abstr. Papers. Amer. chem. Soc. **153**, 1 M (1967)

Kaulla, K. N. von: On an in-vitro mechanism of action of synthetic fibrinolytic agents. Abstr. Papers, Amer. chem. Soc. **155**, 21 N (1968)

Kaulla, K. N. von, MacDonald, T. S.: The effect of heparin on the components of the human fibrinolytic system. Blood **13**, 811—821 (1958)

Kaulla, K. N. von, Smith, R. L.: Urea derivatives as fibrinolysis promoting agents. Proc. Soc. Exptl. Biol. Med. **106**, 530—533 (1961)

Kirschninck, H.: Über einige Inhaltsstoffe von Florideen und ihre Wirkungsrichtungen. Arzneimittel-Forsch. **15**, 947—948 (1965)

Kiseleva, L. N., Romanenko, G. K.: Changes of the blood coagulation and anticoagulation systems under the influence of nicotinic acid. Klin. Med. **44**, 48—50 (1966)

Koestering, H., Koenig, F., Weber, S., Warmann, E., Guerrero, M.: Einfluß von oral und transkutan appliziertem SP 54 auf präformierte Thromben im Tierversuch. Med. Welt (Stuttg.) **24**, 139—140 (1973)

Kokot, F.: Effect of serotonin and 5-hydroxyindoleacetic acid on plasma clearing and fibrinolysis. Patol. Polska **12**, 321—325 (1961)

Kokot, F.: Effect of serotonin on the behavior of euglobulin and serum fibrinolysis and on the blood fibrinogen level in experimental atherosclerosis in pigeons. Patol. Polska **13**, 177—183 (1962)

Kopper, P. H.: Rapid induction of in vivo fibrinolysis with D-gluconyl-L-tyrosine. Nature (Lond.) **211**, 1417 (1966)

Kovacs, I. B., Csalay, L., Csakvary, G.: Antithrombotic and fibrinolytic effect of bencyclane. Arzneimittel-Forsch. **21**, 1553—1556 (1971)

Kraft, E.: The treatment of thromboembolism with drugs which activate endogenous fibrinolysis. Dtsch. med. Mschr. **8**, 63—66 (1963)

Kroll, J.: Influence of bile salts on the lysis of I^{131}-labelled plasma clots in human subcutaneous tissue in vivo. Scand. J. clin. Lab. Invest. **18**, 691—692 (1966)

Kudryashov, B. A., Lyapina, L. A.: Heparin-adrenaline complex as a humoral agent of the blood anticoagulating system. Vopr. Med. Khim. **17**, 46—53 (1971)

Kudryashov,B.A., Lyapina,L.A.: The heparin-urea complex, its physico-chemical properties. Vopr. Med. Khim. **21**, 165—168 (1975)

Kudryashov,B.A., Lyapina,L.A., Moltchanova,L.V., Rustamova,B.A.: On the nature of lytic effect of fibrinogen-heparin and thyroxin heparin complexes on fibrin. Vopr. Med. Khim. **16**, 161—168 (1970)

Kudryashov,B.A., Lyapina,L.A., Zhitnikova,E.S., Obraztsov,V.V.: Formation of the secondary complex of adrenaline-heparin-fibrinogen and its properties. Vopr. Med. Khim. **21**, 65—69 (1975a)

Kudryashov,B.A., Pastorova,V.E., Lyapina,L.A.: The effect of low doses of heparin-urea complex on the aggregation of thrombocytes and fibrinolytic activity of the blood with i.v. injections and in vitro tests. Farmakol. Toksikol. **38**, 441—444 (1975b)

Kumada,T., Abiko,Y.: Enhancement of fibrinolytic and thrombolytic potential in the rat by treatment with an anabolic steroid, furazabol. Thrombos. Haemostas. **36**, 451—464 (1976)

Kuznik,B.I., Basov,V.I., Tsybikov,N.N.: Mechanism of histamine action on the blood coagulability. Farmakol. Toksikol. **35**, 448—452 (1972)

Kwaan,H.C., Brakman,P., Astrup,T.: Enhancement of fibrinolysis and thrombolysis by polysorbate 80 (Tween 80). Experientia (Basel) **23**, 261—262 (1967)

Kwaan,H.C., Lo,R., McFadzean,A.J.S.: On lysis of thrombi experimentally produced within veins. Brit. J. Haemat. **4**, 51 (1958)

Lassman,H.B., Back,N.: Biochemical pharmacology of the fibrinolysin system of the rat. II: The effect of insulin-induced hypoglycemia. J. Pharmacol. exp. Ther. **189**, 327—332 (1974a)

Lassman,H.B., Back,N.: Biochemical pharmacology of the fibrinolysin system of the rat. III: The mechanism of phenformin (1-(β-phenethyl)-biguanide)-induced fibrinolytic activity. J. Pharmacol. exp. Ther. **189**, 333—343 (1974b)

Lassman,H.B., Wilkens,H., Back,N.: Biochemical pharmacology of the fibrinolysin system of the rat. I: The effect of alloxan-induced hyperglycemia. J. Pharmacol. exp. Ther. **189**, 317—326 (1974)

Lazar,G., Toth,A., Karady,I.: Effect of adaptation to histamine and epinephrine on hyperfibrinogenemia induced by histamine and epinephrine. Acta physiol. **41**, 107—112 (1972)

Löfgren,L.: The tissue mast cells, blood-clotting time, and changes in the relative proportions of the white blood cells of guinea pigs during histamine treatment. Acta anat. **26**, 62—80 (1956)

MacNicol,G.P., Douglas,A.S.: Urokinase and non-enzymatic fibrinolytic agents. Scand. J. clin. Lab. Invest. **16** (Suppl. 78), 34—36 (1964)

Magda,K., Szegi,J.: Anti-thrombic effect of monoaminooxidase blocking agents. Gyogyszereszet. **14**, 135—141 (1970)

Mannucci,P.M.: Mechanism of plasminogen activator and factor VIII rise induced by vasoactive drugs. In: Davidson,J.F., Samama,M., Desnoyers,P. (Eds.): Progress in Chemical Fibrinolysis and Thrombolysis, Vol. 1, pp. 109—110. New York: Raven 1975

Mannucci,P.M., Pareti,F.I., Barbi,G.L.: Effect of cyclic AMP and related drugs on plasminogen activator. In: Kaulla,K.N. von and Davidson,J.F. (Eds.): Synthetic Fibrinolytic Thrombolytic Agents. Springfield, Ill.: Thomas 1975

Markwardt,F.: Biochemisch-pharmakologische Grundlagen der antithrombotischen Therapie. Folia haemat. (Lpz.) **103**, 293—312 (1976)

Markwardt,F., Klöcking,H.-P.: Studies on the release of plasminogen activator. Thrombos. Res. **8**, 217—223 (1976)

Markwardt,F., Klöcking,H.-P.: Heparin-induced release of plasminogen activator. Haemostasis **6**, 370—374 (1977)

Meneghini,P.: La shock-vaccino terapia nella cura di un caso di thrombosi traumatica della vena cava inf. Arch. E. Maragliano Pat. Clin. **4**, 771—777 (1949)

Meneghini,P.: Fibrinolytic treatment of thrombo-embolic disease with purified bacterial pyrogens. Acta haemat. (Basel) **19**, 65—81 (1958)

Meneghini,P.: The development of thrombolytic activity. Thrombos. Diathes. haemorrh. (Stuttg.) **6** (Suppl. 1) 217—226 (1961)

Meneghini,P., Morando,G.D.: L'insufficienza venosa post-trombotica. Osservazioni a distanza sul trattamento fibrinolitico-anticoagulante. Minerva Med. **52** 2835—2839 (1961)

Meneghini,P., Piccinini,F.: Attivazione fibrinolytica del sangue da acido da alcool nicotinico. Arch. E. Maragliano Pat. Clin. **14**, 69—74 (1958)

Menon, I. S., Cunliffe, W. J., Weightman, D., Dewar, H. A.: Phenformin and stanozolol in blood fibrinolytic activity. Brit. med. J. **1970** I, 428

Menon, I. S., Kendal, R. Y., Dewar, H. A., Newell, D. J.: Effect of onions on blood fibrinolytic activity. Brit. med. J. **1968** II, 351—352

Milne, W. L., Cohn, S., Pate, R. D.: Role of serotonin in blood coagulation. Amer. J. Physiol. **189**, 470—474 (1957)

Mischenko, V. P., Kuznik, B. I., Bochkarnikov, V. V.: Mechanism of action of vasoactive agents on blood clotting and fibrinolysis. Cor Vasa **14**, 228—238 (1972)

Moschos, C. B., Lehan, P. H., Oldewurtel, H. A., Koroxenidis, G. T.: Studies of clotting and fibrinolysis across the heart: Response to catecholamines infusion. Circulation **32** (Suppl. II) 155 (1965)

Muratova, J., Dlabac, A., Tricka, V., Nemecek, O.: La trimethazone, nouveau dérivé pyrazolidinique doué d'action anti-inflammatoire et antithrombotique. Thérapie **22**, 1265—1272 (1967)

Neri, S., Rossi, G. G., Rossi, F. P. L., Paoletti, P., Panti, A., D'Ayala, V. G.: Effects of bradykinin on coagulation and fibrinolysis. Study in vitro and in vivo. Thrombos. Diathes. haemorrh. (Stuttg.) **14**, 508—518 (1965)

Niewiarowska, M., Wegrzynowicz, Z.: Influence of dicoumarol derivatives on plasma fibrinolytic system. Thrombos. Diathes. haemorrh. (Stuttg.) **3**, 279—285 (1959)

Nilsson, I. M.: Agents stimulating endogenous activators of fibrinolysis: Haemorrhagic and thrombotic diseases. London-New York-Sydney-Toronto: Wiley 1974

Nilsson, I. M.: Phenformin and ethyloestrenol in recurrent venous thrombosis. In: Davidson, J. F., Samama, M., Desnoyers, P. (Eds.): Progress in Chemical Fibrinolysis and Thrombolysis, Vol. 1, pp. 1—12. New York: Raven 1975

Nilsson, I. M., Isacson, S.: Effect of treatment with combined phenformin and ethyloestrenol on the coagulation and fibrinolytic system. J. clin. Pathol. **25**, 638—639 (1972)

Nilsson, I. M., Robertson, B.: Effect of venous occlusion on coagulation and fibrinolytic components in normal subjects. Thrombos. Diathes. haemorrh. (Stuttg.) **20**, 397—408 (1968)

Nityanand, S., Zaidi, S. H.: Experimental pulmonary embolism and arteriosclerosis. Effect of vasospasm. Amer. Heart J. **67**, 529—538 (1964)

Ogston, D.: The effect of phenindione on plasma fibrinolytic activity. Scot. med. J. **6**, 565—566 (1961)

Ohta, G., Takegoshi, T., Ueno, K., Shimizu, M.: Synthesis of androstano (2,3-C) furazans and related compounds. Chem. pharmaceut. Bull. **13**, 1445—1459 (1965)

Olesen, E. S.: A fibrinolytic system in human plasma activated by peptone or acid mucopolysaccharides. Scand. J. clin. Lab. Invest. **13**, 410—415 (1961)

Orlikov, G. A.: Changes in coagulability, heparin level, and fibrinolytic activity of blood during the subcutaneous administration of histamine. Latv. PSR Zinat. Akad. Vestis **6**, 130—133 (1969)

Park, J. K., Lee, P. H.: Effects of lymph and histamine administration on blood coagulation. Proc. Intern. Congr. Hematol. 8 th, Tokyo **3**, 1830—1831 (1960)

Paton, W. D. M.: Histamine release by compounds of simple chemical structure. Pharmacol. Rev. **9**, 269 (1957)

Payling Wright, H., Kubik, M. M., Hayden, M.: Recanalization of thrombosed arteries under anticoagulant treatment. Brit. med. **1953** I, 1021—1023

Ponari, O., Civardi, E., Megha, A., Pini, M., Poti, R., Dettori, A. G.: Effect of alpha and beta blocking drugs on the clotting and fibrinolytic response to venous stasis in man. Brit. J. Haemat. **24**, 463—470 (1973)

Postnov, Y. V., Ananchenko, V. G., Ulitina, P. D.: Effect of disturbances of vascular and connective tissue permeability induced by histamine on some indexes of the physiological blood anticoagulation system under experimental conditions. Arkh. Patol. **26**, 31—38 (1964)

Prino, G., Mantovani, M.: Aspetti farmacologici dell'attivita fibrinolitica dell'Atéroid. Minerva Med. **60** (Suppl. 99), 5015—5022 (1969)

Prino, G., Mantovani, M., Butti, A.: Attivazione della lisi euglobulinica indotta dall'ateroid. Boll. Soc. ital. Biol. sper. **45**, 133—137 (1969)

Rahn, B., Kaulla, K. N. von: Pharmacological induction of fibrinolytic activity in the dog. Proc. Soc. exp. Biol. (N.Y.) **115**, 359—362 (1964)

Rahn, B., Kaulla, K. N. von: Pharmakologische tierexperimentelle Fibrinolyse. Klin. Wschr. 43, 163—169 (1965)

Rasche, H., Hiemeyer, V.: Zur Frage der thrombolytischen Wirkung von Heparin und Nikotinsäure. Med. Klin. 63, 63—65 (1968)

Ray, G., Astrup, T.: Effects of some polysaccharide sulfates and some phosphates on neutral proteases and plasminogen activators. Haemostasis 2, 269—276 (1974)

Raynaud, R., Brochier, M, Griguer, P., Raynaud, P.: Action d'un heparinoide de synthèse (E.S.P.) sur la coagulation. Thérapie 20, 1249—1258 (1965)

Robb, P. M., Santer, G. J., Brown, I. K.: Fibrinolytic activity and D.V.T. Lancet 1974 I, 455

Robertson, B.: Effect of nicotinic acid in health, in thrombotic disease and in liver cirrhosis. Acta chir. scand. 137, 643—648 (1971)

Robinson, G. A. R., Butcher, R. W., Sutherland, E. W.: Cyclic AMP and hormone action. In: Cyclic AMP. New York-London: Academic 1971

Rodionov, Y. Y.: Activation of blood coagulation, caused by renin and angiotensin II. Zdravookhr. Beloruss. 20, 25—27 (1974)

Rodionov, Y. Y., Rodionov, V. Y., Koshelapov, V. I.: Effect of renin and angiotensin on blood coagulation. Dokl. Akad. Nauk SSSR 201, 1504—1506 (1971)

Rosa, A. T., Rothschild, A. M., Rothschild, Z.: Fibrinolytic activity evoked in the plasma of the normal and adrenalectomized rat by cellulose sulphate. Brit. J. Pharmacol. 45, 470—475 (1972)

Roubal, Z., Nemecek, O.: Antiinflammatory compounds exhibiting fibrinolytic activity. J. med. Chem. 9, 840—842 (1966)

Rüegg, M.: Fibrinolysis-enhancing effect and histamine releasing capacity of bisobrin in rats. In: Davidson, J. F., Samama, M., Desnoyers, P. (Eds.): Progress in Chemical Fibrinolysis and Thrombolysis, Vol. 1, pp. 401—405, New York: Raven 1975

Samama, M.: L'activité fibrinolytique induite par le nicotinate de theophylline. C. R. IIè Congrès International d'Angiologie, Darmstadt, 1963

Samama, M.: Oral fibrinolytic therapy. Folia haemat. (Lpz.) 103, 363—371 (1976)

Sandritter, W., Bergerhof, H. D., Kroker, R.: Morphologische Untersuchungen zur Wirkung des Heparins auf experimentelle Ausscheidungsthromben. Frankfurt. Z. Path. 65, 342 (1954)

Sandritter, W., Huppert, M., Schlueter, G.: Zur Frage der Fibrinolyse an experimentellen Gerinnungs- und Ausscheidungsthromben. Klin. Wschr. 36, 651—655 (1958)

Sandritter, W., Schlueter, G., Koeppel, G.: Thrombolyse im Tierexperiment. Untersuchungen mit einem Polysaccharidsulfoester und Streptokinase. Med. Welt (Stuttg.) 51, 2732—2739 (1964)

Sasaki, Y., Takeyama, S.: Inhibition of adrenaline-induced fibrinolysis by alpha-adrenergic blocking agents in the rat. Jap. J. Pharmacol. 22, (Suppl. 120) (1972)

Sasaki, Y., Takeyama, S.: Inhibition of adrenaline-induced fibrinolysis by alpha-adrenergic blocking agents in the rat. Jap. J. Pharmacol. 24, 737—745 (1974)

Schimpf, K., Petry, H. J., Lasch, H. G.: The effect of sympathetic and parasympathetic drugs on the human circulatory system. Dtsch. Arch. klin. Med. 205, 166—175 (1958)

Schneider, C. L., Engstrom, R. M., Miyazaki, Y.: Experimental production of massive vascular stasis stepwise. Fibrination, defibrination, acute cor pulmonale, and panhemostatic depletion. Proc. Intern. Congr. Hematol. 8th, Tokyo 3, 1618—1644 (1960)

Schor, J. M., Steinberger, V., Tutko, E., Aboulafia, S., Pachter, I. J., Jacobsen, R.: Studies with the synthetic fibrinolytic compound EN 1661. In: Schor, J. M. (Ed.): Chemical Control of Fibrinolysis-Thrombolysis, pp. 113—134. New York-London-Sydney-Toronto: Wiley Interscience 1970

Sherry, S.: Hemostatic mechanism and proteolysis in shock. Fed. Proc. 20, 209—218 (1961)

Sherry, S., Lindemeyer, R. I., Fletcher, A. P., Alkjaersig, N.: Studies on enhanced fibrinolytic activity in man. J. clin. Invest. 38, 810—822 (1959)

Shulman, S.: The effects of certain ions and neutral molecules on the conversion of fibrinogen to fibrin. Discussions Faraday Soc. 13, 109—115 (1953)

Sicuteri, F., Giotti, A., Fanciullacci, M., Brunetti, S.: A sulfarated amino acid as a fibrinolytic agent. Cardiov. Res. VI World Congr. Cardiol., 285 (1970)

Singh, J., Oester, Y. T.: Possible effect of nicotine on in vitro human blood coagulation time. Arch. int. Pharmacodyn. 148, 237—242 (1964a)

Singh, J., Oester, Y. T.: Nicotine antagonism with heparin. Possible mode of action on human blood coagulation time in vitro. Arch. int. Pharmacodyn. 149, 354—361 (1964b)

Soulier, J. P., Koupernik, C.: Constance de la fibrinolyse au cours du choc acetylcholinique. Sang 19, 362—369 (1948)

Spampinato, N.: Valutazione dell'attivita fibrinolitica ematica in pazienti trattati con complesso mucopolisaccaridico estrattivo. Minerva Med. 60 (Suppl. 99), 5068—5076 (1969)

Spreafico, P. L., Frandoli, G., Turazza, G.: Fibrinolysis and platelet aggregation in the course of treatment with a combination of p-chlorophenoxyisobutyric acid derivatives in elderly arterosclerotics. Arzneimittel-Forsch. 23, 236—239 (1973)

Stamm, H.: Über die pathologische Aktivierung der Blutfibrinolyse beim Menschen. Geburtsh. Frauenheilk. 24, 1034—1053 (1964)

Stüttgen, G.: Skin irritation, histamine, and blood coagulation. Dermatol. Wschr. 136, 1014—1020 (1957)

Sullenberger, J. W., Anlyan, W. G., Weaver, W. T.: Serotonin in intravascular thrombosis. Surgery 46, 22—29 (1959)

Tanser, A. R.: Fibrinolytic response to oral glucose. Lancet 1966 II, 147—148

Tanser, A. R., Smellie, H.: Observations on adrenaline induced fibrinolysis in man. Clin. Sci. 26, 375—380 (1964)

Tesi, M.: Aspects of clinical methodology in fibrinolytic therapy. In: Davidson, J. F., Samama, M., Desnoyers, P. (Eds.): Progress in Chemical Fibrinolysis and Thrombolysis, Vol. 1, pp. 255—265. New York: Raven 1975

Thomson, W. B., Green, J., Evans, I. L.: The effect of some physiological stimuli on fibrinolytic activity in man measured by the heparin fractionation method. J. clin. Pathol. 17, 341—344 (1964)

Todd, A. S.: The histological localisation of fibrinolysin activator. J. Path. Bact. 78, 281—283 (1959)

Toyoda, K., Shiokawa, Y.: Proteolytic enzyme activity. I: Effect of fatigue on fibrinolysis. Nisshin Igaku 37, 263—267 (1950)

Tsapogas, M. J., Cotton, L. T., Murray, J. G.: The effects of chlorpropamide on intermittent claudication and fibrinolysis. Lancet 1962 I, 1213—1215

Tsitouris, G., Sandberg, H., Bellet, S., Feinberg, L. J., Schraeder, J.: Effects of serotonin on inhibition of the plasmin-plasminogen fibrinolytic system in vitro. J. Lab. clin. Med. 59, 25—39 (1962)

Tudoranu, G., Foni, I., Toporas, P., Creteanu, G., Pavelescu, C.: Chemical anticoagulating agents. Sang 21, 511—514 (1950)

Turazza, G., Gibelli, A., de Nicola, P.: Fibrinolytic action of 7-(2-hydroxy-3-(N-2-hydroxycthyl-amino) propyl)-1,3-dimethylxanthine-pyridine-3-carboxylate (xanthinol nicotinate) and of 3-pyridine acetic acid, alone and associated. Farmaco, Ed. sci. 21, 416—429 (1966)

Vere, D. W., Fearnley, G. R.: Suspected interaction between phenindione and ethyloestrenol. Lancet 1968 II, 281

Verstraete, M.: The position of long-term stimulation of the endogenous fibrinolytic system: Present achievements and clinical perspectives. Thrombos. Diathes haemorrh. (Stuttg.) 34, 613—622 (1975)

Verstraete, M., Amery, A., Maes, H., Vermylen, J.: Influence of chlorpropamide and glucose on fibrinolytic activity. J. Lab. clin. Med. 61, 926—934 (1963)

Wagner, H.: Antagonistic action of histamine and vitamin E on blood coagulation. Ärztl. Wschr. 7, 248—250 (1952)

Wagner-Jauregg, T., Jahn, U., Bürlimann, W.: Fibrinolytische Antirheumatika. Vergleich von Substanzen der Flufenamsäure-Reihe mit Trifluormethyl-Analogen des Azapropazons. Arzneimittel-Forsch. 23, 911—913 (1973)

Walker, I. D., Davidson, J. F.: Long-term fibrinolytic enhancement with anabolic steroid therapy. A five year study. In: Davidson, J. F., Samama, M., Desnoyers, P. (Eds.): Progress in Chemical Fibrinolysis and Thrombolysis, Vol. 3. New York: Raven 1978

Walker, I. D., Davidson, J. F., Young, P., Conkie, J. A.: Plasma fibrinolytic activity following oral anabolic steroid therapy. Thrombos. Diathes. haemorrh. (Stuttg.) 34, 236—245 (1975a)

Walker, I. D., Davidson, J. F., Young, P., Conkie, J. A.: Effect of anabolic steroids on plasma antithrombin III, α_2 macroglobulin and α_1 antitrypsin levels. Thrombos. Diathes. haemorrh. (Stuttg.) 34, 106—114 (1975b)

Wasantapruek, S., Von Kaulla, K. N.: A serial microfibrinolysis test and its use in rats with liver by-pass. Thrombos. Diathes. haemorrh. (Stuttg.) **15**, 284—292 (1966)

Weiner, M., De Crinis, K., Redisch, W., Steele, M. J.: Influence of some vasoactive drugs on fibrinolytic activity. Circulation **19**, 845—848 (1959)

Weiner, M., Redisch, W., Steele, J. M.: Occurrence of fibrinolytic activity following administration of nicotinic acid. Proc. Soc. exp. Biol. (N.Y.) **98**, 755—761 (1958)

Weinland, G., Weinland, W. L.: The influence of acetylcholine and histamine on blood coagulation. Dtsch. Z. Nervenheilk. **163**, 125—130 (1949)

Wenzel, D. G., Singh, J.: Effect of nicotine and epinephrine on in vivo coagulation time in rabbits. J. pharm. Sci. **51**, 875—878 (1962)

Wilson, W., Fostiropoulos, G.: Observations on the use of nicotinic acid to induce in vivo fibrinolytic activity. Amer. J. med. Sci. **238**, 591 (1959)

Winther, O.: Testosteron and blood fibrinolytic activity. Lancet **1965 I**, 823

Winther, O.: Testosteron und fibrinolytische Aktivität. Vorläufige Mitteilung. Med. Welt (Stuttg.) **21**, 1180—1181 (1965 b)

Yamazaki, H., Sano, T., Odakura, T., Takeuchi, K., Matsumura, T., Hosaki, S., Shimamoto, T.: Appearance of thrombogenic tendency induced by adrenaline and its prevention by adrenergic blocking agent, nialamide and pyridinolcarbamate. Thrombos. Diathes. haemorrh. (Stuttg.) **26**, 251—263 (1971)

Yoshizaki, T.: Effects of cholinergic drugs and their blockers on adrenaline release from rat adrenal. Biochem. Pharmacol. **24**, 1401—1405 (1975)

Zunz, E.: The action of some hormones on the coagulation of blood. Ann. Bull. Soc. roy. Sci. Med. Nat. Bruxelles, **1—2**, 1—25 (1935)

Fibrinolytically Active Enzymes

Plasmin

K. C. ROBBINS

A. Plasminogen, the Zymogen Precursor of Plasmin

I. Preparation

Plasminogen, the zymogen precursor of plasmin, can be separated from mammalian plasmas, serums, and enriched plasma fractions (e.g., fractions III and III$_{2,3}$) by an affinity chromatography method with either L-lysine-substituted-Sepharose (DEUTSCH and MERTZ, 1970; ROBBINS and SUMMARIA, 1976) or polyacrylamide (RICKLI and CUENDET, 1971), and either p-aminobenzamidine-substituted Sepharose (HOLLEMAN et al., 1975) or n-butyl p-aminobenzoate-substituted Sepharose (ZOLTON and MERTZ, 1972). Heparin influences the affinity of human plasminogen for L-lysine-substituted Sepharose, and inhibits its elution by ε-aminocaproic acid (HATTON and REGOECZI, 1976). These zymogen preparation can also be prepared by ion-exchange and gel-filtration methods (ROBBINS and SUMMARIA, 1970; WALLÉN and WIMAN, 1970), and the affinity chromatography preparations can be further purified to homogeneity by both ion-exchange chromatography and gel-filtration methods (ROBBINS et al., 1975). Human native (Glu-plasminogen), and partially degraded (Lys-plasminogen) zymogens, have been prepared and characterized; the hydrodynamic properties of these forms are summarized in Table 1. Both forms of the zymogen contain different multiple isoelectric forms (WALLÉN and WIMAN, 1972; SUMMARIA et al., 1972; SUMMARIA et al., 1973a; ROBBINS and SUMMARIA, 1973; SUMMARIA et al., 1976), and they both differ in their hydrodynamic properties (Table 1), amino acid compositions (ROBBINS and SUMMARIA, 1970; ROBBINS and SUMMARIA, 1976), and NH$_2$-terminal sequences (WALLÉN and WIMAN, 1970; ROBBINS et al., 1972; ROBBINS et al., 1973b; WALTHER et al., 1974; SUMMARIA et al., 1975). The Lys-zymogen is a proteolytically altered Glu-zymogen, from which a small peptide(s) of molecular weight 1000–2000 is removed from the NH$_2$-terminal portion of the molecule by limited proteolysis (ROBBINS et al., 1975). Two major affinity chromatography forms, 1 and 2, have been isolated and characterized from both the human Glu- and Lys-zymogen forms by gradient elution from a L-lysine-substituted Sepharose column with a linear gradient of ε-aminocaproic acid (SUMMARIA et al., 1976). Glu-plasminogen can be converted to Lys-plasminogen by plasmin digestion (CLAEYS et al., 1973; VIOLAND and CASTELLINO, 1976). Met$_{69}$-plasminogen (WALLÉN and WIMAN, 1975) and Val$_{79}$-plasminogen (RICKLI and OTAVSKY, 1973) have been described in urokinase-activation mixtures. A low molecular weight form of human plasminogen has been prepared by limited proteolysis with pancreatic elastase (SOTTRUP-JENSEN et al., 1977). A low molecular weight form of sheep plasminogen has been prepared by limited proteolysis with sheep plasmin (PAONI and CASTELLINO, 1975).

Table 1. Hydrodynamic properties of human plasminogen, plasmin, and plasmin-derived heavy (A) and light (B) chains

	Plasminogen				Plasmin		Plasmin-derived chains			
	Native	$\bar{v}$[b]	Degraded[a]	$\bar{v}$	Native	$\bar{v}$	Heavy (A)	$\bar{v}$	Light (B)	$\bar{v}$
Molecular Weight										
1. Ultracentrifugation										
Yphantis method	92000[c] 92000[d]	0.706	90000[c] 83000[d]	0.709	81000[c]	0.713	69000[p] (Glu-2) 61500[p] (Lys-2)	0.703 0.703	24500[d] (Val-)	
absorption optics	83800[e]	0.709	82400[e] 81000[f]	0.714 0.715	76500[e] 75400[f]	0.714 0.715	57200[q] (Lys-) 48800[f] (Lys-)	0.720 0.715	25700[q] (Val-)	0.720
2. Gel filtration	87000[c] 90000[g]		86000[c] 105000[g]		76000[c]					
3. Acrylamide gel-dodecyl sulfate electrophoresis	93000[h] 93000[i] 92250[j] 90800[k] 87000[l] 91000[m] 93600[n] (Glu-1) 91600[n] (Glu-2)		86000[h] 89100[i] 84000[j] 84300[k] 80000[l] 87300[m] 89400[n] (Lys-1) 87900[n] (Lys-2)				68700[n] (Glu-1) 67000[n] (Glu-2) 64400[n] (Lys-1) 63300[n] (Lys-2) 60000[s] (Lys-) 55000[l] (Lys-)		24000[j] (Val-) 26000[l] (Val-)	
Sedimentation coefficients $s^0_{20,w}$(S)	5.0[e] 5.1[c] 5.7[i]		4.4[e] 4.8[c] 4.2[f] 4.5[i]		4.3[e] 4.3[c] 3.9[f]		2.3[q] (Lys-) 2.8[r] (Lys-) 3.9[p] (Lys-) 4.4[p] (Glu-)		1.4[q] (Val-)	
Frictional coefficients f/f^0	1.54[e] 1.50[c]		1.63[e] 1.56[c]		1.64[e] 1.55[c]					
Isoelectric points pI (major)	6.2, 6.3, 6.4, 6.6[o] 6.2, 6.4, 6.5, 6.6[k] 6.0, 6.1, 6.2, 6.4[g] 6.2, 6.3, 6.4, 6.6[n] (Glu-1) 6.4, 6.6[n] (Glu-2)		6.7, 7.2, 7.5, 7.8, 8.1[o] 6.6, 6.7, 7.1, 7.7, 8.0[k] 6.7, 7.2, 7.5[n] (Lys-1) 7.5, 7.8, 8.1[n] (Lys-2)		7.4, 7.7[t]		4.9[o] (Lys-)		5.8, 5.9, 6.0[o] (Val-)	

Immobilized forms of plasminogen have been prepared (RIMON and RIMON, 1974; CHIBBER et al., 1974).

II. Physical and Chemical Properties

The physical and chemical properties of human plasminogen and plasmin have been summarized in recent reviews (ROBBINS and SUMMARIA, 1970; ROBBINS and SUMMARIA, 1976). Some of these properties are summarized in Table 1; the physical and chemical properties of rabbit plasminogen and plasmin have been summarized in a recent review (CASTELLINO and SODETZ, 1976).

III. Primary Structure of Human Plasminogen

1. NH$_2$-Terminus (Glu$_1$-Lys$_{77}$)

The complete amino acid sequence of the NH$_2$-terminus of human plasminogen Glu$_1$-Lys$_{77}$ has been determined (Table 2A) (WIMAN and WALLÉN, 1975a); the NH$_2$-terminus contains two disulfide bonds, Cys$_{30}$-Cys$_{55}$ and Cys$_{35}$-Cys$_{43}$ (WIMAN, 1973). This part of the molecule appears to contain both activator (urokinase)- and plasmin-sensitive bonds, Lys$_{63}$-Ser, Arg$_{68}$-Met (WIMAN and WALLÉN, 1975a). It also contains a specific site (seven residues), Ala$_{45}$-Lys$_{51}$, which in the intact molecule interacts with a component of the heavy(A) chain (WALLÉN and WIMAN, 1975). There are a large number of Arg- and Lys-peptide bonds in this portion of the molecule. The development of Lys-plasminogen from Glu-plasminogen, differing in molecular weight by 1000–2000 (see Table 1), could involve the cleavage of a number of these

---

Footnotes to Table 1

[a] Met- and Lys-forms.
[b] Partial specific volume.

References

[c] SJÖHOLM et al., 1973.
[d] VIOLAND and CASTELLINO, 1976; BAJAJ and CASTELLINO, 1977; partially reduced and carboxymethylated.
[e] ROBBINS et al., 1975.
[f] BARLOW et al., 1969.
[g] WALLÉN and WIMAN, 1972.
[h] WIMAN and WALLÉN, 1973.
[i] CLAEYS and VERMYLEN, 1974.
[j] RICKLI, 1975; partially reduced and carboxymethylated.
[k] COLLEN et al., 1975.
[l] WALTHER et al., 1974; completely reduced and carboxymethylated.
[m] THORSEN and MÜLLERTZ, 1974.
[n] SUMMARIA et al., 1976; completely reduced and carboxymethylated.
[o] SUMMARIA et al., 1972; SUMMARIA et al., 1973a; completely reduced and carboxymethylated.
[p] GONZALEZ-GRONOW et al., 1977; partially reduced and carboxymethylated.
[q] SUMMARIA et al., 1967; completely reduced and carboxymethylated.
[r] SUMMARIA et al., 1971b; completely reduced and carboxymethylated.
[s] RICKLI and OTAVSKY, 1975; partially reduced and carboxymethylated.
[t] ROBBINS and SUMMARIA, 1973.

Table 2. Primary structure of human plasminogen partial sequences

---

A. NH$_2$-terminus[a] (Glu$_1$-Lys$_{77}$)
   Glu-Pro-Leu-Asp-Asp-Tyr-Val-Asn-Thr-Gln-Gly-Ala-Ser-Leu-Phe-Ser-Val-Thr-Lys-lys-
   Gln-Leu-Gly-Ala-Gly-Ser-Ile-Glu-Glu-Cys-Ala-Gln-Ala-Lys-Cys-Glu-Glu-Asp-Glu-Glu-
   Phe-Thr-Cys-Arg-Ala-Phe-Gln-Tyr-His-Ser-Lys-Glu-Gln-Glu-Cys-Val-Ile-Met-Ala-Glu-
   Asn-Arg-Lys-Ser-Ser-Ile-Ile-Arg-Met-Ser-Asp-Val-Val-Leu-Phe-Glu-Lys-

B. *Sequence around sensitive* Arg$_{560}$-*Val activation peptide bond*[b]   UK
   -Cys-Gly-Lys-Pro-Gln-Val-Glu-Pro-Lys-Lys-Cys-Pro-Gly-Arg$\perp$Val-Gly-Gly-Cys-Val-
   Ala-His-Pro-His-Ser-Trp-Pro-Trp-

C. *Sequence around active center serine of light (B) chain*[c]
   -Ser-Cys-Gln-Gly-Asp-Ser*-Gly-Gly-Pro-Leu-Val-Cys-Phe-Glu-Lys-Asp-Lys-Tyr-

D. *Sequence around active center histidine of light (B) chain*[d]
   -His$_{25}$-Phe-Cys-Gly-Gly-Thr-Leu-Ile-Ser-Pro-Glu-Trp-Val-Leu-Ser-Ala-Ala-His*-Cys-Leu-

---

References
[a] WIMAN and WALLÉN, 1975a.
[b] WIMAN and WALLÉN, 1975b; SOTTRUP-JENSEN et al., 1975.
[c] GROSKOPF et al., 1969b.
[d] ROBBINS et al., 1973a.

bonds, including Lys$_{63}$-Ser and Arg$_{68}$-Met, with the release of some peptide material, and with the residual peptides still attached to the molecule. In acrylamide gel-dodecyl sulfate electrophoresis, these residual peptides are removed, and then Lys-plasminogen has the same molecular weight as Lys-plasmin (see Table 1). The NH$_2$-terminal 12-residue sequence of rabbit plasminogen is identical to the human sequence (CASTELLINO et al., 1973). In the cat sequence, Glu$_1$ is replaced by Asp$_1$, in the bovine sequence, Glu$_1$-Pro is replaced by Asp$_1$-Leu, and in the dog sequence, the NH$_2$-terminus is blocked (ROBBINS et al., 1973b).

2. Heavy(A) Chain (Lys$_{78}$-Arg$_{560}$)

The amino acid sequence of the heavy(A) chain portion of human plasminogen has been reported (CLAEYS et al., 1976; MAGNUSSON et al., 1976; LEE and LAURSEN, 1976; SOTTRUP-JENSEN et al., 1978). The amino acid sequence of a large cyanogen-bromide fragment (122 residues) (WIMAN and WALLÉN, 1975b) and a chymotryptic fragment (38 residues) (SOTTRUP-JENSEN et al., 1975) containing the activation site peptide bond "Arg$_{560}$-Val" was determined. A portion of this sequence is shown in Table 2B, which contains the first 24 residues of the light(B) chain with a COOH-terminal Met$_{24}$. Seventeen of the disulfide bonds are in this part of the molecule (the position of 34 Cys-residues has been determined). The heavy(A) chain contains five cringle-like structures similar to those found in bovine prothrombin, in which 20 amino acid positions are identical. Two oligosaccharide groups have been found in this part of the molecule; a glucosamine-based oligosaccharide is attached to Asn$_{288}$, and is present in about one-half of the molecules, and a galactose-based oligosaccharide is attached to Thr$_{345}$, and varies in carbohydrate composition. There appears to be more than one lysine-binding site on the heavy(A) chain (WALLÉN and WIMAN, 1975; SOTTRUP-JENSEN et al., 1978; WIMAN and WALLÉN, 1977). These bindings sites are probably NH_2-terminal to Val_{442}, since a large fragment prepared from an elastase-digest of plasminogen, of molecular weight approximately 38000 containing approximately 350 residues, and starting with Val_{442}, does not adsorb to L-lysine-substituted Sepharose. The heavy(A) chain also contains a benzamidine-binding site that appears to be different from the lysine-binding site (HOLLEMAN et al., 1975). The 4-NH_2-terminal residue sequences of the isolated human and rabbit heavy(A) chains are identical; in the dog sequence, Lys_{78}-Val_{79} is replaced by Arg_{78}-Ile_{79}, and in the cat and bovine sequences, Val_{79} is replaced by Ile_{79} (ROBBINS et al., 1973 b).

3. Light(B) Chain (Val_{561}-Asn_{790}, or Val_1-Asn_{230})

Portions of the amino acid sequence of the light(B) chain of human plasminogen have been determined. The NH_2-terminal 24-residue sequence of the human light(B) chain has been determined (Val_1-Met_{24}) (ROBBINS et al., 1973 b; WIMAN and WALLÉN, 1975 b); the NH_2-terminal 21-residue sequences of isolated cat, dog, rabbit, and bovine light(B) chains were found to be homologous with this sequence, and they contained fourteen identical residues (ROBBINS et al., 1973 b). The evolutionary changes in this portion of the molecule appear to be in the pairs of basic residues at positions 8 and 10, and 20 and 21, and in the pairs of neutral residues at positions 16 and 17. In the bovine light(B) chain, Val_1 is replaced by Ile_1 and Val_{17}, or Ile_{17}, is replaced by Ser_{17}. Cys_5 was determined to be the interchain disulfide bond connecting the heavy(A) and light(B) chains of human plasmin.

The isolated light(B) chain contains the active center of plasmin (SUMMARIA and ROBBINS, 1976 b); a single DFP-sensitive residue (SUMMARIA et al., 1967 b) and a single TLCK-sensitive histidine residue (GROSKOPF et al., 1969 a; ROBBINS et al., 1973 a) is located on this chain of the enzyme. The partial 18-residue amino acid sequence of a tryptic peptide containing the active center serine residue was determined (Table 2C) (GROSKOPF et al., 1969 b) and found to be homologous with the active center serine sequences determined for other serine proteases (HARTLEY, 1970). The partial NH_2-terminal 20-residue amino acid sequence of a large COOH-terminal cyanogen bromide fragment, of approximately 205 residues, of the light (B) chain containing the active center histidine residue ("histidine loop") was determined (Table 2D) (ROBBINS et al., 1973 a). It was found to be homologous to the "histidine loop" sequences of other serine proteases (HARTLEY, 1969).

Apparently, four intrachain disulfide bonds are found in the light(B) chain (SOTTRUP-JENSEN et al., 1978) and are located in the same positions as four of the intrachain disulfide bonds in chymotrypsin (HARTLEY, 1969). Using the chymotrypsin numbering system for this chain, these bonds are probably Cys_{42}-Cys_{58}, Cys_{136}-Cys_{201}, Cys_{168}-Cys_{182}, and Cys_{191}-Cys_{220}. Two interchain disulfide bridges have been reported from sequence analysis connecting the light(B) chain to the heavy(A) chain (SOTTRUP-JENSEN et al., 1978); one interchain disulfide bond had been previously reported by chemical methods (ROBBINS et al., 1977). One interchain disulfide bridge is probably Cys_{20} (chymotrypsin numbering) or Cys_5, of the light(B) chain that connects to Cys_{557} of the heavy(A) chain. This "disulfide loop" contains the essential Arg_{560}-Val bond, which is cleaved during activation of plasminogen, and the activation site "Arg_{560}-Val" loop contains 7 residues between the Cys-residues, 4 residues (Val-Val-Gly-Gly) are COOH-terminal, and 3 residues (Pro-Gly-

Arg) are NH_2-terminal to the essential activation site peptide bond. The second interchain disulfide bridge is probably Cys_{122} (chymotrypsin numbering system), or Cys_{107}, of the light(B) chain, which connects to Cys_{547} of the heavy(A) chain, which is fourteen residues NH_2-terminal to the essential activation site peptide bond. In chymotrypsin, Cys_{122} of the B chain is connected to Cys_1 of the A chain (HARTLEY, 1969).

A functionally active human plasmin-derived light(B) chain has been isolated containing three carboxymethylated cysteines (SUMMARIA and ROBBINS, 1976), indicating the cleavage of probably two interchain and one intrachain disulfide bonds. This functionally active light(B) chain contains the streptokinase-binding site of plasminogen (SUMMARIA and ROBBINS, 1976).

IV. Activation of Human Plasminogen

1. Mechanism

The mechanism of activation of human plasminogen, a single-chain zymogen, by specific activators, involves the cleavage of from one to three specific peptide bonds, to form a two-chain enzyme (heavy(A) and light(B) chains) (ROBBINS et al., 1973 b; WIMAN and WALLÉN, 1973; WALTHER et al., 1974; McCLINTOCK et al., 1974; VIOLAND and CASTELLINO, 1976). The major peptide bonds cleaved are: *1*, Arg_{68}-Met; *2*, Lys_{77}-Lys; *3*, Arg_{560}-Val. Two of these peptide bonds (bonds *2* and *3*) cleave at bond (bond *3*) is cleaved when some plasmin inhibitors, e.g. Aprotinin (SUMMARIA et al., 1974; BAJAJ and CASTELLINO, 1977), and in the presence of varying concentrations of lysine and/or ε-aminocaproic acid (WALTHER et al., 1975). Only one peptide bond (bond *3*) is cleaved when some plasmin inhibitors, e.g., Trasylol (SUMMARIA et al., 1975; VIOLAND and CASTELLINO, 1976), leupeptin (SUMMARIA et al., 1977), $α_1$-antitrypsin (SUMMARIA et al., 1977), and antithrombin III plus heparin (SUMMARIA et al., 1977) are present in the activation mixture. Bond *3* is also cleaved when the equimolar human Glu-plasminogen-streptokinase complex converts to the Glu-plasmin-streptokinase complex (SUMMARIA et al., 1975; VIOLAND and CASTELLINO, 1976). The cleavage of the two NH_2-terminal peptide bonds (bonds *1* and *2*) appears to be by formed plasmin after the Arg_{560}-Val bond is cleaved. Lys_{78}-plasmin is formed from Glu-plasminogen after the essential Arg_{560}-Val peptide bonde (bond*3*) is first cleaved by the specific activator, followed by the cleavage of the Lys_{77}-Lys peptide bond. The rate of cleavage of bonds *1* and *2* is faster than the rate of cleavage of bond *3* (WALTHER et al., 1975). Activation with insoluble urokinase results in the formation of Met_{69}-plasmin (and plasminogen) involving cleavage of bonds *1* and *3* (WIMAN and WALLÉN, 1973). In Glu-plasminogen activation systems without inhibitors, the Lys-plasminogen form is rapidly produced before Lys_{78}-plasmin is produced (WALTHER et al., 1974). In Glu-plasminogen activation systems containing protein, or peptide inhibitors, the Glu-plasmin form is produced with little or no Lys_{77}-plasminogen or Lys_{78}-plasmin produced (SUMMARIA et al., 1975; VIOLAND and CASTELLINO, 1976). A des-Lys_{78}-plasmin form (Val_{79}-plasmin) is found in activation mixtures, probably arising from both Lys_{78}-plasminogen and Lys_{78}-plasmin by cleavage of the Lys_{78}-Val peptide bond (ROBBINS et al., 1972). The physiologic form of human plasmin has not as yet been determined. All mammalian plasminogens studied, e.g., cat, dog, rabbit, and bovine zymogens, appear to be activated by urokinase by the same mechanism (SUMMARIA et al., 1973b; SODETZ and CASTELLINO, 1975).

2. Kinetics

Steady state kinetics of activation have been carried out with human plasminogen as the substrate, and with the following as activators: streptokinase (ALKJAERSIG et al., 1958; WOHL et al., 1978), with urokinase (NANNINGA and GUEST, 1968; CHRISTENSEN and MÜLLERTZ, 1977), staphylokinase (KOWALSKA-LOTH and ZAKRZEWSKI, 1975), with equimolar streptokinase complexes of human plasminogen and plasmin (BUCK and BOGGIANO, 1971; WOHL et al., 1978), and the equimolar streptokinase-plasmin-derived light(B) chain complex (WOHL et al., 1978). With urokinase, the conversion of Lys-plasminogen to plasmin was coupled with the plasmin-catalyzed hydrolysis of N-α-benzoyl-L-arginine ethyl ester (at pH 7.8 and 25° C) (CHRISTENSEN and MÜLLERTZ, 1977). The $K_{m(app)}$ value was 40.7 μM, and the k_{cat} value was 2.6/s. With streptokinase, and with the equimolar streptokinase complexes, the conversion of Lys-plasminogen to plasmin was coupled with the plasmin-catalyzed hydrolysis of N-α-carbobenzoxy-L-lysine-p-nitrophenyl ester (at pH 6.0 and 30° C) (WOHL et al., 1978). The $K_{m(app)}$ values were about 1.2 μM, and the k_{cat} values were about 22/s for these activators. The equimolar light(B) chain-streptokinase gave the same $K_{m(app)}$ value but the k_{cat} value was 50.8/s. The $K_{m(app)}$ value for urokinase with this substrate was 2.8 μM and the k_{cat} value was 3.5/s. Glu-plasminogen activation proceeded at one-third the rate of Lys-plasminogen activation with the same $K_{m(app)}$ value.

B. Plasmin

I. Preparation

Different enzyme forms (Glu-plasmin and Lys-plasmin) can be prepared from human plasminogen, depending upon the nature of the zymogen preparation (e.g., Glu- or Lys-forms, affinity chromatography forms 1 and 2, and isoelectric forms), the activator used, and the conditions for activation. The form of plasmin produced in an activation system depends upon a combination of many different factors: the molar ratios of plasminogen to activator, the relative concentrations of glycerol, lysine, and/or ε-aminocaproic acid, the pH, temperature and time of activation, the absence or presence of a plasmin inhibitor, and its relative effectiveness and reversibility. Trace amounts of highly purified activators, e.g., urokinase or streptokinase, are used in activation mixtures to prepare human Lys-plasmin (ROBBINS and SUMMARIA, 1970); the solvent systems usually contain glycerol in order to protect the enzyme from autolysis. Lys-plasmin reference standards are available in 50% glycerol (KIRKWOOD et al., 1975). In the equimolar human Glu-plasminogen-streptokinase complex, the zymogen is activated to Glu_1-plasmin and then to Lys_{78}-plasmin, with the loss of peptides (SUMMARIA et al., 1974; BAJAJ and CASTELLINO, 1977). In the equimolar human Lys-plasminogen-streptokinase complex, the zymogen converts

only to Lys_{78}-plasmin (SUMMARIA et al., 1974). Human Glu_1-plasmin can be prepared by activation of the zymogen with urokinase in the presence of reversible
plasmin inhibitors, e.g., Aprotinin, the basic bovine trypsin-kallikrein inhibitor (KU-
NITZ) (SUMMARIA et al., 1975; VIOLAND and CASTELLINO, 1976), and streptomyces
leupeptin (SUMMARIA et al., 1977) or irreversible plasmin inhibitors, human plasma
α_1-antitrypsin, and antithrombin III plus heparin (SUMMARIA et al., 1977). Degraded
and smaller forms of plasmin have been prepared by autolysis (TAKEDA and NAKA-
BAYASHI, 1974). Immobilized forms of plasmin have also been prepared (CHIBBER et
al., 1974).

II. Physical and Chemical Properties

The physical and chemical properties of human Lys-plasmin have been summarized
in recent reviews (ROBBINS and SUMMARIA, 1970; ROBBINS and SUMMARIA, 1976) and
some of the hydrodynamic properties are summarized in Table 1. Also, the physical
and chemical properties of rabbit plasmin have been summarized in a recent review
(CASTELLINO and SODETZ, 1976 b).

III. Nomenclature

The form of plasminogen that is the reference for nomenclature purposes is the
native human plasminogen (Glu-plasminogen) (JACKSON, 1977). The general numbering and nomenclature system is represented schematically in Table 3.

IV. Assay Methods

Plasmin is a serine protease with trypsinlike specificity (TROLL et al., 1954; SHERRY et
al., 1966; ROBBINS and SUMMARIA, 1970; WEINSTEIN and DOOLITTLE, 1972). It cleaves
proteins and peptides at arginyl and lysyl peptide bonds, and basic amino acid esters,
and amides. The enzyme has a preference for lysyl peptide bonds in some proteins
and in ester substrates. Functional assay methods for the zymogen (after activation)
and the enzyme have been described using protein substrates JOHNSON et al. (ROBBINS
and SUMMARIA, 1970, 1969; SCHMER and KRYS, 1974; ONG and JOHNSON, 1976),
synthetic ester substrates (SHERRY et al., 1966; CHRISTENSEN, 1975) and nitroanilide
substrates (CHRISTENSEN and MÜLLERTZ, 1974; CLAESON et al., 1978). Specific active
site titration methods have been developed to determine the enzyme concentration
in solution (CHASE and SHAW, 1969; CHRISTENSEN and MÜLLERTZ, 1974; COLEMAN
et al., 1976), and to identify the active site in the zymogen (MCCLINTOCK and BELL,
1971; REDDY and MARKUS, 1972; SCHICK and CASTELLINO, 1974). Fluorometric
(BELL et al., 1974; KESSNER and TROLL, 1976), radioimmunoassays (RABINER et al.,
1969), and specific inhibitor assays (GANROT, 1967) have been described. The enzymatic activity in equimolar plasminogen-streptokinase and plasmin-streptokinase
complexes can also be determined (REDDY and MARKUS, 1974; WOHL et al., 1977).
Methods for determining the concentration of zymogen and enzyme have been
described that utilize specific interactions with streptokinase (GAJEWSKI and MAR-
KUS, 1968). Human plasmin reference preparations have been developed (KIRK-
WOOD et al., 1975).

Table 3. Human plasminogen

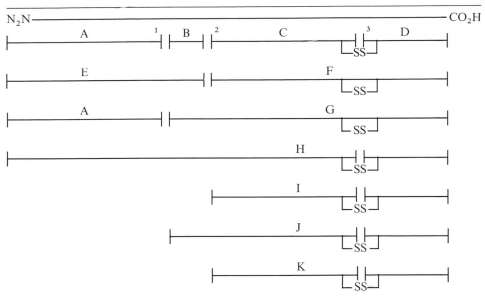

A = Plasminogen Fragment 1 (Res 1–68)
B = Plasminogen Fragment 2 (Res 69–77)
C = Plasmin heavy chain
D = Plasmin light chain
E = Plasminogen Fragment 1 · 2
F = Preplasmin 2
G = Preplasmin 1
H = Meizoplasmin
I = Plasmin
J = Meizoplasmin 1 (des Fragment 1)
K = Plasmin (des Lys_{78})
    I differs from K in that K has amino acid residue Val_{79} as its NH_2-terminals

The concentration of plasminogen in normal human plasma has been determined by different types of methods, i.e., immunochemical, proteolytic, and fibrinolytic, and the results obtained vary with the assay method used. The methods giving the highest values were radioimmunoassay (RABINER et al., 1969) (19–22 mg/100 ml) and affinity chromatography followed by absorbance measurements (ZOLTON et al., 1972) (19–20 mg/100 ml). Functional assays gave lower values: affinity chromatography followed by a solid-phase radioimmunoassay (casein substrate) (SCHMER and KRYS, 1974) (approximately 12 mg/100 ml, corrected to 8 mg/100 ml), fibrinogenolytic-kinetic assay (NANNINGA, 1975) (approximately 7 mg/100 ml). Human plasma contains approx. 2.2 CTA U of plasminogen/ml (SASAHARA et al., 1973), which can be converted to a concentration of approx. 7 mg plasminogen/100 ml, using a specific activity of 30 CTA U of plasminogen/mg protein, the approximate specific activity of pure plasminogen (ROBBINS and SUMMARIA, 1976). The functional assays using whole plasma and measuring plasmin in the presence of different plasmin inhibitors on protein substrates are not quantitative; the use of synthetic substrates for these assays have been described by CLAESON et al. (1978). The concept of complete conversion of plasminogen to the equimolar plasminogen-streptokinase and plasmin-streptokinase complexes with streptokinase and measuring enzyme (or activator) activity is possible (HEIMBURGER, 1975).

V. Kinetic Parameters

Steady state kinetic parameters K_m and k_{cat} (V_{max}) have been determined for human plasmin (SILVERSTEIN, 1973; CHRISTENSEN and MÜLLERTZ, 1974; BELL et al., 1974; REDDY and MARKUS, 1974; SILVERSTEIN, 1975; CHRISTENSEN, 1975; KOSOW, 1975; COLEMAN et al., 1976; WOHL et al., 1977) and rabbit plasmin (SODETZ et al., 1976) and for the equimolar streptokinase complexes with human plasminogen and plasmin (BELL et al., 1974; REDDY and MARKUS, 1974; WOHL et al., 1977), and the equimolar streptokinase-plasmin-derived light (B) chain (WOHL et al., 1977). The K_m values for human plasmin can vary from about 14µM with N-α-carbobenzoxy-L-lysine-p-nitrophenyl ester (at pH 6.0, and 25°–30° C) (SILVERSTEIN, 1973; SILVERSTEIN, 1975; WOHL et al., 1977) to about 6500 µM with N-α-tosyl-L-arginine methyl ester (at pH 8.0 and 30° C) (BROCKWAY and CASTELLINO, 1971), with an intermediate value of about 220–360 µM with N-α-benzoyl-L-arginine ethyl ester (at pH 7.2–7.3 and 25° C) (SILVERSTEIN, 1975; CHRISTENSEN, 1975). The K_m and V_{max} values for the rabbit plasmin affinity chromatography forms 1 and 2 were similar (SODETZ et al., 1976). The k_{cat} value for human plasmin, with N-α-carbobenzoxy-L-lysine-p-nitrophenyl ester, was 22–24/s (at pH 6.0, and 25°–30° C) (SILVERSTEIN, 1973; SILVERSTEIN, 1975; WOHL et al., 1977). The k_{cat}/K_m value for this substrate is about 800 times the k_{cat}/K_m value for N-α-benzoyl-L-arginine ethyl ester (SILVERSTEIN, 1975). In the human plasmin-catalyzed hydrolysis of both N-α-benzoyl-L-arginine-ethyl and -methyl esters (at 25° C) in the pH range of 5.8–9.0, the K_M and k_{cat} values were found to be pH dependent (CHRISTENSEN, 1975). The K_m was pH dependent only in the pH 8.0–9.0 range, and the k_{cat} only in the 6.0–7.0 range. Plasmin catalysis appears to be affected by two ionizing groups, one with a pK equal to 6.5 (perhaps "active site" histidine), and one with a pK equal to 8.4 (perhaps NH_2-terminal valine of the light (B) chain). The K_m value for human plasmin with H-D-valine-L-leucine-L-lysine-p-nitroanilide (at pH 7.4 and 37° C) was 300µM (CLAESON et al., 1978).

The K_m values for various human equimolar plasminogen, plasmin, and plasmin-derived light (B) chain complexes with streptokinase have varied from 14–33 µM with N-α-carbobenzoxy-L-lysine-p-nitrophenyl ester (at pH 6.0 and 30° C) (WOHL et al., 1977). The K_m values for the plasmin-derived light (B) chain and for a plasminogen form with an active site (plasminogen*) were 83 µM, and 42 µM, respectively (WOHL et al., 1977). The k_{cat} values for all of these streptokinase complexes with the same substrate were the same as the k_{cat} value for plasmin, namely 22/s. This indicates that streptokinase (or each of its high molecular weight proteolytically produced forms), which is tightly bound to plasminogen, plasmin, and the plasmin-derived light (B) chain in the complex, has little, if any, effect on the kinetic properties of the enzyme. The k_{cat} value of the plasmin-derived light (B) chain was 2.1/s. With N-α-acetyl-L-lysine-methyl ester (at pH 8.5 and 37° C) and N-α-tosyl-L-argininemethyl ester (at pH 8.0 and 25° C), the K_m and V_{max} values for the equimolar plasmin-streptokinase complex were three times higher than the corresponding values for plasmin and the equimolar plasminogen-streptokinase complex (REDDY and MARKUS, 1974). With N-α-methyl-N-α-tosyl-L-lysine β-napthol ester (at pH 7.0 and 25° C), the K_m and V_{max} values for plasmin and the equimolar plasmin-streptokinase complex were similar (BELL et al., 1974).

The active site of human plasmin and the equimolar streptokinase complexes with plasminogen, plasmin, and the plasmin-derived light (B) chain can be titrated with p-nitrophenyl-p'-guanidinobenzoate (CHASE and SHAW, 1969), which permits the determination of the concentration of active sites (at pH 8.3 and 22°–25° C) (WOHL et al., 1977). This substrate has a very low k_{cat}. This method depends upon the rapid acylation of the enzyme with stoichiometric presteady state release of nitrophenol ("burst" reaction), followed by a very slow deacylation due to the stability of the p-guanidino-benzoyl-plasmin. The active site of human plasmin has also been titrated with N-α-benzoyl-L-arginine-p-nitroanilide (at pH 7.8 and 25° C) using presteady state kinetic methods (CHRISTENSEN and MÜLLERTZ, 1974).

C. Human Plasmin-Derived Heavy (A) and Light (B) Chains

The heavy (A) and light (B) chains of plasmin are located in the NH_2-terminal and COOH-terminal positions, respectively, of the enzyme (ROBBINS et al., 1967; SUMMARIA et al., 1967a). The chains of human plasmin are apparently connected by one (ROBBINS et al., 1967; SUMMARIA et al., 1967a; RICKLI and OTAVSKY, 1975) or two (SOTTRUP-JENSEN et al., 1978) interchain disulfide bonds, which can be selectively cleaved by reducing agents (RICKLI and OTAVSKY, 1975; SUMMARIA and ROBBINS, 1976; GONZALEZ-GRONOW et al., 1977). After reduction of these interchain disulfide bond(s) and carboxymethylation of the sulfhydryl groups, the mixture of partially reduced heavy (A) and light (B) chains can be separated by an affinity chromatography method with a L-lysine-substituted Sepharose column (RICKLI and OTAVSKY, 1975; SUMMARIA and ROBBINS, 1976b; GONZALEZ-GRONOW et al., 1977). The heavy (A) chain is readily adsorbed to the lysine residue of the adsorbent, apparently through the same binding site that is found on the zymogen (RICKLI and OTAVSKY, 1975; WIMAN and WALLÉN, 1977). The light (B) chain is not adsorbed (RICKLI and OTAVSKY, 1975; SUMMARIA and ROBBINS, 1976), and has been prepared as a functionally active component (SUMMARIA and ROBBINS, 1976); the active center, or catalytic site of the enzyme is located on the light (B) chain (SUMMARIA et al., 1967b; GROSKOPF et al., 1969a). The heavy (A) chain is readily eluted from the L-lysine-substituted Sepharose column by ε-aminocaproic acid under conditions similar to those described for the elution of plasminogen. This method has been used to describe and prepare both Glu_1- and Lys_{78}-heavy (A) chains (RICKLI and OTAVSKY, 1975; SUMMARIA and ROBBINS, 1976; GONZALEZ-GRONOW et al., 1977) and the Val_{561}-light(B) chain (SUMMARIA and ROBBINS, 1976). Extensive reduction and alkylation of mammalian plasmins result in a mixture of heavy (A) and light(B) chains that cannot be separated by the specific affinity chromatography method but can be separated by either gel filtration (SUMMARIA et al., 1967b; SUMMARIA and ROBBINS, 1971b; WI-MAN and WALLÉN, 1973; SUMMARIA et al., 1975; SODETZ and CASTELLINO, 1975) or dialysis (GROSKOPF et al., 1969a). The hydrodynamic properties of the human heavy(A) and light(B) chains are summarized in Table 1.

D. Equimolar Plasminogen-Streptokinase, Plasmin-Streptokinase, and Plasmin-Derived Light(B) Chain-Streptokinase Complexes

I. Preparation

Both human plasminogen and plasmin form equimolar complexes with streptoki-nase, an indirect plasminogen activator (ZYLBER et al., 1959; KLINE and FISHMAN, 1961; DAVIES et al., 1964; LING et al., 1965; ROBBINS and SUMMARIA, 1970; ROBBINS and SUMMARIA, 1976; CASTELLINO et al., 1976a). Stoichiometric complexes also are formed with cat, dog, and rabbit plasminogens (SUMMARIA et al., 1974). A series of transformations takes place in the equimolar human plasminogen-streptokinase complex involving both proteins. The first reaction is the formation of an intact complex; plasminogen is immediately transformed into a zymogen with an active site (plasminogen*) without any apparent bond cleavages (McCLINTOCK and BELL, 1971; REDDY and MARKUS, 1972; REDDY and MARKUS, 1973; SCHICK and CASTELLI-NO, 1974; McCLINTOCK et al., 1974; BAJAJ and CASTELLINO, 1977). Plasminogen* is next converted to Glu-plasmin by a single specific bond cleavage (bond 3), and then to Lys-plasmin by one or two additional bond cleavages (bonds 1 and 2) with the liberation of peptides (SUMMARIA et al., 1974; McCLINTOCK et al., 1974; BAJAJ and CASTELLINO, 1977), probably by intermolecular reactions. In the complex, streptoki-nase is specifically cleaved continuously, probably also by intermolecular reactions (limited proteolysis), to give a series of high molecular weight components, each differing in molecular weight by about 4000–5000 (McCLINTOCK et al., 1974; BROCK-WAY and CASTELLINO, 1974; SIEFRING and CASTELLINO, 1976; CASTELLINO et al., 1976a). Four major degraded streptokinase components (SK 1, SK 2, SK 3, and SK 4) have been identified (SUMMARIA et al., 1974; McCLINTOCK et al., 1974; BROCK-WAY and CASTELLINO, 1974; SIEFRING and CASTELLINO, 1976), and two of these components, SK 2 and SK 4 (SK 4′) have been prepared and characterized (BROCK-WAY and CASTELLINO, 1974; SIEFRING and CASTELLINO, 1976). A plasmin-streptoki-nase complex has been isolated containing streptokinase fragment SK 5 of approxi-mately 9000 in molecular weight (SUMMARIA et al., 1971a). Streptokinase fragment SK 2, molecular weight 36000, behaves like native streptokinase in activation of human plasminogen (BROCKWAY and CASTELLINO, 1974). During these transforma-tions all components of the streptokinase molecule appear to be attached to zymo-gen, or zymogen*, or enzyme, in the complex (LING et al., 1967; SUMMARIA et al., 1971a; SUMMARIA et al., 1974; McCLINTOCK et al., 1974).

The functionally active human plasmin-derived light(B) chain also combines stoichiometrically with streptokinase to form a complex (SUMMARIA and ROBBINS, 1976). The binding site for streptokinase in the plasminogen molecule is only on that portion of the molecule COOH-terminal to Arg_{560}-Val, or on the light(B) chain structural component. The heavy(A) chain does not combine stoichiometrically with streptokinase (GONZALEZ-GRONOW et al., 1977). The streptokinase component in this complex goes through similar proteolytic transformations, as is seen in the human plasminogen-streptokinase complex, but not beyond SK 2 (WOHL et al., 1977).

II. Plasminogen Activator Activity

The plasminogen activator activities of equimolar streptokinase complexes with human plasminogen, plasmin and plasmin-derived light(B) chain are dependent upon both the character of the plasminogen component in the complex, and the character, or stage of fragmentation, of the streptokinase component in the complex, SKa-SKf (MARKUS et al., 1976). The plasminogen or plasmin complexes with the highest activator activities are those that contain intact streptokinase, or high molecular weight fragments of this molecule. The activator activities of the plasmin-derived light(B) chain complexes are higher than those found for the zymogen or enzyme complexes (WOHL et al., 1977), with no apparent relationship to the character of the streptokinase moiety, although usually mixtures of SK, SK 1, or SK 2 are found in these light(B) chain complexes. The active center of the activator is located on the plasmin moiety of the complex with both single DFP-sensitive serine and single TLCK-sensitive histidine residues (SUMMARIA et al., 1968; BUCK et al., 1968).

The equimolar human zymogen- or enzyme-streptokinase complex is the most active plasminogen activator of the mammalian complexes; the plasminogen species, e.g., cat and dog, which are not readily activated by streptokinase and form equimolar complexes with streptokinase, have low human and bovine plasminogen activator activities (SUMMARIA et al., 1974). In all of the mammalian plasminogen-streptokinase complexes studied, the proteolytic fragmentation of streptokinase appears to be identical, but the rate of fragmentation appears to be different for each species (SUMMARIA et al., 1974). Those species of plasminogen that cannot be activated by streptokinase, e.g., bovine plasminogen, do not react to form a complex, apparently due to the lack of a binding site for streptokinase in the COOH-terminal or light(B) chain portion of the zymogen.

E. Limited Proteolysis of Protein Substrates

Limited proteolysis of human fibrinogen, a three-chain molecule, by human plasmin results in the formation of the major plasmic fragments X, Y, D, and E, as well as major peptide fractions P 1 and P 2, with two fragment D species and one fragment E species coming from a single fibrinogen molecule (PIZZO et al., 1972; BUDZYNSKI et al., 1974; MIHALYI et al., 1976). The molecular weights for fibrinogen and fragments X, Y, D, and E, are approximately 340000, 240000, 145000, 92000, and 50000, respectively, with the fragment D species showing a great deal of heterogeneity. The peptide fractions P 1 and P 2 have molecular weights of about 27000 and 18000, respectively. A peptide fragment H, which could be peptide P 2, of approximate molecular weight of 20000, appears early in the plasmic cleavage of fibrinogen, non-cross-linked and cross-linked fibrin, originating from the Aα-chain (HARFENIST and CANFIELD, 1975). The plasmic degradation of cross-linked fibrin results in a fragment

D with a molecular weight of about 184000 (FERGUSON et al., 1975). Four early plasmin peptide bond attack points have been located in a 38-residue midsection piece of the Aα-chain of human fibrinogen, which has one of the two α-chain cross-linking acceptor sites. This piece of chain is adjacent to and overlapping with one of the two molecular weight peptides, probably P 2, that is released during plasmin digestion and contains the second α-chain crosslinking acceptor site (TAKAGI and DOOLITTLE, 1975). This peptide, which could also be fragment H, is rich in hydrophilic residues, especially serine, glycine, and proline, and a low content of hydrophobic residues.

Human growth hormone retains its biologic activity after limited proteolysis by human plasmin (LI and GRÁF, 1974). Specific cleavages occur at Arg_{134}-Thr and Lys_{140}-Glu with liberation of a hexapeptide, and the two fragments are connected by a single disulfide bond at Cys_{53}-Cys_{165}. The two fragments, after reduction and alkylation, were found to possess some biologic activity. After recombination by noncovalent forces, the molecule was found to have nearly full biologic activity (LI and BEWLEY, 1976). Limited proteolysis of human placental lactogen (which is homologous to human growth hormone—167 of the 191 amino acids are identical) by human plasmin results in the retention of full biologic activity (RUSSELL et al., 1977); a single peptide bond is cleaved, resulting in two fragments held together by a single disulfide bond, without the liberation of any peptide material. Limited proteolysis of human haptoglobin 1–1 by human plasmin occurs at a single Lys_{128}-Phe bond of the β-chain (HAY et al., 1977).

References

Alkjaersig, N., Fletcher, A. P., Sherry, S.: The activation of human plasminogen. II. A kinetic study of activation with trypsin, urokinase, and streptokinase. J. biol. Chem. **233**, 86—90 (1958)

Bajaj, S. P., Castellino, F. J.: Activation of human plasminogen by equimolar levels of streptokinase. J. biol. Chem. **252**, 492—498 (1977)

Barlow, G. H., Summaria, L., Robbins, K. C.: Molecular weight studies on human plasminogen and plasmin at the microgram level. J. biol. Chem. **244**, 1138—1141 (1969)

Bell, P. H., Dziobkowski, C., Englert, M. E.: A sensitive fluorometric assay for plasminogen, plasmin, and streptokinase. Anal. Biochem. **61**, 200—208 (1974)

Brockway, W. J., Castellino, F. J.: The mechanism of the inhibition of plasmin activity by ε-aminocaproic acid. J. biol. Chem. **246**, 4611—4617 (1971)

Brockway, W. J., Castellino, F. J.: A characterization of native streptokinase and altered streptokinase isolated from a human plasminogen activator complex. Biochemistry **13**, 2063—2070 (1974)

Buck, F. F., Boggiano, E.: Interaction of streptokinase and human plasminogen. VI. Function of the streptokinase moiety in the activator complex. J. biol. Chem. **246**, 2091—2096 (1971)

Buck, F. F., Hummel, B. C. W., De Renzo, E. C.: Interaction of streptokinase and human plasminogen. V. Studies on the nature and mechanism of formation of the enzymatic site of the activator complex. J. biol. Chem. **243**, 3648—3654 (1968)

Budzynski, A. Z., Marder, V. J., Shainoff, J. R.: Structure of plasmic degradation products of human fibrinogen. Fibrinopeptide and polypeptide chain analysis. J. biol. Chem. **249**, 2294—2302 (1974)

Castellino, F. J., Siefring, G. E., Jr., Sodetz, J. M., Bretthauer, R. K.: Amino terminal amino acid sequences and carbohydrate of the two major forms of rabbit plasminogen. Biochem. Biophys. Res. Commun. **53**, 845—851 (1973)

Castellino, F. J., Sodetz, J. M.: Rabbit plasminogen and plasmin isozymes. In: Lorand, L. (Ed.): Methods in Enzymology, Vol. 45, pp. 273—286. New York: Academic Press 1976

Castellino, F. J., Sodetz, J. M., Brockway, W. J., Siefring, G. E., Jr.: Streptokinase. In: Lorand, L. (Ed.): Methods in Enzymology, Vol. 45, pp. 244—257. New York: Academic Press 1976a

Chase, T., Jr., Shaw, E.: Comparison of the esterase activities of trypsin, plasmin, and thrombin on Guanidinobenzoate esters. Titration of the enzymes. Biochemistry 8, 2212—2224 (1969)

Chibber, A. K., Leadbetter, M. G., Mertz, T.: Immobilized human plasmins: preparation and enzymatic properties. Prep. Biochem. 4, 315—330 (1974)

Christensen, U.: PH Effects in plasmin-catalysed hydrolysis of α-N-benzoyl-L-arginine compounds. Biochim. biophys. Acta (Amst.) 397, 459—467 (1975)

Christensen, U., Müllertz, S.: Mechanism of reaction of human plasmin with α-N-benzoyl-L-arginine-p-nitroanilide. Titration of the enzyme. Biochim. biophys. Acta (Amst.) 334, 187—198 (1974)

Christensen, U., Müllertz, S.: Kinetic studies of the urokinase catalysed conversion of NH_2-terminal lysine human plasminogen to plasmin. Biochim. biophys. Acta (Amst.) 480, 275—281 (1977)

Claeson, G., Aurell, L., Karlsson, G., Friberger, P.: Substrate structure and activity relationships. In: Davidson, J. F., M. Samama, P. Desnoyers (Eds.): Progress in Chemical Fibrinolysis and Thrombolysis. Vol. 3. pp. 299—304. New York: Raven Press 1978

Claeys, H., Molla, A., Verstraete, M.: Conversion of NH_2-terminal glutamic acid to NH_2-terminal lysine human plasminogen by plasmin. Thrombos. Res. 3, 515—523 (1973)

Claeys, H., Sottrup-Jensen, L., Zajdel, M., Petersen, T. E., Magnusson, S.: Multiple gene duplication in the evolution of plasminogen. Five regions of sequence homology with the two internally homologous structures in prothrombin. FEBS Letters 61, 20—24 (1976)

Claeys, H., Vermylen, J.: Physico-chemical and proenzyme properties of NH_2-terminal glutamic acid and NH_2-terminal lysine human plasminogen. Influence of 6-aminohexanoic acid. Biochim. biophys. Acta (Amst.) 342, 351—359 (1974)

Coleman, P. L., Latham, H. G., Jr., Shaw, E. N.: Some sensitive methods for the assay of trypsin-like enzymes. In: Lorand, L. (Ed.): Methods in Enzymology, Vol. 45, pp. 12—26. New York: Academic Press 1976

Collen, D., Ong, E. B., Johnson, A. J.: Human plasminogen: In vitro and in vivo evidence for the biological integrity of NH_2-terminal glutamic acid plasminogen. Thrombos. Res. 7, 515—529 (1975)

Davies, M. C., Englert, M. E., deRenzo, E. C.: Interaction of streptokinase and human plasminogen. I. Combining of streptokinase- and plasminogen observed in the ultracentrifuge under a variety of experimental conditions. J. biol. Chem. 239, 2651—2656 (1964)

Deutsch, D. G., Mertz, E. T.: Plasminogen: purification from human plasma by affinity chromatography. Science 170, 1095—1096 (1970)

Ferguson, E. W., Fretto, L. J., McKee, P. A.: A re-examination of the cleavage of fibrinogen and fibrin by plasmin. J. biol. Chem. 250, 7210—7218 (1975)

Gajewski, J., Markus, G.: A new method for plasminogen standardization. Thrombos. Diathes. haemorrh. (Stuttg.) 20, 548—554 (1968)

Ganrot, P. O.: On the determination of molar concentration of plasmin and plasmin inhibitors. Acta chem. scand. 21, 595—601 (1967)

Gonzalez-Gronow, M., Violand, B. N., Castellino, F. J.: Purification and some properties of the Glu- and Lys-human plasmin heavy chains. J. biol Chem. 252, 2175—2177 (1977)

Groskopf, W. R., Hsieh, B., Summaria, L., Robbins, K. C.: Studies on the active center of human plasmin. The serine and histidine residues. J. biol. Chem. 244, 359—365 (1969a)

Groskopf, W. R., Summaria, L., Robbins, K. C.: Studies on the active center of human plasmin. Partial amino acid sequence of a peptide containing the active center serine residue. J. biol. Chem. 244, 3590—3597 (1969b)

Harfenist, E. J., Canfield, R. E.: Degradation of fibrinogen by plasmin. Isolation of an early cleavage product. Biochemistry 14, 4110—4117 (1975)

Hartley, B. S.: Homologies in serine proteinases. Phil. Trans. roy. Soc. Lond. [B] 257, 77—87 (1970)

Hatton, M. W. C., Regoeczi, E.: The effect of heparin on the affinity chromatography of human plasminogen. In: Peeters, H. (Ed.): Protides of the Biological Fluids—23 Colloquium, pp. 545—549. Oxford-New York: Pergamon Press 1976

Hay, R. E., Kurosky, A., Bowman, B. H.: Limited proteolysis of haptoglobin from different species by human plasmin. Fed. Proc. **36**, 825 (1977)

Heimburger, N.: Plasminogen assay: a review and evaluation of various methods. In: Davidson, J. F., Samama, M. M., Desnoyers, P. C. (Eds.): Progress in Chemical Fibrinolysis and Thrombolysis, Vol. 1, pp. 173—179. New York: Raven Press 1975

Holleman, W. H., Andres, W. W., Weiss, L. J.: The relationship between the lysine and the p-aminobenzamidine binding sites on human plasminogen. Thrombos. Res. **7**, 683—693 (1975)

Jackson, C. M.: Recommended nomenclature of blood clotting zymogens and zymogen activation products of the International Committee on Thrombosis and Haemostasis. Thrombos. Hemostas. **38**, 567—577 (1977)

Johnson, A. J., Kline, D. L., Alkjaersig, N.: Assay methods and standard preparations for plasmin, plasminogen and urokinase in purified systems. Thrombos. Diathes. haemorrh. **21**, 259—272 (1969)

Kessner, A., Troll, W.: Fluorometric microassay of plasminogen activators. Arch. Biochem. Biophys. **176**, 411—416 (1976)

Kirkwood, T. B. L., Campbell, P. J., Gaffney, P. J.: A standard for human plasmin. Thrombos. Diathes. haemorrh. (Stuttg.) **34**, 20—31 (1975)

Kline, D. L., Fishman, J. B.: Proactivator function of human plasmin as shown by lysine esterase assay. J. biol. Chem. **236**, 2807—2812 (1961)

Kosow, D. P.: Kinetic mechanism of the activation of human plasminogen by streptokinase. Biochemistry **14**, 4459—4465 (1975)

Kowalska-Loth, B., Zakrzewski, K.: The activation by staphylokinase of human plasminogen. Acta Biochim. Polon. **22**, 327—339 (1975)

Lee, H.-M., Laursen, A.: The primary structure of human plasminogen: characterization and alignment of the cyanogen bromide peptides. FEBS Letters **67**, 113—118 (1976)

Li, C. H., Bewley, T. A.: Human pituitary growth hormone: Restoration of full biological activity by noncovalent interaction of two fragments of the hormone. Proc. nat. Acad. Sci. (Wash.) **73**, 1476—1479 (1976)

Li, C. H., Gráf, L.: Human pituitary growth hormone: Isolation and properties of two biologically active fragments from plasmin digests. Proc. nat. Acad. Sci. (Wash.) **71**, 1197—1201 (1974)

Ling, C.-M., Summaria, L., Robbins, K. C.: Mechanism of formation of bovine plasminogen activator from human plasmin. J. biol. Chem. **240**, 4213—4218 (1965)

Ling, C.-M., Summaria, L., Robbins, K. C.: Isolation and characterization of bovine plasminogen activator from a human plasminogen-streptokinase mixture. J. biol. Chem. **242**, 1419—1425 (1967)

Magnusson, S., Sottrup-Jensen, L., Petersen, T. E., Dudek-Wojciechowska, G., Claeys, H.: Homologous "kringle" structures common to plasminogen and prothrombin. Substrate specificity of enzymes activating prothrombin and plasminogen. In: Ribbons, D. W., Brew, K. (Eds.): Proteolysis and Physiological Regulation, Vol. 11, pp. 203—235. New York: Academic Press 1976

Markus, G., Evers, J. L., Hobika, G. H.: Activator activities of the transient forms of the human plasminogen-streptokinase complex during its proteolytic conversion to the stable activator complex. J. biol. Chem. **251**, 6495—6504 (1976)

McClintock, D. K., Bell, P. H.: The mechanism of activation of human plasminogen by streptokinase. Biochem. Biophys. Res. Commun. **43**, 694—702 (1971)

McClintock, D. K., Englert, M. E., Dziobkowski, C., Snedeker, E. H., Bell, P. H.: Two distinct pathways of the streptokinase-mediated activation of highly purified human plasminogen. Biochemistry **13**, 5334—5344 (1974)

Mihalyi, E., Weinberg, R. M., Towne, D. W., Friedman, M. E.: Proteolytic fragmentation of fibrinogen. I. Comparison of the fragmentation of human and bovine fibrinogen by trypsin or plasmin. Biochemistry **15**, 5372—5381 (1976)

Nanninga, L. B.: Molar concentrations of fibrinolytic components, especially free fibrinolysin, in vivo. Thrombos. Diathes. haemorrh. (Stuttg.) **33**, 244—255 (1975)

Nanninga, L. B., Guest, M. M.: Activity-pH relationship and Michaelis constants during activation of profibrinolysin and during fibrinogenolysis. Thrombos. Diathes. haemorrh. (Stuttg.) **19**, 492—498 (1968)

Ong, E. B., Johnson, A. J.: Protamine, a substrate for thrombolytic agents and enzymes of similar specificity. Anal. Biochem. **75**, 568—582 (1976)

Paoni, N. F., Castellino, F. J.: Isolation of a low molecular weight form of plasminogen. Biochem. Biophys. Res. Commun. **65**, 757—764 (1975)

Pizzo, S. V., Schwartz, M. L., Hill, R. L., McKee, P. A.: The effect of plasmin on the subunit structure of human fibrinogen. J. biol. Chem. **247**, 636—645 (1972)

Rabiner, S. F., Goldfine, I. D., Hart, A., Summaria, L., Robbins, K. C.: Radioimmunoassay of human plasminogen and plasmin. J. Lab. clin. Med. **74**, 265—273 (1969)

Reddy, K. N. N., Markus, G.: Mechanism of activation of human plasminogen by streptokinase. Presence of active center in streptokinase-plasminogen complex. J. biol. Chem. **247**, 1683—1694 (1972)

Reddy, K. N. N., Markus, G.: Further evidence for an active center in streptokinase-plasminogen complex. Interaction with pancreatic trypsin inhibitor. Biochem. Biophys. Res. Commun. **51**, 672—679 (1973)

Reddy, K. N. N., Markus, G.: Esterase activities in the zymogen moiety of the streptokinase-plasminogen complex. J. biol. Chem. **249**, 4851—4857 (1974)

Rickli, E. E.: Human plasminogen: A summary of studies on its isolation, characterization and activation mechanism. Immunochemistry **12**, 629—632 (1975)

Rickli, E. E., Cuendet, P. A.: Isolation of plasmin-free human plasminogen with N-terminal glutamic acid. Biochim. biophys. Acta (Amst.) **250**, 447—451 (1971)

Rickli, E. E., Otavsky, W. I.: Release of an N-terminal peptide from human plasminogen during activation with urokinase. Biochim. biophys. Acta (Amst.) **295**, 381—384 (1973)

Rickli, E. E., Otavsky, W. I.: A new method of isolation and some properties of the heavy chain of human plasmin. Europ. J. Biochem. **59**, 441—447 (1975)

Rimon, A., Rimon, A.: Immobilized components of the plasmin system. In: Salmona, M., Saronio, C., Garattini, S. (Eds.): Insolubilized Enzymes, pp. 135—141. New York: Raven Press 1974

Robbins, K. C., Bernabe, P., Arzadon, L., Summaria, L.: The primary structure of human plasminogen. I. The NH_2-terminal sequences of human plasminogen and the S-carboxymethyl heavy (A) and light (B) chain derivatives of plasmin. J. biol. Chem. **247**, 6757—6762 (1972)

Robbins, K. C., Bernabe, P., Arzadon, L., Summaria, L.: The primary structure of human plasminogen. II. The histidine loop of human plasmin light (B) chain active center histidine sequence. J. biol. Chem. **248**, 1631—1633 (1973a)

Robbins, K. C., Bernabe, P., Arzadon, L., Summaria, L.: NH_2-terminal sequences of mammalian plasminogens and plasmin S-carboxymethyl heavy (A) and light (B) chain derivatives. A reevaluation of the mechanism of activation of plasminogen. J. biol. Chem. **248**, 7242—7246 (1973b)

Robbins, K. C., Boreisha, I. G., Arzadon, L., Summaria, L.: Physical and chemical properties of the NH_2-terminal glutamic acid and lysine forms of human plasminogen and their derived plasmins with an NH_2-terminal lysine heavy (A) chain. Comparative data. J. biol. Chem. **250**, 4044—4047 (1975)

Robbins, K. C., Summaria, L.: Human plasminogen and plasmin. In: Perlman, G. E., Lorand, L. (Eds.): Methods in Enzymology, Vol. 19, pp. 184—199. New York: Academic Press 1970

Robbins, K. C., Summaria, L.: Isoelectric focusing of human plasminogen, plasmin, and derived heavy (A) and light (B) chains. Ann. N.Y. Acad. Sci. **209**, 397—404 (1973)

Robbins, K. C., Summaria, L.: Plasminogen and plasmin. In: Lorand, L. (Ed.): Methods in Enzymology, Vol. 45, pp. 257—273. New York: Academic Press 1976

Robbins, K. C., Summaria, L., Hsieh, B., Shah, R. J.: The peptide chains of human plasmin. Mechanism of activation of human plasminogen to plasmin. J. biol. Chem. **242**, 2333—2342 (1967)

Russell, J., Katzhendler, J., Kowalski, K., Schneider, A. B.: Limited plasmin cleavage of human placental lactogen: Preparation of an active modified hormone. Abstracts 59th Ann. Meeting of the Endocrine Soc. p. 111 (1977)

Sasahara, A. A., Hyers, T. M., Cole, C. M., Ederer, F., Murray, J. A., Wenger, N. K., Sherry, S., Stengle, J. M.: The urokinase pulmonary embolism trial. A national cooperative study. Circulation **47** (Suppl. II), 33—37 (1973)

Schick, L. A., Castellino, F. J.: Interaction of streptokinase and rabbit plasminogen. Biochemistry **12**, 4315—4321 (1973)

Schick, L. A., Castellino, F. J.: Direct evidence for the generation of an active site in the plasmino-gen moiety of the streptokinase-human plasminogen activator complex. Biochem. Biophys. Res. Commun. **57**, 47—54 (1974)

Schmer, G., Krys, J.: A solid-phase radioassay for plasminogen in human plasma. J. Lab. clin. Med. **83**, 153—163 (1974)

Sherry, S., Alkjaersig, N., Fletcher, A. P.: Activity of plasmin and streptokinase-activator on sub-stituted arginine and lysine esters. Thrombos. Diathes. haemorrh. (Stuttg.) **16**, 18—31 (1966)

Siefring, G. E., Jr., Castellino, F. J.: Interaction of streptokinase with plasminogen. Isolation and characterization of a streptokinase degradation product. J. biol. Chem. **251**, 3913—3920 (1976)

Silverstein, R. M.: The plasmin-catalyzed hydrolysis of N-α-CBZ-L-lysine-p-nitrophenyl ester. Thrombos. Res. **3**, 729—736 (1973)

Silverstein, R. M.: The determination of human plasminogen using N-α-CBZ-L-lysine-p-nitro-phenyl ester as substrate. Anal. Biochem. **65**, 500—506 (1975)

Sjöholm, I., Wiman, B., Wallén, P.: Studies on the conformational changes of plasminogen in-duced during activation to plasmin and by 6-aminohexanoic acid. Europ. J. Biochem. **39**, 471—479 (1973)

Sodetz, J. M., Castellino, F. J.: The mechanism of activation of rabbit plasminogen by urokinase. J. biol. Chem. **250**, 3041—3049 (1975)

Sodetz, J. M., Violand, B. N., Castellino, F. J.: A kinetic characterization of the rabbit plasmin isozymes. Arch. Biochem. Biophys. **174**, 209—215 (1976)

Sottrup-Jensen, L., Zajdel, M., Claeys, H., Petersen, T. E., Magnusson, S.: Amino acid sequence of activation cleavage site in plasminogen: Homology with "pro" part of prothrombin. Proc. nat. Acad. Sci. (Wash.) **72**, 2577—2581 (1975)

Sottrup-Jensen, L., Claeys, H., Zajdel, M., Petersen, T. E., Magnusson, S.: The primary structure of human plasminogen: Isolation of two lysine-binding fragments and one "mini"-plasminogen (M.w. 38000) by elastase-catalyzed specific limited proteolysis. In: Davidson, J. F., M. Samama, P. Desnoyers, (Eds.): Progress in chemical fibrinolysis and thrombolysis, Vol. 3. pp. 191—209, New York: Raven Press 1978

Summaria, L., Arzadon, L., Bernabe, P., Robbins, K. C.: Studies on the isolation of the multiple molecular forms of human plasminogen and plasmin by isoelectric focusing methods. J. biol. Chem. **247**, 4691—4702 (1972)

Summaria, L., Arzadon, L., Bernabe, P., Robbins, K. C.: Isolation, characterization, and compari-son of the S-carboxymethyl heavy (A) and light (B) chain derivatives of cat, dog, rabbit, and bovine plasmins. J. biol. Chem. **248**, 6522—6527 (1973 b)

Summaria, L., Arzadon, L., Bernabe, P., Robbins, K. C.: The interaction of streptokinase with human, cat, dog, and rabbit plasminogens. The fragmentation of streptokinase in the equi-molar plasminogen-streptokinase complexes. J. biol. Chem. **249**, 4760—4769 (1974)

Summaria, L., Arzadon, L., Bernabe, P., Robbins, K. C.: The activation of plasminogen to plasmin by urokinase in the presence of the plasmin inhibitor Trasylol. The preparation of plasmin with the same NH₂-terminal heavy (A) chain sequence as the parent zymogen. J. biol. Chem. **250**, 3988—3995 (1975)

Summaria, L., Arzadon, L., Bernabe, P., Robbins, K. C., Barlow, G. H.: Characterization of the NH₂-terminal lysine forms of human plasminogen isolated by affinity chromatography and isoelectric focusing methods. J. biol. Chem. **248**, 2984—2991 (1973 a)

Summaria, L., Boreisha, I. G., Arzadon, L., Robbins, K. C.: Activation of human Glu-plasmi-nogen to Glu-plasmin by urokinase in presence of plasmin inhibitors. Streptomyces leupeptin and human plasma α₁-antitrypsin and antithrombin III (plus heparin). J. biol. Chem. **252**, 3945—3951 (1977)

Summaria, L., Hsieh, B., Groskopf, W. R., Robbins, K. C., Barlow, G. H.: The isolation and charac-terization of the S-carboxymethyl β (light) chain derivative of human plasmin. The localiza-tion of the active site on the β (light) chain. J. biol. Chem. **242**, 5046—5052 (1967 b)

Summaria, L., Hsieh, B., Robbins, K. C.: The specific mechanism of activation of human plasmi-nogen to plasmin. J. biol. Chem. **242**, 4279—4283 (1967 a)

Summaria, L., Ling, C.-M., Groskopf, W. R., Robbins, K. C.: The active site of bovine plasminogen activator. Interaction of streptokinase with human plasminogen and plasmin. J. biol. Chem. **243**, 144—150 (1968)

Summaria, L., Robbins, K. C.: Isolation of a human plasmin-derived, functionally active, light (B) chain capable of forming with streptokinase an equimolar light (B) chain-streptokinase complex with plasminogen activator activity. J. biol. Chem. **251**, 5810—5813 (1976)

Summaria, L., Robbins, K. C., Barlow, G. H.: Dissociation of the equimolar human plasmin-streptokinase complex. Partial characterization of the isolated plasmin and streptokinase moieties. J. biol. Chem. **246**, 2136—2142 (1971a)

Summaria, L., Robbins, K. C., Barlow, G. H.: Isolation and characterization of the S-carboxymethyl heavy chain derivative of human plasmin. J. biol. Chem. **246**, 2143—2146 (1971b)

Summaria, L., Spitz, F., Arzadon, L., Boreisha, I. G., Robbins, K. C.: Isolation and characterization of the affinity chromatography forms of human Glu- and Lys-plasminogens and plasmins. J. biol. Chem. **251**, 3693—3699 (1976)

Takagi, T., Doolittle, R. F.: Amino acid sequence studies on the α-chain of human fibrinogen. Location of four plasmin attack points and a covalent cross-linking site. Biochemistry **14**, 5149—5156 (1975)

Takeda, Y., Nakabayashi, M.: Physicochemical and biological properties of human and canine plasmins. J. clin. Invest. **53**, 154—162 (1974)

Thorsen, S., Müllertz, S.: Rate of activation and electrophoretic mobility of unmodified and partially degraded plasminogen. Effects of 6-aminohexanoic acid and related compounds. Scand. J. clin. Invest. **34**, 167—176 (1974)

Troll, W., Sherry, S., Wachman, J.: The action of plasmin on synthetic substrates. J. biol. Chem. **208**, 85—93 (1954)

Violand, B. N., Castellino, F. J.: Mechanism of the urokinase-catalyzed activation of human plasminogen. J. biol. Chem. **251**, 3906—3912 (1976)

Wallén, P., Wiman, B.: Characterization of human plasminogen. I. On the relationship between different molecular forms of plasminogen demonstrated in plasma and found in purified preparations. Biochim. biophys. Acta (Amst.) **221**, 20—30 (1970)

Wallén, P., Wiman, B.: Characterization of human plasminogen. II. Separation and partial characterization of different molecular forms of human plasminogen. Biochim. biophys. Acta (Amst.) **257**, 122—134 (1972)

Wallén, P., Wiman, B.: On the generation of intermediate plasminogen and its significance for activation. In: Reich, E., Rifkin, D. B., Shaw, E. (Eds.): Proteases and Biological Control. Cold Spring Harbor Conferences on Cell Proliferation, Vol. 2, pp. 291—303. New York: Cold Spring Harbor Lab. 1975

Walther, P. J., Hill, R. L., McKee, P. A.: The importance of the preactivation peptide in the two-stage mechanism of human plasminogen activation. J. biol. Chem. **250**, 5926—5933 (1975)

Walther, P. J., Steinman, H. M., Hill, R. L., McKee, P. A.: Activation of human plasminogen by urokinase. Partial characterization of a pre-activation peptide. J. biol. Chem. **249**, 1173—1181 (1974)

Weinstein, M. J., Doolittle, R. F.: Differential specificities of thrombin, plasmin, and trypsin with regard to synthetic and natural substrates and inhibitors. Biochim. biophys. Acta (Amst.) **258**, 577—590 (1972)

Wiman, B.: Primary structure of peptides released during activation of human plasminogen by urokinase. Europ. J. Biochem. **39**, 1—9 (1973)

Wiman, B., Wallén, P.: Activation of human plasminogen by an insoluble derivative of urokinase. Structural changes of plasminogen in the course of activation to plasmin and demonstration of a possible intermediate compound. Europ. J. Biochem. **36**, 25—31 (1973)

Wiman, B., Wallén, P.: Structural relationship between "glutamic acid" and "lysine" forms of human plasminogen and their interaction with the NH_2-terminal activation peptide as studied by affinity chromatography. Europ. J. Biochem. **50**, 489—494 (1975a)

Wiman, B., Wallén, P.: Amino-acid sequence of the cyanogen-bromide fragment from human plasminogen that forms the linkage between the plasmin chains. Europ. J. Biochem. **58**, 539—547 (1975b)

Wiman, B., Wallén, P.: The specific interaction between plasminogen and fibrin. A physiological role of the lysine binding site in plasminogen. Thrombos. Res. **10**, 213—222 (1977)

Wohl, R. C., Arzadon, L., Summaria, L., Robbins, K. C.: Comparison of the esterase and human plasminogen activator activities of various activated forms of human plasminogen and their equimolar streptokinase complexes. J. biol. Chem. **252**, 1141—1147 (1977)

Wohl, R. C., Summaria, L., Arzadon, L., Robbins, K. C.: Steady state kinetics of activation of human and bovine plasminogens by streptokinase and its equimolar complexes with various activated forms of human plasminogen. J. biol. Chem. **253**, 1402—1407 (1978)

Zolton, R. P., Mertz, E. T.: Studies on plasminogen. X. Isolation of plasminogen by affinity chromatography using sepharose-butesin. Canad. J. Biochem. **50**, 529—527 (1972)

Zolton, R. P., Mertz, E. T., Russell, H. T.: Assay of human plasminogen in plasma by affinity chromatography. Clin. Chem. **18**, 654—657 (1972)

Zylber, J., Blatt, W. F., Jensen, H.: Mechanism of bovine plasminogen activation by human plasmin and streptokinase. Proc. Soc. exp. Biol. (N.Y.) **102**, 755—761 (1959)

Fungal Proteases

W. H. E. Roschlau

Introduction

Living organisms are traditionally divided into plants and animals, even after the study of microscopic life demonstrated the existence of groups of organisms that represent transitional beings which cannot be assigned dogmatically to either kingdom; for in some of their characteristics they may resemble plants, but in others they may be more like animals. An example of such diversity of form are the *fungi*, whose evolution—whether from algae by loss of chlorophyll (plants), or from pre-protozoa (animals)—is still the subject of debate. Thus, while the fungi might properly be regarded as a separate kingdom, they are by tradition plants of the division Mycota, which is subdivided into classes, orders, families, genera, and species on the basis of morphology and reproductive processes.

To define fungi in a general way is hardly possible if one considers the infinite variety of this form of life. However, with the exception of the slime molds (the Myxomycetes) which are ameboid bodies without cell walls, there are certain morphologic features that are common to most or all true fungi: they have no chlorophyll, they possess true nuclei in their cells, they have cell walls containing cellulose and/or chitin, they reproduce by means of spores, and most possess some kind of sexual mechanism. Fungi usually grow as multicellular thread-like, branching bodies (filaments) which intertwine to form networks (mycelium). They are thus distinguished from the yeasts which are unicellular organisms. The multicellular filaments of fungi are capable of growth, and fragments from almost any part of a fungus can give rise to a new individual. There is usually little differentiation between somatic structures; the mycelium of higher fungi, however, is capable of division of labor.

In their natural environment, *parasitic* fungi obtain their nutrients on the surface or within a living host, while *saprophytic* fungi grow on dead organic matter which they decompose. Most fungi, however, can sustain themselves on dead material such as artificial or synthetic media. While different fungi have different optimal nutritional requirements, some can subsist on almost any organic matter, and the ability to utilize available food substances is governed to a large extent by the enzymes a fungus is capable of producing. These enzymes are heterogeneous mixtures with very broad spectra of activity and specificity, conferring on certain fungi a considerable measure of adaptability. Examples of such omnivorous fungi are *Penicillium* species and *Aspergillus* species, the common green and black molds.

There are said to be about 100000 species of mycota. Of specific importance to man, however, are the pathogenic species causing most of the plant diseases in economic crops as well as a variety of mycotic infections in man and animals, and the nonpathogenic species that are used in fermentation processes required for the preparation of certain foodstuffs, in the production of organic acids and vitamins, and for the manufacture of many antibiotic drugs. Thus, while it was known for many years that fungi produce substances and mixtures of enzymes (antibiotics, amylases, collagenases, proteases, peptidases, etc.) of potential or proven industrial and medicinal value, their systematic study was complicated by the enormous number and variety of strains, the complexity of fungal enzymes, and the difficulties in isolation, separation and purification of activities. Since fungal proteases rarely have a single specific action, such proteases as have been isolated are classified according to the pH optimum of the major component on casein, gelatin, or hemoglobin substrates as acidic, neutral, or alkaline protease. Thus, acidic proteases have been obtained from various *Aspergillus* species (*A. niger*, *A. awamori*, *A. saitoi*, *A. oryzae*), neutral proteases from *A. oryzae*, *A. sojae*, *Rhizopus*, *Penicillium*, and *Trichothecium* species, and alkaline proteases from *A. oryzae, A. ochraceus*, some other types of *Aspergilli*, and from *Penicillium* species.

Interest in the exploration of fungal proteases as fibrinolytic agents for the treatment of thrombosis awakened with the report by STEFANINI and MARIN (1958) on the screening of 160 nonpathogenic fungi for fibrinolytic activity, and the identification of two strains of *A. oryzae* as the most likely producers of a high-activity and relatively fibrin-specific proteolytic enzyme. Once stimulated, this work was followed up by a number of investigators, resulting in the production, characterization, and biological evaluation of three proteases (of which the two preparations from *A. oryzae* are considered to be identical) that are now in varying stages of clinical study:

A1. Strain *A. oryzae* B-1273
Principal investigator: R. BERGKVIST, AB Astra, Södertälje, Sweden. Enzyme known as: Protease I, Astra 1652, brinase, brinastrase.

A2. Strain *A. oryzae* B-1273 WA-12 Connaught
Principal investigators: A. L. TOSONI et al., Connaught Medical Research Laboratories, University of Toronto, Canada[1]. Enzyme known as: CA-7, brinase, brinolase.

B. Strain *A. ochraceus* Wilhelm 1079 (IMET PA 126)
Principal investigators: H. TÖPFER et al., VEB Arzneimittelwerk Dresden, German Democratic Republic. Enzyme known as: Ocrase.

Work has also been published on proteases other than from *Aspergillus*, and clinical evaluation of the thrombolytic properties of these enzymes may be expected:

C. Strain *Trichothecium roseum* LINK et FR. "D"
Principal investigators: G. W. ANDREENKO et al., Faculty of Soil Science and Biology, Moscow State University, Moscow, USSR. Enzyme known as: Tricholysin.

D. Strain *Armillaria mellea* ACC 3253, ACC 3659 (FPRL 6H)
Principal investigators: D. BROADBENT et al., Imperial Chemical Industries Limited, Macclesfield, England. Enzyme known as: AM protease.

The commitment to explore fungal enzymes and to carry the investigation through its successive stages of development, was shown to require substantial investments in manpower and in research and production facilities over long periods of time, progressive input from a variety of biomedical specialties, and a receptive clinical community.

The search for promising strains usually began with the screening of known species, which have been obtained from fungus collections of one or the other governmental, industrial, or scientific agencies. STEFANINI and MARIN (1958), for example, screened 160 fungi to find four producers; KOCH (1974) reported on the screening of 200 fungi of which 11 had fibrinolytic activity; and ANDREENKO et al. (1974) examined 207 variants of strain *T. roseum* before deciding on a maximum producer of fibrinolytic activity. KOCH (1974) recommended that successful cultures should, if possible, be subjected to selective breeding in an effort to increase production of a specific (and often inducible) activity and to adapt the strain to more favorable or convenient temperature and pH optima. Another possibility to increase yields and specificity of activity may be through mutation by chemical or physical means, which has been done successfully at the Connaught Medical Research Laboratories with *A. oryzae* B-1273 to yield variants WB-7 and WA-12 Connaught (TOSONI and GLASS, 1963; Connaught Medical Research Laboratories, 1972).

---

[1] Since 1972: Connaught Laboratories Limited, Willowdale, Ontario, Canada.

Once an activity had been demonstrated, and a product of highest possible purity had been obtained, pharmacologic and toxicologic examination was indicated at the earliest possible time in order to avoid the inadvertent development (and associated expenditures) of products with pharmacologically identifiable adverse effects or clinically objectionable characteristics. The early rejection of questionable products and the exploration of alternative strains was likely to be more prudent than to persist and invest in attempts to "purify" a product that presented obvious pharmacologic and toxicologic difficulties.

The cumulative experience with fungal proteases to date has shown that initial expectations for substances with selective *fibrinolytic* activity have not yet been realized; the presently available enzymes, which are highly purified and homogeneous, are rather broad-spectrum *proteolytics*. However, the pharmacologic, toxicologic, and hematologic investigations of the agents were encouraging despite the lack of desired absolute substrate specificity, and therapeutic trials held promise. At this point in time it may be too early, however, to consider fungal proteases as interchangeable alternatives to plasminogen activators. They have not yet been evaluated on the scale and under the conditions of streptokinase and urokinase trials, and their efficacy may differ from that of endogenous plasmin. Therapeutic indications emerge, however, in which fungal proteases appear to be equal or superior to plasminogen activators by virtue of their rapidity of action and the predictability of lytic effects. Fungal proteases may also enjoy popularity in the future for reasons of economy: their cost of manufacture is low, and their availability is virtually unlimited when produced on an industrial scale.

A. Proteases from Aspergillus oryzae

The enzymes of *A. oryzae* were studied by several workers in widely differing localities, and methods of their isolation and purification had been described before their fibrinolytic properties and therapeutic potential were recognized and exploited.

CREWTHER and LENNOX (1950) reported on the successful preparation and crystallization of a protease from *A. flavus-oryzae* 492-2795, which they considered to be equal to trypsin with respect to gelatin digestion, and slightly more active than papain in the digestion of hemoglobin. The preparation was assumed to contain two proteolytic enzymes.

SPECHT (1957) established the presence of three protease components in surface cultures of *A. oryzae*, which he characterized by hemoglobin hydrolysis as an acidic proteinase (pH optimum 3.0–3.5), a middle component (pH optimum 4.5–5.1), and a neutral proteinase (pH optimum about 7.0).

The variety of proteinases in cultures of *A. oryzae*, their inhibition by inhibitors in natural products, and the presence of amylase and peptidases was also described by Japanese investigators (MATSUSHIMA, 1955; SATO and AKATSUKA, 1959; SAWASAKI, 1960; MISAKI et al., 1961, 1970; MATSUSHIMA and SHIMADA, 1962, 1965; AKATSUKA and SATO, 1963a, b; YASUI, 1964).

A major alkaline proteinase of *A. oryzae*, Aspergillopeptidase B, was isolated in homogeneous form and characterized by SUBRAMANIAN and KALNITSKY (1964a, b). NORDWIG and JAHN (1966) studied the specificity of a neutral *A. oryzae* protease, which they found to be quite different from pronase-, trypsin-, and chymotrypsin-like enzymes. They considered it to be a collagenase with *Clostridium*-collagenase specificity.

Strain *A. oryzae* E.I. 212 from the collection of the East India Pharmaceutical Works, Calcutta, was examined by KUNDU et al. (1968) and was found to produce a protease with quite different substrate specificities than those reported for other strains. And an alkaline protease from *A. oryzae* NRRL 2160 (Northern Regional Research Laboratories, Peoria, Ill.) was produced by KLAPPER et al. (1973a, b). It was well studied and characterized by its growth conditions, activity profile, inhibition, and molecular weight. None of these investigators, however, suggested the possible use of the enzymes in fibrinolysis.

The isolation and purification of a protease from *A. oryzae* for the purpose of developing a *clinical thrombolytic agent* was accomplished by four collaborating groups of workers (STEFANINI and coworkers, Boston, Mass., USA; TRUANT and coworkers, Worcester, Mass., USA; BERGKVIST, Södertälje, Sweden; and TOSONI and coworkers, Toronto, Canada) during the late 1950s and early 1960s. It was the first fungal protease to be developed for this specific purpose, and it appears to have been the stimulus and prototype for systematic research into the specific relevance to medicine of fungal enzymes.

Since much of the work on other fibrinolytic fungal proteases was subsequently based on the published experience with *A. oryzae* enzyme, its development deserves a description in detail.

I. Isolation, Purification, and Chemical Characteristics

1. Aspergillin O (Stefanini and Coworkers, USA)

Based on the observations of CREWTHER and LENNOX (1950), who had described a crystalline protease from *A.oryzae*, STEFANINI and MARIN (1958, 1963) screened cultures of 160 nonpathogenic fungi for fibrinolytic activity. The cultures were obtained from a variety of institutions and consisted of *Absidia, Alternaria, Aspergillus, Blastomyces, Candida, Chaetomium, Circinella, Conidiobulus, Cryptococcus, Cunninghamella, Epidermophyton, Epicoccum, Geotrichum, Gliocladium, Helicostylum, Histoplasma, Hormodendrum, Microsporum, Mucor, Mycophyton, Myrothecium, Neurospora, Nocardia, Penicillium, Philophora, Phycomyces, Piptocephalis, Pleurotus, Pyrenochaeta, Rhizopus, Sartorya, Scopulariopsis, Sporotrichum, Syncephalastrum, Thamnidium, Trichoderma, Trichophyton, and Zygorhynchus.*

When transferred to liquid medium (7.2 g sucrose, 3.6 g dextrose, 1.23 g $MgSO_4$ crystals, 13.69 g KH_2PO_4, 2.0 g KNO_3, and 1000 ml H_2O), the cultures showed luxuriant growth. After 6 days of incubation at room temperature the cultures were filtered, a precipitate was formed by the addition of 95% alcohol, and the precipitate was resuspended in saline.

Fibrinolytic activity of extracts was assayed in a system containing 0.2 ml fresh human or bovine platelet-poor plasma and 0.2 ml of fungal extract. The mixture was clotted with 0.2 ml thrombin solution ($= 20$ NIH units), incubated at 37° C, and observed for lysis 12 h later. Direct fibrinolytic activity of fungal extracts was tested on heated Astrup-Müllertz plates prepared with bovine or human fibrinogen. In addition, digestion of casein and egg albumin was studied.

Of 160 nonpathogenic fungi the extracts of four were found to lyse human or bovine fibrin clots and to destroy human and bovine fibrin plates. These were two strains of *A.oryzae* (B-82i and B-1273), one strain of *A.flavus* (B-4m), and one strain of *Absidia coerulea* (D-101). Quantitative comparison of lytic activities of the extremely impure extracts indicated that *A.oryzae* B-1273 gave best overall results with good activity against human plasma clots and human fibrin, poor activity against bovine fibrin and casein, and no activity against egg albumin. One ml of extract from B-1273 was found to be equivalent to 8 µg of trypsin on casein, and to approx. 250 µg of trypsin on human fibrin.

Recognizing *A.oryzae* B-1273 (from the culture collection of the US Quartermaster Research and Development Center, Department of the Army, Natick, Mass.,

USA) as a potential source of potent and relatively selective fibrinolytic material, STEFANINI's group proceeded with attempts to increase the yield of production and to purify the active principle (STEFANINI et al., 1959). In 1959, HORACE and STEFANINI described the conditions and requirements for optimal production of "mold fibrinolysin" from A. oryzae, assigning the name "Aspergillin O" to the substance to distinguish it from the spore pigment Aspergillin of A. niger. Significantly improved yields of active substance were obtained by the addition of Zn^{++}, Fe^{++}, and Mn^{++} to the original medium and a pH shift towards alkalinity.

With the identification of A. oryzae B-1273 as the most promising producer of one or more enzymes with relatively specific fibrinolytic activity (STEFANINI and MARIN, 1963), the discoverers were confronted with the task of developing methods of production and purification with which large quantities of enzyme could be obtained for characterization and biochemical and pharmacologic investigation. However, a program of this scope appeared to be beyond the means of STEFANINI and his collaborators.

Since subsequent developments are inadequately reflected in the chronological order of publication of later work, or are not on public record, a brief mention of intervening events appears to be appropriate:

At some time in 1959, STEFANINI assigned the development rights of Aspergillin O to Research Corp., New York, USA, who issued an exclusive license for large-scale production to Astra Pharmaceuticals, Inc., Worcester, Mass., USA. Attempts were made to culture the mold and to develop industrial techniques of manufacture (TRUANT and NORDSTROM, 1963). This led in time to the involvement and licensing of AB Astra, Södertälje, Sweden (the parent of Astra Pharmaceuticals, USA).

At approximately the same time (1959), STEFANINI was approached independently by scientists from Connaught Medical Research Laboratories, University of Toronto, Canada, with an offer of fermentation expertise, which he accepted by assigning the development rights also to Connaught. The inevitable licensing conflict, when eventually recognized, was amicably resolved when Astra (USA) extended their exclusive rights to Connaught (Canada), followed by a long-term collaborative agreement between Astra (USA), Astra (Sweden), and Connaught (Canada) for the partly integrated development and production of a common enzyme.

STEFANINI's contributions to the production of A. oryzae protease ceased with the beginning of industrial research. It was at about that time that the writer became associated with the enzyme's development and engrossed in the pharmacologic exploration of fungal proteases and their possible exploitation in clinical medicine.

2. Protease I, Brinase, Brinastrase (Bergkvist, Sweden)

The publications by BERGKVIST (1963a–d, 1966) describe in depth the approach to the rational exploration of the complex of A. oryzae proteases, starting with the premise that the substances searched for were more likely *proteolytic* enzymes rather than fibrinolytic material which STEFANINI had considered to be nonprotein in nature.

a) Preparation of Crude Enzyme

Using STEFANINI's original culture of A. oryzae B-1273, BERGKVIST (1963a) obtained enzymes by submerged culture on a protein- and carbohydrate-rich medium (1–1.5% proteins from soybean or peanut meal, 2–4% carbohydrate, magnesium and phosphorus salts, pH 6.5–7.0). As soon as maximum spore formation occurred, i.e., when all proteolytic enzymes could be recovered from the medium (3–4 days), the products were harvested by filtration of the culture.

Concentration of the proteins in the filtrate was by precipitation with tannin (3.0 g of tannin per liter of filtrate at pH 5.5). The copious precipitate was centrifuged and washed in acetone to remove tannin, and it was dried in vacuum. Recovery of proteolytic activity was 80–100% of the activity of the original culture filtrate (BERGKVIST, 1963a). The chief factors determining the effectiveness of precipitation of the proteases were found to be the tannin concentration (at least 3 mg/ml of filtrate), the pH (maximum recovery at pH 5.0–6.0), and the temperature (20° C). The dried powder retained its proteolytic activity for more than a year, it was easily soluble in water, and it allowed the preparation of protease solutions with more than 2000 times the activity of the original filtrate (also described by TRUANT and NORDSTROM, 1963).

b) Determination of Proteolytic Activity

BERGKVIST (1963a) employed casein, hemoglobin, and gelatin substrates. Based on the Kunitz assay of trypsin, which measures digestion products by their ability to absorb ultraviolet light after precipitation of undigested protein with trichloroacetic acid, a solution of 15 g of casein in 500 ml of water, pH 7.4, was used. Assays of caseinase activity were performed in a system of 3 ml casein solution and 3 ml enzyme solution in 0.2 M phosphate buffer pH 7.4. By comparing the optical density of the pre-incubation mixture with that of the mixture after 30 min of incubation at 37° C, a measure of hydrolysis was obtained. Proportionality between the degree of hydrolysis and the quantity of enzyme present in the mixture was achieved by adjusting the amount of enzyme to give an initial optical density (OD) between 0.050 and 0.500 at 280 mμ with 1 cm quartz cuvettes in a Zeiss spectrophotometer. One caseinolytic unit (CU) was arbitrarily assigned to the amount of enzyme that produced an increase in OD of 1.000 at 280 mμ in 30 min of incubation at 37° C.

Hemoglobinase activity was determined on a substrate consisting of 36 g urea, 10 ml 22% hemoglobin, 8 ml 1 N NaOH, and 72 ml H_2O, preincubated for 30–60 min, and mixed with a solution containing 4 g urea in 10 ml 1 M KH_2PO_4. Following similar steps as described for caseinase determinations, optical densities of pre- and post-incubation filtrates were compared, the difference being a measure of hemoglobinase activity. Gelatinase activity was estimated by measuring gelatin viscosity reduction after 5 min of incubation at 37° C of a 5% gelatin solution containing the enzyme.

When testing the protease mixture produced by A. oryzae on a variety of protein substrates, the rates of hydrolysis differed over a wide range of pH values (Fig. 1). BERGKVIST concluded that the broad pH maximum on gelatin indicated the presence of more than one enzyme, which was also reflected in the hydrolysis rate on casein and in the digestion of denatured hemoglobin. It became apparent that for valid activity comparisons the pH range for optimal enzyme stability needed to be determined. As shown in Figure 2, the enzymes were stable at room temperature over a range of pH 4.0–7.0, and they were irreversibly destroyed on both sides of this pH range.

In addition to determining pH optima, BERGKVIST obtained further information on the probable number of different proteases in the crude substance by measuring the effect of pH on inactivation. Inactivation at pH 3.0 and 9.0 (chosen in order to inactivate the enzymes with very different time courses) exhibited a stepwise course when plotted against time, indicating the presence of three proteolytic enzymes in the crude preparation.

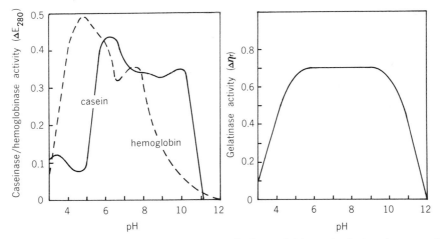

Fig. 1. pH activity of *A. oryzae* proteases on casein, hemoglobin, and gelatin substrates. *Caseinase activity* = rate of hydrolysis of 1.5% casein after incubation for 30 min at 37° C; *hemoglobinase activity* = rate of hydrolysis of 2% urea denatured hemoglobin after incubation for 10 min at 37° C; both expressed as increase in optical density of trichloroacetic acid filtrate. *Gelatinase activity* = reduction in relative viscosity of 5% gelatin after incubation for 5 min at 37° C. After BERGKVIST (1963 a)

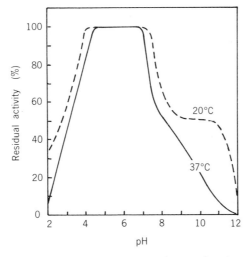

Fig. 2. pH stability of *A. oryzae* proteases. Enzyme mixture of various pH incubated for 30 min at 20° C or 37° C and tested for caseinase activity. After BERGKVIST (1963 a)

c) Differential Analysis of Proteases

The complexity of the protease preparation was demonstrated by continuous electrophoretic separation at three different pHs, giving distribution patterns as illustrated in Figure 3. This confirmed the presence of three proteases at pH 4.5 and 6.0, and the denaturation of one protease at pH 8.5. The results of electrophoretic separation are summarized in Table 1.

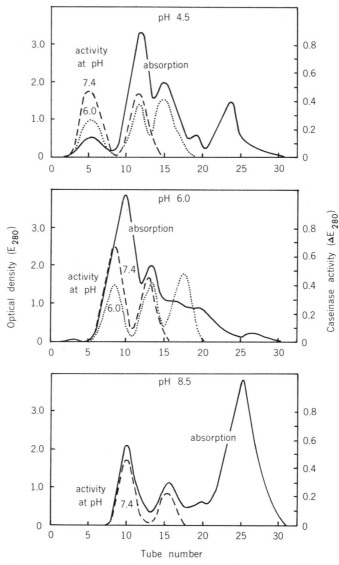

Fig. 3. Distribution patterns for separation of proteins in crude protease mixture from *A. oryzae* by continuous electrophoresis at 3 different pHs. After Bergkvist (1963a)

For separation and isolation of the three proteases, Bergkvist (1963a) then employed column chromatography on DEAE-cellulose buffered with 0.01 *M* phosphate buffer at pH 6.0. Eight distinct protein peaks were obtained, of which three possessed caseinolytic activity (Fig. 4). These were named proteases I, II, and III, having a combined proteolytic activity of about 85–90% of that originally applied to the column. When calculated from the ion exchange chromatography data, the amounts of the protease fractions were: protease I = 28%, protease II = 24%, and protease III = 48% of total proteolytic activity.

Table 1. Separation of proteases from *A. oryzae* by continuous electrophoresis at pH 4.5, 6.0, and 8.5. Caseinase activity determined at pH 6.0 and 7.4 and expressed in % of total activity. (After BERGKVIST, 1963a)

	Protease I		Protease II		Protease III	
Caseinase activity at pH	6.0	7.4	6.0	7.4	6.0	7.4
Electrophoresis at pH 4.5	29.0	66.0	23.5	34.0	47.5	—
pH 6.0	28.5	65.0	24.0	35.0	47.5	—
pH 8.5	—	65.0	—	35.0	—	—

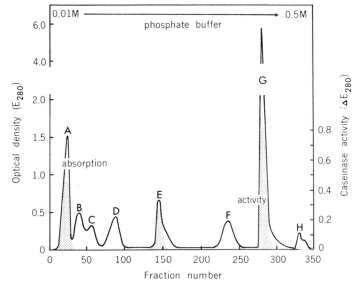

Fig. 4. Chromatography of crude protease mixture from *A. oryzae* on DEAE-cellulose buffered with 0.01 M phosphate buffer pH 6.0. 2.0 g of dialyzed material in 15 ml of buffer applied to column, fraction volume 5.0 ml, 4° C. *Peak A* = protease I (28% of total activity), *peak E* = protease II (24% of total activity), *peak G* = protease III (48% of total activity). After BERGKVIST (1963a)

d) Separation of Proteases

A different—and large-scale—separation was accomplished by BERGKVIST (1963a) with a multistage batch procedure on CM-cellulose at pH 5.5, 4.5, and 3.0 respectively, which caused selective and quantitative adsorption of the different proteases on CM-cellulose from which the active material was eluted (protease I at pH 5.5, protease II at pH 4.5, and protease III at pH 3.0). The relative purity of these fractions was demonstrated by DEAE-cellulose chromatography, which indicated that the highly purified protease I contained only small amounts of two inactive proteins. Proteases II and III, while also considerably purified, still contained other components (Fig. 5).

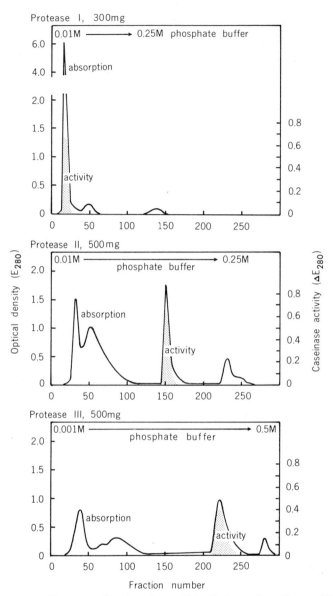

Fig. 5. Chromatograms of protease fractions from CM-cellulose adsorption on DEAE-cellulose columns buffered with 0.01 M phosphate buffer pH 6.0. Fraction volume 5.0 ml, 4° C. After BERGKVIST (1963a)

e) Properties of Proteases

The properties of purified proteases I, II, and III of *A. oryzae* were examined by BERGKVIST (1963b) in studies of their action on protein and synthetic substrates, by identifying pH and temperature optima, and by studying their inhibition. Protease I also was crystallized with acetone treatment of a concentrated solution. The results

Table 2. Some properties of proteases produced by *A. oryzae*. Strong inhibition (+) or no inhibition (−). (After BERGKVIST, 1963b)

Property	Protease		
	I	II	III
pH optima on: casein	8.2	6.8	—
denatured hemoglobin	7.6	6.8	4.3
gelatin	9.0—9.5	6.3	4.5
tosyl arginine methyl ester	8.5	—	—
Temperature optimum, °C	50	50	45
pH stability	5.0—8.5	4.5—10.5	3.0—6.3
Inhibition by: Na-laurylsulfonate	+	—	+
laurylamine	+	+	+
L-cysteine	−	+	−
ethylenediaminetetraacetic acid	−	+	−
ε-aminocaproic acid	−	−	−
soybean trypsin inhibitor	−	−	−

of these investigations are summarized in Table 2, allowing the conclusion that a crude filtrate of cultures of *A. oryzae* yields three distinct proteases that can be separated, isolated almost quantitatively, and highly purified. Of these, proteases I and II had pH optima and pH stability within physiologically acceptable limits, while protease III appeared not to warrant further investigation as a potential human thrombolytic agent.

Although the ultimate substrates for a potential thrombolytic agent should ideally be fibrin and fibrinogen, BERGKVIST (1963c) chose to retain the caseinolytic method as the primary assay in all studies, and to standardize proteases I and II in caseinolytic units (CU). When compared with trypsin, both proteases and crystalline trypsin assayed at about 15 CU per mg.

In order to distinguish between proteases I and II, and to identify the protease with the most desirable characteristics, BERGKVIST (1963c) determined their activities on fibrin and fibrinogen substrates. Possible relative specificities were demonstrated on formed fibrin clots in the presence of protease. By plotting enzyme concentration against clot lysis time (Fig. 6), protease I was revealed to have much higher fibrinolytic activity than protease II, although both had about the same caseinolytic activity per unit weight. The clearly greater fibrinolytic activity of protease I was confirmed on Astrup-Müllertz fibrin plates (Fig. 7), which also showed the lack of plasminogen activator properties of the proteases when tested on heated and unheated plates (where the activity on heated plates was higher than expected due to the easier degradation of heat-denatured proteins).

Fibrinogenolysis was examined by incubating the proteases with human fibrinogen at 25° C and testing for residual clottable fibrinogen upon addition of small amounts of thrombin. These tests (Fig. 8) showed that protease II attacked fibrinogen more rapidly than did protease I.

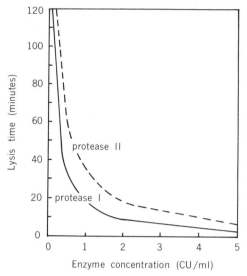

Fig. 6. Fibrinolytic activity of proteases I and II. Lysis time of clots made from 0.25% human fibrinogen estimated at pH 7.4 and 37° C. After BERGKVIST (1963c)

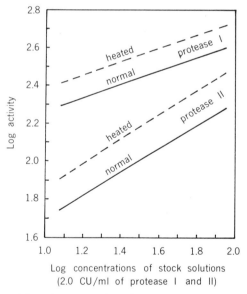

Fig. 7. Fibrinolytic activity of proteases I and II on normal and heated Astrup-Müllertz fibrin plates, incubated for 18 h at 32° C. After BERGKVIST (1963c)

On the basis of these investigations, BERGKVIST concluded that protease I constituted a substance with potential therapeutic value as a thrombolytic agent. The designation "protease I" was retained throughout the subsequent period of pharmacologic and clinical investigation until the drug was released for clinical use under the names brinase and brinastrase.

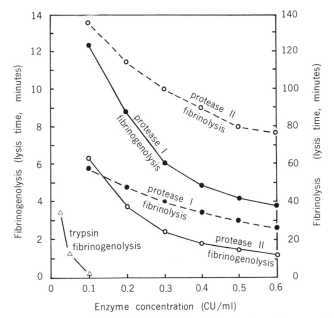

Fig. 8. Fibrinogenolytic and fibrinolytic activity of proteases I and II. *Fibrinogenolysis* = time (in min) of incubation (at 25° C) of human fibrinogen (0.5%) and enzyme required to make human fibrinogen unclottable with thrombin. *Fibrinolysis* = time (in min) of incubation (at 25° C) of human fibrinogen-enzyme-thrombin clots to lyse completely. After BERGKVIST (1963c)

3. CA-7, Brinase, Brinolase (Tosoni and Coworkers, Canada)

Concurrently with the production and purification of *A. oryzae* enzymes by BERG-KVIST, work proceeded independently at the Connaught Medical Research Laboratories, University of Toronto, Canada.

a) Preparation of Crude Enzyme

Following a period of experimentation with various media for optimal growth conditions, TOSONI and GLASS (1963) found that the growth of *A. oryzae* B-1273 (and later WB-7 and WA-12, strains developed by ultraviolet irradiation in the Connaught Laboratories) could be enhanced to yield substantial, i.e., commercial, quantities of crude enzymes by adding "corn-steep liquor" (a byproduct in the preparation of corn starch, containing substantial amounts of lactic acid), α-hydroxy acids (e.g., glycerin) and α-keto acids at acid pH, and to grow the mold in deep-culture at 35° C. This medium was adapted to industrial fermentation techniques, and large quantities of crude enzyme were successfully prepared in 2000 and 10000 liter batches. The resulting enzyme-containing broth was filtered and precipitated with lignin, which is unaffected by the presence of trace amounts of iron in mild-steel fermenters (IVES and TOSONI, 1967), or with tannic acid when stainless-steel fermenters were used. Following acetone washing and drying, the crude enzyme substance could then be stored indefinitely as a dry powder. This crude material was of relatively low activity, similar to BERGKVIST's crude enzyme mixture and somewhat

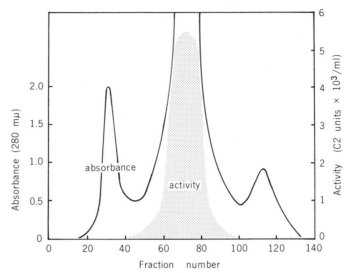

Fig. 9. Gel filtration of crude pretreated enzyme from *A. oryzae* on Sephadex G-50 (4.0 g in 35 ml, 0.5 M sodium acetate buffer pH 5.0, fraction volume 20 ml, 4° C). Column eluted with dist. water adjusted to pH 5.0 with dilute HCl. Total fibrinolytic activity before chromatography = 1.35×10^6 C2 U; activity of combined fractions 65–83 following chromatography = 1.01×10^6 C2 U (yield = 75%). From Roschlau and Ives (1974)

analogous to Stefanini's end product. It was designated "Aspergillin O" to distinguish it from the purified product.

b) Purification of Enzyme

The crude precipitate was purified by treating a solution with a chelating agent, followed by batch treatment with Sephadex G-25 at 4° C to remove salts and impurities and to reduce the volume. The solution was then passed through a column of Sephadex G-50 at 4° C and was eluted with very dilute hydrochloric acid (Ives and Tosoni, 1967; Roschlau and Ives, 1974). The major protein constituent containing all activity (Fig. 9) was treated with charcoal to remove color, sterilized by filtration, measured into vials, and freeze-dried (Table 3).

The highly purified freeze-dried enzyme maintained stability for more than a year, after which time it slowly began to lose activity due to autolysis. In order to extend the stability of the enzyme for unlimited shelf life at room temperature, small amounts of heat-treated human albumin (200 mg per gram of purified enzyme) were added before lyophilization (Tosoni et al., 1970; Roschlau and Ives, 1974). Electrophoretic examination of stabilized enzyme showed that the albumin was to a large extent destroyed before freeze-drying and that the resultant mixture of peptides and enzyme formed stable complexes. Stabilization became standard procedure in the commercial production of *A. oryzae* enzyme in Canada.

The enzyme was code-named CA-7, and although the methods of preparation differed from those described by Bergkvist (1963a) for protease I, the products were nearly identical by physical and chemical characteristics. (The need for stabilization of the Canadian-produced enzyme may indicate a somewhat higher degree of purity

Table 3. Representative data on preparation of CA–7 from lignin and tannin crude enzyme. (After IVES and TOSONI, 1967)

Stage in purification	Type of sample	Quantity	Potency in C2 U[a]	Total C2 U ($\times 10^6$)	% Yield	
					Stepwise	Overall
Lignin crude enzyme	Powder	196.0 g	210/mg	41.2	—	—
Solution, filtration, dialysis, concentration	Solution	500.0 ml	35400/ml	17.7	43	43
Sephadex G − 25, Sephadex G − 50	Solution	625.0 ml	14800/ml	9.3	52.5	22.5
Freeze-drying	Powder	9.2 g	990/mg	9.1	98	22
Tannin crude enzyme	Powder	219.0 g	300/mg	65.7	—	—
Solution, filtration, dialysis, concentration	Solution	485.0 ml	52000/ml	25.2	38	38
Sephadex G − 25, Sephadex G − 50	Solution	3000.0 ml	5100/ml	15.3	61	23
Freeze-drying	Powder	12.1 g	1150/mg	13.9	91	21

[a] 1 C2 U = fibrinolytic activity of 1 µg of Connaught house standard C2.

than BERGKVIST's product.) Throughout the developmental period the Canadian-produced protease was known as "CA-7." Since its release for clinical use the non-proprietary names brinase and brinolase have been assigned.

c) Determination of Fibrinolytic Activity

The methods of assay used by the Canadian workers consisted of the ASTRUP-MÜLLERTZ fibrin plate (ROSCHLAU, 1964) and of a fibrin-suspension assay developed by DYER and KADAR (1964). In the latter assay finely divided powder of human or bovine fibrin (particle size approx. 5 µ diameter) was suspended in Tris buffer pH 7.4 in a concentration of 1 mg/ml. When enzyme solution was added in the proportion of 1 part of enzyme to 2 parts of fibrin suspension, the turbidity of the mixture was approx. 20% light transmittance at 620 mµ in a Coleman Universal spectrophotometer. Incubation of the mixture at 37° C in a shaking water bath allowed fibrinolysis to proceed at a rapid pace, indicated by a clearing of turbidity. Turbidity of the digest was again measured after 15 min incubation, and the activity of an enzyme solution was calculated from the difference in light-transmittance of pre- and post-incubation samples (DYER and KADAR, 1964). The fibrin suspension assay provided a more accurate estimate of fibrinolytic activity than did other methods employing fibrin as substrate, since well-defined end points were obtained by use of spectrophotometric measurements. The method was since modified (ROSCHLAU and MILLER, 1970) to adapt it also to the measurement of fibrinolytic rate reactions and to the determination of fibrinolytic enzyme inhibitors.

In recognition of fibrin being the more rational (i.e., specific) substrate for a fibrinolytic enzyme, and in reliance on precise measurements of fibrinolytic activity, the Canadian enzyme was standardized in fibrinolytic units of activity by assigning an arbitrary value of 1000 units to the activity of 1 mg of a house standard C2.

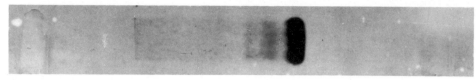

Fig. 10. Electrophoresis pattern of brinolase. Sepraphore III cellulose acetate strip in Gelman apparatus, using 0.01 *M* ammonium acetate buffer pH 7.0, 25 V/cm for 1 h. Stained with 0.5% amido black. From Roschlau and Ives (1974)

d) Characterization of Purified Enzyme

The purified enzyme was characterized by a variety of methods (Ives and Tosoni, 1967; Roschlau and Ives, 1974). Electrophoresis on cellulose acetate strips (Fig. 10) indicated that minor impurities remained even after extensive purification, and they could not be entirely removed. The faint minor bands on cellulose acetate strips may in fact be isozymes (Roschlau and Ives, 1974), since ultracentrifuge analysis gave a single symmetrical peak with an indicated molecular weight of approx. 22000.

The amino acid analysis of purified enzyme is shown in Table 4, from which a molecular weight of 20130 is calculated. Since neither cysteine nor cystine could be demonstrated, it is likely that the molecule consists of a single polypeptide chain.

Maximum acitivity on tosyl arginine methyl ester (TAME) occurred at pH 7.9–8.1 (Fig. 11). As was also shown by Bergkvist with protease I, the enzyme is irrever-

Table 4. Amino acid composition of brinolase.[a] (From Roschlau and Ives, 1974)

Amino acid	Content μM/5 mg	Assuming 11 Leucines	Rounded
Lysine	2.035	13.0	13
Histidine	0.66	4.2	4
Arginine	0.46	2.9	3
Aspartic acid	3.635	23.1	23
Threonine	2.01	12.8	13
Serine	3.33	21.2	21
Glutamic acid	2.395	15.2	15
Proline	0.78	5.0	5
Glycine	3.655	23.3	23
Alanine	4.55	29.0	29
Cystine	none detected		
Valine	2.54	16.1	16
Methionine	0.165	1.0	1
Isoleucine	1.625	10.4	10
Leucine	1.725	11.0	11
Tyrosine	0.84	5.3	5
Phenylalanine	0.79	5.0	5
Tryptophan[b]			2
Total number of residues			199
Mol wt			20130

[a] 5 mg of brinolase hydrolyzed at 110° C for 16 h. Content figures are the average of two runs. Composition calculated on the basis of there being 11 leucine residues.
[b] Tryptophan determined by spectrophotometric methods.

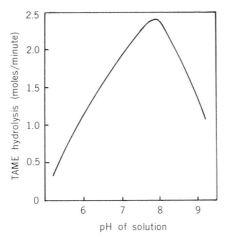

Fig. 11. pH dependence of brinolase activity against tosyl arginine methyl ester (TAME). Substrate: 4 ml of 0.1 M TAME solution of varying pH. Enzyme: 0.05 ml of a 1.0 mg/ml aqueous solution of brinolase (= 50 C2 U). Reaction velocity determined over first 5 min of reaction time. From ROSCHLAU and IVES (1974)

sibly inactivated below pH 4.0 and above pH 10. The determination of maximum reaction rates (ROSCHLAU and IVES, 1974) demonstrated that the enzyme appears to be most active against cystine derivatives and only slowly active against glutamine and asparagine. This activity can be inhibited by the addition of alcohol, but there is still appreciable hydrolysis in the presence of up to 10% of ethyl alcohol.

4. Comparison of Swedish and Canadian Enzymes

It was pointed out earlier that the development of *A. oryzae* enzymes was a collaborative effort of American, Canadian, and Swedish workers, that the approaches to the problems of isolation, preparation, and purification differed from each other in several aspects, but that the finally obtained materials of clinical purity were practically identical under all conditions of assay of fibrinolytic, fibrinogenolytic, caseinolytic, and esterolytic activity. The enzymes are considered to be interchangeable for these reasons, although the Canadian product contains a stabilizing agent (heat-treated human albumin) added in the final stage of the manufacturing process.

However, since the Swedish enzyme (protease I, brinase, brinastrase) is standardized in caseinolytic units by a modification of the method of Kunitz (17 CU per mg at pH 7.4), and the Canadian enzyme (CA-7, brinase, brinolase) is standardized in fibrinolytic units (1000 C2 U per mg at pH 7.4), and since it became the custom to cite dosages of brinastrase in units of weight but those of brinolase in units of fibrinolytic activity, there exists a certain amount of unfortunate confusion in the literature. For purposes of comparison, therefore, the following activity relationship exists between the two enzymes:

1 mg of substance (brinastrase or brinolase)

=   17 CU (brinastrase, Sweden),
= 1000 C2 fibrinolytic U (brinolase, Canada).

In view of the identity of products, it is therefore deemed permissible (and indeed necessary for the purpose of discussion) to treat both enzymes as a common entity. The task will be simplified by using henceforth the designation "Aspergillin O" for the *crude*, nonpurified enzyme mixture from the growth of *A. oryzae* B-1273 (described by STEFANINI and coworkers and used as starting material for both the Canadian and Swedish processes of manufacture), the name "brinase" whenever common characteristics of the *purified* enzymes are discussed, and to reserve the individual names "brinastrase" (Sweden) and "brinolase" (Canada) for those occasions that require identification of the manufacturer. [2]

II. Biological and Pharmacologic Properties

1. Inhibition by Plasma and Serum

The description of biological effects of brinase requires a prior discussion of the inhibitory properties of plasma and serum. It has long been known that normal serum will neutralize the activity of many proteolytic enzymes (BERGKVIST, 1963 d), and the inhibition by serum of trypsin, chymotrypsin, and plasmin has been thoroughly investigated. Mammalian blood also inhibits brinase to varying degree, the extent of this inhibition depending as much on the species as on the individual.

BERGKVIST (1963 d) studied serum inhibition of brinase by using casein and human fibrin as substrates. As shown in Figures 12 and 13, the activities of brinase, chymotrypsin, and trypsin were remarkably different in the presence of human serum, the inhibitory effects on trypsin and chymotrypsin being far greater than on brinase.

The rate of inhibition of brinase by serum was found to vary with temperature (Fig. 14), from which BERGKVIST concluded that it might be a two-stage process: an immediate inhibition independent of temperature followed by a second reaction that is highly temperature-dependent. BERGKVIST proposed the presence of two inhibitory substances in human serum, which were subsequently called "rapid" and "slow" inhibitor. It was suggested that the "rapid" inhibition is a reversible process, presumably by substrate competition with the inhibitor for the enzyme. Figure 15 shows clear competition between the serum components and the fibrin substrate for the active site of the enzyme, supporting the conclusion that the reaction is reversible.

The presence of two types of inhibitors for brinase was confirmed by BERGKVIST after continuous flow paper electrophoresis of human serum and testing the fractions for antiproteolytic activity. It was found that the "rapid" inhibitor migrated with the α_1-globulins and the "slow" inhibitor with the α_2-globulins, which was very similar to the inhibition by serum of plasmin. Since the reactions of serum inhibitors with both brinase and plasmin were profoundly affected by the presence of a protein substrate, and the inhibition by the α_1-inhibitor ("slow") did not progress further in the presence of substrate whereas the inhibition by the α_2-inhibitor ("rapid") was

---

[2] On the recommendation of the United States Adopted Names Council, and by agreement of the manufacturers, both enzymes were initially named brinase. The US Adopted Names Council at a later date recommended a change to brinolase in order to avoid possible prescribing errors relating to other proprietary preparations. While this change was made for the enzyme manufactured and used in North America, the name brinase continued to be applied to the European product. Brinolase has since been registered in Canada under the name Connbrinolase.

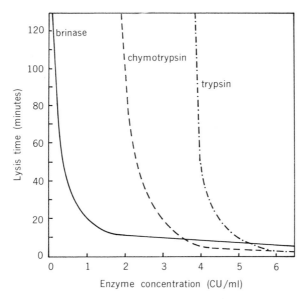

Fig. 12. Clot lysis in presence of human serum by brinase, chymotrypsin, and trypsin. Lysis time for clots made from 0.5% human fibrinogen and 0.2 ml of human serum per ml estimated at pH 7.4 and 37° C. After BERGKVIST (1963 d)

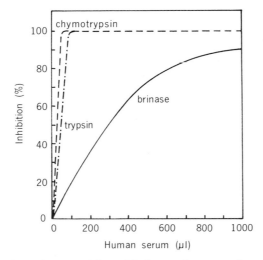

Fig. 13. Inhibition of caseinase activity of brinase, chymotrypsin, and trypsin by varying amounts of human serum, determined by rate of hydrolysis of 1.5% casein at pH 7.4 after incubation for 30 min at 37° C. Final volume of reaction mixture was 6.0 ml, and 1.0 CU of each protease was used in all estimations. Increase in optical density of trichloroacetic acid filtrate was used as a measure of proteolytic activity. Percent inhibition was calculated from difference in activity between partially inhibited enzyme and same amount of enzyme incubated with buffer alone. After BERGKVIST (1963 d)

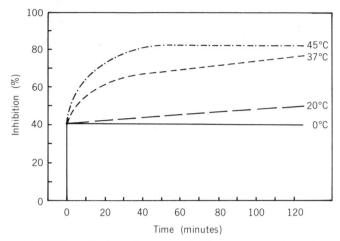

Fig. 14. Percent inhibition of brinase by serum at different temperatures. Inhibition of fibrinolytic activity of 2.0 CU of enzyme was estimated. At zero time, 0.2 ml of human serum was added to each sample, and residual activity was estimated after different times of incubation. From Bergkvist (1963 d)

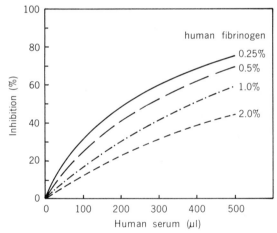

Fig. 15. Effects of different concentrations of fibrin on inhibition of brinase by "rapid" inhibitor of serum. Clots were made from 0.25%, 0.5%, 1%, and 2% human fibrinogen. Inhibition of 2.0 CU of enzyme by human serum was estimated at pH 7.4 and 37° C. Controls were run with serum replaced by buffer. From Bergkvist (1963 d)

reversible by an increase in substrate, Bergkvist (1963 d) proposed that a complex between brinase and the "rapid" (α_2-globulin) inhibitor may serve as a transport form or reservoir of the enzyme in blood, free enzyme being released in the presence of fibrin clots. The inhibitor complex was also seen to act as a physiologic protector by (a) preventing immediate enzyme degradation, and (b) protecting other plasma proteins from brinase attack.

Concurrently and independently, Stefanini and Karaca (1963) examined the serum inhibition of Aspergillin O on Astrup-Müllertz fibrin plates containing

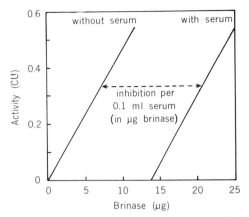

Fig. 16. Inhibition of brinase by human serum. From LINDVALL et al. (1969)

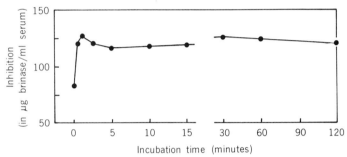

Fig. 17. Influence of incubation time on inhibition of brinase activity by human serum. From LINDVALL et al. (1969)

varying additions of human serum. They found that the addition of serum to the fibrinogen solution prior to its clotting with thrombin inhibited the activity of the crude enzyme in direct relation to the serum volume.

Using a viscosimetric method with gelatin as substrate, LINDVALL et al. (1969) expanded on the work of BERGKVIST and confirmed the presence of two inhibitory fractions in serum by electrophoretic separation and heat treatment.

Total inhibitors were assayed by incubating increasing amounts of brinase in 0.9 ml Tris buffer and 0.1 ml serum at 35.5° C for 30 min, and measuring the remaining activity on gelatin. The relationship between the remaining activity and the amount of enzyme was linear, with parallel displacement of the response curve from that without serum (Fig. 16), the difference being a measure of inhibition of brinase activity by serum.

Enzyme-inhibitor complex formation was studied in serum incubated with brinase for varying periods of time, indicating that complexes formed immediately as shown in Figure 17. Inhibition of the enzyme (i.e., complex formation) was proportional to the amount of serum up to 0.6 ml of serum per ml of incubation mixture (Fig. 18).

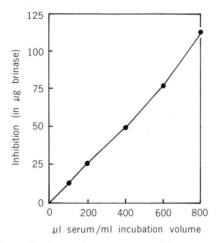

Fig. 18. Inhibition of brinase by increasing amounts of human serum per ml of incubation volume after heating at 35.5° C for 5 min. From LINDVALL et al. (1969)

Electrophoretic separation of human serum by LINDVALL et al. yielded two main inhibitors, the one migrating immediately behind albumin while the other migrated more slowly. Analysis of these fractions showed that the rapidly migrating inhibitor corresponded to a trypsin-inhibitor and ought to be identical with α_1-antitrypsin. The slowly migrating component, on the other hand, was found also to inactivate plasmin.

Since the trypsin-inhibitor may be inactivated by heating to 60° C, total inhibitory activity may be separated into its main components by heat treatment. Applying this method, LINDVALL et al. found that serum of healthy subjects contained varying amounts of both heat-labile and heat-stable brinase inhibitors (Table 5), with a range of total inhibitors from 106 to 202 µg of brinase per ml of serum (mean = 146 µg ± 22 SD), of which approx. 40% were heat-labile (anti-trypsin) inhibitor and 60% were heat-stable (anti-plasmin) inhibitor. Thus there was shown to be considerable overlap of inhibitor activity and specificity. LINDVALL et al. concluded that rapid complex formation will occur between brinase and its inhibitors in vivo. But, since one of the inhibitors is common to brinase and plasmin, they proposed that the affinity of brinase for the plasmin inhibitor may deprive this of the opportunity to inhibit physiologically activated plasmin in vivo, thus indirectly generating plasmin activity by complexing its inhibitor. This mechanism is advanced as partial explanation of the thrombolytic effects of brinase at doses below the inhibitor level of the individual (cf. Sects. III and IV).

The potential but variable inhibition of brinase activity in whole circulating blood of animals and man was examined by BERGKVIST and SVÄRD (1964), ROSCHLAU (1964, 1965, 1971a), GIERING and TRUANT (1966), and JÜRGENS et al. (1970) amongst others. The fundamental importance of enzyme inhibition as a determinant of attainable fibrinolytic effects on the one hand, and as a safeguard against excessive proteolysis on the other, was recognized, and tests were developed for the measurement of brinase inhibition and for the prediction of optimal thrombolytic dosage in animals and man (cf. Sect. VII).

Table 5. Brinase inhibitors of 17 healthy persons. (From LINDVALL et al., 1969)

Subject	Inhibitor value corresponding to µg of brinase per ml of serum		
	Total	Heat-labile	Heat-stable
A. M.	131	78	53
P. S.	106	43	63
A. H.	139	73	66
G. L.	149	72	77
O. M.	158	80	78
A. O.	156	67	89
L. L.	162	73	89
P. E.	153	62	91
R. S.	154	62	92
A.-G. D.	148	51	97
L. S.	152	38	114
K. O.	167	44	123
H. S.	202	69	133
B. E.	120	54	66
S. L.	116	48	68
J. C.	141	60	81
T. R.	135	48	87
$\bar{X} \pm$ SD	146 ± 22	60 ± 13	86 ± 22
Range	$106 - 202$	$38 - 80$	$53 - 133$

In studies on rabbits and cats, BERGKVIST and SVÄRD (1964) correlated administered dosage of brinase with serum-inhibitor activity, pharmacologic-hematologic events, and attainable lysis of artificial venous thrombi. The inhibitory activity of serum was determined with the method of BERGKVIST (Sect. VII/1). A typical experiment is shown in Figure 19. Each injection of brinase lowered serum-inhibitor activity abruptly, followed by a slow recovery to a level below the pre-injection value. On the assumption that the irreversible inhibitor may possibly be an enzyme that destroys brinase, BERGKVIST and SVÄRD proposed that upon injection brinase reacted with both the reversible and the irreversible inhibitors, thus decreasing the total amount of available inhibitors. Partial return of inhibitor activity was thought to occur after reactivation of the irreversible inhibitor following destruction of bound brinase, while the reversible brinase-inhibitor complex remained in circulation. About 40 CU of brinase per kg of cat were required to reduce total inhibitors to about 10% of pretreatment values, and a further 10 CU per kg resulted in free proteolytic activity in the blood.

While studying the behavior of inhibitors in the dog, ROSCHLAU (1964, 1965, 1971 a) measured total brinase inhibitors as "protease resistance" (cf. Sect. VII/2, Table 14), from which was developed a dose-prediction test. It was found that the normal range of brinase inhibitors in the dog lay between 50 and 115 inhibitor or TTR ("test tube requirement") units (mean = 82 TTR U $\pm$ 15.8 SD) (Fig. 20), indicating a great variability between individuals. Species differences were also shown to be significant when comparing the dog inhibitor data with those of healthy human

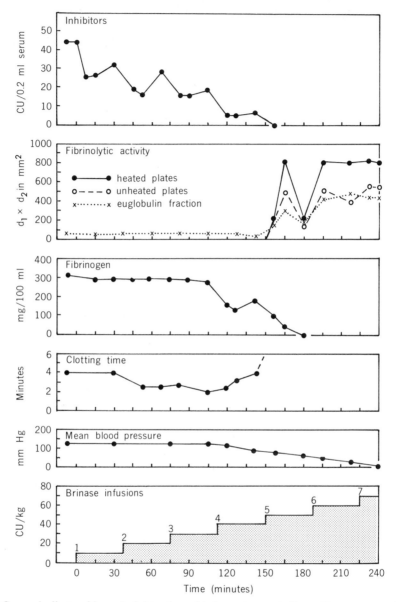

Fig. 19. General effects of i.v. administration of brinase to a cat. From BERGKVIST and SVÄRD (1964)

subjects of the study by ROSCHLAU (Table 6) which gave a mean of 113 TTR U, and that of LINDVALL et al. (Table 5) showing a mean of 146 µg (or TTR U).

The importance of inhibitor (protease resistance) determinations became apparent when brinase was administered systemically to dogs in experimental thrombolytic therapy (ROSCHLAU, 1964, 1965, 1971a). It was found that too "low" a dose will likely be thrombolytically ineffective, while too "high" a dose may cause side-effects

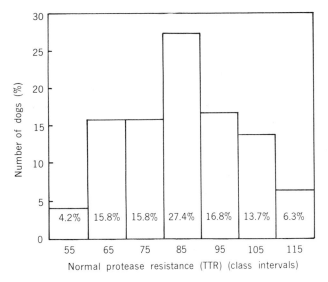

Fig. 20. Frequency distribution of normal protease resistance in 95 dogs. This is an approximately normal distribution, illustrating need for individualized dosage of brinase: animals to right will require (and tolerate) larger doses than animals to left. From ROSCHLAU (1965)

Table 6. Protease resistance in sample of healthy human volunteers. All determinations made at same time of day on 3 consecutive days. (From ROSCHLAU, 1965)

Volunteer (Sex)	Protease resistance (TTR units)[a]			
	Day 1	Day 2	Day 3	Mean
J. H. (m)	105	110	105	107
B. M. (m)	135	135	140	137
N. P. (m)	110	130	110	117
R. H. (m)	110	110	110	110
T. H. (m)	135	135	135	135
H. R. (m)	135	130	135	133
P. N. (m)	140	135	130	135
M. B. (m)	125	145	150	140
H. T. (m)	140	130	140	137
P. S. (m)	125	135	135	132
H. J. (m)	110	120	115	115
J. H. (f)	135	135	135	135
C. H. (f)	135	135	135	135
J. L. (f)	150	140	145	145
H. D. (f)	130	125	135	130
J. C. (f)	150	155	150	152
Mean of the day	129	132	131	131

[a] Method described in Sect. VII/2.

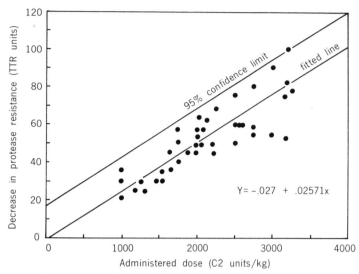

Fig. 21. Plot of relationship of administered dosage of brinase to decrease in protease resistance in 46 dogs. Seven different production lots of brinase were used. From ROSCHLAU (1965)

from free proteolytic activity. Thus, an "optimal" dose needed to be titrated for each individual based on the measurement of prevailing inhibitor levels before enzyme administration. A linear regression of protease resistance (inhibitor level) in dependence on administered dosage was established (Fig. 21) and was tested statistically (Table 7). From this was developed a dose-prediction test having as its target a post-treatment protease resistance value of 30 TTR U (Fig. 22). This target had been chosen by trial and error, since it represented a sufficiently adequate posttreatment inhibitor level to safeguard against inhibitor depletion and side-effects, but allowed optimal enzymatic activity for the attainment of demonstrable experimental thrombolysis.

Table 7. Analysis of variance of decrease in protease resistance (slopers of relationships and positions of responses of seven lots of brinase are are compared; data of 46 dogs from Fig. 21). From ROSCHLAU (1965).

	d.f.	S.S.	M.S.	F
Total	45	16 348.4	12 716.9	
Slope	1	12 716.9	63.92	147
Difference in adjusted means (common slope)	6	383.5	79.13	1
Difference between slopes	6	474.8	86.66	1
Deviation from lines with seperate slopes	32	2 773.2		

The standard error of estimate is $\sqrt{(86.66)} = 9.3$ TTR units.

Conclusions:

1. The different lots do not give significantly different slopes
2. The different lots do not give significantly different adjusted means
2. The *y*-intercept determined from all observations is not significantly different from zero

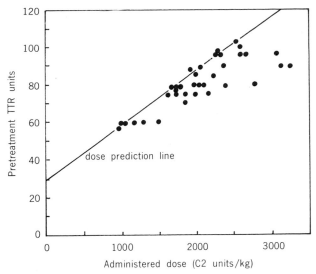

Fig. 22. Scattergram of brinase doses required to lower protease resistance of dogs to approx. 30 TTR units. Doses were predicted from pretreatment protease resistance value of each dog *(ordinate)* as previously established by trial and error *(diagonal line)*. Predictions frequently found to be low, and additional small doses of brinase were required to bring posttreatment protease resistance to 30 TTR units. *No overdoses were predicted.* From ROSCHLAU (1965)

The levels of total, heat-labile, and heat-stable inhibitors of brinase (LINDVALL et al., 1969) have also been studied by JÜRGENS et al. (1970) in eight patients suffering from a variety of thrombotic manifestations to whom brinase has been administered by repeated infusions of 150 mg per patient. The total pretreatment inhibitor values were found to vary from 119 to 202 µg brinase per ml of plasma (mean = 172 µg), that of heat-labile inhibitor from 46 to 97 µg/ml (mean = 78 µg, or 45% of total inhibitor), and that of heat-stable inhibitor from 68 to 105 µg/ml (mean = 95 µg, or 55% of total inhibitor). These findings demonstrated slightly elevated total inhibitor levels over those in healthy young adults (cf. Tables 5 and 6), although the differences between samples were not statistically significant.

Following infusion of 150 mg brinase on several occasions, inhibitor levels were reduced as shown in the example in Figure 23. It was observed that in all patients studied, the decrease in total inhibitors after the first infusion was essentially due to a decrease in the heat-stable (i.e., antiplasmin) inhibitor, which remained low thereafter. The heat-labile (i.e., antitrypsin) inhibitor was only slightly affected from the first infusion, but it reacted more strongly in subsequent treatments, being restored between treatments to approximate pretreatment levels. JÜRGENS et al. concluded that the heat-labile inhibitor may undergo rapid resynthesis while the heat-stable inhibitor does not quite recover its original concentration. In vivo there appeared to exist a preference for enzyme-inhibitor complex formation between the heat-stable antiplasmin and brinase as opposed to complex formation between brinase and antitrypsin, lending support to the hypothesis advanced by LINDVALL et al. (1969) that the complexing of antiplasmin by brinase may allow the persistence of physio-

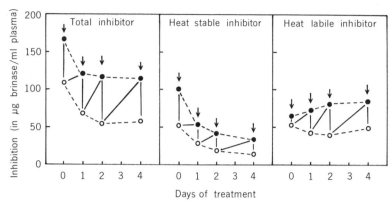

Fig. 23. Inhibitor changes in man after infusions of 150 mg brinase. Inhibitor level before (●) and after (○) treatment. *Arrows* indicate days of treatment. From JÜRGENS et al. (1970)

logically activated plasmin in the circulation, thus contributing substantially to the fibrinolytic state.

In an effort to elucidate the possible effects of brinase on plasma constituents involved in the conversion of plasminogen to plasmin, KIESSLING and SVENSSON (1970) treated purified plasminogen with brinase and obtained plasminogen fractions by gel filtration. These cleaved products of purified plasminogen could still be activated to plasmin. However, plasma treated with brinase and fractionated by gel filtration did not yield active plasminogens. The authors concluded that a complex was formed between brinase and an unidentified plasma protein, by which the enzyme lost about 60–90% of its activity on casein (a high molecular weight substrate), but that it retained its activity on low molecular weight substrates. Since the behavior of brinase was thus analogous to the activity of plasmin when complexed with its inhibitor α_2-macroglobulin, KIESSLING and SVENSSON suggested α_2-macroglobulin as the protein which forms a complex with brinase, one mole of the macroglobulin binding one mole of the enzyme.

2. Pharmacokinetics

The distribution and fate of brinase in the body were studied by BERGKVIST (1966) with ^{131}I-labeled enzyme. Following i.v. injection of 15 CU (i.e., 1.2 µCi ^{131}I) per kg into cats, it was found that the main part of the injected dose (about 70–80%) was cleared quite rapidly, but some radioactivity persisted in the circulation for a rather long time. One process with a half-life of about 25 min, and another with a more variable half-life of 150–300 min, were encountered. The persistence of labeled brinase was assumed by BERGKVIST to represent brinase complexed with the reversible inhibitor in serum.

BERGKVIST also concluded from these experiments that a certain amount of injected enzyme was adsorbed onto pre-existing clots: experimental venous clots removed from the animals 3 h after labeled brinase administration contained between 0.35 and 4.2% (mean = 1.7%) of the injected radioactivity.

Table 8. Tissue distribution of brinase in the cat 4 h after i. v. injection, as determined by ^{131}I radio-activity following exsanguination. (From BERGKVIST, 1966)

Tissue	Weight g	Total C.p.m.	C.p.m. per g	Total injected activity %
Liver	105	59885	570	7.0
Spleen	11	5090	463	0.6
Kidneys	31	20073	648	2.3
Stomach	27.5	35805	1302	4.2
Heart	13.5	2727	202	0.3
Lungs	22.5	11590	515	1.3
Thyroid	0.5	5330	10660	0.6
Urine	52	284856	5478	33.0

The tissue distribution of ^{131}I-labeled brinase 4 h after injection into cats (BERGKVIST, 1966) showed highest specific activity in thyroid, urine, and stomach. Obviously, brinase was excreted by the kidneys, as the urine contained between 25 and 35% of the injected activity within a 4-h period. BERGKVIST suggested that brinase was metabolized, and that the radioactivity in thyroid, stomach, and urine was most likely due to breakdown products (Table 8).

3. Proteolysis

a) Fibrin

In the course of their early investigations of Aspergillin O, STEFANINI et al. (1962) compared the fibrinolytic activity of trypsin and Aspergillin O in vivo in dogs. The authors gained the general impression that, in small doses, both trypsin and Asper-gillin O accelerated the clotting mechanism without significant fibrinolytic activity. At dose levels in the fibrinolytic range, however, trypsin activated plasmin and destroyed antiplasmin, accompanied by a destruction of antithrombin and an accel-eration of thrombin generation, severe hypofibrinogenemia, incoagulability of the blood, and complete breakdown of the clotting mechanism. Aspergillin O, on the other hand, induced significant fibrinolysis with less evidence of acceleration of clotting, less sustained depression of fibrinogen, and a depression (rather than accel-eration) of thrombin generation. Trypsin and Aspergillin O were thus shown by STEFANINI et al. to be strikingly dissimilar at equipotent fibrinolytic and caseinolytic dosage in their effects on coagulation proteins, with Aspergillin O seemingly being the "better" agent.

The potent fibrinolytic activity of brinase was demonstrated quantitatively on human and bovine fibrin by BERGKVIST (1963c), ROSCHLAU (1964), DYER and KA-DAR (1964), OGSTON and OGSTON (1968), and ROSCHLAU and MILLER (1970). It was shown that brinase hydrolysed human and bovine fibrin in any one of a variety of assay systems, and that it was not an activator of plasminogen (Figs. 7, 8, 24, 25). DYER and KADAR (1964) compared the qualitative fibrinolytic activities of brinase and plasmin (Fig. 25), suggesting that the hydrolysis of human fibrin by brinase possibly proceeds in a fashion similar to that of plasmin as demonstrated by the

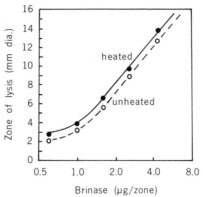

Fig. 24. Standard curves of brinase on heated and unheated Astrup-Müllertz bovine fibrin plates. Fifty plates run for each curve. After Roschlau (1964)

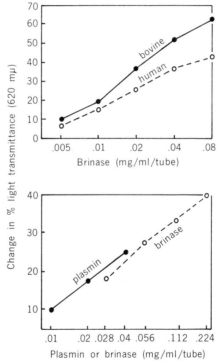

Fig. 25. *(Above)* Changes in turbidity of suspensions of human and bovine fibrin incubated with various levels of brinase. Mixtures were incubated at 37° C for 15 min at pH 8.0. *(Below)* Comparison of fibrinolysis of human fibrin suspension by plasmin and brinase. Both reactions were incubated at 37° C for 15 min at pH 7.4. After Dyer and Kadar (1964)

similarity between slopes of the respective dose-response curves. Ogston and Ogs-ton (1968) compared caseinolytically equipotent amounts of plasmin and brinase on human plasma clots in the presence and absence of serum, concluding that lysis produced by brinase and plasmin was similar in the absence of serum, while the

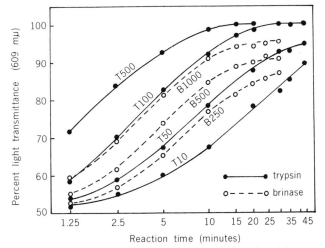

Fig. 26. Changes in turbidity of bovine fibrin suspension produced by trypsin and brinase in buffer at pH 7.4, incubated at 37° C. $T=$N.F.U. of trypsin per ml buffer, $B=$C 2 U of brinase per ml buffer. Modified method of DYER and KADAR (1964). After ROSCHLAU and MILLER (1970)

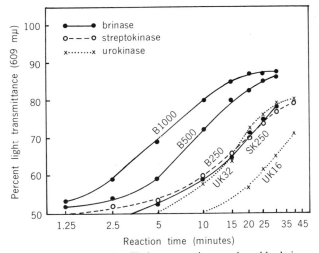

Fig. 27. Changes in turbidity of bovine fibrin suspension produced by brinase, streptokinase, and urokinase in serum, incubated at 37° C. $B=$C 2 U of brinase per ml serum, SK = Christensen U of streptokinase per ml serum, $UK=$Ploug U of urokinase per ml serum. Modified method of DYER and DAKAR (1964). After ROSCHLAU and MILLER (1970)

presence of serum had a greater inhibitory effect on brinase than on plasmin. ROSCH-LAU and MILLER (1970) compared the fibrinolytic activity of brinase with that of trypsin and plasmin (activated with streptokinase and with urokinase), confirming qualitative similarities in the mechanism of action of the different enzymes (Figs. 26, 27).

Comparative studies on the degradation of cross-linked and non-cross-linked human fibrin clots by plasmin, trypsin, chymotrypsin, and brinase were carried out by Gormsen and Feddersen (1974). Fibrin clots with either no or complete γ-dimerization and α-polymerization were degraded by the enzymes, and the degradation products in the supernatants were characterized by crossed agarose immuno-electrophoresis and sodium dodecyl sulphate polyacrylamide electrophoresis. The main degradation products from digestion of non-cross-linked and cross-linked fibrin by trypsin, chymotrypsin, and brinase were found to be closely related to those appearing after plasmin digestion, as indicated by the appearance of D-antigenic fragments (approx. mol wt 80000 from non-cross-linked fibrin, and mol wt 170000, i.e., double-D, from cross-linked fibrin) and E-antigenic fragments (approx. mol wt 50000 from both kinds of fibrin) during the initial steps of degradation with all enzymes. However, all D-antigenic fragments disappeared after extended or repeated degradation by trypsin, chymotrypsin, and brinase. The heterogeneity of D-fragments, especially from brinase and chymotrypsin digestion, corresponded to that found after fibrinogenolysis with the enzymes (Gormsen et al., 1973). Core fragments E, which are said to correspond to the N-terminal disulphide knot of Blombäck and are plasmin-resistant, became electrophoretically heterogeneous upon extended digestion with trypsin, chymotrypsin, and brinase with development of partial antigenicity against plasmin-produced core fragments E. The authors concluded that plasmin, trypsin, chymotrypsin, and brinase had similar cleavage pathways on non-cross-linked and cross-linked fibrin until the appearance of terminal core fragments E, which were resistant to further plasmin degradation but yielded polypeptides below mol wt 50000 when treated extensively or repeatedly with trypsin, chymotrypsin, and brinase.

b) Fibrinogen

The effects of brinase on fibrinogen were observed early during experimental evaluation of the enzyme (Bergkvist, 1963c, Fig. 8; Bergkvist and Svärd, 1964, Fig. 19; Monkhouse et al., 1964, Figs. 28, 29). More recent studies by Hessel and Blombäck (1973), by Donati et al. (1973), and by Gormsen et al. (1973) of the action of the enzyme on fibrinogen have shown that there are fundamental differences between plasmin and brinase in the specificity of bond cleavage and the production of degradation products.

Donati et al. (1973) administered ^{125}I-fibrinogen (100 µCi) to patients 2 days before brinase therapy. Following brinase infusion, fibrinogen complexes and fragments were demonstrated by gel filtration in the plasma of these patients. Such complexes, however, did not occur during comparable streptokinase therapy. In vitro incubation of normal plasma with brinase in concentrations similar to those obtained in vivo also produced complexes and fragments of fibrinogen, the complexes being comparable to those from very low concentrations of thrombin.

Hessel and Blombäck (1973) studied the effects of brinase on the γ-chain of human fibrinogen by means of two-dimensional peptide mapping, comparing brinase with trypsin and plasmin. Following incubation of substrate and enzymes, a lyophilisate was prepared from the supernatant digest and was subjected to electrophoresis and paper chromatography. The peptide spots were visualized with ninhydrin stain, after which they could be submitted to amino acid analysis. Trypsin, which splits on the carboxy-terminal side of arginine and lysine residues, gave rise to

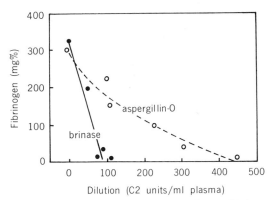

Fig. 28. Effects of brinase and Aspergillin O (crude) on plasma fibrinogen levels in vitro. After
MONKHOUSE et al. (1964)

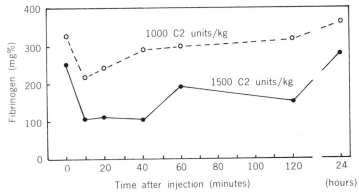

Fig. 29. Effects of brinase on blood fibrinogen levels following i.v. infusions in dogs. After MONK-
HOUSE et al. (1964)

seven fragments; plasmin, which splits on the carboxy-terminal end of lysine, gave
rise to five fragments; while brinase gave rise to many more fragments. The authors
concluded that brinase appears to be very nonspecific on the γ-chain of fibrinogen,
and that its spectrum of activity was likely to include plasma proteins other than
fibrinogen.

GORMSEN et al. (1973) used immunoelectrophoresis to demonstrate fibrinogen-
related antigens following digestion by brinase, trypsin, and chymotrypsin. It was
shown that the fragments obtained after nonexhaustive digestion with these enzymes
appeared immunologically identical with those from plasmin digestion. However,
after sustained digestion, especially with brinase and chymotrypsin, further degradation was obtained with the appearance of fragments with significantly lower molecular weight (< 50000) than the end products (E-fragments) of plasmin digestion (cf.
GORMSEN and FEDDERSEN, 1974). These fragments retained some E-antigenic properties, suggesting that brinase is capable of producing a variety of low molecular
weight peptides from fibrinogen whose biological activities might be different from
those of plasmin digestion.

Nyman (1975) investigated the changes in the fibrinogen molecule after brinase infusions into patients. It was found that the enzyme caused variable reductions in fibrinogen levels without, however, significantly affecting clottable protein. Sodium dodecyl sulfate polyacrylamide gel electrophoresis showed slower polymerization of reduced fibrinogen, which was associated with a splitting of the Aα-chain, and which occurred even without excessive lowering of brinase inhibitors. Reduced cross-linked fibrin showed an electrophoretic pattern indicating total cross-linking of the α- and γ-chains. Presumed formation of fibrin monomers was demonstrated by positive ethanol gelation tests, which could not be prevented by concomitant heparinization of patients. A band corresponding to the γ-dimer, and similar to that seen in disseminated intravascular clotting, was found upon electrophoresis of heat-precipitated fibrinogen.

Although fibrin polymerization was slowed by the action of brinase on the Aα-chain of fibrinogen, hemostasis was not clinically impaired. This was attributed by Nyman to the normal cross-linking of both chain fragments.

Gaffney et al. (1975) examined the fibrinogenolytic activity of brinase and confirmed the rapid digestion of human fibrinogen in vitro to aggregable degradation products in the molecular size range of 310000–230000. The susceptibility of fibrinogen polypeptide chains to brinase attack was in the order Aα, γ, Bβ, and lysis of the Bβ-chain appeared to be the rate-limiting step in the conversion of the higher molecular weight fragments to the core fragments D_{br} and E_{br}. Since the NH_2-terminal tyrosine was conserved during fibrinogen digestion, and D-dimer fragments appeared only briefly during lysis of totally cross-linked fibrin, the authors suggested that brinase attacks primarily the carboxy end of the γ-chain. Cross-linked α-chains of fibrin, while resistant to plasmin attack, were found to be vigorously digested by brinase.

In the plasmas of cancer patients being treated with brinase, Gaffney et al. found degraded fibrinogen (lacking intact Aα-chains) and aggregates. These aggregates contained some cross-linked γ-chains (γ-γ-dimers), which suggested that brinase in vivo had both lytic and coagulant properties. When clotted with thrombin, these plasmas contained no cross-linked α-chains.

Positive plasma ethanol gelation tests were attributed by the authors to the presence of aggregable high molecular weight fragments as observed during in vitro lysis of fibrinogen by brinase.

c) Other Natural Proteins and Synthetic Substrates

The early work by Stefanini et al. (1962) and by Bergkvist (1963b) had demonstrated the activity of brinase on casein, gelatin, and urea-denatured hemoglobin, from which several assay methods have been developed.

Hessel and Blombäck (1973) have shown considerable activity on human albumin, obtaining a great number of peptide spots from two-dimensional peptide-mapping of 4-h brinase-albumin digests.

The most commonly used synthetic substrate of brinase was tosyl arginine methyl ester (TAME), which was utilized for assay purposes at various stages of production (Roschlau and Ives, 1974).

4. Hemostasis

Digestion of coagulation proteins by brinase may cause interference with hemostatic mechanisms, which manifests itself as a coagulation defect and as reduced adhesiveness and aggregability of blood platelets.

a) Coagulation

The effects of Aspergillin O on some components of the coagulation system were first reported by MARIN et al. (1961) and by KARACA et al. (1962b, c). Using both in vitro and in vivo techniques, it was indicated that all effects were concentration-dependent, and that "high" doses of crude enzyme generally delayed the generation of thrombin and diminished the activity of clot accelerators, together with moderate fibrinogenopenia. Owing to the extreme impurity of Aspergillin O, however, quantitative dose-effect relationships and the differentiation of enzyme effects from those of impurities were impossible to establish.

The coagulation effects of the purified enzyme were investigated by MONKHOUSE et al. (1964) who studied the responses of recalcified clotting time, plasma fibrinogen, prothrombin, thrombin clotting times, and antithrombin activity both in vitro and in vivo.

When adding brinase to citrated dog plasma in concentrations varying from 0.5 to 100 C2 U (0.5–100 µg) per ml of plasma and measuring the recalcified clotting times in intervals therafter, there was considerable variation in enzyme effects depending on dose and time of incubation. Low doses of brinase initially decreased recalcified clotting times, while high doses prolonged the recalcified clotting times to incoagulability (Fig. 30). The clot-promoting effects of small doses of brinase were confirmed in similar studies by OGSTON and OGSTON (1968).

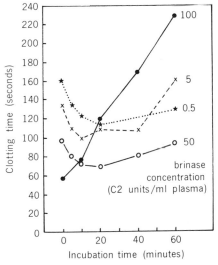

Fig. 30. Recalcified clotting times of citrated dog plasma at intervals following addition of varying amounts of brinase. Incubation at 37° C; enzyme concentrations in C2 U/ml plasma. After MONKHOUSE et al. (1964)

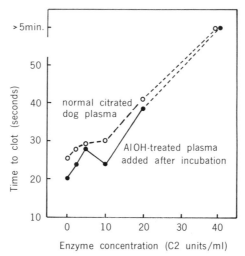

Fig. 31. Effect of incubation of plasma with brinase in vitro for 30 min on one-stage prothrombin clotting times. After MONKHOUSE et al. (1964)

The action of brinase on prothrombin was measured by one-stage prothrombin times of plasma following incubation with increasing amounts of enzyme. In other experiments, fresh aluminum hydroxide-treated plasma was added to the system after incubation to assure sufficient fibrinogen and accelerator factors without altering the prothrombin concentration. As shown in Figure 31, prothrombin times increased to more than 60 sec when the enzyme concentration reached 40 C 2 U (40 μg) per ml of plasma. A more direct study with prothrombin prepared from beef plasma showed a greatly accelerated conversion to thrombin in the presence of calcium, with brinase acting much like tissue thromboplastin. Thrombin generation decreased with increasing enzyme concentration, however, and larger concentrations of enzyme inhibited thrombin generation. Antithrombin activity, i.e., the activity in plasma causing progressive enzymatic inactivation of thrombin, was found by MONKHOUSE et al. to be destroyed by brinase (Fig. 32).

From this work the authors concluded that brinase acts on a number of coagulation proteins, and that its thromboplastic-like activity has an initial clot-promoting effect which is overbalanced by a progressively destructive action on prothrombin, thrombin, and fibrinogen. Prothrombin appeared to be the more sensitive plasma constituent, and all effects were strictly dependent on enzyme concentration.

OGSTON and OGSTON (1968) studied the coagulant properties of brinase and reported that fibrin was formed in plasma upon addition of brinase, but that this fibrin formation was not as rapid as from the addition of thrombin. Heparin did not prevent brinase-induced clotting, and adsorption with aluminum hydroxide gel did not affect the amount and rate of fibrin formation. The authors concluded that brinase acted directly on fibrinogen to produce fibrin rather than by inducing the formation of thrombin. OGSTON and OGSTON therefore considered brinase to be an unsuitable thrombolytic agent because lysis of plasma clots will likely not take place without concomitant destruction or conversion to fibrin of the surrounding plasma fibrinogen.

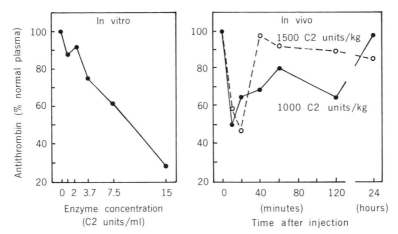

Fig. 32. *(Left)* Decrease in antithrombin activity of defibrinated plasma with increasing amounts of brinase added in vitro. *(Right)* Effect on antithrombin activity in dog following i.v. injection of brinase. After MONKHOUSE et al. (1964)

In vivo studies by BERGKVIST and SVÄRD (1964) and by ROSCHLAU (1964) demonstrated dose-dependent coagulant/anticoagulant effects in experimental animals. A slight acceleration of whole blood clotting accompanied the administration of "small" doses of brinase that reduced inhibitor levels somewhat but did not produce detectable fibrinolysis. When doses were increased and inhibitors were reduced to obtain fibrinolytic activity in the blood, the whole blood clotting time lengthened. Blood became incoagulable upon exhaustion of brinase inhibitors (cf. Fig. 19).

b) Platelet Function

Early observations on the effect of brinase on platelet function were made by JÜRGENS (1966b), SVÄRD (1966), BYGDEMAN (1967), and DE NICOLA et al. (1967).

JÜRGENS (1966b) described a method to determine spontaneous platelet aggregation—essentially the clumping of platelets in platelet-rich plasma (PRP) with subsequent filtration through glass sand—which allowed the determination of platelet aggregates by differential pre- and post-aggregation platelet counts.

Intravenous infusions of 120 and 150 mg of brinase in 5% levulose solution into 28 patients resulted in dose-dependent reductions of spontaneous platelet aggregation, with maximal effects noted about 4 days after treatment (Fig. 33). A continuous depression of spontaneous platelet aggregation was obtained by JÜRGENS with infusions of brinase every 4–6 days (Fig. 34), where the fluctuations in platelet aggregability were relatively small. Concurrently with measurements of platelet aggregation, JÜRGENS studied the effects of brinase on some coagulation factors. Thrombelastograms, heparin tolerance tests, and recalcification times remained unchanged, while isolated prothrombin, thromboplastin times (Quick) and factor VII changed to varying degrees (Fig. 35). These coagulation responses occurred during the hours following brinase infusions and had mostly terminated 6–8 h later, thus occurring prior to the demonstrable effects on platelets. The author suspected that the platelet effects of

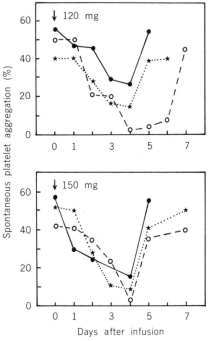

Fig. 33. Effects of single i.v. doses of 120 and 150 mg brinase on spontaneous platelet aggregation (3 patients). From Jürgens (1966b)

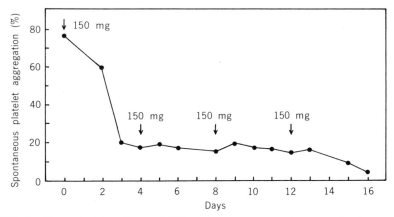

Fig. 34. Effects of repeated i.v. doses of 150 mg brinase on spontaneous platelet aggregation. From Jürgens (1966b)

brinase may have been due to the appearance of fibrinogen degradation products (FDP).

Svärd (1966) studied the effects of brinase on rabbit platelets in vitro. Platelets were either washed or unwashed, and aggregation was measured by Born's turbidimetric technique. Washed platelets were found to aggregate on addition of brinase

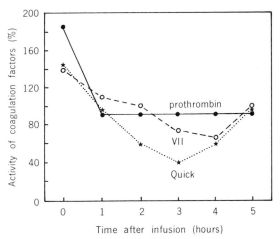

Fig. 35. Post-infusion effects of a single i.v. dose of 180 mg brinase on Quick time, factor VII and isolated prothrombin. From JÜRGENS (1966b)

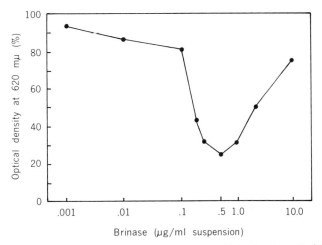

Fig. 36. Effect of brinase on aggregation of washed rabbit platelets. Ca⁺⁺ added to stirred platelet suspension 0.5 min before enzyme. OD observed 10 min after enzyme addition. From SVÄRD (1966)

and calcium ions, the aggregation being equivalent to that produced by adenosine diphosphate (ADP) at optimal concentration (Fig. 36). "Low" and "high" concentrations of enzyme produced only very slight changes. The effects were found to be calcium-dependent and could be inhibited with tosyl arginine ethyl ester (TAEE). At concentrations below 0.1 µg/ml of platelet suspension, brinase caused only very slight aggregation, and these platelets were subsequently found to be less responsive to ADP aggregation. This inhibitory effect on washed platelets (Fig. 37) was reversible by addition of fibrinogen to the inhibited system, restoring full aggregability to the platelet suspension.

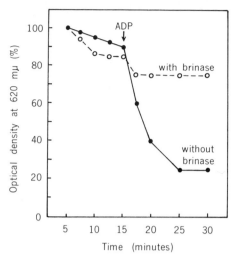

Fig. 37. Inhibition of ADP-induced aggregation of washed rabbit platelets by brinase. Ca^{++} added to stirred suspension at 4.5 min, brinase (0.001 μg/ml) or buffer at 5 min, and ADP (16 μg/ml) at 15 min. After SVÄRD (1966)

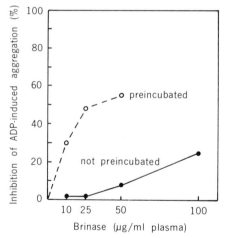

Fig. 38. Inhibition of ADP-induced aggregation of unwashed rabbit platelets by brinase. Samples of PRP were either preincubated with enzyme at room temperature for 5 min before aggregation with ADP (4 μg/ml), or enzyme was added to PRP simultaneously with ADP. After SVÄRD (1966)

The effects of brinase on unwashed platelets in PRP were different in that higher concentrations of enzyme were required, and only inhibition of aggregation was observed (Fig. 38). SVÄRD proposed that brinase affected platelets probably via a two-stage reaction of which the first stage might be an alteration of the platelet membrane with release of platelet fibrinogen, and that fibrinogen is likely to occupy a key position in the process of platelet aggregation and inhibition.

BYGDEMAN (1967) studied the effects of brinase in vitro on human platelets by means of ADP adhesion and aggregation (Figs. 39, 40), thus confirming the observa-

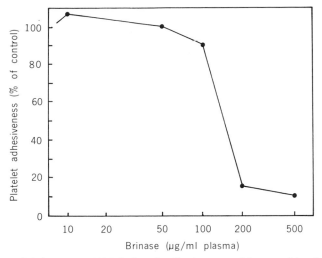

Fig. 39. Effect of brinase on ADP-induced adhesiveness of human blood platelets in vitro. ADP=0.15 µg/ml plasma. Mean of 7 experiments. From BYGDEMAN (1967)

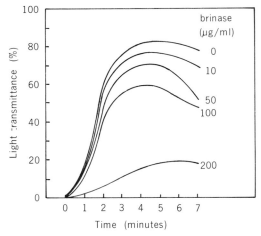

Fig. 40. Effect of brinase on ADP-induced aggregation of human blood platelets in vitro. ADP = 0.2 µg/ml plasma. After BYGDEMAN (1967)

tions by SVÄRD (1966) that the enzyme could counteract ADP-induced aggregation of rabbit platelets, but noting that the concentrations of enzyme required for human platelet inhibition were about double those required for rabbit platelet inhibition. Reflecting on the relatively low doses of enzyme required by JÜRGENS (1966b) to induce inhibition of spontaneous platelet aggregation in patients, BYGDEMAN suggested that the inhibitory effects may be due to induced changes in plasma composition, and possibly an accumulation of FDP.

De NICOLA et al. (1967) correlated platelet inhibitory effects of brinase with corresponding increases in fibrinolytic activity in 18 patients receiving doses ranging from

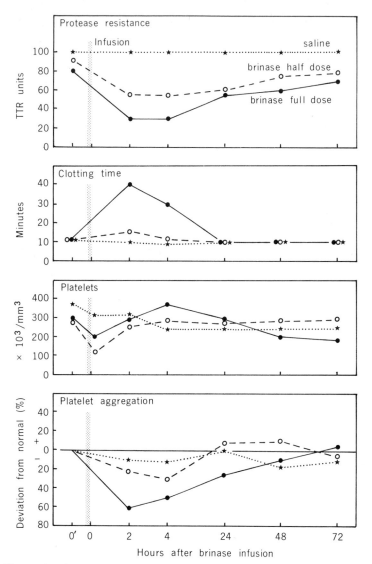

Fig. 41. Effects of brinase infusions on selected parameters in dog. *Drug concentration* = 250 C2 U/ml saline. *Rate of infusion* = 2500 C2 U/min. *Full dose* = calculated to reduce protease resistance to 30 TTR U (="thrombolytic dose," mean for 4 dogs = 1940 C2 U/kg). *Half dose* = $^1/_2$ thrombolytic dose (mean for 4 dogs = 990 C2 U/kg). *Saline control* = equivalent volume of saline without enzyme. Inhibition of ADP-induced platelet aggregability: full dose = 60%, half dose = 30%. From ROSCHLAU and GAGE (1972 b).

52 to 156 mg per patient. It was found that inhibition of ADP-induced platelet aggregation, considerable increases in fibrinolytic activity, and prolongation of prothrombin times resulted in dependence on the doses of enzyme infused, with consistent and reproducible changes occurring at doses exceeding 100 mg/patient. thus confirming the data obtained by JÜRGENS (1966 b).

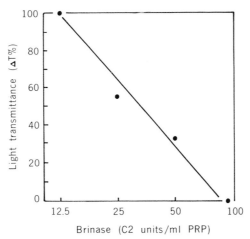

Fig. 42. In vitro inhibition of dog platelet aggregation by brinase. Mean responses of 5 dog plasmas (1 ml PRP incubated with 0.1 ml brinase solution for 30 min at 37° C, then aggregated with 1.0 μg ADP), blanks without brinase = 100% ΔT. From ROSCHLAU and GAGE (1972 b)

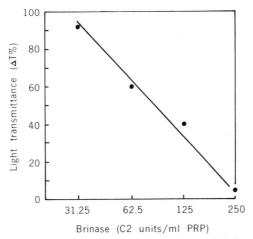

Fig. 43. In vitro inhibition of human platelet aggregation with brinase. Mean responses of 10 human plasmas (conditions as in Fig. 42, but aggregated with 250 μg collagen), blanks without brinase = 100% ΔT. From ROSCHLAU and GAGE (1972 b)

These investigations indicated a key role for fibrinogen in the inhibition of platelet function by brinase. This was further examined by ROSCHLAU and GAGE (1972 a, b) and by ROSCHLAU et al. (1975). Platelet aggregation was studied in PRP by means of a turbidimetric method in a platelet aggregometer, using ADP and collagen as aggregating stimuli. In vivo administration of brinase to dogs showed dose-dependent inhibition of ADP-induced aggregation that reached its maximum 2–4 h following enzyme infusion and lasted for about 1–2 days (Fig. 41). This dose dependency was also shown in vitro in dog and human PRP preincubated with brinase and aggregated with ADP or collagen (Figs. 42, 43). When plasma fibrinogen was di-

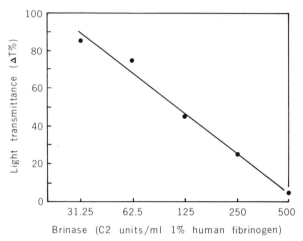

Fig. 44. In vitro inhibition of human platelet aggregation by brinase-produced human fibrinogen degradation products (FDP). Mean responses of 3 human plasmas in duplicate aggregated with 250 μg collagen, blanks without FDP = 100% *ΔT*. *Abscissa* shows amounts of brinase incubated for 30 min at 37° C with 1 ml of 1% purified fibrinogen, of which 0.5 ml was combined with 0.5 ml PRP for aggregation. From ROSCHLAU and GAGE (1972 b)

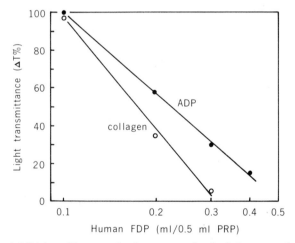

Fig. 45. In vitro inhibition of human platelet aggregation by brinase-produced human fibrinogen degradation products (FDP). Mean responses of 2 human plasmas in duplicate aggregated with 0.5 μg ADP and 250 μg collagen, blanks without FDP = 100% *ΔT*. *Abscissa* shows increments of FDPs derived from incubation for 30 min at 37° C of 1 ml of 1% purified fibrinogen with 500 C2 U of brinase. Increments adjusted to 0.5 ml with incubated enzyme-free fibrinogen and combined with 0.5 ml PRP for aggregation. From ROSCHLAU and GAGE (1972 b)

gested with varying doses of brinase and the digests were added to fresh PRP, inhibition of platelet aggregation was obtained in dependence on the amounts of generated FDP. FDPs produced from purified human fibrinogen gave similar results irrespective of the aggregating stimulus (Figs. 44, 45).

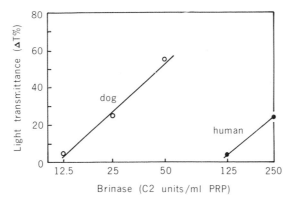

Fig. 46. In vitro aggregation of human and dog platelets with brinase. Mean responses of 5 dog and 10 human plasmas. Human platelets require 10 times higher doses than dog platelets for aggregation. From ROSCHLAU and GAGE (1972 b)

The platelet aggregating properties of brinase in dog and human PRP are shown in Figure 46, confirming earlier reports by SVÄRD (1966). Platelets subjected to the action of brinase concentrations of 100 and 200 C2 U (µg) per ml of PRP revealed no morphologic damage attributable to direct proteolysis when examined by electron microscopy, although aggregation was inhibited by 55% and 85% respectively.

ROSCHLAU and GAGE (1972 b) concluded that systemic infusions of brinase in dogs caused transient formation of microaggregates (shown by brief falls in platelet counts immediately following enzyme infusions, cf. Fig. 41), followed at once by dose-dependent inhibition of platelet aggregability for various periods of time. The inhibition of platelet function and the concomitant dose-dependent anticoagulant effects of brinase were attributed to the appearance of FDPs, and a mechanism similar to that in the dog was proposed for the responses of human platelets observed by JÜRGENS (1966 b) and by DE NICOLA et al. (1967, 1974) (Fig. 47).

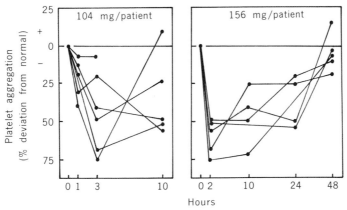

Fig. 47. Inhibition of ADP-induced platelet aggregation in patients following infusions of 104 and 156 mg of brinase per patient. ADP = 42 µg/ml patient's PRP. Platelet aggregability in percent deviation from patient's pretreatment response. After DE NICOLA et al. (1974)

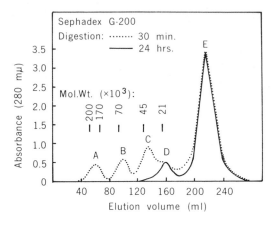

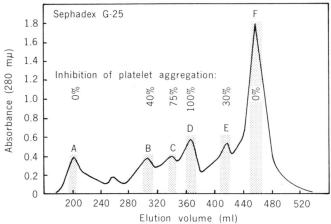

Fig. 48. *(Above)* Gel filtration of brinase-fibrinogen digests on Sephadex G-200. *Digests:* 250 C 2 U (= 250 μg) of brinase/ml 1% human fibrinogen incubated at 37° C for 30 min and 24 h. *Eluant:* 0.1 M Tris-HCl buffer pH 7.4 with 0.5 M NaCl and 0.003 M EDTA. *Mol wt markers:* blue dextran (200000), human γ-globulin (170000), human serum albumin (70000), egg albumin (45000), soybean trypsin inhibitor (21000). *30-min digest:* Fragments X, Y and intermediates *(peak A)*, fragment D *(peak B)*, fragment E *(peak C)*, low-molecular-weight proteins *(peak E)*. *24-h digest:* Residual brinase activity and probable fragment E split products *(peak D)*, low-mol-wt proteins *(peak E)*. Platelet-inhibitory activity identified in fractions of lowest mol wt (< 10000). *(Below)* Brinase-fibrinogen digest (62.5 C2 U of enzyme/ml 1% human fibrinogen, incubated for 24 h at 37° C) on Sephadex G-25 medium (fractionation range = mol wt 5000–1000). *Eluant:* deionized dist. water pH 7.4. Peak fractions pooled as indicated, freeze-dried and quantitatively reconstituted, and used in platelet aggregation tests in a concentration of 20 mg/ml PRP. Maximal inhibition of platelet aggregation obtained with fraction D (apparent mol wt 2500). From ROSCHLAU et al. (1975)

In view of the strong implications of brinase-produced FDPs in platelet inhibition, ROSCHLAU et al. (1975) digested human fibrinogen with brinase in vitro and obtained split products by column chromatography that were similar to those obtained by plasmin digestion (Fig. 48). Maximal platelet inhibitory activity was found to reside in the low molecular weight fractions from maximal fibrinogenolysis, which may be nonantigenic peptides appearing during the elaboration of fibrinogen fragment E. Comparison of the biological activities of brinase-produced peptides with plasmin-degraded low molecular weight fibrinogen peptides of SOLUM et al. (1973) showed remarkable quantitative and qualitative similarities when tested under comparable conditions in vitro, even though their source in the fibrinogen molecule and the cleavage sites may differ. However, since systemic fibrinolytic activity induced with plasmin rarely showed platelet inhibition to the extent observed with brinase, ROSCHLAU et al. (1975) raised the question whether the brinase-fibrinogen peptides can be regarded as the only and specific mediators of platelet inhibition. They calculated that the available circulating fibrinogen would hardly be sufficient to produce the required amounts of peptides (as indicated from in vitro studies) to account for the observed effects on platelet aggregation with clinical fibrinolytic doses of brinase in vivo, implying that the peptide deficit needs to be made up from nonfibrinogen proteins susceptible to brinase (but not to plasmin) cleavage. The most likely source of additional peptides is serum albumin, which is readily degraded by brinase (HESSEL and BLOMBÄCK, 1973), and whose peptides have strong anti-aggregating properties (ROSCHLAU, 1977).

5. Physicochemical Effects

SAWYER (1975) reported some effects of brinase on the physicochemical characteristics of the cardiovascular system of dogs and rabbits after comparing the actions of brinastrase, brinolase and Thrombolysin (streptokinase/human plasmin mixture) on the following: (a) the electrophoretic mobility of canine erythrocytes and platelets; (b) the alterations of the vascular intimal surface charge as determined by electro-osmosis and streaming potentials; (c) the alterations in platelet and erythrocyte adhesion characteristics; (d) the histologic appearance of rabbit blood vessels; (e) the appearance of canine blood vessels as demonstrated by scanning electron microscopy; and (f) the changes in blood coagulability as determined by various standard methods.

Brinastrase administered in a dose of 2 mg/kg, and brinolase in a dose of 1 mg/kg, were found to increase the net negative surface charge of the vascular intima. The electrophoretic mobility of blood platelets and erythrocytes was altered by an initial increase in the surface negativity followed 2 days later by a return to normal (i.e., a biphasic response). Platelet adhesion to metal surfaces and to the vascular endothelium was reduced, and histologic examination of hyperlipidemic rabbit blood vessels indicated reduced fat infiltration with minimal destruction of the vascular wall. All of these physicochemical effects of brinase were found to be comparable to the overall effects of Thrombolysin when administered in comparable dosage.

6. Kininogenesis

From early investigations of brinase in experimental animals (BERGKVIST and SVÄRD, 1964; ROSCHLAU, 1964, 1966) it became apparent that the enzyme affected systemic blood pressure to varying degrees depending on the size of the dose, the concentration, the speed of administration, and the circulatory competency of the subject. The cardiovascular effects of brinase have subsequently been studied, show-

GUINEA-PIG 410 G

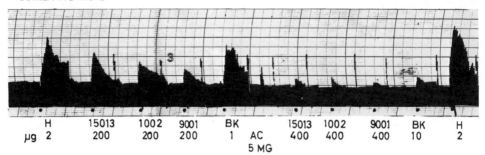

	H	15013	1002	9001	BK		15013	1002	9001	BK	H
	μg 2	200	200	200	1	AC	400	400	400	10	2
						5 MG					

Fig. 49. Bronchoconstriction in guinea-pig. Bronchoconstrictory effects of histamine *(H)*, brady-kinin *(BK)* and various batches of brinase of both Swedish *(15013)* and Canadian *(1002, 9001)* manufacture are compared, and antagonistic effect of acetylsalicylic acid *(AC)* shown. From Svärd (1974)

ing the formation of bradykinin-like peptides from the administration of enzyme doses that overwhelm or exceed the inhibitor level of the respective individual.

Freedman (1969) and Freedman and Roschlau (1970) investigated the kinino-genic properties of brinase, the spectrum of induced vascular effects, and possible means of pharmacologic modification of protease-induced hypotension. Blood pressure responses in the dog to infusions of brinase and of bradykinin were found to be qualitatively similar and quantitatively dose-related, the diastolic pressure falling most quickly and severely, followed in time by transient augmentation of pulse pressure, reflex tachycardia and hyperventilation, and accompanied by capillary hyperpermeability.

Svärd (1972, 1974) demonstrated falls in blood pressure in rabbits when brinase doses approached almost complete depletion of inhibitors. This hypotension was attributed to the formation of vasoactive peptides, and it was dependent on intact enzyme activity. Inactivation of the protease by incubation at 60° C completely abolished the blood pressure effects. Using guinea-pig bronchoconstriction as a model parameter, Svärd (1974) compared the effects of intravenously administered brinase, histamine, and bradykinin. The effects of bradykinin and some closely related peptides may be antagonized by acetylsalicylic acid, and Svärd showed that this antagonism extended to brinase but not to histamine (Fig. 49), from which was concluded that the rapid injection of brinase caused local excess of enzyme over inhibitors, leading to the formation of bradykinin-like substances with bronchoconstrictor activity.

Since hypotensive episodes were commonly observed in experimental animals when brinase was administered at too rapid a rate of infusion or too high a concentration, and also when inhibitors became depleted from administration of overdoses, possible pharmacologic reversal of brinase-induced hypotension was attempted. Roschlau et al. (1969) titrated dogs with infusions of excessive doses of protease until inhibitors were exhausted, incoagulability of the blood was obtained, free proteolysis was demonstrated by hepatocellular damage (estimated by determinations of serum transaminase), and capillary hyperpermeability (estimated by determinations of hematocrit) and severe hypotension occurred. Control animals died from irreversible hypotension and cardiovascular failure before eventual hemorrhagic sequelae

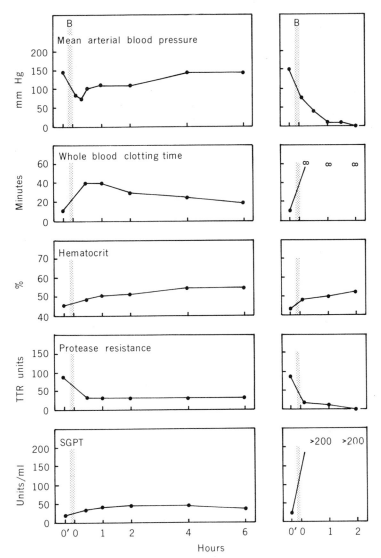

Fig. 50. *(Left)* Mean values of selected parameters of 5 dogs treated with "optimal" doses of brinase, individually calculated to lower protease resistance to 30 TTR U. B = brinase infusion. *(Right)* Same parameters of 5 dogs treated with "lethal" doses of brinase, individually calculated to lower protease resistance to 0 TTR U (i.e., inhibitor depletion). From ROSCHLAU et al. (1969)

from free proteolysis had time to develop (Fig. 50). Attempts to modify brinase-induced hypotension consisted of pretreatment with β-adrenergic blocking agents, which allowed the survival of "lethal" doses of brinase (Fig. 51). Established hypotension responded to long-acting sympathomimetics (such as metaraminol bitartrate, a noncatecholamine, Fig. 51). In this manner the persistent vasomotor collapse from "lethal" doses of brinase was modified, gaining time to correct eventual coagulation defects with replacement therapy.

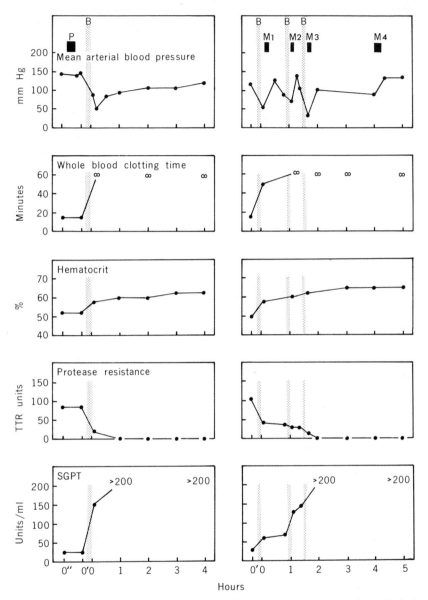

Fig. 51. *(Left)* Mean values of selected parameters of 3 dogs that survived "lethal" doses of brinase (as in Fig. 50, *right*) after pretreatment with β-adrenergic blocker. P = propranolol hydrochloride, 1 mg/kg; B = individually calculated dose of brinase to lower protease resistance to 0 TTR U. *(Right)* Same parameters of 3 dogs that received divided doses of brinase *(B)* to lower protease resistance progressively, and treated with metaraminol bitartrate to control brinase-induced hypotension. Metaraminol bitartrate: $M_1 = 70$ µg/kg, $M_2 = 70$ µg/kg, $M_3 = 250$ µg/kg, $M_4 = 300$–500 µg/kg. M_4 administration was determined by magnitude of secondary hypotension and was given in varying dosages to restore normotension. From ROSCHLAU et al. (1969)

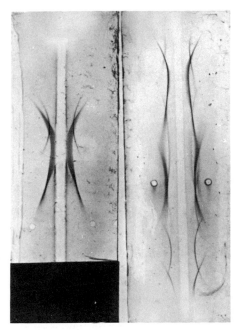

Fig. 52. Immunoelectrophoretic patterns of purified brinase *(Left)* and crude Aspergillin O *(Right)*. From SVÄRD (1974)

7. Antigenicity

Brinase, a protein with a molecular weight of about 20000, must be suspected to be a potential antigen. Several attempts have therefore been made to study immunogenicity and antigenicity of the enzyme. Precipitating antibodies of the IgG class may be produced in rabbits and guinea-pigs only after intense immunization employing Freund's complete adjuvant, and in vivo experiments in guinea-pigs sensitized and subsequently challenged with near-toxic doses of brinase did not demonstrate anaphylaxis (SVÄRD, 1974; Connaught Medical Research Laboratories, unpublished reports). The immunoelectrophoretic patterns from brinase and Aspergillin O, run against a hyperimmune rabbit serum, are shown in Figure 52. When comparisons were made in guinea-pigs between brinase and human γ-globulin, the incidence of anaphylactoid reactions of any kind was 5% with brinase and 40% with γ-globulin. Since only low-titered antisera were obtained even after intense immunization, brinase must be regarded as a very low immunogen with practically no antigenic properties (SVÄRD, 1974).

8. Toxicity

The acute intravenous LD_{50} of brinase in mice is about 25 mg/kg (25000 C2 U/kg) (ROSCHLAU, 1971a; SVÄRD, 1974). The side-effects of brinase in animals and man can uniformly be attributed to proteolysis of substrates other than fibrin. The dominant symptomatology was found to be hypocoagulability owing to lysis of some coagulation proteins (e.g., fibrinogen, prothrombin), hemoconcentration consequent to increased capillary permeability, and hypotension of varying intensity (both due to kinin formation). Proteases in general participate in the formation of several kinins with peripheral actions such as vasodilatation, capillary leakage, contraction of smooth muscle, bronchoconstriction, and pain. Hydrolysis of coagulation proteins by brinase may lead to aberrations in the clotting process depending on plasma titer and on concurrent promoting and inhibiting factors. In the blood, brinase is normally held in balance by combination with inhibitors circulating with the α-globulins. However, when administered too rapidly or in excess of inhibitors, brinase will indiscriminately attack other than specific substrates, giving rise to a variety of clinical symptoms. The acute toxicity of brinase is thus inversely proportional to its inhibition in blood, and several studies have demonstrated the enzyme's safety on the one hand, and its propensity to cause toxic effects on the other, in relation to its state of inhibition.

ROSCHLAU (1966) investigated acute brinase-related toxicity in 36 dogs. All animals carried experimental arterial occluding thrombi, to be lysed with single systemic administrations of protease. Doses were individually calculated from the pretreatment inhibitor level (protease resistance) to lower protease resistance to various target levels at which thrombolysis occurred. At no time were inhibitors depleted. The important variables that were judged to be objective indicators of toxic effects were the whole blood clotting time, systolic blood pressure, hematocrit, serum glutamic pyruvic transaminase, and the autopsy findings (i.e., evidence of extravasation) after sacrifice 24–72 h later.

To obtain blood levels of enzyme with predictably thrombolytic effects, circulating inhibitors needed to be reduced but not depleted (ROSCHLAU, 1964). The optimal single dose to achieve this balance was found in the dog to be that amount of enzyme which lowered protease resistance to about 30 TTR U. Smaller doses were not predictably thrombolytic, while larger doses led to exhaustion of inhibitors and free proteolysis (ROSCHLAU, 1964). As shown in Figure 53, toxicity from intravenous injections of brinase into dogs was directly related to the intensity of induced proteolytic activity. Posttreatment inhibitor levels below 30 TTR U were accompanied by significantly greater toxicity than were levels above 30 TTR U. This was confirmed in a separate study by ROSCHLAU and TOSONI (1965), in which brinase treatments with a protease resistance target of 40 TTR U were without side-effects.

The dependence of brinase toxicity on its inhibition by blood inhibitors has also been demonstrated experimentally by ROSCHLAU et al. (1969) and by FREEDMAN and ROSCHLAU (1970), and additional evidence was provided by other investigators in the course of experimental and clinical thrombolysis with the protease. Thus, acute toxicity data varied from one species to another, and in some instances within the same species. This variability was shown to be a consequence of significant fluctuations in the levels of protective serum inhibitors characteristic of different species and individuals (ROSCHLAU, 1971a). The fundamental importance of optimal inhibitor neutralization with administered brinase for the attainment of thrombolytic efficacy, and the avoidance of acute toxic side-effects, was thus recognized and formed the basis for the formulation of various treatment schemes in the clinical therapeutic use of the enzyme.

Interactions of brinase with radio-opaque dyes used in angiography were examined by FRISCH et al. (1970, 1971) after it had been observed clinically (LUND et al.,

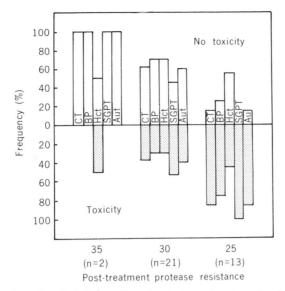

Fig. 53. Distribution of toxic brinase effects in 36 dogs at various levels of inhibitor reduction (posttreatment protease resistance = 35, 30, and 25 TTR U). *CT* = whole blood clotting time; *BP* = systolic blood pressure; *Hct* = hematocrit (reflecting hemoconcentration); *SGPT* = serum glutamic pyruvic transaminase (reflecting liver damage); *Aut* = gross extravasation at autopsy. *Criteria for toxicity:* Clotting time > 60 min; blood pressure fall > 25%; hematocrit increase > 25%; SGPT > 50 units; autopsy grossly pathologic. After Roschlau (1966)

1968 b) that thrombolytically effective intra-arterial infusions of brinase, when combined with arteriography, caused local intra-arterial aggregation of cellular elements which occasionally impaired collateral flow and microcirculation, accompanied by leakage of contrast medium from small vessels. Experimental thrombi were produced in both femoral arteries of dogs, and one side was treated with intra-arterial injections of brinase alone while the contralateral side received alternating injections of brinase and Urografin 60%. The combination of enzyme and contrast medium caused proximal enlargement of thrombi which could only be removed with subsequent instillations of pure brinase, and edematous changes were observed in the tissues adjacent to arteries treated with the combination of agents. None of these effects could be demonstrated in thrombosed vessels receiving brinase without contrast medium, or in nonthrombosed vessels receiving the combination of drugs. Permeability changes, therefore, were attributed to the interaction of brinase and radio-opaque medium when given together or in rapid succession in the presence of vascular obstruction. Interactions no longer occurred when the agents were administered separately in intervals of 1 h or more (FRISCH, 1974).

The acute lethal effects of brinase were studied by administering intentional overdoses of enzyme by slow infusion to anesthetized dogs until death occurred (ROSCHLAU, 1966, and unpublished; ROSCHLAU et al., 1969; FREEDMAN and ROSCHLAU, 1970). Immediately upon depletion of inhibitors the blood became incoagulable, the blood pressure fell to extremely (i.e., nonfunctional) values, brief compensatory tachycardia and hyperventilation occurred, serum transaminase rose to levels indicative of severe hepatocellular damage, and the animals expired from vasomotor collapse. Upon autopsy the most striking finding in all cases was the absence of overt hemorrhages into body cavities. Extravasation, when observed, consisted of hematoma-like discolorations in the walls of the gallbladder and urinary bladder, the serosa of ileum and cecum, and sometimes the root of the mitral valve together with pulmonary petechiae and atelectases. The cause of death of animals from acute overdosage of brinase, therefore, could not be attributed to hemorrhage but was found to be due to the explosive intravascular liberation of highly vasoactive substances leading to cardiovascular collapse.

While most of the acute toxic effects of brinase were investigated in anesthetized animals, Roschlau (unpublished) and Roschlau and Tosoni (1965) also studied the reactions of a small number of unanesthetized dogs to systemic infusions of thrombolytic doses of the enzyme. Despite dose-dependent changes in coagulation parameters and occasional hypotensive episodes, none of the animals exhibited signs of distress during treatment, or gross pathologic changes upon sacrifice several days or weeks later. Infusions repeated in daily or weekly intervals were also tolerated without outward side-effects if individual doses were calculated to avoid inhibitor depletion. There was, however, the occasional vomiting, diarrhea, and micturition (the latter provoked by the volumes of infusion fluid) shortly after completion of an infusion indicative of smooth muscle stimulation. Other kinin-mediated responses (e.g., pain, bronchoconstriction) were not observed.

Chronic toxicity studies in animals (Roschlau, 1971a) did not show significant alterations in blood chemistry, hematology, or urinalysis. Electrocardiograms did not vary from pretreatment controls, gross pathologic changes were not observed, and no indications of drug-induced lesions were found following evaluation of histopathology. The chronic toxicity data, which were accepted as evidence of the drug's profile for licensing purposes by governmental agencies (Connaught Medical Research Laboratories, 1965, 1970, 1972), indicated a lack of cardiac, hepatic, and renal effects from repeated administrations of brinase as long as serum inhibitors were not allowed to become exhausted. A summary of brinase side-effects is given in Table 9.

Table 9. Brinase side-effects commonly observed in experimental animals. (From Roschlau, 1971a)

Parameter	Low dose: Plasma inhibitors not affected	Therapeutic dose: Plasma inhibitors partly neutralized	Overdose: Plasma inhibitors depleted
Coagulation	Hypercoagulable (transient)	Slightly hypocoagulable (2–3 times normal clotting time)	Incogulable (transient)
Platelets	Hyperaggregable (transient)	Hypoadhesive - hypoaggregable (ADP, collagen)	
Cardiovascular	None	None	Hypotension (transient)
Hepatotoxicity	None	None	SGPT elevation (transient)
Other	None	None	Late pyrexia; late GI hypermotility

III. Experimental Thrombolysis

1. In Vitro Experiments

The thrombolytic efficacy of brinase was studied by ROSCHLAU (1964) by suspending 24-h-old blood clots of about 0.5 g in solutions of brinase and of urokinase-activated plasmin of similar activity. During incubation at 37° C, the clots suspended in brinase retained their shape, structure, and consistency throughout the process of lysis, losing weight by a melting-away process from the periphery toward the center. In contrast, clots suspended in plasmin solution acquired a jelly-like consistency and disintegrated. The internal disintegration of clots in plasmin solution was attributed to activation of clot plasminogen by excess urokinase. It was concluded that the mechanism of clot lysis by brinase was a surface action and not an activation of clot plasminogen.

In a study of thrombolysis by activation of plasminogen and by direct proteolysis, SCHMIDT (1965, 1966a, b) examined the mode of action of brinase in a system using retracted whole blood clots, either suspended on wires or lying on the bottom of tubes containing 2 ml of autologous serum or saline, to which varying doses of streptokinase or brinase were added, followed by incubation at 37° C for observation of qualitative and quantitative lysis. SCHMIDT demonstrated that clots lying on the bottom of tubes could not be lysed with brinase doses of up to 1000 C2 U, while suspended clots lysed completely within 4 h of incubation with 1000 C2 U of protease. Plasminogen activation with streptokinase caused only partial lysis of suspended clots, whether incubated in saline or in serum, while brinase caused lysis irrespective of the medium employed.

SCHMIDT concluded from these experiments that plasminogen activation with streptokinase, or the direct addition of plasmin, will lyse only those portions of retracted whole blood clots that are rich in erythrocytes with scanty fibrin, while parts of the thrombus with compact fibrin masses and strong retraction were resistant to the action of streptokinase or plasmin. In contrast, similar clots treated identically with brinase were shown to lyse completely from the surface down, independent of thrombus structure.

In simulation of in vivo thrombolysis, SCHMIDT subjected intra-vitally formed thrombi obtained from embolectomies to similar in vitro conditions. The results indicated that naturally grown intravascular thrombi responded to streptokinase with partial lysis in dependence on thrombus structure, while brinase caused complete dissolution.

ALBERT (1973) employed thrombelastography to demonstrate the mechanism of clot lysis by brinase. To citrated whole blood were added varying amounts of protease, the blood was recalcified, and small amounts of thrombin were added. Clotting and lysis were displayed in a thrombelastogram. The results indicated that high doses of brinase completely prevented clotting of recalcified, thrombinized blood when incorporated into the forming thrombus. Lower doses of the enzyme caused rapid thrombolysis, the speed being directly proportional to the concentration of incorporated brinase. In analyzing the thrombelastograms, ALBERT concluded that the lysis of thrombi containing brinase within their mass proceeded with diminishing speed as enzyme was consumed during the reaction.

When added to preformed clots by layering, brinase was shown to cause frontal lysis depending on the surface area of the clot and the concentration of enzyme. Comparing internal and frontal lysis patterns, ALBERT showed that complete dissolution of 0.6 ml blood clots was obtained in the thrombelastograph by internal lysis in less than 1 h with 50 C2 U, and by frontal lysis in approx. 2 h with 1000 C2 U and in 3–4 h with 500 C2 U.

2. In Vivo Experiments

The thrombolytic efficacy and potential clinical usefulness of brinase was investigated in several animal species by a variety of methods. Systemic as well as local application of the enzyme succeeded in lysing experimental thrombi, and the side-effects produced by such therapy were judged to be acceptable when viewed in the light of attainable thrombolytic results.

a) Systemic Administration

Working with the *crude* preparation, MARIN et al. (1961) studied the thrombolytic activity of Aspergillin O on experimental venous thrombi produced by sodium morrhuate in 70 dogs. The authors obtained recanalization of vessels thrombosed for 24–48 h, as demonstrated by venography. The administration of lytic doses of Aspergillin O was accompanied by falls in plasma fibrinogen levels, reduced activity of some other coagulation factors (notably prothrombin and labile and stable factors), and a delay in the production of thrombin. It was concluded that the combined effects of Aspergillin O may indeed be interesting enough to warrant further investigation.

In vivo studies of the *purified* enzyme began with the work of BERGKVIST and SVÄRD (1964) in cats and of ROSCHLAU (1964) in dogs.

BERGKVIST and SVÄRD produced femoral vein clots in anesthetized cats by several techniques such as injection of thrombin, sodium morrhuate, or homologous serum, and also with electric current and heat. In most experiments, however, thrombin was used, and the ability of brinase to lyse these clots of varying age was estimated by conventional X-ray techniques.

When subjecting venous clots that were 2, 6, 24, 48 and 72 h old to single i.v. injections of brinase, lysis was found to be complete in most animals with 2-h clots and some of the 6- and 24-h clots. No clear-cut dissolution was evident with clots older than 48 h. Control cats receiving saline solution gave no evidence of lysis or recanalization. BERGKVIST and SVÄRD observed a dose-dependent decrease in serum inhibitor activity (cf. Fig. 19) and attributed the pattern of responses to the existence of two different inhibitors which needed to be depressed to a certain level at which fibrinolytic activity in the animal's blood became apparent. A dose-dependent effect on coagulation was noted, beginning with a shortening of clotting times with low doses of brinase, followed by hypo- and incoagulability of the blood as brinase doses were increased. The blood pressure was shown to fall as blood levels of the enzyme rose toward fibrinolytic levels.

Although there were variations in the capacity of the serum inhibitor system of a normal cat population, and the doses of brinase ought to have been individualized for each animal, these variations were found to be small and the cats were treated with standard doses of 35 CU (approx. 2 mg) per kg, sufficient to give an effect, yet below the inhibitor level. These animals did not present pathologic findings upon sacrifice. Once the level of inhibitors was surpassed, however, hemorrhagic lesions of varying severity were observed.

ROSCHLAU (1964, 1972a) and ROSCHLAU and TOSONI (1965) produced thrombi in the femoral arteries and jugular veins of dogs by scarification of the intima. The presence of occlusive thrombi was confirmed by inspection and flow measurements 24 h later, and treatment with systemic i.v. infusions of brinase was initiated under anesthesia. Thrombolysis was assessed by measuring the re-establishment of arterial blood pressure and by visual measurement of venous thrombi.

The variations in serum inhibitor levels of dogs were found to be significant (cf. Fig. 20), which required individualization of dosage to obtain thrombolysis without toxicity. A dose-prediction test based on the measurement of total brinase inhibitors was developed[3] (ROSCHLAU, 1964, 1965), with which it became possible to administer brinase to dogs with safety and efficacy. The results of a large number of dog experiments indicated that under optimal conditions recanalization of vessels may be achieved within a few hours of commencing systemic therapy. The individual single dose of protease required for thrombolytic effects was found to be that amount of enzyme which lowered protease resistance to about 30 TTR U. At autopsy a few days after brinase treatments no clots could be detected in the majority of arteries, although intima lesions from scarification were always present. In some instances small thrombi adhering to the intima lesion were found, indicating incomplete lysis. These remnants invariably consisted of platelet deposits which did not respond to enzymatic digestion. In control experiments with saline infusions instead of brinase, spontaneous clot lysis was not observed.

These experiments revealed a set of fundamental restrictions of brinase administration, which have since been shown to apply in concept also to systemic administration to humans. In the dog:

1. The enzyme needed to be diluted, preferably not exceeding a concentration of 0.25 mg ($=250$ C2 U) per ml of diluent.

2. The rate of infusion needed to be adjusted to a uniform 2.5 mg ($=2500$ C2 U $= 10$ ml of the above dilution) per minute.

3. Infusions should preferably be made into large veins in order to assure instant contact of enzyme and inhibitors.

4. The total dose needed to be individually calculated, on the basis of pretreatment inhibitor levels and body weight, to obtain a reduction of serum inhibitors (protease resistance) to approx. 30 TTR U.

The side-effects observed during single intravenous infusions of thrombolytically effective doses of brinase were entirely dependent on the rapidity and degree of induced proteolytic activity. They consisted of brief periods of hypercoagulability in the initial minutes of infusion followed at once by a reversible prolongation of clotting times to approx. 3–4 times normal, and of a slight reversible decline in blood pressure to about 90% of normal (Fig. 54).

The apparent difficulties of management arising from such single-dose therapy were minimized (ROSCHLAU and TOSONI, 1965) by repeated administrations of

---

[3] See Section VII/2.

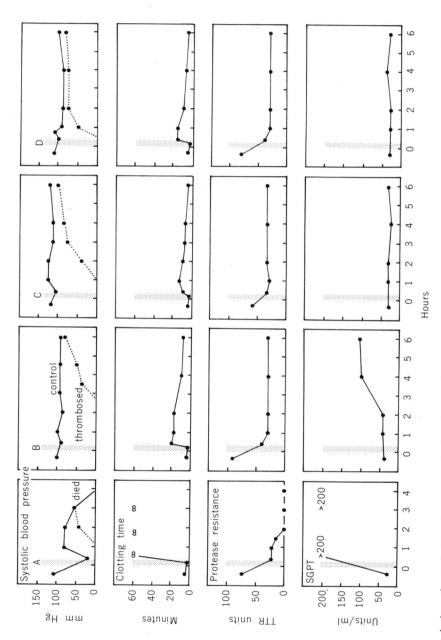

Fig. 54. Relation of systolic blood pressure, clotting time, and serum transaminase to protease resistance in 4 dogs with arterial thrombi. *A* and *B* : 2000C2 U of brinase per kg irrespective of pretreatment protease resistance, causing death of one animal in whom dose was excessive. *C* and *D* : Individualized dosage calculated from pretreatment protease resistance (*C* = 1000 C 2 U/kg, *D* = 1800 C 2 U/kg), obtaining thrombolysis without toxicity. After ROSCHLAU (1964)

smaller doses of brinase (target protease resistance = 40 TTR U instead of 30 TTR U, allowing a higher posttreatment inhibitor level) for several days. The lytic effects of repeated smaller doses were comparable to those after intensive single-dose therapy, and owing to the conservation of inhibitors, the side-effects on coagulation and blood pressure were almost entirely avoided.

The results of ROSCHLAU (1964) and of ROSCHLAU and TOSONI (1965) were confirmed in the dog by HUANG et al. (1969) using similar techniques of thrombus formation, dose prediction, and dosage. However, the thrombi were made radio-opaque by incorporating a radio-opaque substance (Steripaque) during clot formation, and the dissolution was followed continuously by X-ray visualization. The authors succeeded in lysing 3-day-old clots within an hour of infusion of calculated doses of brinase.

GIERING and TRUANT (1966) studied the quantitative in vivo dissolution of autologous preformed clots in dogs. Blood was withdrawn from the animals and allowed to clot around a specially constructed polyethylene tubing to which the clots adhered firmly. After incubation for 3 h and clot retraction, the entire structure was weighed and inserted into the jugular vein of the same dog via the internal maxillary vein. The animals were then treated systemically with fixed doses of brinase and heparin (the latter required to prevent initial clot extension during brinase infusion), after which the clots were retrieved, reweighed, and the extent of lysis was quantitated. The authors demonstrated the variability of lysis in dependence on serum inhibitor levels of individual animals on the one hand, and the attainment of significant lysis without the need for depletion of inhibitors on the other.

b) Local Administration

In efforts to improve the effectiveness of brinase on types of thrombi that were found to be refractory to systemic thrombolytic therapy, and to avoid systemic side-effects completely, ROSCHLAU and FISHER (1966) attempted the lysis of 24-h-old venous and arterial occluding thrombi produced by scarification of the intima in anesthetized dogs with local applications of the enzyme in the near vicinity of the occlusions.

Brinase solutions were prepared to contain 1000 C2 U (1 mg) per ml of saline, and 2-ml portions were injected into the thrombosed vessels via one of the tributaries (veins) or branches (arteries), to be repeated at 5–10-min intervals until clot dissolution occurred under direct vision. The experiments were carried out in the presence and absence of circulating blood, and with or without heparin added to the enzyme solution or given prior to or after brinase instillations.

Injections of 2000 C2 U of brinase into thrombosed veins caused immediate extension of the clot, to be followed by lysis of the primary thrombus and the secondary clot only upon subsequent applications of enzyme. Anticoagulation of the animals was therefore required. Addition of 50 U of heparin to each 1000 C2 U of brinase prevented secondary clotting, and intravenous thrombi were rapidly lysed by approx. 10000 C2 U of enzyme given in four or five divided doses 5–10 min apart. Recanalized vessels remained patent during 24 h of observation, at which time their appearance was normal. When blood was excluded from the vessel segments during brinase instillations, the enzyme requirements were less because of the absence of enzyme inhibitors, but rethrombosis was observed 24 h after therapy.

Arterial thrombolysis occurred more quickly and with less enzyme than did lysis of venous thrombi. The treated vessels were patent and essentially normal 24 h later, except for the occasional subendothelial transverse striation attributed to vessel distension during enzyme instillation into occluded arteries. Exclusion of blood allowed thrombolysis to proceed at about the same pace with the same dose requirements. However, intimal damage was present when blood was excluded, as indicated by subendothelial hematomas of varying extent; rethrombosis was not observed.

The authors concluded that small doses of brinase had demonstrable clot-promoting effects that needed to be counteracted with heparin if the full lytic potential of brinase on preformed thrombi was to be realized. The results gave clear evidence of enzyme inhibition when circulating blood was allowed to enter the thrombosed vessel segments to compete with locally instilled brinase, as shown by the lesser dose requirements for thrombolytic effects in the absence of circulating blood. Slight enzymatic attack on the vessel walls in the absence of inhibitors occurred, which in veins caused rethrombosis 24 h after lysis of primary thrombi. There were no systemic toxic effects. When compared with systemic dose requirements, the local doses were between one-fourth and one-third of systemic doses of similar thrombolytic efficacy.

PARKER and BOYD (1968) treated anesthetized dogs with direct pulmonary artery infusions of brinase in an effort to demonstrate the safety of this procedure. The animals did not carry pulmonary thrombi or emboli, and indications of the enzyme's thrombolytic efficacy under these conditions were not obtained. Brinase infusions were carried out at various concentrations and rates, and the authors confirmed the general constellation of systemic side-effects and toxicity as described by ROSCHLAU (1964, 1966) for intravenous infusions in dependence on the degree of protease resistance (inhibitor) neutralization. It was concluded by PARKER and BOYD that direct pulmonary artery infusions of brinase in dogs can be carried out without risk of dangerous side-effects provided that the maximum allowable dose (as predicted by the protease resistance test of ROSCHLAU) is not exceeded and the enzyme is well diluted.

In their study of the interaction of brinase and radio-opaque dyes, FRISCH et al. (1970, 1971) treated experimentally produced arterial thrombi in anesthetized dogs with intra-arterial injections of brinase in dosages ranging from 2 to 10 mg (1 mg/ml at intervals of 5 min). Thrombolytic results were estimated by palpation, distal arterial pulse pressure, and photography, and it was shown that recanalization of 4-day-old arterial thromboses may be obtained within 1 h with repeated doses of brinase to a total of about 4 mg per vessel. The appearance of vessels after thrombolysis (inflammatory changes and destruction of intima, media hemorrhages) was attributed to the lesions caused by prior thrombus formation, and not to the direct effects of the enzyme.

CUTHBERTSON and GILFILLAN (1971) described the use of brinase for recanalization and maintenance of patency of chronically indwelling arterial catheters in non-anesthetized rhesus monkeys. Catheters were filled with a solution of heparin (1000 U/ml) and brinase (1000 C2 U/ml) prior to use for periodic blood pressure measurements, and, when clotted during periods of idleness, occlusions were cleared promptly with instillations of concentrated brinase solutions for 1 h. This regimen allowed the continued use of implanted catheters in the awake monkey for periods of up to 22 months.

IV. Other Experimental Proteolytic Uses

1. Tissue Culture

Brinase has been investigated for use in tissue culture by SABINA et al. (1963). The enzymatic dispersion of established cell lines (bovine kidney, monkey kidney epithelium, human carcinoma and amnion, mouse fibrosarcoma) cultivated on glass with trypsin and brinase was compared, showing that all cell lines responded favorably to treatment with brinase while some lines failed to grow when they were released from the glass with trypsin. Luxuriant primary cultures from fresh tissues were established using brinase as the dispersing agent, and after many consecutive passages, cells subcultured by brinase treatment rather than by scraping, were similar both in morphology and in rate of division. From this was concluded that brinase may be used to advantage to start primary cultures and to prepare subcultures of cell lines that are usually damaged by trypsin.

2. Enzymatic Zonulysis in Ophthalmology

The use of brinase to facilitate lens extraction in cataract surgery was investigated in rabbits by LEWANDOWSKI et al. (1974) and in Cynomolgus monkeys (*Macaca fascicularis*) by PROMPITAK et al. (1974) and PROMPITAK and CHISHOLM (1974). This thorough and extensive work was stimulated by clinical experience with enzymatic zonulysis using α-chymotrypsin, which had gained popularity in adult surgery, and the observation that in young patients its effects were less clear-cut because of incomplete digestion of zonules and posterior lens-vitreous attachments.

In a series of double-blind trials in anesthetized rabbits LEWANDOWSKI et al. (1974) instilled 1 ml of α-chymotrypsin (150 U/ml) into the posterior chamber of one eye and 1 ml of brinase (50 or 100 C2 U/ml) into the other, to be followed 6 min later by intracapsular cataract extraction using sliding technique with cryophake and counter-pressure. The facility of lens extraction was judged either to be equal with both enzymes or to favor one or the other. Criteria for comparison were the extent of zonulysis, the facility of separation of lens-vitreous attachments, and the amount of vitreous loss.

Evaluating the results by sequential analysis, the authors determined that lens extraction was facilitated in favor of both dose levels of brinase at the 95% confidence levels. The rabbits were observed for a period of 4 weeks postoperatively and were then sacrificed. The eyes were processed for histopathologic examination.

All animals treated with α-chymotrypsin developed some measure of vitreous loss and retinal detachment, but no major wound disruptions occurred. The 100 C2 U dose of brinase caused severe clinical uveitis in most rabbits, which was least pronounced with the 50 C2 U dose. When compared with chymotrypsin, brinase caused less frequent loss of vitreous. The authors concluded that, in the rabbit, brinase was significantly more effective in facilitating lens extraction than was α-chymotrypsin at a dose of 150 U/ml.

In a search for a substance which consistently and safely breaks the lenticulo-vitreous attachment in children, PROMPITAK et al. (1974) investigated brinase in Cynomolgus monkeys with techniques of intracapsular lens extraction similar to the rabbit study of LEWANDOWSKI et al. Using only one eye of each of a pair of monkeys, one received 1 ml of brinase (100 C2 U) and the other 1 ml of α-chymotrypsin (150 U). The facility of lens extraction was evaluated double-blind by the ease of zonular rupture, the adherence of vitreous to the posterior lens capsule, and the occurrence of vitreous loss. The monkeys were followed postoperatively for 3–7 weeks, they were examined twice a week by fundoscopy and for intraocular pressure, and the eyes were enucleated thereafter for histophathologic examination.

The data from sequential analysis showed that 100 C2 U of brinase were better than 150 U of α-chymotrypsin in facilitating lens extraction at the 95% confidence level. Vitreous loss occurred once in nine eyes treated with brinase, but in four of nine eyes treated with α-chymotrypsin. Clinical observations during the postoperative periods showed that brinase was no more toxic to the monkey eye than was α-chymotrypsin. No toxic effects on ocular tissues were observed with either enzyme.

A more detailed toxicity study with brinase was performed by PROMPITAK and CHISHOLM (1974) in an effort to determine the concentration at which toxic effects may occur in the monkey eye. Brinase was used to facilitate lens extraction in concentrations of from 100 to 6400 C2 U per ml, using the same operative techniques as before and following the animals for 2 weeks postoperatively. Vitreous loss occurred infrequently with brinase concentrations as high as 400 C2 U/ml. Concentrations of 800 C2 U/ml and above caused vitreous loss in all eyes. Conjunctival injection was present and cleared more slowly with higher enzyme concentrations. All corneas were clear, and anterior uveitis when present diminished in the 2nd week. All corneas healed well, with slight vacuolization of corneal endothelial cytoplasm. This occurred with equal frequency in untreated (sham-operated) eyes as well as after α-chymotrypsin treatment. It was concluded that brinase concentrations up to 400 C2 U/ml caused no complications that could be attributed to the enzyme while significantly facilitating intracapsular lens extraction in the monkey.

V. Clinical Thrombolysis [4]

1. Systemic Infusion

The first attempts to administer *A. oryzae* enzyme to man were made by KARACA et al. (1962a) who treated 102 patients with Aspergillin O, of which 45 infusions in 20 patients with disseminated carcinomatosis, lymphoma, leukemia, and cerebral and coronary occlusions were reported in detail. The doses of Aspergilin O (crude enzyme) ranged from 4 mg/kg to 14 mg/kg in concentrations of 1 mg/ml saline. Owing to the impurity of Aspergillin O, a comparison of its fibrinolytic activity with that of the purified enzyme brinase cannot be made, and the order of magnitude of the employed dosage cannot be assessed.

Intravenous infusions were begun with an initial speed of 1 mg/min, which was gradually increased to 4 mg/min if no hypotension developed. Visual in vitro clot lysis as an indicator of induced fibrinolytic activity, when present, was greatest at the end of an infusion and lasted for about 1 h, thrombin formation was delayed for about the same period, the recalcified clotting time was slightly accelerated, and the platelet count fluctuated about the normal. The clotting time in siliconized test tubes was significantly shortened. Plasma fibrinogen decreased moderately with little relationship between the dose of Aspergilling O, the fibrinogen changes, and the occurrence of clot lysis. All changes reverted to normal over a period of 3–24 h.

In addition to occasional hypotension, two cases developed fever during or within 4 h after infusion. Nausea, vomiting, and diarrhea were observed in one case. Extravasation of enzyme caused edema of the injection site in four cases, but no bleeding manifestations were encountered.

---

[4] Several clinical trials are in progress at the time of writing.

It is apparent that the intravenous administration of impure Aspergillin O to man was remarkably well tolerated, although the doses administered were small by present standards, as indicated by the clot-promoting effects noted in all patients and the apparent absence of clinically demonstrable effects in those patients with established thrombosis. Other than mentioning whole blood clot lysis and increased esterase activity of serum, KARACA et al. gave no indication of therapeutic results.

The purified enzyme brinase received its first clinical evaluation by JÜRGENS (1966a, unpublished personal communications), who identified the principal characteristics and effects of the purified enzyme in man and indicated methods of its use. To about 50 patients suffering from a variety of thrombotic disorders or complications, brinase was administered in doses ranging from 150–210 mg per patient, infused i.v. in a volume of 500 ml of 5% levulose within 60–90 min. This dose range had been determined by JÜRGENS during studies of inhibitor levels and was found to neutralize brinase inhibitors sufficiently in most patients without causing their depletion. In addition, however, JÜRGENS determined individual inhibitor levels in patients for dose adjustments during therapy. The overall incidence of side-effects was low and was primarily related to the speed of infusion and the concentration of enzyme solution.

JÜRGENS' cases consisted of 10 arterial thromboses, 4 patients with superficial thrombophlebitis, 4 patients with thrombophlebitis migrans, 5 deep-vein thromboses, 2 subclavian thromboses, 3 patients with post-thrombotic syndrome, and 21 patients with retinal vein thrombosis. Two patients received brinase for preoperative thrombosis prophylaxis.

The results of JÜRGENS' study were astonishingly good, although poorly documented and often assessed by ambiguous methods of clinical observation. However, notwithstanding the superficial nature of therapeutic evaluation, the trial indicated the range of tolerated dosage and the absence of sensitization reactions in patients receiving multiple infusions over extended periods of time. One patient who received an overdose of 350 mg reacted with incoagulability, depletion of plasma fibrinogen, and signs of kinin activation (nausea, diarrhea, involuntary micturition and defecation, retrosternal and abdominal pain, and pain in the kidney region without hema-

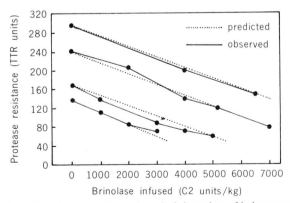

Fig. 55. Regression of protease resistance by administration of brinase to 4 patients with greatly varying pretreatment inhibitor levels, indicating requirement for individualized dosage of enzyme. (--------) predicted on basis of dose-prediction tests; (———) measured during enzyme infusions. ROSCHLAU (1972b)

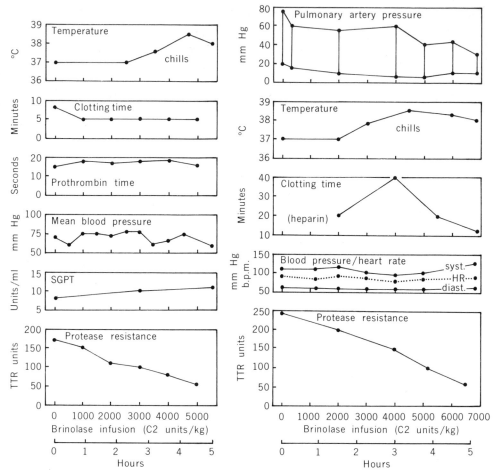

Fig. 56. *(Left)* Systemic brinase treatment of acute retinal vein thrombosis. Only side-effect febrile reaction at completion of treatment. Marginally useful vision restored 3 days after therapy. *(Right)* Pulmonary embolism treated with brinase by pulmonary artery catheterization. Febrile reaction toward completion of infusion. Pulmonary artery pressure normalized during therapy; complete resolution of extensive pulmonary obstructions (visualized by scan and arteriography) 3 days after therapy. ROSCHLAU (1972b)

turia). The patient recovered completely within 1 day after infusion of 500 ml fresh frozen plasma. Accidental perivascular injection has caused pronounced and painful edema, which was successfully treated with prednisolone.

    For unknown reasons JÜRGENS did not pursue the investigation, but his reports stimulated others to look at brinase as a clinical thrombolytic agent. ROSCHLAU (1968, 1971a, 1972b) treated a few isolated cases of retinal vein thrombosis and pulmonary embolism, mainly for the purpose of correlating the protease-resistance test and dose-prediction between dog and man, with emphasis primarily on the clinical pharmacology of the agent and secondarily on attainable thrombolytic results. Based on the principles evolved in the dog, the protease-resistance test was

Table 10. Nonrecent peripheral arterial disease treated with repeated intravenous infusions of brinase. (After FRISCH, 1974)

Patient (Age)	Duration	Brinase infusions	Claudication distance[a]		Systolic blood pressure (mm Hg)					
			Pre-treatment	Post-treatment	Arm[b]		Right leg[c]		Left leg[c]	
					Pre-	Post-	Pre-	Post-	Pre-	Post-
1 (57)	1 year	4 weekly	100 m	1600 m	128	138	102	110	92	80
2 (58)	1.5 years	4 weekly	200 m	1600 m	180	172	92	108	102	136
3 (64)	5 years	4 weekly	30 m	250 m	150	143	88	126	74	72
4 (54)	6 months	4 weekly	60 m	1600 m	150	119	165	152	98	110
5 (57)	2.5 years	3 daily	500 m	1600 m	170	152	162	182	90	152
6 (69)	2 years	3 daily	300 m	500 m	128	130	0	68	82	85
7 (70)	2.5 years	3 daily	100 m	1600 m	155	150	76	90	90	120
8 (74)	1.5 years	3 daily	100 m	500 m	165	132	75	76	10	110
9 (74)	2 months	7 daily	25 m	300 m	164	145	0	88	0	120
10 (65)	1 year	6 daily	20 m	1600 m	120	108	0	165	0	70
11 (83)	1 year	5 daily	100 m	200 m	150	150	30	108	130	110
12 (62)	2 years	7 daily	20 m	75 m	130	150	40	92	0	88
13 (53)	2 years	3 daily	50 m	200 m	180	120	70	70	100	100
14 (52)	2 months	6 daily	30 m	100 m	122	122	40	58	25	42
15 (64)	2 years	2 daily	50 m	200 m	130	140	40	90	0	70
16 (50)	6 months	2 daily	100 m	1600 m	190	130	0	120	110	130

[a] Claudication distance before and after brinase treatment as estimated by walking under normal conditions until appearance of disabling pain.
[b] Arm pressure = systemic pressure.
[c] Blood pressure cuff placed around calf; recording by Doppler probe over posterior tibial artery.

adapted for human use, and a method of dose prediction was developed for the safe administration of thrombolytically effective dosage (Fig. 55). The relationship between administered dosage and reduction of protease resistance, the absence of significant side-effects during controlled administration of the enzyme, and the attainment of in vivo thrombolysis were confirmed (Fig. 56).

FITZGERALD and collaborators employed systemic brinase therapy in chronic peripheral artery obstruction (FITZGERALD et al., 1972; FITZGERALD and FRISCH, 1973, 1974; FRISCH, 1974). A series of 16 patients with clinically established histories of intermittent claudication on the basis of chronic occlusive disease of the lower limbs were treated with i.v. brinase, 100 mg in 200 ml saline, over a period of 1 h (= 1.5 mg/min). This dosage was chosen as it could be expected to reduce but not deplete systemic brinase inhibitors. Repeated infusions were given once a week for 4 weeks to four patients, and daily for 2–7 days to 12 patients. All patients had arterial obstuctions confirmed by arteriography, and the changes occurring during and after brinase treatment were assessed by continuous-wave ultrasound scanning and DOPPLER recording of peripheral blood pressure in the affected limbs.

When assessed by the improvement in claudication distance, the treatments were highly successful (Table 10). In addition, in eight limbs previously absent pedal pulses returned during the course of brinase infusions. In most patients the blood pressures in the two limbs responded individually, indicating that the changes in blood pressure were indeed an effect of the enzyme on local circulation and not a reflection of systemic effects.

There were no coagulation or liver function abnormalities during the treatment periods. Brinase inhibitors as assessed by the viscosimetric method of LINDVALL et al. (1969) were lowered but not depleted, antiplasmin titers were gradually reduced, and fibrin/fibrinogen split products appeared in plasma, reaching a maximum 4–6 h after infusions. Fibrinogen showed a slight decrease subsequent to treatment but remained within normal limits. Side-effects were not observed since inhibitors were not excessively reduced by the applied doses of enzyme, and no evidence of antigenicity was obtained.

The prompt and marked improvement in exercise tolerance in patients with a long history of intermittent claudication, the increased systolic blood pressure in the affected limbs, the recurrence of previously absent pedal pulses, and the improved pulse pressure transmission times along the diseased arterial segments were attributed by FITZGERALD and FRISCH (1973) to the lysis by brinase of poorly organized thrombus accumulated on top of areas of atheroma, thus restoring functional hemodynamics in the areas supplied by that part of the arterial system.

FITZGERALD and FRISCH (1975) have since extended this study to 44 patients with chronically obstructed peripheral arteries. Twenty of these patients were claudicants (stage II), and 24 had rest pain or gangrene (stage III or IV). Individual dosage requirements were calculated from the level of brinase inhibitors in plasma, measured with the method of KIESSLING (1973, cf. Sect. VII), as reported by FRISCH et al. (1975) and modified by NYMAN and DUCKERT (1975). Some patients were anticoagulated with warfarin during and following brinase therapy, and the follow-up period extended from 6 months to 3 years.

The treatments resulted in good clinical improvement in 11 of 20 stage II patients (pretreatment arm-leg pressure gradient $= 88 \pm 41$ mm Hg), in 10 of 12 stage III patients (pretreatment pressure gradient $= 108 \pm 43$ mm Hg), and in 6 of 12 stage IV patients (pretreatment pressure gradient $= 129 \pm 45$ mm Hg). A post-treatment pressure gradient of 44 ± 27 mm Hg was recorded in the patients responding to brinase therapy (27 of 44), while those patients who failed to show clinical improvement retained a higher gradient of 81 ± 49 mm Hg. The authors found good agreement between these pressure gradient measurements, the simultaneous continuous-wave ultrasound scanning data for documentation of occluding or stenosing arterial lesions, and the clinical response to brinase therapy. They concluded that significant reductions in the severity of arterial lesions were achieved.

A similar study was reported by EKESTRÖM et al. (1975) and by LUND et al. (1975) who treated 35 patients with chronic peripheral arterial disease, of which 27 were on the basis of arteriosclerosis and 8 were obstructions of other etiology. Twenty of these patients received i.v. infusions of brinase, the dosage calculated on the basis of brinase plasma inhibitors with the method of KIESSLING. Five patients received the enzyme intra-arterially during vascular surgery, to be followed with intravenous infusions postoperatively. In 10 patients the treatments were discontinued for unrelated reasons. All patients were anticoagulated with dicumarol and/or heparin.

After initial arteriography the response to treatment was assessed by peripheral blood pressure measurements, dynamic fluorescein angiography, and electromagnetic flow measurements. Twenty of the 25 completed treatments resulted in clinical improvement. After preoperative intra-arterial instillation of brinase an increased blood flow in the superficial femoral artery was recorded. The arm-leg pressure gradient of 112 ± 24 mm Hg before brinase treatment was reduced to 49 ± 20 mm Hg in patients with arteriosclerotic obstructions showing clinical improvement (while there was no change in clinical failures), and nonarteriosclerotic occlusions responded with an arm-leg pressure gradient of 32 ± 21 mm Hg. Fluorescein angiography indicated improved microcirculation. There were no bleeding complications.

The intravenous dosage of brinase in the studies of FITZGERALD and FRISCH (1975), EKESTRÖM et al. (1975) and LUND et al. (1975) was based on the routine determination of the brinase-inhibitor capacity of plasma measured with the azocollagen technique of KIESSLING. FRISCH et al. (1975a, b) have evaluated this method in 355 brinase treatments and reported good correlation between the predicted lowering of plasma inhibitors and the determined post-infusion values. Individual dose requirements could thus be calculated for the attainment of fibrinolytic activity, and free proteolysis through inhibitor depletion was avoided.

2. Local Perfusion

The rapid thrombolytic effects of local administration of brinase to dogs (ROSCHLAU and FISHER, 1966) have been utilized for the recanalization of occluded hemodialysis shunts, recanalization of occluded indwelling cannulae and catheters, lysis of arterial thrombi by intra-arterial instillation of brinase, and intra-articular instillation in arthritic joint hydrops.

a) Cannula Declotting

Hemodialysis cannula declotting with brinase was developed to satisfy the clinical need for a rapidly and reliably acting agent in acute emergency situations. KESSEL et al. (1968), PERRY (1968) and ROSCHLAU (1968) explored the enzyme's usefulness in small numbers of patients with acutely clotted arterial and venous cannulae of SCRIBNER shunts, and established treatment schemes for large-scale clinical trials. They also defined the mode of action of the enzyme and the probable side-effects when used in this condition, and they provided a basis for therapeutic expectations. Further contributions to the evaluation of brinase in clotted hemodialysis shunts were made by EGAN (1969), ROSCHLAU (1971a, b, 1972b), SHIMIZU et al. (1971), PEDRONI et al. (1972), ALBERT et al. (1972), ALBERT (1973), FRISCH (1972, 1974), and DE NICOLA et al. (1974).

In general, repeated instillations at brief intervals of small amounts of brinase into occluded shunt implants resulted in rapid recanalization independent of the patient's brinase-inhibitor level. Laboratory control of systemic fibrinolysis and coagulation, titration of dosage, and monitoring of patients for extended periods of time (as usually required in systemic fibrinolytic therapy) were found to be unnecessary. The dosage of enzyme for recanalization of hemodialysis shunts by local application was shown to be less than $^1/_{10}$ th of the dose that would be required for comparable thrombolytic effects if the enzyme were administered systemically. The amounts of brinase escaping into the general circulation were insignificant, systemic inhibitors were not affected, and systemic toxicity has not been shown. The local side-effects

Table 11. Declotting of hemodialysis shunt cannulae with brinase. Collaborative trial in Canadian artificial kidney centers.[a] (From ROSCHLAU, 1971b)

	Arteries		Veins		Total	
	No.	%	No.	%	No.	%
Total number of treatments	78	100	212	100	290	100
Recanalization:	60	77	144	68	204	70
Complete (blood flow restored to pre-clotting rate and volume)	*(51)*	*(65)*	*(127)*	*(60)*	*(178)*	*(61)*
Partial (functional blood flow at less than pre-clotting rate and volume)	*(9)*	*(12)*	*(17)*	*(8)*	*(26)*	*(9)*
Failure (requiring surgical revision of shunt):	18	23	68	32	86	30
Side-effects:						
Local vascular pain	13	16	72	34	85	29
Hypersensitivity/allergenicity syndromes					4	1.4
Other systemic reactions					5	1.7

[a] Shunt life extended by an average of 6 (0–18) months

encountered during hemodialysis declotting were mainly attributable to local kinin activation (i.e., transient pain) and to the occasional perivascular leakage of enzyme from deteriorated implant sites (i.e., edema, erythema). Clinical trials with significant numbers of patients (Table 11), of whom many were treated intermittently over periods exceeding 1 year, showed that sensitization reactions occurred infrequently.

For lysis of occluded hemodialysis shunts, 2–5 ml of brinase solution containing 1 mg/ml saline (= 1000 C2 U/ml, 17 caseinolytic U/ml) were instilled into the occluded cannula. After 5–10 min the solution was aspirated, and if recanalization had not been achieved the instillation was repeated with fresh brinase solution. In the majority of cases patency of the shunt was obtained within 20–40 min with total amounts of 5–15 mg of brinase, variously documented by angiography, flow measurements, etc.

This concentration of brinase has frequently caused transient pain in the injected vessels, whereupon ROSCHLAU (1971b) proposed a reduction in concentration to 0.5 mg (500 C2 U) per ml. Furthermore, the observation by ROSCHLAU and FISHER (1966) of the clot-promoting properties of small doses of brinase has led ROSCHLAU (1971 b) to advocate the addition of small amounts of heparin to the brinase solution. Thus, two variations of dosage recommendations were established:

FRISCH (1972, 1974) — European Trial Data: 1.0 mg brinastrase per ml saline, instilled in portions of 2–5 ml until recanalization occurs.

ROSCHLAU (1971b) — Canadian Trial Data: 0.5 mg (500 C2 U) brinolase and 25 U heparin per ml saline, instilled in portions of 2–5 ml until recanalization occurs.

The results of clinical trials in 558 shunt occlusions are summarized in Tables 11 and 12. All patients had acutely clotted shunts that resisted declotting by conventional means of irrigation and clot extraction, requiring surgical shunt replacement for resumption of adequate dialysis. Although the results differed somewhat between the European and the Canadian trials, assumed to be due to differences in patient

Table 12. Local instillation of brinase into totally occluded external hemodialysis shunts. Immediate treatment results in European and Canadian trials[a]. (From FRISCH, 1974)

Study	Brinase solution[b]	Total number of treatments	Recanalization (%)		Failure (%)
			Complete	Partial	
European	1 mg/ml (1000 C2 U)	268	76	14	10
Canadian	0.5 mg/ml (500 C2 U) plus heparin	290	61	9	30

[a] Criteria for evaluation: Complete recanalization = blood flow restored to pre-clotting values. Partial recanalization = blood flow at less than pre-clotting value, dialysis possible. Failure = surgical relocation of shunt required.

[b] See text.

selection, enzyme concentration, and treatment techniques, the procedure has been widely accepted for routine use in dialysis centers.

Recanalization of occluded indwelling catheters and cannulae with brinase has been reported by HARTZELL and HOLMDAHL as quoted by FRISCH (1974). One to 5 ml of enzyme solution containing 1 mg/ml saline was injected into the cannula or the infusion tubing, resulting in recanalization in less than 10 min. Significant side-effects were not observed, but some patients reported a tingling sensation at the cannula site.

b) Intra-arterial Instillation

LUND et al. (1968 a, b) treated acute occlusions of the femoral and popliteal arteries with intra-arterial administration of brinase. The enzyme concentration consisted of 1 mg/ml, and doses of 50–100 mg were deposited in 10 ml portions near the obstruction by intra-arterial catheterization. The response was assessed by repeated arteriography, indicating that rapid partial or complete canalization of occlusions could be obtained within 1 h. In a detailed and well-documented case study, LUND et al. (1968 a) described the progressive recanalization of completely thrombosed femoral and popliteal arteries with restoration of peripheral circulation. Concomitant side-effects were due to permeability changes induced by the interaction of X-ray contrast medium and brinase when administered alternatingly in rapid succession for demonstration of progressive lytic changes by arteriography (LUND et al., 1968b; FRISCH et al., 1971; cf. Sect. II/6). Omission of repeated arteriography during thrombolysis by intra-arterial brinase administration in subsequent studies (LUND and FRISCH, as quoted by FRISCH, 1974) prevented these local side-effects. Owing to the relatively low doses of enzyme required for recanalization of vessels by direct perfusion, systemic side-effects were not observed.

NYMAN et al. (1974, 1975) described the local administration of brinase to 9 and 16 patients with recent arterial occlusions of the lower limbs, all confirmed by arteriography. Treatments were conducted with daily infusions, by polyethylene catheterization, of 50–200 mg brinase (50 mg brinase and 500 U heparin/40 ml/h) depending on the fibrinogen level and the results of brinase-inhibitor assays. Between brinase infusions the patients received continuous heparin. Brinase inhibitors were measured by the method of AMUNDSEN et al. (1973, Sect. VII/3), and daily pre- and postinfusion coagulation tests consisted of Quick time, prothrombin time, factors II, V, VII and X, fibrinogen, and ethanol gelation test.

In three out of nine patients with thrombotic occlusions, hemodynamically good blood flow was restored, but only relatively fresh occlusions were recanalized with 5–10 daily treatments. In three of four patients with embolic occlusions, lysis was obtained with two or three daily treatments. The results of this investigation are summarized in Table 13, excluding three patients in whom arteriographic controls were not obtained.

Side-effects were judged to be minor in the 13 patients of Table 13. They consisted of local pain (7 patients), transient elevation of serum transaminase (2), abdominal pain (1), fever over 38° C (1), epidermolysis (1), and erythema (1). However, in 3 patients excluded from the table because of incomplete assessment more marked side-effects occurred, such as limb-swelling and hematomas, most likely to be attributed to perivascular leakage of enzyme. Observed coagulation and hematologic changes consisted of a lowering of fibrinogen levels and positive ethanol gelation tests after brinase infusions, other parameters being unaffected.

In assessing the use of brinase, NYMAN et al. emphasized that successful lysis of arterial occlusions may only be expected in the presence of a large, accessible fibrin component. However, when comparing the results of their study with those of ROSCHLAU and FISHER (1966) in the dog, the authors felt that the efficacy of brinase in the human was less than in the dog, which they attributed to differences in inhibitors between these species. In addition, the authors were unable to show a correlation between systemic inhibitor neutralization and local thrombolytic activity. Systemic inhibitor determinations were thus incapable of predicting the proportions of free and bound brinase at the site of infusion, which may in some instances have caused side-effects from free proteolysis in ischemic limbs where blood flow (and the availability of inhibitors) was impaired.

c) Intra-articular Instillation

As quoted by FRISCH (1974), KAGSTAD and TISELIUS used brinase as an aid in the aspiration of highly viscous and fibrinous synovial fluid in arthritic hydrops of the knee joint. Thirty min after intra-articular instillation of 15–20 mg brinase in a concentration of 1 mg/ml, the aspiration of previously highly viscous joint fluid could be achieved, and the regularly present fibrin-lining of arthritic joints was removed or significantly reduced. In consequence, the refilling interval was prolonged, but a transient local hyperthermic reaction frequently accompanied the procedure.

VI. Other Clinical Uses

1. Inhibition of Platelet Aggregation

JÜRGENS (1966 b) administered brinase to 28 patients for the purpose of inhibition of blood platelet aggregation. Doses of 120 and 150 mg per patient were dissolved in 500 ml of 5% levulose and were infused i.v. over a period of 1 h. This caused a substantial decrease in spontaneous platelet aggregation which persisted for several

Table 13. Local infusions of brinase in 9 thrombotic and 4 embolic arterial occlusions of the lower limb (From NYMAN et al., 1975)

Patient	Localization of proximal end of occlusion	Age of occlusion (days)	Angiographic results[a]	Hemodynamic results (a.d.p./a.t.p.)[b] Before	After	Total dose of brinase (mg)	No. of treatments (days)	Inhibitors[c] (U/ml) Before	After
Thrombotic occlusions									
1	A. fem. sup.	24	0	0/65	30/75	300	4	4.1	0.7
2	A. fem. sup.	60	0	0/0	0/0	250	2	8.8	4.2
3	A. poplitea	1	++	0/60	100/135	400	5	6.8	2.8
4	A. poplitea and A. iliaca	1 5 years	0	0/0	0/85	450	5	3.4	0.7
5	A. fem. sup.	7	0	0/0	0/60	1050	11	6.3	5.1
6	A. fem. sup.	4	++	70/75	190/195	550	10	5.9	3.1
7	A. fem. sup.	3	(+)	60/0	80/0	950	15	4.7	2.3
8	A. fem. sup.	30	0	50/90	65/70	600	11	4.0	1.7
9	Tr. communis	10	++	0/45	10/100	650	9	7.6	4.9
Embolic occlusions									
10	A. poplitea sin.	1	+++	100/125	175/200	300	3	5.7	2.7
	A. fem. prof. sin.	1	+++						
	A. poplitea dex.	8	0	95/95	100/110				
	A. fem. prof. dex.	8	+						
11	A. poplitea	1	++	65/0	140/140	200	2	Not determined	
12	A. poplitea	1	++	0/55	110/100	1150	18	9.1	1.6
13	Tr. communis	1	0	95/95	115/115	450	6	Not determined	

[a] Arteriography, graded 0 (no change) to +++ (complete recanalization).
[b] Peripheral blood pressure, arteria dorsalis pedis/arteria tibialis posterior, mm Hg, Doppler method.
[c] Method of AMUNDSEN et al. (1973).

days (cf. Sect. II/3/b). Even considerably smaller doses (e.g., 60 mg/patient) occasionally produced this effect. The maximal response usually occurred 4 days after a single infusion, with return to normal platelet aggregability by the 6th day (Fig. 33). Continuous depression of spontaneous aggregation was achieved with repeated infusions of 150 mg of brinase every 4–6 days (Fig. 34). Concomitant changes in the coagulation system (Fig. 35) were transient and preceded the effects on blood platelets. No systemic toxicity was encountered.

A similar study was made by DE NICOLA et al. (1967, 1974) in 18 female patients aged 37–75 years and suffering from arteriosclerosis and its complications. Brinase was administered by i.v. infusions in doses of 52, 105 or 156 mg/patient, dissolved in 150–250 ml saline, and given over 1–2 h. However, while JÜRGENS had measured sponatenous platelet aggregation, DE NICOLA et al. induced aggregation with adenosine diphosphate (ADP), which led to somewhat different results. Inhibition of ADP-induced aggregation occurred rapidly, with return to pretreatment activity 24–48 h later (Fig. 47). This difference in response between JÜRGENS and DE NICOLA et al. was attributed to differences in aggregation methods. The effects were dose-dependent and were accompanied by an increase in fibrinolytic activity and by a transient prolongation of the prothrombin and recalcification times. No significant immediate or delayed side-effects were observed.

The demonstration of inhibition of platelet aggregation by intravenous infusions of nontoxic doses of brinase, however, has not generated much interest in the enzyme's clinical use for this purpose. Orally effective drugs with greatly reduced risks of acute toxic side-effects have since been recognized and were extensively evaluated, placing brinase into a lesser position of importance for clinical inhibition of platelet function. The presumed mechanisms of inhibition had been described (Sect. II/3/b) as being mediated by secondary small molecular weight peptides from the enzymatic degradation of fibrinogen and possibly other plasma proteins.

2. Chemotherapy of Malignant Disease

In several studies of the probable effects of brinase on the course of malignant disease, THORNES and his collaborators have investigated the enzyme's properties for inhibition of metastatic spread. As described by O'MEARA (1958) and by O'MEARA and JACKSON (1958), the thromboplastic activity of cancer tissue is many times greater than that of normal tissue, and the inhibitors of fibrinolysis, the antiplasmins, are increased in patients with cancer (THORNES et al., 1967). These were the initial principal reasons for attempting to inhibit thromboplastic activity of human cancer tissue and to decrease antiplasmins (i.e., enhance endogenous fibrinolytic activity) with brinase.

O'BRIEN et al. (1968) attempted to lower serum antiplasmin levels in 14 cancer patients with 42 i.v. infusions of brinase, the maximum number of infusions to a single patient being 7. The doses were calculated from, and therapy was monitored by the protease-resistance test of ROSCHLAU. The average dose was 205 mg of protease, and the higher the dose the greater and more lasting was the effect produced. It was shown (Fig. 57) that the dose-dependent lowering of brinase inhibitors (protease resistance) was accompanied by approximately parallel changes in antiplasmin values, and that these effects could be maintained for considerable lengths of time with

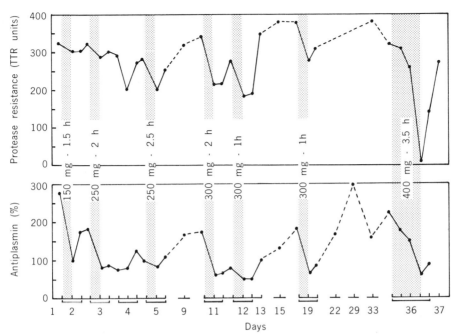

Fig. 57. Effect of repeated brinase infusions on antiplasmin levels and protease resistance in patient with cancer. From O'BRIEN et al. (1968)

repeated infusions of brinase. Fibrinogen levels were depressed with doses over 200 mg/patient, the whole blood clot lysis time was shortened, the prothrombin time was increased, but the whole blood-clotting time was not affected unless brinase doses were excessive. Polymorphonuclear leukocytosis developed during brinase infusions and lasted for 24 h. Side-effects were variable and dose-dependent, consisting of occasional flushing and warmth of face and extremities, drowsiness, tachycardia, sweating, nausea, and diarrhea. Severe back pain developed in two cases with vertebral metastases Elek-Ouchterlony immunodiffusion tests in agar, carried out in one case 2 months after therapy, showed precipitating antibodies to brinase. No patient deteriorated as an immediate result of therapy, one case of advancing myeloma with paraplegia was improved, but the symptomatic improvement in all other treated patients was inconclusive.

Based on the observation that both plasmin and brinase have direct effects on cancer cells in vitro, THORNES (1968) showed that, when added in vitro to the whole blood of patients with myeloid leukemia, brinase reduced the number of immature cells by 40% over a period of 4 h, and that a 30% reduction may be obtained in vivo in the same patients with the infusion of 150 mg of protease. THORNES (1968) proceeded to treat seven patients with leukemia (one acute myeloid, three chronic myeloid, one chronic lymphatic, one acute „stem cell", one acute monocytic) confirmed by bone-marrow biopsy. Protease infusions were given in repeated daily doses of 50–150 mg per patient in 200 ml saline over 60 min to lower excessively high antiplasmin levels to approx. 50% of an arbitrary „normal". The immature cells in

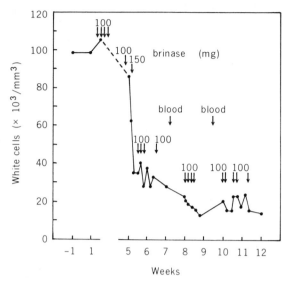

Fig. 58. White blood cell counts in relation to brinase therapy (as indicated) in patient with chronic lymphatic leukemia diagnosed 12 months before and not responding to methotrexate and prednisone. Antiplasmin levels lowered from 780% to 55% during brinase infusions. From THORNES (1968)

the peripheral circulation were reduced to varying degree by each infusion (Fig. 58), and no effects were observed on normal cells and blood platelets. THORNES concluded that the action of brinase was directed primarily toward immature cells, that it did not affect healthy normal white blood cells, and that its activity appeared to be potentiated in vivo. The feeling of well-being induced by protease was similar to that resulting from administrations of other fibrinolytic agents. One case of anaphylaxis was encountered without, however, influencing protease activity.

Thus, THORNES (1970) found that brinase had a similar cytotoxic effect as plasmin, and that excessively high antiplasmin levels in acute human leukemias (usually 10 times „normal") may be reduced to 50% of normal by brinase therapy, resulting in the removal of leukemia cells from the circulation. Compared with L-asparaginase, brinase was found to inhibit the growth of both asparagine-sensitive and insensitive leukemia cells in culture, and that it attacked endoplasmic reticulum and mitochondria first and nuclear and cell membranes later.

A case of acute leukemia treated with brinase had a rapid and unexplained reduction in white blood cell count following blood transfusion, which led THORNES et al. (1970) to search for cytotoxic antibodies against leukocytes and leukemia cells. The antibodies found in four patients were autoantibodies against the patients' own cells and were active only in the presence of complement. They were therefore classified as complement-dependent cytotoxic autoantibodies. The ability of brinase to stimulate the formation of cytotoxic autoantibodies was considered by THORNES et al. to be a useful property in antileukemic therapy.

The results obtained in relapsed cases have stimulated THORNES and collaborators to investigate brinase therapy as the initial treatment of leukemia in 25 patients

(15 acute, 10 chronic). Protease was given intravenously in daily dosage of 100–250 mg/patient for adults and 2.5 mg/kg for children. Dose requirements were individually estimated by the protease-resistance test of ROSCHLAU. It was found that the more abnormal the cells in the blood of the patients the more dramatic was the fall in the leukemic cell counts. Initial infusions were the most effective. Blast cells in the peripheral blood were removed within 1 h, but they reappeared 24 h later since short-term therapy did not affect the bone marrow. In chronic leukemia the white cell counts were reduced by as much as 74000/mm^3 in 1 h, and cell rupture without apparent destruction of cell contents was observed. Patients in whom autocytotoxic antibodies could be demonstrated went into remission for varying lengths of time and were successfully controlled with further brinase treatments or anticoagulants or steroids and cytotoxic agents.

The role of brinase-provoked autocytotoxic antibodies was further investigated by THORNES et al. (1972) in three children and three adults. Autocytotoxicity was found to be transient, lasting from 3–15 days, but repeated courses of brinase, whether given alone or in combination with antileukemic drugs, produced further autocytotoxic antibodies. Remission was obtained in three of five patients on combination therapy and in one patient with acute myeloblastic leukemia who received only brinase.

THORNES et al. (1972) proposed that brinase may be a valuable adjunct in the treatment of leukemia because: (1) it lowers antiplasmin levels and allows the host's own plasmin to act unopposed in a directly cytotoxic fashion; (2) it produces autocytotoxic antibodies against leukemic cells that appear to be inactive against the patient's own lymphocytes; (3) it interferes with cell membrane permeability (SMYTH et al., 1971, 1975), thus making leukemic cells more accessible to the antibody; (4) the cells of the erythroid series seem not to be involved, but in the absence of autocytotoxicity the number of circulating platelets and polymorphonuclear leukocytes are increased; (5) it is compatible with other drugs in combined chemotherapy; and (6) rare anaphylactoid reactions are controllable and do not interfere with the fibrinolytic activity of brinase.

VII. Clinical Control of Therapy

1. Brinase Inhibitor Assay (Bergkvist, 1963d; Bergkvist and Svärd, 1964)

Freshly drawn venous blood is allowed to clot in glass tubes at room temperature. After 2 h the blood is centrifuged and the serum is pipetted off. To 0.2 ml of serum are added 2.0 caseinolytic units of brinase in Tris buffer and the final volume is adjusted to 0.7 ml with Tris buffer. Then 0.2 ml of human fibrinogen solution (2.5%) and 0.1 ml of bovine thrombin solution (100 NIH units/ml) in Tris buffer are added, which produces a plasma clot. The clotted tube is incubated at 37° C to produce lysis, the end point of lysis being the time required for all air bubbles trapped in the meshwork of the clot to rise to the surface. Mixtures containing buffer in place of serum serve as controls.

A dose-response curve is constructed by plotting enzyme concentrations (in caseinolytic units) against lysis times of clots containing the same amount of fibrin as used in the determination of inhibitors. The difference between the proteolytic activity in the presence of serum and that in the presence of buffer represents the units of brinase inhibited by the amount of serum used.

The inhibitor level is defined as the amount of brinase (in caseinolytic units) inhibited by 0.2 ml of serum under specified conditions.

2. Protease Resistance Test (Roschlau, 1964, 1965, 1971 a, 1972 b)

Developed for use as a bedside test to predict dosage and to monitor brinase therapy (Table 14). *Preparation:* Increasing amounts of brinase (from 0–300 C2 U in increments of 20 C2 U in aliquots of 0.1 ml Tris buffer pH 7.4) are placed in sets of 16 test tubes (13 × 100 mm). Bovine thrombin (5 NIH U/0.1 ml Tris buffer) is added to each tube. The sets are prepared in quantity, freeze-dried, and reconstituted with 0.2 ml distilled water before use.
Use: Into each reconstituted tube of a 16-tube set, 1.0 ml of fresh whole blood is pipetted, resulting in immediate clotting. Upon incubation for 10 min at 37° C, lysis of varying extent occurs, depending on the brinase concentration in individual tubes. The end point is the tube in the set in which the enzyme content slightly exceeds the inhibitor level of the blood, expressed as lysis of varying degree (i.e., all tubes with enzyme content below the end point will remain clotted, and all tubes above the end point will be lysed after 10 min of incubation). The inhibitor level (protease resistance) is expressed in C2 U of brinase activity required to overcome the blood inhibitor concentration (= test tube requirement = TTR).

Conversion of the TTR value to the total circulating blood (for convenience the body weight) allows the approximate estimation of dosage to attain a desired target reduction of systemic brinase inhibitors. The test is robust, and it also gives an indirect measure of clottable fibrinogen in the blood by the presence and firmness of a clot in tube No. 1 which contains no brinase.

Table 14. Protease resistance test (brinase inhibitor assay) for rapid estimation of systemically administered dosage. (After ROSCHLAU, 1971 a)

Method: Prepare 16 test tubes (13 × 100 mm) containing

Tube No.	1	2	3	4	5	6	7	8	9	10	11	12	13	14	15	16
C2 U of brinase	0	20	40	60	80	100	120	140	160	180	200	220	240	260	280	300
NIH U of thrombin	5	5	5	5	5	5	5	5	5	5	5	5	5	5	5	5

Tubes prepared in quantity and freeze-dried. Stability at 4° C approx. 2 years. Reconstituted with 0.2 ml distilled water before use.

Test: 1 ml of whole blood added to each tube and incubated for 10 min at 37° C.
End point: The first tube in the series showing lysis.
Recorded value: TTR Units ("test tube requirement" units of brinase in equilibrium with brinase inhibitors in the blood).
Dose prediction: By conversion table in C2 Units/kg body weight.

3. Photometric Determination of Inhibitors on Chromogenic Substrate (Amundsen et al., 1973; Svendsen and Amundsen, 1973)

A synthetic chromogenic tripeptide-amide is used as substrate, with a high susceptibility for plasmin and brinase. The substrate is cleaved at high rates, yielding chromogenic *p*-nitroaniline, which can be detected by spectrophotometric methods. Preincubation of enzyme with microliter quantities of plasma and subsequent determination of substrate cleavage allows the accurate detection of inhibitory capacity in plasma. The method is quick, sensitive, and simple, the reaction can be stopped at any time after incubation, and it is well suited for automation.

Method (NYMAN and DUCKERT, 1975):

	Standard	Test
Tris-imidazole buffer, pH 8.2	0.6 ml	0.55 ml
Brinase (0.1 caseinolytic U/ml)	0.4 ml	0.4 ml
Plasma (diluted 1:5)	—	0.05 ml

Incubated for 5 min, after which 0.25 ml of each incubation mixture are mixed with 0.25 ml of substrate solution (1 mM [0.681 mg/ml] of N-Benzoyl-*l*-phenylalanyl-*l*-valyl-*l*-arginine-*p*-nitroanilide HCl [*S-2160*, AB Bofors, Sweden] in water) and 2.0 ml buffer, and read at O.D. 405 mμ at 25° C.

Calculation:

$$\frac{O.D._{,standard} - O.D._{,test}}{0.01} = \text{brinase-inhibition in substrate U/ml plasma.}$$

4. Photometric Determination of Inhibitors on Azocollagen Substrate (Kiessling, 1973; Frisch et al., 1975 a, b)

Plasma is incubated with varying amounts of brinase. An insoluble substrate, azocollagen, is added and the reaction is terminated by filtration after 5 min of incubation. Free proteolytic activity (i.e., amounts of brinase in excess of inhibitor capacity of the plasma) induces liberation of azo dye from the azocollagen complex, which is read in a spectrophotometer. The inhibitor capacity of the plasma is calculated as micromoles per liter of plasma, expressed as brinase activity.

Method (as modified by NYMAN and DUCKERT, 1975):

A brinase stock solution containing 10 CU per ml is prepared, from which dilutions are made with water for a standard curve (0.1–1.5 CU/ml) and for the inhibitor test (1.0 CU/ml).

	Standard	Test
Tris-imidazole buffer, pH 8.2	0.8 ml	0.75 ml
Brinase (1.0 caseinolytic U/ml)	0.2 ml	0.2 ml
Plasma (diluted 1:2)	—	0.05 ml

Incubated for 5 min at 25° C, after which 0.5 ml of each incubation mixture is mixed with 25 mg Hide Powder Azure (Calbiochem, USA) and 4.5 ml buffer containing 0.1% Triton X-100. This mixture is incubated for 15 min at 37° C, filtered, and the color intensity of the filtrate is read at 595 mμ. The corresponding brinase activity is read from a standard curve.

Calculation:

$\text{Brinase}_{standard} - \text{Brinase}_{test} \times 40 = \text{brinase-inhibition in caseinolytic U/ml plasma.}$

5. Critique of Tests

Systemic therapy with brinase requires the determination of circulating inhibitors, a reliable method of predicting individual dosage to avoid unintentional depletion of inhibitors, a means of monitoring the progressive inhibitor neutralization during brinase infusions for eventual dose adjustments, and a posttreatment inhibitor determination to indicate that treatments were adequate. An inhibitor assay, therefore, needs to be rapid and relatively simple, the results must be reproducible and reliable for the purpose, and preferably interchangeable between laboratories.

The inhibitor assay of BERGKVIST employs serum, the preparation of which is time-consuming and rules out the use of the assay during enzyme infusions for the monitoring of inhibitor neutralization and dose adjustments. The determination of end points is subjective, which might introduce a certain variability of results between individual users. When employed only as a pre- and posttreatment inhibitor test under standardized conditions, preferably performed by the same individual at all times, the assay is a reliable test of total brinase inhibitors in both animals and man.

The protease-resistance test of ROSCHLAU is a rapid method of total inhibitor determination in whole blood. The test was designed as a bedside method with minimal demands on equipment and technical expertise, and it was shown to predict optimal dosage of enzyme based on C2 U/kg body weight (Figs. 55, 56). Although the test was developed in the dog where it was shown to predict enzyme doses with accuracy, exposing less than 5% of animals to the risk of "overdose" (the variability being due largely to gross disproportions in body weight and blood volume of some of the dogs) (Figs. 21, 22), it was easily adapted for human use. However, its reliability as a

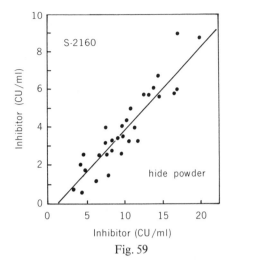
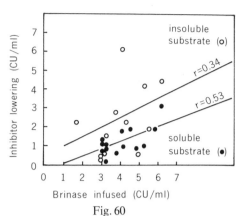

Fig. 59   Fig. 60

Fig. 59. Correlation between brinase inhibitor values obtained with a soluble substrate (*S-2160*, N-Benzoyl-*l*-phenylalanyl-*l*-valyl-*l*-arginine-*p*-nitroanilide HCl, AB Bofors, Sweden; AMUNDSEN et al., 1973) and an insoluble substrate (Hide Powder Azure, Calbiochem, USA; modified from KIESSLING, 1973). From NYMAN and DUCKERT (1975)

Fig. 60. Dose prediction for brinase. Correlation between infused amount of brinase (in CU/ml plasma) and observed reduction of circulating inhibitors (CU/ml plasma) using insoluble (Hide Powder) and soluble substrates (S-2160, Fig. 59). After NYMAN and DUCKERT (1975)

routine inhibitor test needs still to be demontrated in a large patient population (ROSCHLAU and SUTTON, 1977).

The tests of AMUNDSEN and of KIESSLING (modified) were evaluated by NYMAN and DU-CKERT (1975) in order to compare the results obtained with a soluble substrate with those of an insoluble substrate, and to assess the value of both methods in respect to brinase dose-prediction. The insoluble substrate was found to give values that were 2–3 times higher than those obtained with the soluble substrate (Fig. 59). The inhibitor response to infused brinase showed corresponding differences between assay methods as well as great individual variations (Fig. 60). NYMAN and DUCKERT observed that the soluble substrate was the more convenient assay, with satisfactorily reproducible results for practical purposes. They were disturbed by the fact that both methods showed poor dose-response correlation in vivo, which did not allow the accurate prediction of dosage. For the individual patient, however, both methods provided a guide for avoiding overdosage of brinase.

It is suggested that presently available brinase-inhibitor assays are specialized tests whose usefulness is in large measure determined by the expertise of interpretation of results applied to individual patients. All tests provide a measure of pretreatment inhibitor levels from which approximate individual doses may be calculated as long as a predetermined margin of safety is provided. Possible factors contributing to the observed variability in obtaining inhibitor reductions to predetermined target levels may be: (1) individually different relative concentrations of the two known brinase inhibitors (LINDVALL et al., 1969); (2) enzyme binding to noncirculating inhibitors (NYMAN and DUCKERT, 1975); (3) distribution of brinase into compartments other than plasma (SVÄRD and BERGKVIST, personal communication, 1962); and (4) gross disproportionality between body weight and plasma volume in individual patients (FREEDMAN and ROSCHLAU, 1970). Because of these nonmethodologic factors, which seem on occasion to outweigh the inherent errors or deficiencies of the respective tests, the objective spectrophotometric methods of AMUNDSEN and of KIESSLING appear not to offer significant advantages over the tests of BERGKVIST and of ROSCHLAU, which depend on subjective interpretation of results.

B. Protease From Aspergillus ochraceus

Following the report by STEFANINI and MARIN (1958) on the isolation of a fibrinoly-tic protease from *A. oryzae*, considerable interest was awakened in the examination of other strains of fungi for the eventual isolation and production of therapeutic thrombolytic enzymes. In the mid-1960s, a group of scientists at the VEB Arzneimit-telwerk Dresden, German Democratic Republic (BÄRWALD et al., 1969; TÖPFER et al., 1969) succeeded in developing a protease from *A. ochraceus*, which has since been evaluated successfully as an experimental thrombolytic agent under the name ocrase.

I. Isolation, Purification and Chemical Characteristics

The screening of 158 strains of *Alternaria, Aspergillus, Botrytis, Chaetomium, Fusar-ium, Gliocladium, Mucor, Myrothecium, Penicillium, Pullularia, Rhizopus, Scopular-iopsis, Stachybotrys*, and *Trichoderma* from the culture collection of VEB Arzneimit-telwerk Dresden for proteolytic activity identified 36 strains as prolific caseinase producers. Cultivation of strains on modified CZAPEK-DOX agar medium with casein at 25° C, and later in shake culture under pH-control, showed *A. ochraceus* Wilhelm 1079 (IMET[5] PA 126) to be the source of an extracellular alkaline protease with promising fibrinolytic characteristics (BÄRWALD et al., 1969, 1974; TÖPFER et al., 1969).

1. Preparation of Crude Enzyme

As described by BÄRWALD et al. (1969, 1974) and by TÖPFER et al. (1971a, b), the crude enzyme was obtained by deep culture of the mold. Fermentation occurred in two steps, of which the first was designed to obtain sufficient mycelium to start the main culture. Spores were transferred to a medium consisting of glucose, "corn-steep liquor" and $CaCO_3$ at pH 4.5–5.5. After 48 h the mycelium was harvested and the main culture was inoculated.

When grown on a medium of lactose, glucose, soya meal, KH_2PO_4, KCl, $MgSO_4$ and $FeSO_4$ at pH 4.5 and 25° C in stainless steel fermenters, the culture filtrate, after 6 days, showed a proteolytic activity in excess of 7 Kunitz caseinolytic U/ml (Fig.61). BÄRWALD et al. (1969, 1974) found that the proteolytic activity of filtrates was greatest when organic nitrogen was supplied as heat-treated soya meal, providing 1.8% total nitrogen for an activity of approx. 10 caseinolytic U/ml, and that other organic nitrogen—or inorganic nitrogen—was entirely unsuitable for protease production from *A. ochraceus*.

After 6 days of fermentation the culture filtrate was precipitated with tannic acid, washed with acetone, and dried to obtain crude protease with an activity of about 1 caseinolytic U/mg.

2. Purification of Enzyme

The crude enzyme was purified by ion exchange chromatography and gel filtration (TÖPFER et al., 1969, 1971a, b; TÖPFER and PIESCHE, 1974). A solution of crude protease (1 caseinolytic U/mg) of pH 6.8 was centrifuged at 15000 g and was run

---

[5] Institut für Mikrobiologie und Experimentelle Therapie, Jena, GDR

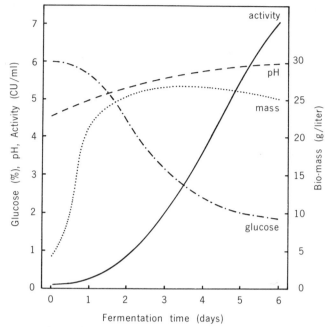

Fig. 61. Crude protease formation by *A. ochraceus* in stainless steel fermenters of 63 l capacity. From BÄRWALD et al. (1974)

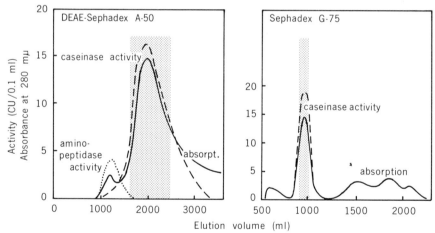

Fig. 62. *(Left)* Chromatography of crude *A. ochraceus* protease on DEAE-Sephadex A-50, buffered with 0.1 *M* ammonium acetate buffer pH 6.8. *(Right)* Gel chromatography of partly purified product (active fractions of Fig. 62, *left*) on Sephadex G-75. Activity of starting material = 1 CU/mg; activity of final product = 16 CU/mg. From TÖPFER et al. (1971 a)

through DEAE-Sephadex A-50 at 4° C, to be eluted with 0.1*M* ammonium acetate buffer pH 6.8. The fractions of highest caseinolytic activity were collected and precipitated with ethanol. The yield from 75 g of crude protease was approx. 5 g with a proteolytic activity of about 10 caseinolytic U/mg (Fig. 62, *left*).

Table 15. Purification of alkaline protease from *A. ochraceus*. (From Töpfer and Piesche, 1974)

Stage in purification	Quantity (g protein)	Total activity (CU)[a]	Specific activity (CU/mg)[a]	Concentration
Culture filtrate (10 l)	400	80 000	0.2	1
Tannin precipitation	30	60 000	2.0	10
Chromatography, DEAE-Sephadex A-50	3.5	42 000	12.0	60
Chromatography, Sephadex G-75	1.5	24 000	16.0	80

[a] Caseinolytic units (Kunitz).

After centrifugation at $5000\,g$, this partly purified enzyme was rechromatographed on Sephadex G-75 at $4°$ C and eluted with distilled water. The protease-containing fractions were collected and freeze-dried, yielding approx. 1.5–2.0 g from 5 g of starting material, with a proteolytic activity of about 15–16 caseinolytic U/mg (Fig. 62, *right*). A typical purification is shown in Table 15. Standardized to contain 15 caseinolytic U/mg substance, the material was distributed as ocrase[6] for characterization and experimental preclinical and clinical evaluation.

3. Characterization of Purified Enzyme

Töpfer et al. (1971 b) and Töpfer and Piesche (1974) characterized the purified protease by electrophoresis, and by determinations of pH optima, temperature stability, molecular weight, and inhibition of activity.

When run on cellulose acetate strips and on polyacrylamide gel (Fig. 63), the enzyme was shown to be homogeneous. One or two faint bands appearing in polyacrylamide gel electrophoresis were considered by Töpfer and Piesche to be artefacts from possible damage to the enzyme during processing. The isoelectric point was determined at pH 6.1–6.3. (It is of interest that brinase from *A. oryzae* gave a similar picture on cellulose acetate strips [Roschlau and Ives, 1974; cf. Fig. 10], showing one or two faint secondary bands which were considered to be products of autolysis rather than impurities.) The molecular weight of ocrase was found to be approx. 25 000 when determined by gel filtration on Sephadex G-75.

Optimal activity of ocrase occurred at pH 8.0, and optimal stability was observed between pH 6.0 and 7.0 in dependence on calcium ion concentration (Fig. 64). Calcium ions were also found to stabilize the enzyme during dialysis, while EDTA accelerated its inactivation.

The highest reaction velocity occurred at $50°$ C, with rapid loss of activity at higher temperatures (Fig. 65). Enzyme solutions were stable at temperatures below $40°$ C, retaining maximal activity for 24 h at $4°$ C and pH 6.0.

Comparison of ocrase and trypsin on tosyl arginine methyl ester (TAME) showed trypsin to be about 5 times as active on this trypsin-specific substrate. However, when tested on fibrin plates for fibrinolytic activity, ocrase was 5 times more active than trypsin; and the protease had about twice the activity of trypsin on casein.

---

[6] Nonproprietary name recommended by World Health Organization.

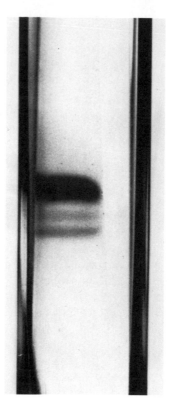

Fig. 63. Polyacrylamide gel electrophoresis of ocrase. Ampholine (LKB Producter, Sweden) pH 3–10; 0.2% H_2SO_4 (anode); 0.4% ethanolamine (cathode); 200–400 V, 4° C, 5–6 h. Stained with amido black 10 B. From Töpfer and Piesche (1974)

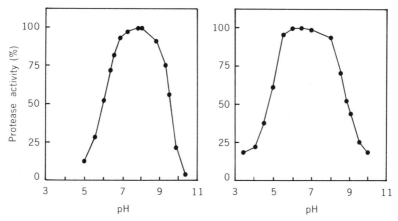

Fig. 64. Ocrase activity in dependence on pH. (Left) pH optimum on 1.5% casein substrate, Britton-Robinson buffer 0.04 M, incubated for 30 min at 37° C. Absorbance of trichloroacetic acid filtrate at 280 mµ. (Right) pH stability after incubation of enzyme in Britton-Robinson buffer 0.04 M of respective pH for 3 h at 37° C. Determination of residual activity on casein substrate at pH 8.0. From Töpfer et al. (1971 b)

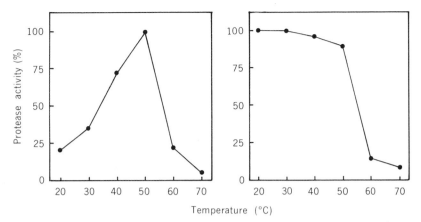

Fig. 65. Ocrase activity in dependence on temperature. *(Left)* Temperature optimum on 1.5% casein substrate, Britton-Robinson buffer $0.04\,M$, pH 6.0, incubated for 10 min at respective temperature. Absorbance of trichloroacetic acid filtrate at 280 mµ. *(Right)* Temperature stability after incubation of enzyme in Britton-Robinson buffer $0.04\,M$ pH 6.0, for 10 min at respective temperature. Determination of residual activity on casein substrate at pH 8.0. From Töpfer et al. (1971 b)

Ocrase activity was strongly inhibited by potato inhibitor, trypsin inhibitor from *Hirudo medicinalis*, ovomucoid from egg albumin, and serum, while soybean trypsin inhibitor and beef lung proteinase inhibitor had practically no inhibitory activity. Strong inactivation was also obtained with the heavy metals Mn^{++}, Ag^+, Cu^{++}, Cd^{++}, Cr^{+++}, Zn^{++}, Hg^{++}, Fe^{+++}, and Co^{++}.

The inhibition of caseinolytic enzyme activity by $10^{-5}M$ concentrations of diisopropylfluorophosphate (DFP) and phenylmethylsulfonylfluoride (PMSF) characterized ocrase as a serine enzyme. The presence of disulfide bridges was shown, while essential SH-groups could not be demonstrated (Töpfer and Piesche, 1974).

II. Biological and Pharmacologic Properties

1. Inhibition

The biological inhibition of ocrase activity (as distinct from inactivation) by various known inhibitor substances was studied by Teisseyre et al. (1974). It was shown that the commonly used plasmin inhibitors Trasylol and soybean trypsin inhibitor (SBTI) were ineffective, but that potato inhibitor in high concentration was able to reduce ocrase activity (Fig. 66, *left*).

Teisseyre et al. also showed the inhibition of ocrase by serum (Fig. 66, *right*). This effect occurred almost immediately, since the degree of inhibition did not differ between enzyme samples preincubated with serum for 1 min or for 10 min (cf. Fig. 17 for brinase). This effect was ascribed to an interaction with α_2-macroglobulins in analogy to brinase inhibition.

The inhibitory activity of serum from different species was investigated by Klöcking and Markwardt (1971 a), who determined the loss of activity of ocrase in serum on bovine fibrin. The results in Table 16 were obtained in a test system

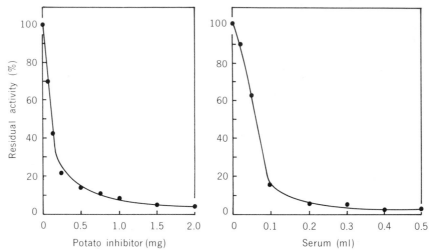

Fig. 66. *(Left)* Inhibition of ocrase by potato inhibitor. Enzyme concentration = 20 μg/ml. Inhibitor added, casein added 5 min later, incubated for 30 min at 37° C. Perchloric acid–soluble peptides measured by spectrophotometry. *(Right)* Inhibition of ocrase by serum. Enzyme concentration = 20 μg/ml. Conditions as above. From TEISSEYRE et al. (1974)

Table 16. Inhibition of fibrinolytic activity of ocrase by serum of different species. (From KLÖCKING and MARKWARDT, 1971a)

Species	Inhibition (%)
Rabbit	34
Dog	38
Mouse	55
Rat	57
Human	61

consisting of 0.2 ml bovine fibrinogen (25 mg/ml Tris buffer), 0.1 ml ocrase (800 μg/ml), and 0.1 ml serum, to which was added 0.1 ml thrombin solution (50 NIH U/ml) to clot. The percent inhibition was determined from the lysis times of samples with and without addition of serum.

2. Proteolysis

a) Fibrin and Fibrinogen

The fibrinolytic activity of ocrase was examined in vitro by KLÖCKING and MARKWARDT (1971 a). Using normal and heated Astrup-Müllertz fibrin plates, the authors demonstrated fibrinolysis on both types of substrate and concluded that ocrase acts directly rather than by activation of plasminogen.

In other experiments, increasing amounts of ocrase were added to citrated plasma, which was then clotted with thrombin, incubated at 37° C, and the lysis time was

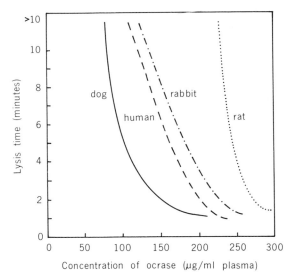

Fig. 67. Lysis of plasma clots by various concentrations of ocrase incubated at 37° C. From KLÖCKING and MARKWARDT (1971 a)

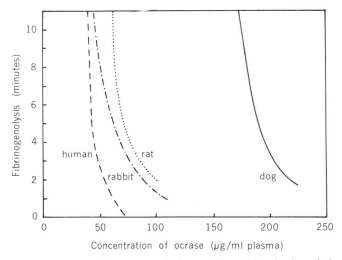

Fig. 68. Plasma fibrinogenolysis by ocrase. *Ordinate:* Time of incubation of plasma and enzyme required to render plasma incoagulable with thrombin. From KLÖCKING and MARKWARDT (1971 a)

measured. Figure 67 shows the dependence of lysis of plasma clots of different species on the concentration of inhibitors in the respective plasmas. Thus, a 5 min lysis time was obtained with 100 µg of ocrase per ml of dog plasma, 160 µg/ml human plasma, 180 µg/ml rabbit plasma, and 240 µg/ml rat plasma.

Fibrinogenolytic effects of ocrase, which were indicated by prolongations of thrombin clotting times of plasmas containing the enzyme, were further investigated

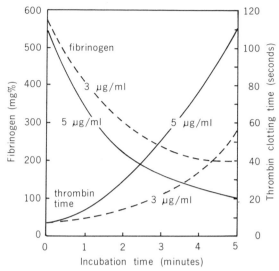

Fig. 69. Hydrolysis of bovine fibrinogen by ocrase at two dose levels, expressed as reduction of fibrinogen and prolongation of thrombin clotting time. From KLÖCKING and MARKWARDT (1971 a)

by KLÖCKING and MARKWARDT (1971 a) in a system measuring residual clottability after incubation of citrated plasma with ocrase. The time after which no clot could be formed with thrombin was considered to be the fibrinogenolysis time (Fig. 68). This effect on fibrinogen was also shown in an isolated system employing purified bovine fibrinogen incubated with the enzyme for varying lengths of time (Fig. 69).

TEISSEYRE et al. (1974) examined the proteolytic effects of ocrase on fibrin and fibrinogen, both in a purified system and in plasma, where it was generally found that much higher concentrations of enzyme were required for proteolysis in plasma or serum due to the presence of inhibitors.

Figure 70 shows the proteolysis of purified fibrinogen, and of plasma and serum proteins by ocrase. The enzyme concentration for hydrolysis of 2% fibrinogen was 70 µg/ml, and that for plasma and serum was 1 mg/ml. The authors concluded from these findings that ocrase had considerable activity on plasma proteins in addition to its fibrinolytic and fibrinogenolytic effects, which should confer a decisive importance upon the inhibitory barrier of plasma when ocrase is used in the living organism.

Fibrinogenolysis was found by TEISSEYRE et al. to occur in plasma with relatively low enzyme concentrations. Using ^{131}I-labeled fibrinogen added to plasma, the authors demonstrated a progressive escape of radioactivity into the liquid phase in dependence on the time of incubation and on the concentration of enzyme (Fig. 71).

The actions of ocrase and of plasmin were compared in a purified system, and the proteolytic effects were evaluated by measuring radioactivity. As shown in Figure 72, ocrase released more soluble peptides from both fibrinogen and fibrin than did plasmin, indicating that more peptide bonds are broken by ocrase. Similar experiments with stabilized and nonstabilized fibrin (Fig. 73) showed that plasmin dissolved stabilized fibrin at a slower rate than nonstabilized fibrin, while ocrase had almost the same rate of hydrolysis on both types of fibrin.

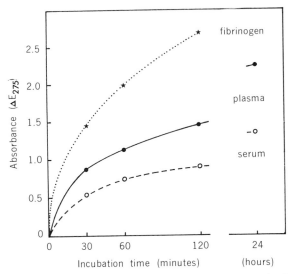

Fig. 70. Proteolysis of purified fibrinogen, plasma, and serum proteins by ocrase. Enzyme concentrations: for 2% fibrinogen solution = 70 µg/ml; for plasma and serum = 1 mg/ml. Measured as increase in light absorbance of perchloric acid-treated samples. From TEISSEYRE et al. (1974)

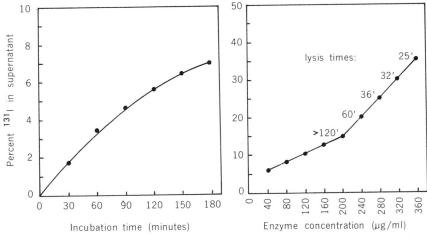

Fig. 71. Proteolysis of ^{131}I-labeled fibrinogen by ocrase, measured as percent radioactivity detected in supernatant after perchloric acid precipitation. *(Left)* As function of incubation time. Enzyme concentration = 60 µg/ml. *(Right)* As function of enzyme concentration. Incubation time = 60 min. Lysis times of samples indicated. From TEISSEYRE et al. (1974)

When studying the products formed during digestion of fibrinogen, TEISSEYRE et al. noted further dissimilarities between ocrase and plasmin. For example, it was found that exhaustive digestion with ocrase produced peptides that bore no electrophoretic resemblance to plasmin products, being almost identical whether produced from fibrinogen, fibrin, or stabilized fibrin.

The products of fibrinogen degradation by ocrase were studied for their anticoagulant activity. It appeared that very low doses of ocrase had negligible clot-promot-

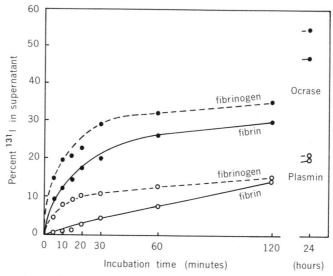

Fig. 72. Comparison of ocrase and plasmin proteolysis of purified fibrinogen and fibrin. Enzyme concentrations: ocrase = 175 µg/ml; plasmin = 60 µg/ml; added prior to clot formation. Measurements as in Fig. 71. After TEISSEYRE et al. (1974)

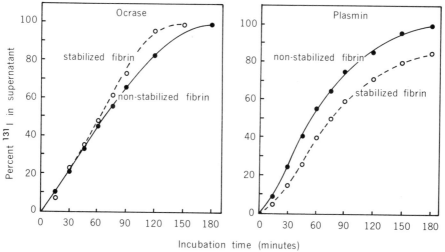

Fig. 73. Comparison of ocrase *(left)* and plasmin *(right)* thrombolysis on stabilized and non-stabilized fibrin. Enzyme concentrations: ocrase = 350 µg/ml; plasmin = 125 µg/ml; into which preformed clots were immersed. Measurements as in Fig. 71. After TEISSEYRE et al. (1974)

ing activity, while ocrase-produced fibrinogen digestion products inhibited fibrinogen-fibrin conversion and thus acted as anticoagulants (Fig. 74). This effect was similar to that produced by plasmin digestion products.

TEISSEYRE et al. (1974) concluded that ocrase degraded fibrinogen further than plasmin, and that it was apparently less specific in its fibrinolytic effects. While this may be considered to be a disadvantage in the clinical use of the enzyme, its pro-

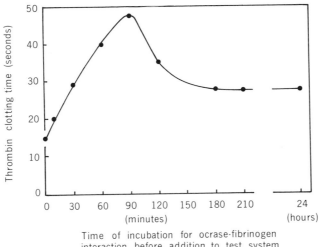

Fig. 74. Anticlotting effects of ocrase-produced fibrinogen degradation products. Test system: 0.4 ml plasma, 0.05 ml fibrinogen-ocrase mixture incubated for the times shown on *abscissa*, 0.1 ml thrombin (50 NIH U/ml). After Teisseyre et al. (1974)

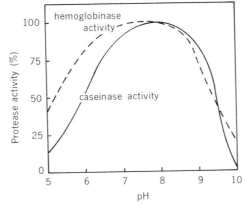

Fig. 75. Caseinase and hemoglobinase activity of equipotent amounts of ocrase at varying pH. From Töpfer et al. (1971a)

nounced thrombolytic activity on stabilized *and* nonstabilized fibrin may be viewed as a practical advantage over plasmin since in vivo thrombolysis involves primarily stabilized fibrin clots.

b) Other Natural Proteins

The activity of ocrase on casein, gelatin, and hemoglobin was studied by Töpfer et al. (1971a), who demonstrated considerable proteolysis in dependence on pH (Fig. 75). These properties of the enzyme were utilized for various assay purposes during production and purification.

3. Hemostasis

a) Coagulation

Klöcking and Markwardt (1971 a) assessed the effects of ocrase on prothrombin. They found that plasma which had been rendered incoagulable by incubation with ocrase regained its clottability with thrombin when exogenous fibrinogen was added. This indicated that nonfibrinogen coagulation factors were likely not affected to a significant degree.

Quantitative analysis of prothrombin levels in ocrase-treated plasma showed that significant changes in prothrombin did not occur with enzyme doses up to 200 µg/ml plasma incubated for 15 min at 37° C (Klöcking and Markwardt, 1971 a).

The ability of ocrase to activate the clotting system was also investigated by Klöcking and Markwardt (1971 a). A direct, thrombin-like activity could not be shown in human, dog, and rat citrated plasma. However, citrated rabbit plasma clotted in dependence on protease concentration. The threshold concentration of ocrase to initiate clotting of citrated rabbit plasma was about 40 µg/ml, and increasing enzyme doses up to 120 µg/ml shortened clotting times progressively. Further increases of enzyme produced fibrinogenolytic effects which overbalanced the clot-promoting activity, leading to eventual incoagulability when enzyme levels approached 200 µg/ml.

The coagulation of recalcified plasma, on the other hand, was accelerated in all plasma species investigated by Klöcking and Markwardt (Fig. 76). Thus, maximal acceleration of clotting occurred in dog plasma with 60 µg/ml, in human plasma with 80 µg/ml, and in rabbit and rat plasma with 160 µg/ml. The reductions of recalcified clotting times were about 50% in human and dog plasma, 25% in rat plasma, and

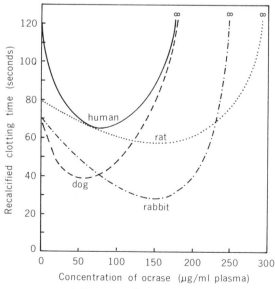

Fig. 76. Effect of ocrase on recalcified clotting times of various plasma species. From Klöcking and Markwardt (1971 a)

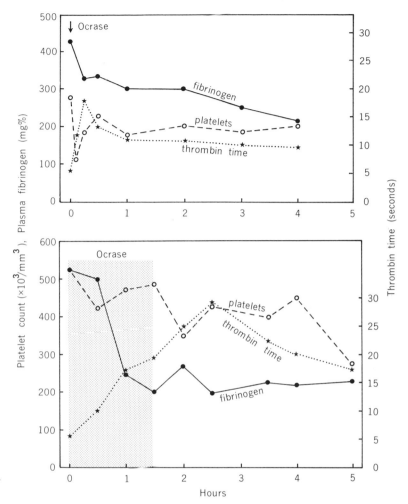

Fig. 77. Responses of selected coagulation parameters following infusions of ocrase into anesthetized rabbits. *(Above)* Single injection of 5 mg/kg (approx. 15 mg/animal). *(Below)* Slow infusion of 0.125 mg/kg/min. (31.5 mg/animal). From KLÖCKING and MARKWARDT (1971 b)

75% in rabbit plasma. Increases of enzyme concentrations resulted in incoagulability. The authors concluded that ocrase had significantly less coagulant activity than other proteolytic enzymes, e.g., trypsin.

The in vivo effects of ocrase on coagulation were studied by KLÖCKING and MARKWARDT (1971 b) in anesthetized rabbits and dogs. Single i.v. infusions of 5.0 mg/kg rabbit caused brief, transient falls in platelet counts, progressive lowering of plasma fibrinogen levels, and transient prolongations of thrombin times (Fig. 77). Thrombelastogram tests showed no significant abnormalities. The same qualitative changes in coagulation parameters were observed if infusions of ocrase were given at about twice the dose but at a slower rate over a longer period of time. However, the quantitative changes were more pronounced and of longer duration (Fig. 77). Plasma

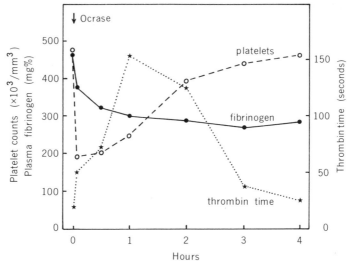

Fig. 78. Responses of selected coagulation parameters following single injection of 2.5 mg ocrase/kg in anesthetized dog. From KLÖCKING and MARKWARDT (1971 b)

clots showed spontaneous lysis approx. 60–200 min after the start of infusions, and thrombelastograms gave prolonged reaction times after 1–4 h.

The effects of single i.v. infusions of ocrase (2.5 mg/kg) in dogs (Fig. 78) were similar to those obtained in rabbits, with a more rapid reversal of platelet count and thrombin time changes. Thrombolytic activity was demonstrated by spontaneous plasma clot lysis during the 4 h following single ocrase doses of 2.5 mg/kg.

Table 17. Inhibition by ocrase of thrombus formation in jugular veins and carotid arteries of rats. Venous clots produced by serum injections and ligation; arterial thrombi produced by electric-current intima damage. (From KLÖCKING et al., 1974)

No. of rats	Ocrase[a] (mg/kg i.v.)	Rats developing thrombi		p[b]
		No.	%	
Venous clots				
30	—	30	100	—
20	5.0	19	95	NS
10	10.0	3	33	0.05
19	15.0	3	16	0.01
Arterial thrombi				
16	—	16	100	—
20	2.5	16	80	NS
20	5.0	13	65	0.05
31	10.0	1	3.2	0.01

[a] Administered 10 min before serum injection (veins) or electric-current application (arteries).
[b] Statistical significance by χ^2-test.

Inhibition of thrombus formation by ocrase was demonstrated in rats by KLÖCK-ING et al. (1974). The normally occurring clotting of veins within 10 min of injection of activated human serum and ligation of vessel segments was prevented following systemic pretreatment with ocrase in 67% of animals with 10 mg/kg, and in 84% of animals with 15 mg/kg (Table 17). Arterial thrombosis was induced by electric-current intima damage of carotid arteries, resulting in 100% thrombosis in untreated rats. Pretreatment with 5 mg ocrase/kg reduced the incidence of thrombus formation by 35%, and 10 mg/kg prevented thrombosis almost completely (Table 17). The results of both investigations were further documented by KLÖCKING et al. by flow measurements and vessel temperature recordings.

b) Platelet Function

The effects of ocrase on blood platelets were examined in vitro by HOFFMANN (1971) with the turbidimetric method of Born. Human platelets in platelet-rich plasma (PRP) or in washed suspension were aggregated with 0.4 µg ADP/ml PRP, or with 1.0 NIH U thrombin/ml platelet suspension. Concentrations of ocrase were between 0.1 and 100 µg/ml.

Preincubation of washed human platelets suspended in Tyrode's solution with various doses of ocrase resulted in dose-dependent inhibition of thrombin aggregation (Fig. 79). The inhibition was independent of the length of incubation time, with maximal effects occurring in all experiments after 3 min of preincubation of platelets with the enzyme. Inhibition was less pronounced, however, when platelets were suspended in defibrinated plasma, which was attributed by HOFFMANN to the presence of ocrase inhibitors in plasma and to substrate competition from plasma proteins.

The linearity of absorbance curves during preincubation of platelets with the enzyme before aggregation with thrombin or ADP indicated to HOFFMANN that ocrase had no platelet-aggregating properties of its own in dose ranges between 0.1 and 100 µg per ml of human platelet suspension. However, these findings may apply only to human platelets, since specific tests of platelet aggregation by ocrase, using different platelet species, have not been reported. For example, the aggregating properties of brinase were shown by SVÄRD (1966) in washed rabbit platelet suspensions in the presence of Ca^{++} (maximal aggregation with 0.5 µg brinase/ml, Fig. 36), and in dog and human PRP by ROSCHLAU and GAGE (1972b) who found dose-dependent aggregation with 12–50 µg brinase/ml dog PRP and 125–250 µg brinase/ml human PRP (Fig. 46). Comparison of the brinase data of SVÄRD and of ROSCHLAU and GAGE indicate significant species differences in platelet aggregability, with human PRP responding least to the aggregation with brinase. The inability of ocrase to aggregate human platelets at doses between 0.1 and 100 µg/ml (HOFFMANN, 1971) must therefore be regarded as appylying specifically to this species and dose range. That ocrase has the potential to cause transient formation of microaggregates suggests itself from the experiments of KLÖCKING and MARKWARDT (1971b), who reported steep but reversible falls in total platelet counts in rabbits and dogs immediately following single infusions of the enzyme (cf. Figs. 77, 78). These in vivo data are in agreement with those reported by ROSCHLAU and GAGE (1972b) for brinase.

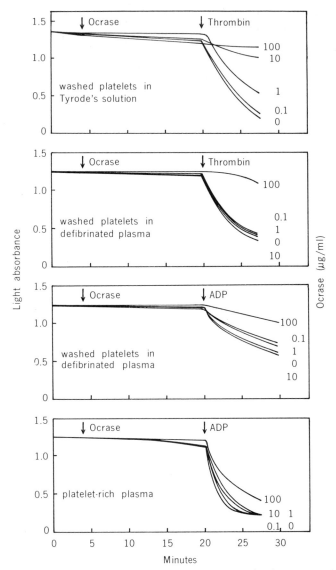

Fig. 79. Inhibition of platelet aggregation by ocrase. Human platelet preparations preincubated with enzyme for 17 min at 18° C and aggregated with thrombin (1.0 NIH U/ml) or ADP (0.4 μg/ml). Method of Born. After HOFFMANN (1971)

ADP-induced aggregation of washed human platelets in defibrinated plasma was also inhibited by high doses of ocrase. However, these effects varied considerably with the type of platelet preparation, the inhibition being least pronounced in human PRP (Fig. 79).

In vivo tests of platelet inhibition were conducted by HOFFMANN (1971) in anesthetized rabbits receiving 2.5 mg ocrase per kg by ear vein. Inhibition of aggregation was observed immediately following ocrase infusions and lasted for at least 6 h

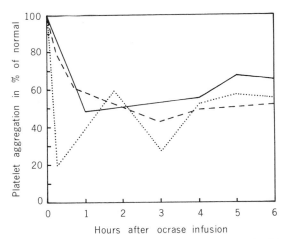

Fig. 80. In vivo inhibition by ocrase of rabbit platelets aggregated with ADP (0.4 µg/ml PRP). Pretreatment aggregation = 100%. Ocrase = 2.5 mg/kg. Results of 3 individual experiments. From HOFFMANN (1971)

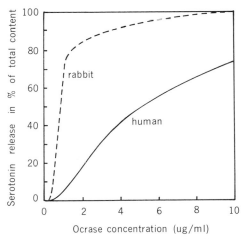

Fig. 81. Serotonin release from rabbit and human platelets by ocrase. Platelet suspensions in Tyrode's solution incubated with enzyme for 10 min at pH 7.2 and 37° C. From HOFFMANN (1971)

(Fig. 80). The enzyme dose employed did not markedly affect the coagulation system during the test period.

The release of platelet biogenic amines (serotonin) by ocrase is shown in Figure 81. The release reaction was found to be species-specific, with rabbit platelets responding most readily to low doses of the enzyme. HOFFMANN interpreted these data as indicating that ocrase altered the platelet membrane, rendering platelets inaggregable despite release of platelet nucleotides and biogenic amines. Functional damage of platelets was not observed.

4. Toxicity

The acute toxicity of ocrase was investigated by KLÖCKING et al. (1974) in mice, rats, and rabbits. The LD_{50} in mice was 27.5 mg/kg by i.v. infusion and 17.6 mg/kg by the i.p. route. Oral doses of up to 1.0 g/kg were without toxicity. The LD_{50} in rats was 17.0 mg/kg by both the i.v. and i.p. routes; and in the rabbit, 7.0 mg/kg from i.v. injection.

KLÖCKING et al. (1974) reported some pharmacodynamic observations with ocrase on isolated organs. It was found that the enzyme was without effect (neither inhibitory nor potentiating) on the acetylcholine contraction of frog skeletal muscle when used in concentrations of up to 5.0 µg/ml of frog-Ringer-solution.

Concentrations of up to 200 µg/ml of Tyrode's solution had no effect on barium chloride-, carbachol-, or histamine-induced spasms of the isolated guinea-pig ileum.

The isolated perfused frog heart responded with dose-dependent negative inotropy following perfusion with 1.5–10.0 µg ocrase per 2 ml frog-Ringer-solution. A similar effect occurred in the isolated guinea-pig heart in a Langendorff preparation. Adrenaline (0.05 ml, 1×10^{-5} g/ml) reversed the negative inotropic action of ocrase.

Systemic blood pressure effects of the enzyme were studied by KLÖCKING et al. (1974) in urethane-anesthetized rabbits. It was shown that rapid injection of 2.5–5.0 mg ocrase/kg into the cannulated jugular vein lowered carotid artery pressure by approx. 60 mm Hg. This response was biphasic, with normalization of pressure about 20 min later.

III. Experimental Thrombolysis

1. In Vitro Experiments

As described by KLÖCKING and MARKWARDT (1971a) in experiments with native human thrombi obtained from autopsies, ocrase caused partial or complete lysis in dependence on enzyme concentration and incubation time. For example, thrombi suspended in 8 ml of protease solution at 37° C lysed completely within 6 h in the presence of 100 µg of protease per ml. Lower enzyme concentrations caused corresponding partial lysis, while thrombi in saline remained unaffected during incubation.

2. In Vivo Experiments

Most of the investigations of the thrombolytic effects of ocrase in the living animal were conducted by KLÖCKING and MARKWARDT (1971b), NOWAK (1972), BIESELT et al. (1974), KLÖCKING et al. (1974), and SEDLARIK et al. (1976), MARKWARDT et al. (1977).

a) Systemic Administration

KLÖCKING and MARKWARDT (1971b) demonstrated the systemic thrombolytic efficacy of ocrase in anesthetized mice. Intravenous thrombi were produced by direct-current lesions in the ear veins, from which about 80% of animals developed permanent thrombi which were visualized under a dissecting microscope 2 h after production. In 20% of cases the thrombi lysed spontaneously, and these animals were excluded from further study.

Table 18. Thrombolysis with ocrase in the ear vein of mice. (From KLÖCKING and MARKWARDT, 1971b)

No. of mice with ear vein thrombi	Time of treatment after thrombosis (8 mg ocrase/kg i.v.)	Thrombolysis after 24 h		
		Complete	Partial	None
22	2 h	2	10	10
22	2 h and 6 h	15	4	3
34	2 h and 20 h	14	12	6

Animals with 2 h thrombi were divided into three groups (Table 18) and received standard doses of 8 mg of ocrase per kg at 2 h, 2 and 6 h, or 2 and 20 h following thrombosis. The results of thrombolysis were assessed 24 h after the start of treatment by inspection and photography.

As shown in Table 18, a single application of protease appeared not to be sufficient to cause complete lysis. If ocrase was given twice, however, thrombolysis occurred with high frequency, favoring the shorter rather than the longer interval between infusions.

b) Local Administration

Artificial thrombi were produced by injection of sclerosing agents and thrombin in the semi-ligated femoral arteries of anesthetized dogs (KLÖCKING and MARKWARDT, 1971b). One day later, the thrombi were inspected, palpated, and measured externally, followed by direct intra-arterial application of ocrase (1 mg/ml/min) for 30 min into the vicinity of the obstruction. Treatment results were documented by photography.

In experiments on six dogs, the local instillation of ocrase caused a marked reduction in thrombus size about 10 min after the start of infusions, followed by complete recanalization after about 30 min with a total enzyme dose of 30 mg/animal.

NOWAK (1972) performed experiments in rabbits. Artificial thrombi were induced in the abdominal aorta by rinsing a ligated 3 cm segment with a 4% silver nitrate solution. Occlusive thrombi formed within 4 h. When infused locally with 1 mg ocrase/ml/min, partial recanalization occurred in about 10 min, and after 20 min complete disappearance of thrombi was observed.

Using artificially thrombosed brachial arteries of dogs, NOWAK infused protease in concentrations of 2 mg/ml/min and obtained partial lysis after 4 or 5 min, to be followed by complete recanalization about 15 min later.

BIESELT et al. (1974) explored the feasibility of using ocrase for the recanalization of clotted hemodialysis shunts. The authors implanted polyethylene Scribner-type shunts into the femoral artery and vein of 13 dogs. The initial patency and eventual clotting of the implants was checked periodically by angiography for about 10 days.

Thrombosis occurred spontaneously and regularly in varying time intervals, involving the whole length of the implants. Eleven thrombosed shunts were then treated by local intravascular instillations of ocrase (1 mg/ml) until recanalization occurred. The maximal dose required for this procedure was 2.5 mg/kg, and the

Table 19. Lysis with ocrase of experimental shunt occlusions in the dog. (After BIESELT et al., 1974)

Dog No.	Days until clotted[a]	Ocrase infused (mg)[b]	Thrombolysis		SGOT (U)		SGPT (U)	
			Obtained	in min	Pre	Post	Pre	Post
1	12	40	Yes	45	18	20	15	10
2	10	40	Yes	30	25	28	10	18
3	10	25	Yes	30	28	8	13	9
4	5	20	Yes	30	22	18	11	10
5	5	30	Yes	45	6	10	6	5
6	6	35	Yes	35	10	53	8	24
7	14	60	No	60	8	9	2	8
8	5	30	Yes	30	8	9	10	12
9	4	25	Yes	30	16	19	4	18
10	9	35	Yes	45	19	79	9	52
11	9	35	Yes	30	23	62	20	41

[a] The time required for individual shunts to thrombose spontaneously.
[b] 1 mg/ml infused slowly at the thrombus until recanalization occurred.

average duration of therapy was 30–40 min (Table 19). The treatments were tolerated without significant side-effects or toxicity. There was a general tendency toward moderate hypocoagulability (as evidenced by reductions of plasma fibrinogen levels and platelet counts, and prolongation of thrombin times), without clinical manifestations of bleeding. Accelerated clotting was not observed.

The lysis of thrombi up to 14 days old was studied by SEDLAŘIK et al. (1976) in 15 dogs receiving ocrase by local infusion. Occluding thrombi were produced in the femoral artery by direct-current stimulation and were confirmed by arteriography. After 3, 6 or 14 days the vessels were cannulated near the occlusion, and ocrase was infused in a concentration of 1 mg/2.5 ml saline. As shown in Table 20, complete recanalization of vessels was obtained in all animals but one that carried one of the 2-week-old thrombi. The required doses of enzyme (0.67–2.86 mg/kg) were without systemic side-effects and caused only minor fluctuations in fibrinogen levels and platelet counts. The authors considered the successful lysis of old thrombi with ocrase to be of significant clinical importance.

IV. Other Experimental Uses

Ocrase was used by UHLENBRUCK et al. (1972) to study incomplete erythrocyte antibodies by means of agglutination reactions. One volume of freshly washed red cells was incubated for 30 min at 37° C with 5 volumes of 0.1% ocrase solution pH 7.0, after which the cells were again washed and used in agglutination tests in 1% suspension.

It was found that several different agglutinins (such as Anti-Rh_0, Anti-A_{HP}, lectins, snail extracts) did not react with untreated human, bovine and gallinacean erythrocytes, i.e., they were "incomplete", but that they agglutinated enzyme-treated cells. UHLENBRUCK et al. showed that this effect was due to an action of the protease on the cell surface by demonstrating and measuring glycoprotein-bound neuraminic

Table 20. Lysis of experimental arterial thrombi in dogs by local application of ocrase. (After SEDLAŘÍK et al., 1976)

Dog No.	Weight (kg)	Age of thrombus (days)	Ocrase dose (mg)			Thrombolysis		Fibrinogen (mg %)		Platelet count (×10³/mm³)	
			Total	mg/kg	mg/kg/min	Obtained	in min	Before	After[a]	Before	After[a]
1	30	3	20	0.67	0.022	Complete[b]	30	277	226	245	200
2	30	3	20	0.67	0.022	Complete	30	207	194	110	100
3	23	3	20	0.87	0.029	Complete	30	207	264	77	120
4	21.5	3	20	0.93	0.031	Complete	30	315	279	125	106
5	20	3	20	1.0	0.04	Complete	25	245	185	114	78
6	21	6	25	1.19	0.025	Complete	45	233	226	125	133
7	24.5	6	30	1.22	0.027	Complete	45	220	157	165	155
8	20.5	6	35	1.71	0.049	Complete	35	295	200	220	180
9	26	6	35	1.35	0.039	Complete	35	295	257	165	165
10	23	6	30	1.30	0.043	Complete	30	235	225	181	120
11	14	14	40	2.86	0.064	Complete	45	271	110	168	160
12	22.5	14	45	2.0	0.025	Complete	80	270	263	83	48
13	22	14	60	2.73	0.046	Partial[c]	60	352	264	132	128
14	18	14	40	2.22	0.028	Complete	80	298	210	171	160
15	19.5	14	25	1.28	0.037	Complete	35	295	220	105	149

[a] Determined 10 min after completion of infusion.
[b] Complete recanalization determined by angiography.
[c] Incomplete recanalization on angiogram.

acid in the supernatant (85.2 µg/ml human packed cells; 91.6 µg/ml bovine packed cells). Similar results had also been obtained by the authors with brinase and with pronase. The authors considered fungal proteases to be valuable tools for the exploration of cell membrane structure and the variable topographic arrangement of blood group and transplantation antigens on cell surfaces.

V. Clinical Thrombolysis

The effects of ocrase in the human were studied by VOGEL et al. (1974), who also conducted a preliminary clinical trial in patients with thromboembolic disease.

1. Coagulation

In preparation of the use of ocrase in humans, VOGEL et al. examined the effects of the enzyme on several coagulation parameters in vitro. Immunoelectrophoretic studies showed the presence of two fibrinogen split products after incubation of human fibrinogen with the protease. Low concentrations of ocrase shortened the partial thromboplastin times and thrombin times, while higher doses led to a prolongation of these parameters. There were some individual variations of response within the general trends, which were attributed by VOGEL et al. to the variable inhibition of ocrase by individual plasmas. The effects on partial thromboplastin time and thrombin time were not influenced by lack of factors VIII and IX or by low platelet counts.

2. Determination of Dosage

An in vitro protease-resistance test (modified method of ROSCHLAU) was developed by VOGEL et al., in which 1-ml aliquots of citrated blood were mixed with increasing quantities of ocrase solution and clotted with thrombin (20 NIH U/ml). Following incubation for 10 min at 37° C, the protease concentration sufficient to lyse the blood clot was determined.

The screening of 160 blood samples from healthy blood donors as well as from patients with a variety of diseases showed considerable variation of ocrase resistance between a low of 150 µg/ml and a high of 300 µg/ml (cf. Tables 5 and 6, Figs. 55–57 for brinase).

3. Therapeutic Use

The compatibility of ocrase was first tested by VOGEL et al. in 21 healthy volunteers. Protase was injected i.v. in doses of 0.06–0.6 mg/kg, and the electrocardiogram and coagulation parameters were monitored.

Nine persons tolerated the injections without side-effects. Minor symptoms such as flushing, rising heat, burning at the injection site, and lacrimation occurred in 10 volunteers. Two cases responded with deeper reddening of the face, while one subject developed a localized edema at the injection site. There was no hypotension and no change in electrocardiograms. The repeated administration of the same dose to three of these individuals was tolerated in the same manner.

Ten other volunteers received infusions of 0.66–1.0 mg ocrase/kg over 2 h. The doses were below the individual inhibitor levels as determined by the ocrase-resis-

Table 21. Results of ocrase infusions in 17 patients with thromboembolic disease. (From VOGEL et al., 1974)

Patient No.	Diagnosis	Ocrase dose/patient	Result[a]
1	Peripheral artery occlusion	1 × 80 mg	0
2	Peripheral artery occlusion	2 × 80 mg	0
3	Peripheral artery occlusion	3 × 80 mg	0
4	Peripheral artery occlusion	3 × 80 mg	0
5	Peripheral artery occlusion	3 × 80 mg	+
6	Peripheral artery occlusion	5 × 80 mg	+ +
7	Peripheral artery occlusion	3 × 100 mg	+ +
8	Peripheral artery occlusion	3 × 100 mg	+
9	Peripheral artery occlusion	4 × 80 mg	+ +
10	Endangiitis obliterans	10 × 80 mg	0
11	Retinal artery occlusion	3 × 80 mg	+ + +
12	Pelvic vein thrombosis	3 × 80 mg	+ + +
13	Pelvic vein thrombosis	3 × 80 mg	+ + +
14	Pelvic vein thrombosis	4 × 80 mg	+ + +
15	Pelvic vein thrombosis	6 × 80 mg	+ +
16	Pelvic vein thrombosis	5 × 100 mg	+
17	Pelvic vein thrombosis	4 × 100 mg	+ + +

[a] Results: 0 = no change from pretreatment condition; + = slight clinical improvement; + + = significant clinical improvement; + + + = complete clinical restitution.

tance test. Three of these subjects responded with minor subjective symptoms, while one case developed urticaria that necessitated discontinuing the infusion. The reaction was controlled with calcium thiosulfate and antihistaminics. Coagulation parameters remained within normal limits.

VOGEL et al. proceeded to treat 17 patients with thromboembolic disease (six pelvic vein thromboses, one occlusion of the central retinal artery, one endangiitis obliterans, and nine peripheral artery occlusions of arteriosclerotic origin). The clinical diagnosis was confirmed in all cases by oscillography, plethysmography, and angiography. Although the trial was admittedly small, tentative and experimental, VOGEL et al. showed (Table 21) that peripheral arterial occlusions did not respond well to systemic therapy. On the other hand, the treatments of 5 out of 6 pelvic vein thromboses and the retinal artery occlusion were highly successful, resulting in complete restitution.

Observed side-effects were less frequent or pronounced than in the volunteer subjects of the preclinical study. Phlebitic irritation occurred in two cases, and in four patients with pelvic vein thromboses the body temperature rose to 38° C. The fever was interpreted by VOGEL et al. as being a possible consequence of thrombolysis, since it occurred only in those patients in whom the treatment was clinically successful (see also ROSCHLAU, 1972b, Fig. 56). The failure to obtain clinical results in peripheral artery occlusions was attributed by VOGEL et al. to the incurably advanced state of disease in these patients, whose atherosclerotic vessels had previously been refractory to any other form of therapy. VOGEL et al. considered ocrase to be well-tolerated and, within the limits of the study, to possess extraordinary efficacy.

C. Protease from Trichothecium Roseum

Research in the Soviet Union showed the existence of fibrinolytically active proteases in cultures of a number of *Actinomyces* species (EGOROV and ARAKELOVA, 1972; EGOROV et al., 1972a, b). ANDREEVA et al. (1972) studied proteolytic enzymes from different strains of *Penicillium lilacinum*, and PRUDLOV et al. (1973) described the production of proteases by *Fusarium graminearum* and by *Alternaria* species.

A. *oryzae* was briefly examined by ANDREENKO and STRUKOVA (1966), after which the ANDREENKO group began a systematic investigation of the mold *Trichothecium roseum* Link (ANDREENKO et al., 1968, 1971, 1974), resulting in the fibrinolytic enzyme, tricholysin.

I. Isolation and Purification

ANDREENKO et al. (1974) examined 207 strains of *T. roseum*, of which 80% were found to be proteolytically active, and some also showed fibrinolytic activity. Maximal fibrinolysis was obtained with *T. roseum* "D."

The degree of activity of *Trichothecium* cultures was determined by the choice of culture medium, the highest activity occurring when the mold was grown on a synthetic medium with 2% carbohydrate, gelatin, and peptone. It was shown that enzyme production occurred with two maxima (Fig. 82), the first peak at 48 h accompanied by an intensive growth of mycelium, and the second peak at 96 h preceding lysis of the fungus. ANDREENKO et al. concluded from this activity pattern that the first maximum was most likely due to an exoenzyme, while the second was the result of endoprotease production.

The culture filtrate was concentrated by precipitation with cold acetone, followed by drying *in vacuo* over concentrated sulfuric acid. The water-soluble component was then further purified by gel filtration on Sephadex G-100 (Fig. 83) and the fractions with highest activity were lyophilized, yielding about 500 mg of active material from one liter of culture filtrate. The final product was a homogeneous substance with high fibrinolytic activity, and it was named tricholysin.

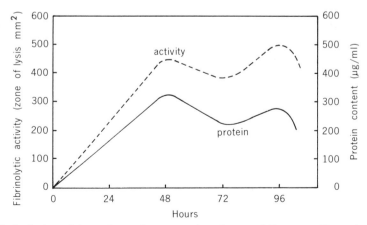

Fig. 82. Fibrinolytic activity and protein content in cultures of *T. roseum*. From ANDREENKO et al. (1974)

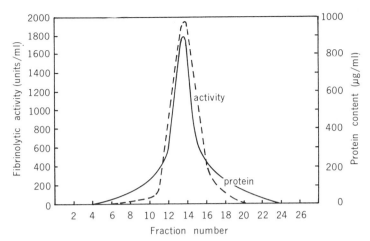

Fig. 83. Gel filtration of *T. roseum* on Sephadex G-100. From ANDREENKO et al. (1974)

The stability of the enzyme extended over 2–3 months when stored in the dry form at $-20°$ C, and solutions remained active at temperatures up to $50°$ C. The pH stability lay between pH 5.0 and 8.0, with a pH optimum at 7.0.

II. Biological Properties

1. Fibrinolysis

In vitro experiments by ANDREENKO et al. (1974) showed that small amounts of tricholysin added to rat plasma caused rapid lysis of plasma clots. Higher concentrations prevented clotting. When injected i.v. into rats in a dose of 15 mg/ml/180 g rat (Fig. 84), in vivo fibrinolytic activity was elevated 10 min after injection, but it returned to pretreatment levels 2 h later. Antiplasmin levels were significantly elevated, and plasma fibrinogen was reduced. When administered repeatedly to rats at intervals of 1–2 h, the fibrinolytic activity remained elevated for about 4 h, and in vitro fibrin clots were lysed.

Although prepared by roughly the same methods, some variations in physiologic responses were observed with different preparations (tricholysin 1 and 2, both obtained by acetone precipitation and Sephadex G-100 treatment, Fig. 84). These variations were attributed by ANDREENKO et al. to slightly different degrees of purity.

2. Thrombolysis

ANDREENKO et al. (1974) produced experimental thrombi in rats that were subsequently treated with i.v. injections of tricholysin, presumably 15 mg/ml/180 g rat. Most of the thrombi in 41 animals were partly or completely lysed within 3–6 h with "therapeutic" doses, while none of five control rats showed spontaneous thrombolysis.

An interesting observation during these experiments was the lack of correlation between fibrinolytic and thrombolytic efficacy of one of the tricholysin preparations.

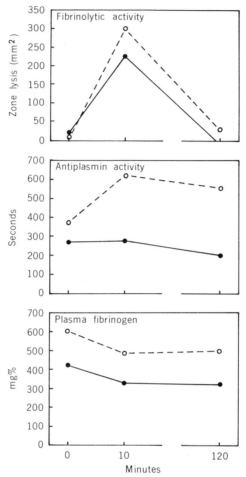

Fig. 84. Fibrinolytic activity, antiplasmin activity, and response of plasma fibrinogen in rats following i. v. administration of 15mg/ml/180g rat of tricholysin 1 (●———●) and tricholysin 2 (○ - - - - - ○). After ANDREENKO et al. (1974)

When precipitated with alcohol instead of acetone during production, the agent retained its high fibrinolytic activity but lost all of its thrombolytic properties.

In animals receiving two or three injections of enzyme, as well as in those treated with "therapeutic" doses that caused lysis of experimental thrombi, toxic reactions were not observed. These favorable preliminary findings should lend encouragement to the Soviet authors to proceed with the systematic development of the enzyme.

D. Protease from Armillaria mellea

In 1973, BROADBENT et al. of Imperial Chemical Industries Ltd., Macclesfield, England, obtained patents on the production of a fibrinolytic fungal protease from the fruiting body of the basidiomycete, *Armillaria mellea*.

The authors had found that the mature fruiting body, or cap, of the fungus which grows parasitically or saprophytically on trees in the United Kingdom and elsewhere is the source of enzymic substances having fibrinolytic and fibrinogenolytic activity. Of about 140 varieties of *A. mellea* collected and screened during 1969, approx. 50 were found to produce the enzyme. Strains ACC 3659 (FPRL 6H, Ministry of Technology, Forest Products Research Laboratories, Princes Risborough, Aylesbury, Buckinghamshire, England) and ACC 3253 ("*Armillaria mellea*," Centraalbureau voor Schimmelcultures, Baarn, Netherlands) were chosen as source material for enzyme production.

I. Isolation, Purification, and Chemical Characteristics

As described by BROADBENT et al. (1973), the mature fruiting bodies were homogenized in cold water, and the resulting mixture was separated by filtration to obtain aqueous extracts. Alternatively, the mycelium of *A. mellea* was grown on a nutrient medium by surface culture, and the mycelium was used for further processing.

Unwanted proteins in the aqueous extract were removed by precipitation with organic solvents. The activity of the enzyme-containing extract was precipitated and was partially purified by cation-exchange chromatography on carboxymethylcellulose, after which the activity-containing fractions were concentrated by pressure dialysis.

This crude enzyme preparation was purified by column chromatography on Sephadex G-75, the eluate containing the enzyme was concentrated by pressure dialysis, it was freeze-dried, and it was identified as AM protease. The enzyme had a high thermal stability and was stable over a pH range of 4.0–9.0.

Characterization showed AM protease to be essentially homogeneous by sedimentation and electrophoretic criteria. It behaved as a single component in the ultracentrifuge and on passage through Sephadex G-150, and its molecular weight was estimated at approx. 30000. Upon electrophoresis in polyacrylamide gel the protease migrated as a single component with γ-globulin. The N-terminal amino acid was found to be isoleucine.

AM protease readily degraded casein at pH 7.0, which was found to be much less, however, than the digestion produced by trypsin, chymotrypsin, or plasmin. There was little degradation of serum albumin or γ-globulin, but fibrinogen was extensively degraded. Synthetic esters used for the characterization of trypsin- and chymotrypsin-like enzymes were not susceptible to AM protease degradation, but it acted on the β-chain of oxidized insulin with the appearance of tyrosine, lysine, and leucine, which differentiated the protease from trypsin and chymotrypsin.

II. Biological Properties

BROADBENT et al. (1973) and COTTON and WALTON (1973) have studied the thrombolytic usefulness of AM protease in a wide range of models in analogy to the earlier investigations of other fungal proteases.

COTTON and WALTON (1973) infused solutions of AM protease into rabbits, rats, and monkeys to assess the effects on coagulation and fibrinolysis. It was found that prolongations of thrombin, prothrombin, and partial thromboplastin times occurred, lasting 4–6 h from single infusions. Immediate side-effects were not observed, but large doses appeared to cause transient peripheral vasoconstriction. Repeated doses did not produce anaphylaxis, and animals were still alive 1 year following enzyme administrations.

The inhibition of AM protease by plasma of various species including man, and the estimation of required fibrinolytic dosage, was described by BROADBENT et al. (1973). When measured by prolongations of clotting times, optimal plasma activity was obtained with loading doses of 0.05–5.0 mg/kg/h, to be followed by intermittent maintenance doses of approx. 10% of the initial dose for the next 2 h, and then decreasing to less than 1% of the loading dose every 2–3 h. In this way sustained plasma activity was obtained. The need for reductions in the size and rate of administration of doses required to maintain activity over prolonged periods of time was attributed to a fall-off in the rate of return of inhibitors into the circulation.

The plasma fibrinolytic activity of AM protease was assessed by COTTON and WALTON (1973) in plasma of rats following infusion of doses that produced a prolongation of thrombin clotting time to more than 20 min and of prothrombin time to 30–40 sec. The plasmas of these animals caused significant fibrinolysis in vitro.

The authors studied in vivo thrombolysis on arterial thrombi in dogs and monkeys by scarifying the intima and infusing enzyme intermittently 3 h after thrombus formation so as to maintain a measurable increase in fibrinolytic activity without causing hemorrhage. Relatively large doses of enzyme were initially necessary to produce the required activity (as measured by prolongation of clotting times), followed by lower maintenance doses. Low doses of AM protease did not cause a shortening of whole blood clotting times. The assessment of thrombolytic effects was made by quantitatively measuring the reduction in thrombus size after an arbitrary time interval, from which COTTON and WALTON concluded that the enzyme was capable of inducing thrombolysis.

The side-effects of AM protease in animals consisted of occasional minor extravasation when high doses were employed. However, there was frequent myocardial damage and significant elevations in serum glutamic oxalacetic transaminase (SGOT) from therapeutic doses. The reasons for this observation, whether due to a direct action of the enzyme or to impurities, were not yet clarified.

The ability of blood platelets to aggregate with ADP was reduced at a time when the partial thromboplastin time was prolonged. A few hours after protease infusions the platelet count and thrombin-clottable fibrinogen were significantly reduced, these changes occurring when the effects on partial thromboplastin time were in the process of reverting to normal.

Animals that died from intentional or accidental overdoses revealed minor extravasation in the form of punctuate hemorrhages in internal organs, but death was not due to excessive blood loss. Some overdosed animals recovered following infusion of reconstituted bovine plasma.

As cited by COTTON and WALTON (1973), clotted arterial and venous catheters in dogs and rats were cleared with AM protease in over 80% of animals if the obstructions were less than 3 days old.

The enzyme is under further investigation, regarding in particular its isolation, enzymic properties, and effects on fibrinogen and other proteins.

Acknowledgments. The following have kindly assisted in providing additional information on industrial patents and unpublished industrial research, and have reviewed the relevant sections of the manuscript. For *Astra Läkemedel AB, Sweden* (Brinastrase): Dr. E. P. FRISCH and Dr. P. O. SVÄRD, Södertälje, Sweden; for *Connaught Laboratories Ltd., Canada* (Connbrinolase): Dr. A. M. FISHER, Dr. A. L. TOSONI, and Mr. D. G. GLASS, Willowdale, Canada; for *VEB Arzneimittelwerk Dresden, German Democratic Republic* (Ocrase): Dr. H. TÖPFER, Dresden, GDR. Prof. G. W. ANDREENKO, Moscow, USSR, made available additional published information on the development of fungal protease research in the Soviet Union, which was translated for me from the Russian by my graduate student, Mr. M. JUNYK. These contributions helped me to present a hopefully comprehensive picture of current developments, whose progress is necessarily influenced — and in some measure funded — by industrial pharmaceutical interests.

The figures and tables were reproduced or adapted by me from the originals by kind permission of the publishers as follows:

Acta Biologica et Medica Germanica, Volume 26 (1971), 35–44: Figures 67–69, 76, Table 16; *1111–1115:* Figures 62, 75.

Acta Chemica Scandinavica, Volume 17 (1963), 1521–1540: Figures 1–5, Table 1; *1541–1551:* Table 2; *2230–2238:* Figures 6–8; *2239–2249:* Figures 12–15; *Volume 23 (1969), 2165–2174:* Figures 16–18, Table 5.

Acta Physiologica Scandinavica, Volume 60 (1964), 363–371: Figure 19; *Volume 78 (1970), 11–19:* Figure 23.

Angiology, Volume 17 (1966), 882–886: Figure 53.

Blood, Volume 23 (1964), 729–740 (DYER, A. E., KADAR, D.: Fibrin suspension assay for fibrinolytic activity): Figure 25.

Canadian Journal of Biochemistry (National Research Council of Canada), *Volume 45 (1967), 1055–1065:* Table 3.

Canadian Journal of Physiology and Pharmacology (National Research Council of Canada), *Volume 42 (1964), 109–125:* Figures 24, 54; *377–384:* Figures 28–32; *Volume 43 (1965), 741–749:* Figures 20–22, Tables 6, 7; *Volume 47 (1969), 369–376:* Figures 50, 51; *Volume 48 (1970), 61–68:* Figures 26, 27.

Folia Haematologica, Leipzig, Volume 95 (1971), 174–178: Figures 64, 65; *179–186:* Figures 77, 78, Table 18; *187–192:* Figures 79–81; *Volume 101 (1974), 14–21:* Figures 82–84; *22–37:* Figures 9–11, Table 4; *38–44:* Figure 47; *45–62:* Figures 49, 52; *63–82:* Tables 10, 12; *83–90:* Figure 61; *91–98:* Figure 63, Table 15; *99–110:* Figures 66, 70–74; *111–117:* Table 17; *118–124:* Table 19; *125–131:* Table 21.

Lancet, Volume 1 (1968), 173–176: Figure 57; *Volume 2 (1968), 1220–1223:* Figure 58.

Life Sciences, Volume 5 (1966), 1379–1387: Figures 33–35; *Volume 6 (1967), 499–505:* Figures 39, 40.

Scandinavian Journal of Haematology, Volume 3 (1966), 277–289: Figures 36–38.

Thrombosis et Diathesis Haemorrhagica (Stuttgart), Suppl. 46 (1971), 229–241: Tables 9, 14; *Suppl. 47 (1971), 315–323:* Table 11; *Volume 28 (1972), 31–48:* Figures 41–46; *Volume 33 (1975), 221–225:* Figures 59, 60.

References

Akatsuka, T., Sato, M.: Studies on peptidases of *Aspergillus oryzae*. Part II. A survey of dipeptidase and aminopolypeptidase activites of various molds, and a study of mold culture method and enzyme extraction. Agr. biol. Chem. **27**, 71—75 (1963a)

Akatsuka, T., Sato, M.: Studies on peptidases of *Aspergillus oryzae*. Part III. Further studies on the specificities of the purified dipeptidase. Agr. biol. Chem. **27**, 828—835 (1963b)

Albert, F. W.: Brinolase — Thrombolytische Wirkung in vitro und in vivo. Fortschr. Med. **91**, 1165—1167 (1973)

Albert, F. W., Kreiter, H., Leube, G.: Antikoagulantien und Fibrinolytika in der Hämodialysebehandlung. Therapiewoche **22**, 677—692 (1972)

Amundsen, E., Svendsen, L., Vefling, A.: A sensitive photometric method for determination of plasma inhibition towards plasmin and brinase. Abstr. 22, IV. Int. Congr. Thrombos. Haemostas. (1973)

Andreenko, G. W., Maksimova, R. A., Korukova, A. A., Palmova, N. P.: Fibrinolytic activity of *Tri-chothecium roseum* LINK. Proc. Acad. Sci. USSR **179**, 454—456 (1968)

Andreenko, G. W., Orlova, A. S., Maksimova, R. A., Poch, L. I.: Study of the fibrinolytic agent iso-lated from *Trichothecium roseum* LINK culture liquid. J. Biochem. Microbiol. Acad. Sci. USSR **7**, 178—182 (1971)

Andreenko, G. W., Silaev, A. B., Maksimova, R. A., Poch, L. I., Serebrjakova, T. N.: Fibrinolytische und thrombolytische Wirkung von Proteasen einiger Pilzkulturen. Folia haemat. (Lpz.) **101**, 14—21 (1974)

Andreenko, G. W., Strukova, S. M.: Isolation of active protease from *Aspergillus oryzae* culture liquor. Biochem. Acad. Sci. USSR **31**, 477—483 (1966)

Andreeva, N. A., Ushakova, V. I., Egorov, N. S.: Studies on proteolytic enzymes from different strains of *Penicillium lilacinum* THOM with respect to their fibrinolytic activity. Microbiol. Acad. Sci. USSR **41**, 417—422 (1972)

Bärwald, G., Jahn, G., Metzner, B.: Verfahren zur Gewinnung einer alkalischen Protease. DDR-Wirtschafts-Patent No. 79702 (1969)

Bärwald, G., Jahn, G., Volzke, K.-D.: Mikrobiologische Gewinnung einer Protease mit fibrinoly-tischer Wirkung aus *Aspergillus ochraceus*. Folia haemat. (Lpz.) **101**, 83—90 (1974)

Bergkvist, R.: The proteolytic enzymes of *Aspergillus oryzae*. I. Methods for the estimation and isolation of the proteolytic enzymes. Acta chem. scand. **17**, 1521—1540 (1963 a)

Bergkvist, R.: The proteolytic enzymes of *Aspergillus oryzae*. II. Properties of the proteolytic enzymes. Acta chem. scand. **17**, 1541—1551 (1963 b)

Bergkvist, R.: The proteolytic enzymes of *Aspergillus oryzae*. III. A comparison of the fibrinolytic and fibrinogenolytic effects of the enzymes. Acta chem. scand. **17**, 2230—2238 (1963 c)

Bergkvist, R.: The proteolytic enzymes of *Aspergillus oryzae*. IV. On the inhibition of the enzymes by serum. Acta chem. scand. **17**, 2239—2249 (1963 d)

Bergkvist, R.: Process of isolating and separating proteolytic enzymes. U.S. Patent No. 3 281 331 (1966)

Bergkvist, R., Svärd, P. O.: Studies on the thrombolytic activity of a protease from *Aspergillus oryzae*. Acta physiol. scand. **60**, 363—371 (1964)

Bieselt, R., Sedlařik, K., Stanulla, H.: Thrombolyse experimentell erzeugter Shuntverschlüsse. Fo-lia haemat. (Lpz.) **101**, 118—124 (1974)

Broadbent, D., Turner, R. W., Walton, P. L.: Fibrinolytic fungal protease. Canadian Patent No. 921 848 (1973)

Bydgeman, S.: Effect of an *Aspergillus* enzyme on adenosinediphosphate (ADP) induced platelet aggregation and adhesiveness. Life Sci. **6**, 499—505 (1967)

Connaught Medical Research Laboratories: Brinase – New Drug Submission – Department of National Health and Welfare, Canada – June 8, 1965

Connaught Mesical Research Laboratories: Brinase – New Drug Submission – Department of National Health and Welfare, Canada – December 14, 1970

Connaught Medical Research Laboratories: Brinolase – New Drug Submission – Department of National Health and Welfare, Canada – February 15, 1972

Cotton, R. C., Walton, P. L.: A novel fibrinolytic enzyme isolated from the fruiting body of the basidiomycete *A. mellea*. Abstract 24, IV. Int. Congr. Thrombos. Haemostas. (1973)

Crewther, W. G., Lennox, F. G.: Preparation of crystals containing protease from *Aspergillus ory-zae*. Nature (Lond.) **165**, 680 (1950)

Cuthbertson, E. M., Gilfillan, R. S.: Direct measurement of external iliac artery blood flow in the awake unmedicated primate (Rhesus monkey): Effect of sympathectomy. J. Surg. Res. **11**, 18—22 (1971)

De Nicola, P., Cultrera, G., Gibelli, A., Manai, G.: Experimentelle und klinische Untersuchungen mit einer Protease aus *Aspergillus oryzae* (Brinase): Fibrinogen-Turnover, Thrombozytenag-gregation und Verschluß des Scribner-Shunts. Folia haemat. (Lpz.) **101**, 38—44 (1974)

De Nicola, P., Gibelli, A., Turazza, G., Giarola, P.: Influence of an *Aspergillus* enzyme on ADP-induced platelet aggregation and fibrinolysis. Life Sci. **6**, 1233—1244 (1967)

Donati, M. B., Vanhove, P., Claeys, H., Vermylen, J., Verstraete, M.: In vivo and in vitro effect of brinase on plasma fibrinogen: A gel filtration study. Abstract 21, IV. Int. Congr. Thrombos. Haemostas. (1973)

Dyer, A. E., Kadar, D.: Fibrin suspension assay for fibrinolytic activity. Blood **23**, 729—740 (1964)

Egan, E. L.: Local use of protease in haemodialysis clotting problems. J. Irish med. Ass. **62**, 179—180 (1969)

Egorov, N. S., Arakelova, V. A.: Effect of various factors on the activity of proteolytic enzymes of *Actinomyces odorifer* and its mutants. Microbiol. Acad. Sci. USSR **41**, 695 –699 (1972)

Egorov, N. S., Ushakova, V. I., Arakelova, V. A.: Effect of various sources of nitrogen and carbon nutrition on the production of fibrinolytic enzymes in *Actinomyces odorifer* and its mutants. Microbiol. Acad. Sci. USSR **41**, 139—145 (1972a)

Egorov, N. S., Ushakova, V. I., Arakelova, V. A.: Biosynthesis of fibrinolytic enzymes of *Actinomyces* grown in different culture media. Microbiol. Virol., Sci. Proc., Biol. Sci. (USSR), **3**, 89—93 (1972b)

Ekeström, S., Frisch, E. P., Lund, F., Magaard, F.: Brinase treatment of advanced obliterative arterial disease. Abstract 428, V. Int. Congr. Thrombos. Haemostas. (1975)

Fitzgerald, D. E., Frisch, E. P.: Relief of chronic peripheral artery obstruction by intravenous brinase. J. Irish med. Ass. **66**, 3—8 (1973)

Fitzgerald, D. E., Frisch, E. P.: Continuous wave ultrasound evaluation of brinase treatment of chronic arterial obstruction. Angiology **25**, 444—448 (1974)

Fitzgerald, D. E., Frisch, E. P.: C-W ultrasound evaluation of chronic peripheral arterial disease treated by i.v. brinase. Abstract 427, V. Int. Congr. Thrombos. Haemostas. (1975)

Fitzgerald, D. E., Frisch, E. P., Thornes, R. D.: Thrombolytic therapy with brinase of chronic peripheral arterial disease. J. Irish Coll. Phys. Surg. **1**, 123—129 (1972)

Freedman, H. J.: Investigations into the mechanism and the pharmacological modification of protease-induced hypotension in the dog. Thesis, Department of Pharmacology, University of Toronto (1969)

Freedman, H. J., Roschlau, W. H. E.: Some factors influencing the toxicity of thrombolytic enzymes (brinase). Canad. J. Physiol. Pharmacol. **48**, 69—76 (1970)

Frisch, E. P.: Clinical experience with brinase. J. clin. Path. **25**, 553—654 (1972)

Frisch, E. P.: Clinical review on brinase, a protease from *Aspergillus oryzae*. Folia haemat. (Lpz.) **101**, 63—82 (1974)

Frisch, E. P., Blombäck, M., Ekeström, S., Kiessling, H., Lund, F., Magaard, F.: Dosage of i.v. brinase in man based on brinase inhibitor capacity and coagulation studies. Angiology **26**, 557—563 (1975a)

Frisch, E. P., Blombäck, M., Kiessling, H.: Dosage of brinase in man based on determination of brinase inhibitor capacity and coagulation studies. Abstract 429, V. Int. Congr. Thrombos. Haemostas. (1975b)

Frisch, E. P., Hedin, L., Lund, F., Magnusson, G.: Intraarterielle regionale Thrombolyse mit Protease I. Tierexperimentelle Untersuchung über eine mögliche Interferenz mit Röntgenkontrastmittel. Thrombos. Diathes. haemorrh., Suppl. **38**, 231—242 (1970)

Frisch, E. P., Lund, F., Moller, G., Hedin, L., Magnusson, G.: Permeability changes in the dog by repeated arteriography during regional intra-arterial thrombolysis with brinase. VI. Europ. Conf. Microcirculation, Aalborg 1970. Basel: Karger, 1971, pp. 399—403

Gaffney, P. J., Lord, K., Thornes, R. D.: The action of brinase *in vitro* and *in vivo*. Abstract 426, V. Int. Congr. Thrombos. Haemostas. (1975)

Genton, E., Pechet, L.: Thrombolytic agents: A perspective. Ann. intern. Med. **69**, 625—628 (1968)

Giering, J. E., Truant, A. P.: An experimental method for quantitative evaluation of thrombolysis: Effect of CA-7, a protease from *Aspergillus oryzae*. Angiology **17**, 661—669 (1966)

Gormsen, J., Feddersen, C.: Degradation of non cross-linked and cross-linked fibrin clots by plasmin, trypsin, chymotrypsin and brinase. Thrombos. Res. **5**, 125—139 (1974)

Gormsen, J., Feddersen, C., Andersen, R. B.: Degradation of human fibrinogen by brinastrase, trypsin and chymotrypsin. An immunological study. Scand. J. Haemat. **10**, 349—357 (1973)

Hessel, B., Blombäck, M.: Proteolytic action of brinase. Abstract 20, IV. Int. Congr. Thrombos. Haemostas. (1973)

Hoffmann, A.: Über die Beeinflussung von Plättchenfunktionen durch eine Protease aus *Aspergillus ochraceus*. Folia haemat. (Lpz.) **95**, 187—192 (1971)

Horace, J. F., Stefanini, M.: Fibrinolysis III. Nutritional and environmental requirements for optimum production of fibrinolysin from *Aspergillus* (Aspergillin O). Proc. Soc. exp. Biol. (N. Y.) **102**, 201—203 (1959)

Huang, C. L., O'Brien, E. T., Thornes, R. D.: The thrombolytic action of Protease I on experimentally produced venous thrombi in the dog. Irish J. med. Sci. **2**, 379—389 (1969)

Ives, D. A. J., Tosoni, A. L.: Purification of CA-7, a thrombolytic fungal protease. Canad. J. Biochem. **45**, 1055—1065 (1967)

Jürgens, J.: Personal communications (1966a)

Jürgens, J.: Effect of an *Aspergillus* enzyme on platelet aggregation in humans. Life Sci. **5**, 1379—1387 (1966b)

Jürgens, J., Lindvall, S., Magnusson, O., Orth, K.: Proteolytic inhibitors in plasma from man treated with a protease from *Aspergillus oryzae*. Acta physiol. scand. **78**, 11—19 (1970)

Karaca, M., Stefanini, M., Mele, R.: Fibrinolysis VII. Clot lysis, coagulation, and fibrinolytic mechanisms after administration of Aspergillin O (mold fibrinolysin) in man. J. Lab. clin. Med. **59**, 799—814 (1962a)

Karaca, M., Stefanini, M., Mele, R. H., Mossa, A., Soardi, F.: Fibrinolysis VIII. Comparative study *in vitro* of the effects of various proteolytic agents on the blood clotting mechanism of human plasma. J. Lab. clin. Med. **60**, 117—124 (1962b)

Karaca, M., Stefanini, M., Soardi, F., Mele, R.: Fibrinolysis VI. Activity of Aspergillin O (mold fibrinolysin) *in vitro*. Proc. Soc. exp. Biol. (N. Y.) **109**, 301—304 (1962c)

Kessel, M., Bennhold, I., Froese, P.: Untersuchungen über die Wirksamkeit eines neuen fibrinolytischen Enzyms zur lokalen Thrombolyse am Scribner-Shunt. Klin. Wschr. **46**, 1263—1266 (1968)

Kiessling, H.: Personal communication (1973)

Kiessling, H., Svensson, R.: Influence of an enzyme from *Aspergillus oryzae*, Protease I, on some components of the fibrinolytic system. Acta chem. scand. **24**, 569—579 (1970)

Klapper, B. F., Jameson, D. M., Mayer, R. M.: The purification and properties of an extracellular protease from *Aspergillus oryzae* NRRL 2160. Biochim. biophys. Acta (Amst.) **304**, 505—512 (1973a)

Klapper, B. F., Jameson, D. M., Mayer, R. M.: Factors affecting the synthesis and release of the extracellular protease of *Aspergillus oryzae* NRRL 2160. Biochim. biophys. Acta (Amst.) **304**, 513—519 (1973b)

Klöcking, H.-P., Hauptmann, J., Nowak, G.: Tierexperimentelle Untersuchungen mit einer Protease aus *Aspergillus ochraceus*. Folia haemat. (Lpz.) **101**, 111—117 (1974)

Klöcking, H.-P., Markwardt, F.: Über die fibrinolytische Wirkung einer aus *Aspergillus ochraceus* isolierten Protease. Acta biol. med. germ. **26**, 35—44 (1971a)

Klöcking, H.-P., Markwardt, F.: Thrombolytische Wirkung einer Protease aus *Aspergillus ochraceus*. Folia haemat. (Lpz.) **95**, 179—186 (1971b)

Koch, H. A.: Über die fibrinolytische Aktivität von Pilzen aus mikrobiologischer Sicht. Folia haemat. (Lpz.) **101**, 9—13 (1974)

Kundu, A. K., Das, S., Manna, S., Pal, N.: Extracellular proteinases of *Aspergillus oryzae*. Appl. Microbiol. **16**, 1799—1801 (1968)

Lewandowski, R. L., Corey, P. N., Chisholm, L.: Effect of brinolase on lens extraction in rabbits. A double blind study. Canad. J. Ophthal. **9**, 351—354 (1974)

Lindvall, S., Magnusson, O., Orth, K.: On the inhibition of a fibrinolytic enzyme from *Aspergillus oryzae* by serum. Acta chem. scand. **23**, 2165—2174 (1969)

Lund, F., Ekeström, S., Frisch, E. P., Magaard, F.: Thrombolytic treatment with i.v. brinase of advanced arterial obliterative disease of limbs. Angiology **26**, 534—556 (1975)

Lund, F., Hellström, L., Frisch, E. P.: Combined arteriography and regional thrombolytic therapy. Opusc. med. (Stockh.) **13**, 281—290 (1968a)

Lund, F., Hellström, L., Frisch, E. P.: Side effects observed in combined arteriography and regional thrombolytic therapy with protease. Opusc. med. (Stockh.) **13**, 396—403 (1968b)

Markwardt, F., Klöcking, H.-P., Sedlařik, K., Drawert, J.: Tierexperimentelle Untersuchungen zur thrombolytischen Wirkung von Ocrase. Acta biol. med. germ. **36**, 1315 (1977)

Marin, H., Stefanini, M., Soardi, F., Müller, L.: Fibrinolysis V. The thrombolytic and anticoagulant activity of mold fibrinolysin (Aspergillin O) *in vivo*. J. Lab. clin. Med. **58**, 47—59 (1961)

Matsushima, K.: On the naturally occurring inhibitors of *Aspergillus* protease. Part I. Occurrence and distribution of the inhibitors in natural products. J. agr. chem. Soc. Jap. **29**, 883—887 (1955)

Matsushima, K., Shimada, K.: Studies on the proteolytic enzymes of molds. Part XIX. Column chromatography of proteases of *Aspergillus oryzae*. J. agr. chem. Soc. Jap. **36**, 193—197 (1962)

Matsushima, K., Shimada, K.: Effects of EDTA on the alkaline protease of *Aspergillus oryzae*. J. agr. chem. Soc. Jap. **39**, 164—167 (1965)

Misaki, T., Yamada, M., Okazako, T., Sawada, J.: Studies on the protease constitution of *Aspergillus oryzae*. Part I. Systematic separation and purification of proteases. Agr. biol. Chem. **34**, 1383—1392 (1970)

Misaki, T., Yasui, H., Sawada, J., Tanaka, I.: Studies on the acid-stable digestive system. Part V. On the identification, protease and amylase of *Aspergillus oryzae* var. *microsporus* TPR-18. J. agr. chem. Soc. Jap. **35**, 1258—1264 (1961)

Monkhouse, F. C., Daramola, F., Gillespie, R. J.: The action of a proteolytic enzyme from *Aspergillus oryzae* on components of the blood clotting system. Canad. J. Physiol. Pharmacol. **42**, 377—384 (1964)

Nordwig, A., Jahn, W. F.: Spezifitätseigenschaften einer Protease aus *Aspergillus oryzae*. Z. Physiol. Chem. **345**, 284—287 (1966)

Nowak, G.: Fibrinolysis by protease of *Aspergillus ochraceus*. Acta Univ. Carol. [Med. Monogr.] (Praha) **52**, 113—114 (1972)

Nyman, D.: The effect of brinase on fibrinogen *in vivo*. Thrombos. Diathes. haemorrh., **33**, 217—220 (1975)

Nyman, D., Da Silva, M. A., Widmer, L. K., Duckert, F.: Thrombolytische Behandlung arterieller Verschlüsse mit Brinase, einem proteolytischen Enzym aus *Aspergillus*. Schweiz. med. Wschr. **104**, 1865—1867 (1974)

Nyman, D., Da Silva, M. A., Widmer, L. K., Duckert, F.: Local treatment of recent arterial thromboembolic occlusions with brinase. Thrombos. Diathes. haemorrh. **34**, 498—503 (1975)

Nyman, D., Duckert, F.: Assay of brinase inhibitors with soluble and insoluble substrates. Thrombos. Diathes. haemorrh. **33**, 221—225 (1975)

O'Brien, E. T.: The fibrinolytic system in arteriosclerosis. J. Irish med. Ass. **62**, 203—212 (1969)

O'Brien, E. T., Thornes, R. D., O'Brien, D., Hogan, B.: Inhibition of antiplasmin and fibrinolytic effect of protease in patients with cancer. Lancet **1968 I**, 173—176

Ogston, D., Ogston, C. M.: *In vitro* studies on a proteolytic enzyme from *Aspergillus oryzae* (Protease I). Thrombos. Diathes. haemorrh. **19**, 136—144 (1968)

O'Meara, R. A. Q.: Coagulative properties of cancer. Irish J. med. Sci. **394**, 474—479 (1958)

O'Meara, R. A. Q., Jackson, R. D.: Cytological observations in carcinoma. Irish J. med. Sci. **391**, 327—330 (1958)

Parker, J. M., Boyd, J. G.: Safety of Ca-7 (fibrinolytic enzyme) for direct pulmonary artery perfusion. Int. J. clin. Pharmacol. **1**, 545—549 (1968)

Pedroni, G., Giarola, P., Gibelli, A.: Preliminary report on the use of brinase from *Aspergillus oryzae* in cases of arterial venous shunt occlusions. Farmaco **27**, 60—64 (1972)

Perry, A. W.: Treatment of clotting in arterial hemodialysis cannulae with CA-7 (fibrinolytic enzyme derived from *Aspergillus oryzae*). Canad. med. Ass. J. **98**, 762—764 (1968)

Prompitak, A., Chisholm, L.: Brinolase for lens extraction in Cynomolgus monkey (Macaca Fascicularis). A toxicity study. Canad. J. Ophthal. **9**, 360—362 (1974)

Prompitak, A., Corey, P. N., Chisholm, L.: Effect of brinolase on lens extraction in Cynomolgus monkeys (Macaca Fascicularis). A double blind study. Canad. J. Ophthal. **9**, 355—359 (1974)

Prudlov, B., Ushakova, V. I., Egorov, N. S.: Effect of nitrogen sources in the medium on the production of proteolytic enzymes by *Fusarium graminearum* and *Alternaria* species. Microbiol., Acad. Sci. USSR **42**, 203—207 (1973)

Roschlau, W. H. E.: The evaluation in the dog of a proteolytic enzyme derived from *Aspergillus oryzae*. Canad. J. Physiol. Pharmacol. **42**, 109—125 (1964)

Roschlau, W. H. E.: Natural protease resistance to Ca-7 (fibrinolytic enzyme from *Aspergillus oryzae*) in the dog. Canad. J. Physiol. Pharmacol. **43**, 741—749 (1965)

Roschlau, W. H. E.: Systemic toxicity of CA-7 (fibrinolytic enzyme from *Aspergillus oryzae*) in the dog. Angiology **17**, 882—886 (1966)

Roschlau, W. H. E.: Thrombolytic therapy with CA-7, a fibrinolytic enzyme from *Aspergillus oryzae*: A report of two representative cases. Canad. med. Ass. J. **98**, 757—761 (1968)

Roschlau, W. H. E.: Brinase (CA-7). A new fibrinolytic agent. Thrombos. Diathes. haemorrh., Suppl. **46**, 229—241 (1971 a)

Roschlau, W. H. E.: The use of brinase (fibrinolytic enzyme from *Aspergillus oryzae*) in the management of clotting problems in long-term hemodialysis. Thrombos. Diathes. haemorrh., Suppl. **47**, 315—323 (1971 b)

Roschlau, W. H. E.: Thrombolytic properties and side effects of brinase (fibrinolytic enzyme from *Aspergillus oryzae*) in the dog. J. clin. Path. **25**, 635—636 (1972 a)

Roschlau, W. H. E.: Clinical experience with brinolase, a fibrinolytic enzyme from *Aspergillus oryzae*. Circulation **46**, Suppl. II, Abstr. 212 (1972 b)

Roschlau, W. H. E.: Inhibition of platelet aggregation by brinolase degradation products of fibrinogen and serum albumin. Abstracts p. 92, VI. Int. Congr. Thrombos. Haemostas. (1977)

Roschlau, W. H. E., Fisher, A. M.: Thrombolytic therapy with local perfusions of CA-7 (fibrinolytic enzyme from *Aspergillus oryzae*) in the dog. Angiology **17**, 670—682 (1966)

Roschlau, W. H. E., Freedman, H. J., Miller, S. L.: Pharmacological modification of the vascular response to systemically administered thrombolytic enzymes (CA-7). Canad. J. Physiol. Pharmacol. **47**, 369—376 (1969)

Roschlau, W. H. E., Gage, R.: Inhibition of blood platelet aggregation by brinolase (fibrinolytic enzyme from *Aspergillus oryzae*). Abstracts p. 240, III. Int. Congr. Thrombos. Haemostas. (1972 a)

Roschlau, W. H. E., Gage, R.: The effects of brinolase (fibrinolytic enzyme from *Aspergillus oryzae*) on platelet aggregation of dog and man. Thrombos. Diathes. haemorrh. **28**, 31—48 (1972 b)

Roschlau, W. H. E., Gage, R., Lo, H. Y.: Platelet effects of brinolase-produced human fibrinogen degradation products. In: Platelets—Recent Advances in Basic Research and Clinical Aspects. Proc. Int. Sympos. Blood Platelets, Istanbul 1974, 334—340. Excerpta Medica (1975)

Roschlau, W. H. E., Ives, D. A. J.: Review of the biochemistry and coagulation physiology of brinolase (fibrinolytic enzyme from *Aspergillus oryzae*). Folia haemat. (Lpz.) **101**, 22—37 (1974)

Roschlau, W. H. E., Miller, S. L.: New assay of fibrinolytic activity as a continuous rate reaction. Canad. J. Physiol. Pharmacol. **48**, 61—68 (1970)

Roschlau, W. H. E., Sutton, D. M. C.: Brinolase dose prediction with the protease resistance test. Abstracts p. 254, VI. Int. Congr. Thrombos. Haemostas. (1977)

Roschlau, W. H. E., Tosoni, A. L.: Thrombolytic therapy with CA-7 (fibrinolytic enzyme from *Aspergillus oryzae*) in the dog. Canad. J. Physiol. Pharmacol. **43**, 731—740 (1965)

Sabina, L. R., Tosoni, A. L., Parker, R. C.: Preparation of mammalian cell cultures with enzyme from *Aspergillus oryzae*. Proc. Soc. exp. Biol. (N. Y.) **114**, 13—16 (1963)

Sato, M., Akatsuka, T.: Purification of peptidases of *Aspergillus oryzae* and some properties of the purified peptidases. Bull. agr. chem. Soc. Jap. **23**, 465—474 (1959)

Sawasaki, T.: Fractionation of amylases and proteinases in the enzymes of *Aspergillus oryzae*. J. ferment. Ass. Jap. **18**, 607—612 (1960)

Sawyer, P. N.: Effects of various fibrinolytic agents on the physicochemical characteristics of the cardiovascular system. Abstract 425, V. Int. Congr. Thrombos. Haemostas. (1975)

Schmidt, H. W.: Thrombolyse durch Plasminogen-Aktivierung und durch direkte Proteolyse. Arzneimittel-Forsch. (Drug Res.) **15**, 132—135 (1965)

Schmidt, H. W.: Zur Thrombolyse mit verschiedenen Fibrinolytica. I. Untersuchungen an experimentellen menschlichen Nativblutthromben. Klin. Wschr. **44**, 618—621 (1966 a)

Schmidt, H. W.: Zur Thrombolyse mit verschiedenen Fibrinolytica. II. *In vitro*-Untersuchungen an intravital entstandenen menschlichen Thromben. Klin. Wschr. **44**, 621—625 (1966 b)

Sedlařik, K., Perlewitz, J., Klöcking, H.-P.: Lyse experimentell erzeugter arterieller Thromben durch lokale Applikation von Ocrase beim Hund. Folia haemat. (Lpz.) **103**, 117—122 (1976)

Shimizu, A., Trivedi, H., Fay, W. P., Thompson, G. D.: Straight arteriovenous shunt for long-term hemodialysis. J. Amer. Med. Ass. **216**, 645—647 (1971)

Smyth, H., Farrell, D., Thornes, R. D., Hiney, N.: Histochemical effects of the proteolytic enzyme brinase on ascites tumour cells. Irish J. med. Sci. **144**, 312—318 (1975)

Smyth, H., Flahavan, E., Thornes, R. D.: The effects of protease I of *Aspergillus oryzae* (brinase) on membrane permeability and growth of Landschutz ascites tumor cells. Int. J. Cancer **7**, 476—482 (1971)

Solum, N. O., Rigollot, C., Budzyński, A. Z., Marder, V. J.: A quantitative evaluation of the inhibition of platelet aggregation by low molecular weight degradation products of fibrinogen. Brit. J. Haemat. **24**, 419—434 (1973)

Specht, H.: Die Proteinasen des *Aspergillus oryzae*. Naturwissenschaften **44**, 37—38 (1957)

Stefanini, M., Adamis, D. M., Soardi, F., Marin, H. M., Mele, R. H.: Purification of Aspergillin O. Lancet **1959 II**, 443—444

Stefanini, M., Karaca, M.: Natural inhibitors of fungal protease (Aspergillin O). Ann. N. Y. Acad. Sci. **103**, 803—815 (1963)

Stefanini, M., Marin, H. M.: Fibrinolysis I. Fibrinolytic activity of extracts from nonpathogenic fungi. Proc. Soc. exp. Biol. (N. Y.) **99**, 504—507 (1958)

Stefanini, M., Marin, H. M.: Fibrinolytic agents derived from molds and process of making and using same. Canadian Patent No. 669375 (1963)

Stefanini, M., Marin, H. M., Soardi, F., Mossa, A.: Fibrinolysis IX. The comparative activity *in vivo* of trypsin and Aspergillin O (mold fibrinolysin). Angiology **13**, 254—259 (1962)

Subramanian, A. R., Kalnitsky, G.: The major alkaline proteinase of *Aspergillus oryzae*, Aspergillopeptidase B. I. Isolation in homogeneous form. Biochemistry **3**, 1861—1867 (1964a)

Subramanian, A. R., Kalnitsky, G.: The major alkaline proteinase of *Aspergillus oryzae*, Aspergillopeptidase B. II. Partial specific volume, molecular weight, and amino acid composition. Biochemistry **3**, 1868—1874 (1964b)

Svärd, P. O.: The effect of an enzyme preparation from *Aspergillus oryzae* on the aggregation of rabbit platelets *in vitro*. Scand. J. Haemat. **3**, 277—289 (1966)

Svärd, P. O.: Basic biochemical and pharmacological properties of brinase. J. clin. Path. **25**, 633—634 (1972)

Svärd, P. O.: On the pharmacology of brinase, a proteolytic enzyme from *Aspergillus oryzae*. Folia haemat. (Lpz.) **101**, 45—62 (1974)

Svendsen, L., Amundsen, E.: Estimation of plasmin and brinase activities by means of a highly susceptible synthetic chromogenic peptide substrate. Abstract 23, IV. Int. Congr. Thrombos. Haemostas. (1973)

Teisseyre, E., Latallo, Z. S., Kopeć, M.: Studies on the proteolysis of fibrinogen and fibrin by *Aspergillus ochraceus* enzyme as compared to the action of plasmin. Folia haemat. (Lpz.) **101**, 99—110 (1974)

Thornes, R. D.: Inhibition of antiplasmin, and effect of Protease I in patients with leukaemia. Lancet **1968 II**, 1220—1223

Thornes, R. D.: Fibrinolytic therapy of leukemia. Abstract 691, X. Int. Cancer Congr. (1970)

Thornes, R. D.: Fibrinolytic therapy of leukaemia. J. roy. Coll. Surgns. Irel. **6**, 123—128 (1971)

Thornes, R. D., Deasy, P. F., Carroll, R., Reen, D. J., MacDonell, J. D.: The use of the proteolytic enzyme brinase to produce autocytotoxicity in patients with acute leukemia and its possible role in immunotherapy. Cancer Res. **32**, 280—284 (1972)

Thornes, R. D., Lim Hoe Kee, J., Devlin, J. G., MacDonell, J. D.: Complement dependent cytotoxic autoantibodies in patients with acute leukaemia following fibrinolytic therapy with Protease I of *Aspergillus oryzae*. Irish J. med. Sci. **3**, 107—114 (1970)

Thornes, R. D., O'Donnell, J. M., O'Brien, D. J.: The physiology of fibrinolysis: (ii) Antiplasmin. Irish J. med. Sci. **494**, 73—81 (1967)

Töpfer, H., Piesche, K.: Charakterisierung einer alkalischen Protease aus *Aspergillus ochraceus*. Folia haemat. (Lpz.) **101**, 91—98 (1974)

Töpfer, H., Piesche, K., Schäfer, G.: Verfahren zur Isolierung eines fibrinolytischen Enzyms. DDR-Wirtschafts-Patent No. 77175 (1969)

Töpfer, H., Piesche, K., Schäfer, G.: Isolierung und Eigenschaften einer fibrinolytisch aktiven Protease aus *Aspergillus ochraceus*. Acta biol. med. germ. **26**, 1111—1115 (1971a)

Töpfer, H., Piesche, K., Schäfer, G.: Isolierung einer fibrinolytisch aktiven Protease aus *Aspergillus ochraceus*. Folia haemat. (Lpz.) **95**, 174—178 (1971b)

Tosoni, A. L., Glass, D. G.: Production of fibrinolytic material from strains of *Aspergillus*. Canadian Patent No. 671647 (1963)

Tosoni, A. L., Glass, D. G., Ives, D. A. J., Roschlau, W. H. E., Fisher, A. M.: Brinase—A blood-clotlysing enzyme. Abstracts, Joint Conference, American Chemical Society and Chemical Institute of Canada, Toronto, Canada (1970)

Tosoni, A. L., Ives, D. A. J.: Production of high-activity fibrinolytic agents. Canadian Patent No. 671648 (1963)

Tosoni, A. L., Ives, D. A. J.: Production of high-activity fibrinolytic agents. U.S. Patent No. 3140984 (1964)

Truant, A. P., Nordstrom, F. G.: Agents having fibrinolytic activity and process of making same. Canadian Patent No. 665557 (1963)

Uhlenbruck, G., Wetzel, K., Santa Maria, P., Prokop, O.: *Aspergillus ochraceus* Protease: Ein weiteres Enzym zum Nachweis inkompletter Erythrozytenantikörper. Acta. biol. med. germ. **29**, 185—188 (1972)

Vogel, G., Grossmann, K., Huyke, R., Zuber, W.: Klinische und gerinnungsphysiologische Untersuchungen mit einer Protease aus *Aspergillus ochraceus*. Folia haemat. (Lpz.) **101**, 125—131 (1974)

Yasui, T.: Proteolytic enzymes of *Aspergillus oryzae*. Part I. Two kinds of protease produced in a submerged culture. J. agr. chem. Soc. Jap. **38**, 361—366 (1964)

Defibrinogenation with Thrombin-Like Snake Venom Enzymes

K. STOCKER

A. Introduction

I. Specific Defibrinogenation

Disappearance of plasma fibrinogen has been observed in man following the bite of venomous snakes, e.g., *Agkistrodon rhodostoma* (REID and THEAN, 1963), *Bothrops atrox* (GHITIS and BONELLI, 1963), *Crotalus adamanteus* (WEISS et al., 1969), *Crotalus viridis* (MUGNERET, 1973), *Cerastes cerastes* (STRAUB, 1971), *Echis carinatus* (WEISS et al., 1973) and *Vipera russellii* (DE VRIES and COHEN, 1969). Fibrinogen depletion may be a consequence of direct prothrombin activation by the venom *(E. carinatus)*, or of prothrombin activation via activation of factor X *(V. russellii)*, of fibrinogenolysis *(C. cerastes)*, or it may be initiated by a limited proteolytic action of snake venom enzymes, comparable to the action of thrombin on fibrinogen, leading to formation and secondary degradation of fibrin-related material.

The specific removal of plasma fibrinogen by some purified thrombin-like snake venom enzymes proved to be a unique and new principle for anticoagulation and reduction of blood viscosity in prophylaxis and treatment of thrombotic diseases. Whether direct and indirect prothrombin activating enzymes from snake venoms may be used in the same manner is being investigated (KORNALIK and HLADOVEC, 1975).

II. Occurrence of Thrombin-Like Enzymes in Snake Venoms

Proteolytic enzymes, which in vitro convert fibrinogen into fibrin, have been detected in venoms of *crotalidae* and *viperidae* (Table 1). The thrombin-like enzymes have been extracted, purified and characterized from the venoms of *A. acutus* (OUYANG et al., 1971), *A. contortrix contortrix* (HERZIG et al., 1970), *A. rhodostoma* (ESNOUF and TUNNAH, 1967), *Bitis gabonica* (MARSH and WHALER, 1974), *B. atrox* (STOCKER and EGBERG, 1973), *C. adamanteus* (MARKLAND and DAMUS, 1971), *Crotalus horridus* (BONILLA, 1975), and *Trimeresurus gramineus* (OUYANG and YANG, 1974).

The defibrinogenating effect of most of these purified enzymes has been investigated in laboratory animals but extensive pharmacologic studies and clinical trials have been performed on *A. rhodostoma* thrombic protease (generic name: ancrod) and on *B. atrox* thrombic protease (generic name: batroxobin) only. Parenteral administration of ancrod or batroxobin causes the conversion of fibrinogen into a fibrin derivative which is rapidly degraded by a secondary fibrinolytic process and eliminated with the urine. Untoward side-effects during experimental or therapeutic defibrinogenation with ancrod or batroxobin are rare.

Table 1. Snake species producing venom with thrombin-like activity

Species	Authors
Agkistrodon	
A. acutus	OUYANG et al. (1971)
A. bilineatus	DENSON et al. (1972)
A. contortrix contortrix	HERZIG et al. (1970)
A. contortrix mokeson	DENSON et al. (1972)
A. halys blomhoffii	SATO et al. (1965)
A. piscivorus	ESNOUF and TUNNAH (1967)
A. rhodostoma	DIDISHEIM and LEWIS (1956)
Bitis	
B. gabonica	MARSH and WHALER (1974)
Bothrops	
B. alternatus	JANSKY (1950)
B. andianus	STOCKER, unpublished
B. atrox L.	JANSKY (1950); DEVI et al. (1972)
B. atrox asper	STOCKER et al. (1974)
B. atrox (maranhao)	STOCKER et al. (1974), STOCKER and BARLOW (1975)
B. atrox moojeni	STOCKER et al. (1974), STOCKER and BARLOW (1975)
B. bilineatus	VAZ and PEREIRA (1940)
B. castelnaudi	STOCKER, unpublished
B. cotiara	JANSKY (1950); STOCKER et al. (1974)
B. erythromelas	VELLARD (1938)
B. hyoprorus	STOCKER, unpublished
B. jararaca	KLOBUSITZKY and KOENIG (1936)
B. jararacussu	DIDISHEIM and LEWIS (1956)
B. lanceolatus	STOCKER et al. (1974)
B. microphtalmus	STOCKER, unpublished
B. neuwiedii	DIDISHEIM and LEWIS (1956)
Crotalus	
C. adamanteus	MARKLAND and DAMUS (1971)
C. durissus durissus	DENSON et al. (1972)
C. horridus	DENSON (1969)
C. terrificus basilicus	JANSKY (1950)
C. terrificus terrificus	DENSON (1969)
C. viridis helleri	DENSON et al. (1972)
Lachesis	
L. mutus	JANKSY (1950)
Trimesurus	
T. erythrurus	MITRAKUL (1973)
T. flavoviridis	DENSON et al. (1972)
T. gramineus	OUYANG and YANG (1974)
T. okinavensis	ANDERSSON (1972)
T. popeorum	MITRAKUL (1973)
T. purpureo maculata	DENSON (1969)

The pit viper, *A. rhodostoma*, the venom of which is used for the production of ancrod, is found widely distributed, probably in several subspecies in Southeast Asia; *B. atrox*, the pit viper furnishing the batroxobin-containing venom, originates in various forms from South and Central America (HOGE, 1965). Batroxobin deriving from the venom of various *B. atrox* subspecies shows characteristic differences in some physicochemical and biochemical properties (STOCKER et al., 1974; STOCKER and BARLOW, 1975) and even differences in the duration of the in vivo action have been observed (LOPACIUK et al., 1975). Batroxobin for experimental and therapeutic defibrinogenation (Defibrase) is being prepared exclusively from the venom of *B. atrox moojeni (BAmoojeni)*, a subspecies which may be bred in captivity (LELOUP, 1973, 1975).

III. Nomenclature

The Subcommittee on Nomenclature of the International Society on Thrombosis and Haemostasis recommended that thrombin-like snake venom enzymes should be named as thrombic proteases preceded by the Latin name of the species from which they have been isolated, e.g., *B. atrox thrombic protease*. The subcommittee furthermore suggested that these enzymes should be included in the report of the Commission on Enzymes of the International Union of Biochemistry and listed in that report under the generic name, peptide peptidohydrolase (3.4.4); the specific number to be decided by the enzyme commission (BLOMBÄCK, 1973).

The generic names *ancrod* and *batroxobin* have been approved by the World Health Organization for *A. rhodostoma* thrombic protease and for *B. atrox* thrombic protease respectively, the only enzymes being so far in use as defibrinogenating agents in man. However, since a batroxobin-containing drug as well as a laboratory reagent containing this enzyme have been marketed under the registered trade marks *Reptilase* and *Reptilase-Reagent*, and since Reptilase-DEF was a provisional designation for the first batroxobin preparations destined for experimental defibrinogenation, the mark Reptilase was erroneously used as a generic name by several authors. Additional confusion was caused by the fact that, for each defibrinogenating drug, ancrod and batroxobin, three different registered trademarks had to be used. A review on the current nomenclature of ancrod- and batroxobin-containing preparations is given in Table 2.

Table 2. Nomenclature for ancrod and batroxobin

Common name (BLOMBÄCK, 1973)	*A. rhodostoma* thrombic protease	*B. atrox* thrombic protease
Generic name (WHO)	Ancrod	Batroxobin
Registered trademarks for defibrinogenating agents	Arvin Arwin Venacil	Defibrase Defibrol D-Fibrol
Synonyms	Thromboserpentin (COPLEY et al. 1973)	Bothropothrombin (MARX, 1966) Thromboserpentin (COPLEY et al. 1973)
Other than defibrinogenating products containing the enzyme	— —	Reptilase (hemostatic) Reptilase-Reagent

B. Characterization of Ancrod and Batroxobin

I. Physicochemical Properties

I. Ancrod

Ancrod, according to ESNOUF and TUNNAH (1967), is a glycopeptide with a carbohydrate content of more than 20%. As determined by the same authors, ancrod migrates with an electrophoretic mobility of 3.9×10^{-5} V/cm^2/s in moving boundary electrophoresis at pH 7.0, its partial specific volume is 0.69, the sedimentation coefficient (Svedberg) is 3.35 at a protein concentration of 4.86 mg/ml and the diffusion coefficient D_{20} is 4.81×10^{-7} cm^2/s. The molecular weight, as determined by ultracentrifugation, ranged from 37, 410–43, 840, a discrepancy, which, according to the authors, has to be attributed to partial dimerization of the enzyme. The molecular weight as calculated from the amino acid analysis was 30000, whereas the value determined by COLLINS and JONES (1972) by means of gel chromatography was 55000.

The amino acid analysis of ancrod (ESNOUF and TUNNAH, 1967) shows aspartic acid to be the quantitatively most important amino acid constituent, followed by arginine, glycine, and isoleucine.

2. Batroxobin

Reduced and alkylated batroxobin of either *B. atrox* subspecies appears in electrophoresis in sodium dodecyl sulphate containing polyacrylamide gel, carried out according to McDONAGH et al. (1972), after staining with either Coomassie blue or Schiff's reagent, as one single band which characterizes the enzyme as a single-chain glycopeptide. Its carbohydrate content, its molecular weight, and its relative electrophoretic mobility as determined by immunoelectrophoresis, according to STOCKER et al. (1974), show subspecies-dependent differences (Table 3).

The isoelectric point of batroxobin from *BA moojeni* venom is 6.6, as determined by isoelectric focusing and OD$^{1\%}_{1cm}$ 280 nm of the same is 10.5. The amino acid analysis of batroxobin from either *B. atrox maranhao (BA maranhao)* venom or from a mixture of the two subspecies' venoms (HESSEL, 1975) reveals, as for ancrod, aspartic acid to be the major constituent followed by glycine, proline, and isoleucine; the N-terminal amino acid of batroxobin from both subspecies is valine.

II. Enzymatic Properties

1. Specificity

Contrary to thrombin, which converts fibrinogen into fibrin by splitting off the fibrinopeptides A and B, in vitro fibrin formation by either ancrod (EWART et al., 1970), or by batroxobin (BLOMBÄCK et al., 1957; STOCKER and STRAUB, 1970) is initiated by splitting of those Arg-Gly bonds of the Aα-chain which lead to release of fibrinopeptide A, whereas the Bβ-chain remains unaffected.

Prolonged incubation of a N-terminal chain fragment (N-DSK) of fibrinogen with ancrod causes, by cleavage of an Arg-His bond in the α-chain, the release of the heptapeptide Gly-Pro-Arg-Val-Val-Glu-Arg, whereas further action of batroxobin on N-DSK deprived from peptide A,

Table 3. Properties of batroxobin from different *B.atrox (BA)* varieties

	Batroxobin from venom of			Thrombin
	BA asper	BA maranhao	BA moojeni (Defibrase)	
Mol wt, SDS gel electrophoresis				
Reduction prevented	32000	43000	36000	—
Reduced and alkylated	32000	41600	35800	—
Isoelectric point	—	—	6.6	—
$OD_{1\,cm}^{1\%}$ 280 nm	—	—	10.5	—
Relative electrophoretic mobility				
PAA gel, pH 2.5 (BA moojeni = 1.0)	1.2	0.77	1.0	—
Agarose 1%, pH 8.6 (bromophenol blue = 1.0)	—	0.21	0.12	—
Neutral carbohydrate	—	10%	5%	—
Specific activity (batroxobin units per mg protein)	2000	1900	500	—
Inhibition of clotting activity by α_2-macroglobulin				
% clot propagation inhibition by 50 μg α_2-M/ml fibrinogen	—	5.6%	0.5%	—
Clot solubility in monochloroacetic acid 1%	No	Yes	No	No
Retraction of platelet rich plasma clot	No	No	No	Yes
Peptide A release from fibrinogen	Yes	Yes	Yes	Yes
Peptide B release from fibrinogen	No	No	No	Yes
Inhibition by heparin or hirudin	No	No	No	Yes
Inactivation by diisopropylfluorophosphate	Yes	Yes	Yes	Yes
Inactivation by iodoacetamide	No	No	No	Yes

causes, like thrombin, by cleavage of an Arg-Val bond, the release of the tripeptide Gly-Pro-Arg (HESSEL and BLOMBÄCK, 1971). ZAJDEL et al. (1975) detected a degradation product of 27000 daltons of the Aα-chain of bovine fibrinogen following prolonged (24h) digestion with batroxobin, whereas under the same conditions ancrod was found to be unable to produce any electrophoretically detectable fragment of the Aα-chain. This is in contrast to the observations of MATTOCK and ESNOUF (1971) who were able to demonstrate the formation of a fragment of 39000 daltons by only 10 min incubation of prothrombin-free human plasma with ancrod, whereas batroxobin failed to produce any α-chain fragment within this short reaction time. This is to some extent confirmed by WALTER et al. (1975) who demonstrated the formation of a human fibrinogen fragment of 37000 daltons by the action of ancrod, but not by batroxobin of either *BA moojeni* or *BA maranhao* venom. EDGAR and PRENTICE (1973) detected, following 1-h ancrod digestion of human fibrinogen, an Aα-chain fragment of 31000 daltons which was degraded to fragments of 27000, 25000, 16000, and 10000 daltons by further incubation with ancrod. A chain fragment of 39000 remained bound with the clot. The ability of some ancrod preparations to cause complete degradation of Aα-chain of fibrinogen, as reported by PIZZO et al. (1972), might be attributed to a contamination with other venom proteases rather than to a broad specificity of ancrod itself (EWART et al., 1970; HATTON, 1973).

Neither ancrod (BELL et al., 1968a) nor batroxobin (EGBERG, 1973a) significantly affect other clotting factors than fibrinogen and factor XIII. WALTER et al. (1975) demonstrated by measuring the formation of γ-γ dimers and polymers of the α-chain of human fibrinogen, coagulated in the presence of factor XIII by thrombin, ancrod, and batroxobin preparations, that all these enzymes are able to convert the zymogen

Table 4. Amino acid sequences of fibrinopeptide A from man and some laboratory animals (BLOMBÄCK et al., 1966)

17	16	15	14	13	12	11	10	9	8	7	6	5	4	3	2	1	
H-	ALA	ASP	SER	GLY	GLU	GLY	ASP	PHE	LEU	ALA	GLU	GLY	GLY	GLY	VAL	ARG-OH	Man
H-	THR	ASN	SER	LYS	GLU	GLY	GLU	PHE	ILU	ALA	GLU	GLY	GLY	GLY	VAL	ARG-OH	Dog
H-	GLY	ASP	VAL	GLN	GLU	GLY	GLU	PHE	ILU	ALA	GLU	GLY	GLY	GLY	VAL	ARG-OH	Cat
H-ALA	ASP	THR	GLY	THR	THR	SER	GLU	PHE	ILU	*ASP*	GLU	GLY	*ALA*	GLY	*ILU*	ARG-OH	Rat
H-VAL	ASP	PRO	GLY	GLU	SER	THR	PHE	ILU	*ASP*	GLU	GLY	*ALA*	*THR*	*GLY*	ARG-OH		Rabbit
H-	THR	ASP	THR	GLU	PHE	GLU	ALA	ALA	GLY	GLY	GLY	VAL	ARG-OH				Guinea-pig

factor XIII into the active transpeptidase factor XIII$_a$. The speed of factor XIII activation by an equal enzyme dose (NIH thrombin units) decreased in the following order: thrombin → batroxobin *(BA moojeni)* → ancrod → batroxobin *(BA maranhao)*.

GAFFNEY and BRASHER (1974) detected, by following the formation of cross-linked fibrin subunits, a slow activation of factor XIII by ancrod, even when a potential prothrombin activation was abolished by hirudin. However, BELL (1974) reported that ancrod is unable to activate factor XIII and furthermore, STOCKER and BARLOW (1975) also concluded, from the fact that *BA maranhao* batroxobin forms with prothrombin deficient plasma a clot which is soluble in monochloro-acetic acid, that this subspecies batroxobin did not activate factor XIII. McDONAGH and McDONAGH (1975) also failed to demonstrate any activating effect of ancrod and *BA maranhao* batroxobin, whereas *BA moojeni* batroxobin appeared as an activator of factor XIII as measured by the dansyl cadaverine incorporation method according to McDONAGH et al. (1971). The disagreement concerning the effect of thrombin-like snake venom enzymes on factor XIII may be due to differences in sensitivity of the applied methods as well as to impurities in the enzyme preparations tested (EWART et al., 1970; HATTON, 1973; McDONAGH and McDONAGH, 1975).

Ancrod and batroxobin act with a species-dependent preference on plasma and fibrinogen of different mammals (WIK et al., 1972; CSAKO et al., 1975). Thus, coagulation of rabbit fibrinogen takes about 10 times longer than the coagulation of human fibrinogen after addition of equal amounts of batroxobin. According to ASHFORD et al. (1968) the rat requires about 50 times the human dose of ancrod for defibrinogenation. In addition to this species differences in metabolic velocity dependence of ancrod and batroxobin action may be caused by structural differences of fibrinogen. Likewise, the apparently essential part for thrombic enzyme binding between Phe in the 9th position and the C-terminal Arg of the fibrinopeptide A molecule (SVENDSEN et al., 1972) shows particular differences in the rodents, especially in rat and rabbit, as compared with other species (BLOMBÄCK et al., 1966, Table 4).

Neither ancrod (PITNEY et al; 1969a) nor batroxobin (HARDER and STRAUB, 1972) as demonstrated by fibrin plate techniques or by means of the chandler tube (TURPIE et al., 1971), exerts any direct fibrinolytic or plasminogen-activating effect. However, both enzymes have been reported to potentiate plasminogen-activation by urokinase or streptokinase (KWAAN and GRUMET, 1973). Plasmin generated from plasminogen, either by activation with urokinase, streptokinase, heart activator, or human plasma activator, dissolves ancrod or batroxobin-produced fibrin much faster than fibrin formed by thrombin (TURPIE et al., 1971; KWAAN and BARLOW, 1971; ZAJDEL et al., 1975). This increased susceptibility to hydrolysis was also observed when activation of factor XIII in clotting mixtures was inhibited by EDTA (KWAAN et al., 1973). Fibrin formed by ancrod or batroxobin appears as thin filaments in

Table 5. Synthetic substrates cleaved by ancrod and batroxobin

Substrate	Cleavage by		Authors
	Ancrod (a)	Batroxobin (b)	
Benzoyl arginine ethyl ester	Yes	Yes	a) Esnouf and Tunnah (1967) b) Soria et al. (1969)
Tosyl arginine methyl ester	Yes	Yes	a) Esnouf and Tunnah (1967) b) Hohnen (1957)
Lysine methyl ester	No	No	a) Hatton (1973) b) unpublished
Arginine methyl ester	Yes	—	Exner and Koppel (1972)
α-Acetyl arginine methyl ester	Yes	—	Exner and Koppel (1972)
Benzoyl arginine p-nitroanilide	Yes	Yes	a) Collins and Jones (1972) b) unpublished
Benzoyl arginine amide	Yes	—	Collins and Jones (1972)

Table 6. Clotting and amidolytic activity of ancrod, batroxobin, and thrombin

	Clotting activity		Amidolytic activity	
	Plasma clotting[a] units per ml (adjusted)	NIH (thrombin)u[a] per ml	Bz-Phc-Val-Arg-pNA (mU[a] per ml)	Z-Gly-Pro-Arg-pNA (mU[a] per ml)
Human thrombin	20.0	4.2	120	192
Bovine thrombin	20.1	4.1	182	194
B. moojeni (Defibrase)	20.0	8.6	2.8	13.6
Ancrod	20.0	4.1	2.2	1.4

[a] Two Plasma clotting units (PCU) = amount of enzyme contained in 0.1 ml which coagulates 0.3 ml of citrated normal human plasma in 19 ± 0.2 s, 37° C (1 PCU of batroxobin = 1 BU). NIH(thrombin) units determined on bovine fibrinogen using US standard thrombin as a reference. 1 mU (milli unit) = amount of enzyme which hydrolyzes 1 nmol of substrate in 1 min under standard conditions.

electron microscopy, whereas fibrin formed by thrombin appears as thick interlaced fibers (Krause and Zimmermann, 1972; Kwaan and Grumet, 1975).

In contrast to thrombin, ancrod (Brown et al., 1972) and batroxobin (Niewiarowski et al., 1972) do not induce platelet aggregation and release reactions. Both enzymes form, with human platelet-rich plasma, nonretracting clots and batroxobin does not cause any alteration of the platelet ultrastructure (Niewiarowski et al., 1975). It coagulates isolated platelet fibrinogen in vitro but it does not affect the fibrinogen content of platelets in vivo (Johnsson, 1975; Lopaciuk et al., 1975b).

Batroxobin, similarly to thrombin, is capable of activating the clotting mechanism of Limulus polyphemus (Fumarola et al., 1975).

Like thrombin and other serine proteases, ancrod and batroxobin are also capable of hydrolyzing synthetic amino acid esters and amides (Table 5). The limited

Table 7. Amidolytic, esterolytic, and clotting activity of batroxobin *(BA moojeni)* and acetylated batroxobin *(BA moojeni)*

	Batroxobin	Acetylated batroxobin	Loss by acetylation
Plasma clotting units per mg	380	128	66%
Esterolytic activity (BAEE), mU/mg	6500	5900	9%
Amidolytic activity (Z-Gly-Pro-Arg-pNA), mU/mg	258	155	60%

proteolytic action of ancrod and batroxobin may be simulated on low molecular fibrinopeptide A analogues such as dansyl-Gly-Gly-Val-Arg-GlyOMe (CHEN et al., 1972) or the chromogenic simplified peptide A configuration Bz-Phe-Val-Arg-pNA (SVENDSEN et al., 1972). Z-Gly-Pro-Arg-pNA, a highly specific chromogenic substrate for thrombin and batroxobin, which is extremely slowly split by ancrod (Table 6), was built up following the structure of the thrombin- and batroxobin-specific fibrinogen split product Gly-Pro-Arg (HESSEL and BLOMBÄCK, 1971).

Acetylation of batroxobin *(BA moojeni)* results in a parallel reduction of clotting and amidolytic activity as measured on Z-Gly-Pro-Arg-pNA, whereas the esterolytic activity determined on benzoyl arginine ethyl ester is only slightly reduced (Table 7).

2. Activators and Inactivators

Batroxobin-induced coagulation of fibrinogen and cleavage of Z-Gly-Pro-Arg-pNA are accelerated in the presence of imidazole, a compound which may therefore be considered an activator of batroxobin.

Diisopropylfluorophosphate inactivates ancrod (COLLINS and JONES, 1972) as well as batroxobin, characterizing these enzymes as serine proteases.

Neither enzyme is inhibited by polyvalent protease inhibitors such as aprotinin and soybean trypsin inhibitor and, despite their thrombin-like substrate specificity, both enzymes are unaffected by specific thrombin inhibitors such as hirudin, heparin, and antithrombin III. Whereas thrombin is completely inactivated by 15 h incubation at 20° C, pH 7.4, with iodoacetamide 0.1 M, batroxobin under similar conditions preserves its total clotting and amidolytic activity. The activity of batroxobin is moreover not affected by 1 h incubation, at pH 7 and 20° C, with sodium-dodecyl-sulphate 0.01%, whereas thrombin loses its activity by such treatment. Batroxobin, as opposed to thrombin, is not inactivated by concanavalin A (KARPATKIN and KARPATKIN, 1974) and not significantly inhibited by Nα-dansyl-L-arginine-4-ethylpiperidine amide (OKAMOTO et al., 1975). Thrombin inhibitors of the benzamidino type (MARKWARDT et al., 1968) exert only a low inhibitory effect on batroxobin. Both ancrod (EXNER and KOPPEL, 1972) and batroxobin (EGBERG and NORDSTROEM, 1970) are competitively inhibited by tosyl arginine methyl ester. Fibrinogen fragment E was found competitively to inhibit batroxobin (LARRIEU et al., 1972).

Batroxobin is bound to α_2-macroglobulin and loses thereby its clotting activity, whereas its amidolytic activity on the small synthetic substrate Bz-Phe-Val-Arg-pNA remains almost unaffected (EGBERG, 1974). Inhibition of batroxobin by α_1-antitrypsin has been observed by MATSUDA et al. (1975). Inhibition of ancrod by α_2-macroglobulin and maybe antithrombin III was reported by PITNEY and REGOECZI (1970).

3. Stability

Batroxobin remains stable in aqueous solutions in the wide pH range of 2.5–9 for several hours at 20° C. Diluted solutions (20 BU per ml) in physiologic saline, pH 6.5, containing 0.02% of modified gelatine, and 0.3% of chlorobutol, remained stable for more than 2 years at +4° C. A solution of batroxobin in glycerol may be heated for 1 h at 100° C without significant loss of activity.

According to GAFFNEY (1975) a freeze-dried ancrod preparation containing human albumin and phosphate buffer, shows a half-life of 2.7^{12} years at +4° C, as calculated from Arrhenius plots.

III. Immunochemical Properties

Both ancrod and batroxobin are antigenic, and commercially available anti-*A. rhodostoma* serum neutralizes the enzymatic activity of ancrod and forms, with this enzyme, a precipitating complex; in parallel, anti-*Bothrops* serum neutralizes the enzymatic activity of batroxobin and undergoes, with this enzyme, a positive precipitin reaction. However, as demonstrated by BARLOW et al. (1973), ancrod and batroxobin are immunologically distinct proteins; immunodiffusion studies with specific antibodies and the purified enzymes showed no cross reaction between the two proteins.

IV. Assay Methods

The potency of ancrod and batroxobin may be determined by clotting tests using plasma or fibrinogen as a substrate, by measuring the catalytic release of fibrinopeptide A from fibrinogen by N-terminal analysis (JORPES et al., 1958), by following photometrically the release of p-nitroaniline from either Bz-Phe-Val-Arg-pNA (SVENDSEN et al., 1972) or Z-Gly-Pro-Arg-pNA, or by measuring the esterolytic activity of ancrod (COLLINS and JONES, 1972) and of batroxobin (SORIA et al., 1969).

The most commonly used potency assays for ancrod and batroxobin are based on the measurement of the clotting time of either normal human plasma or purified fibrinogen following the addition of the enzyme preparation. Both substrates, purified fibrinogen preparations even more than freshly prepared or freeze-dried normal human plasma, may vary from batch to batch and the reproducibility of the assay is therefore limited. The potency of ancrod (SHARP et al., 1968) as well as of batroxobin (STOCKER and EGBERG, 1973) has also been determined by comparison with thrombin standards. However, each thrombin-like enzyme should, for the following reasons, be assayed against its own reference standard: (a) differences in substrate specificity; (b) species-dependent interaction of thrombin, thrombin-like enzymes, and fibrinogen; (c) different kinetics of the catalyzed reactions; (d) different effect of FDP and variations in ionic strength and pH on ancrod and batroxobin-induced fibrin formation. Reference standards for ancrod and batroxobin are at present being established and will become available through the World Health Organization.

1. Assay on Human Plasma

Citrated human plasma is prepared by adding 9 parts of freshly drawn venous blood to 1 part of sodium citrate solution, 3.8%, and subsequent centrifugation for 30 min at 3000 rpm. A pool obtained from 10 healthy donors is subdivided into 1-ml portions and stored in a frozen state, below $-20°$ C. Fresh or frozen plasma may be substituted by commercially available lyophilized citrated normal human plasma (Citrol, Dade, Miami, Florida, USA).

Citrated human plasma, 0,3 ml, is preincubated for 2 min at 37° C; 0.1 ml batroxobin diluted with the vehicle of the test sample is added and the time from the enzyme addition to clot formation is recorded. Two batroxobin units represent that amount of enzyme, contained in 0.1 ml, which coagulates 0.3 ml of citrated human plasma in 19 ± 0.2 s. A standard curve is obtained by plotting the log of the clotting time vs. the log of the enzyme concentration. The potency of an unknown batroxobin sample can be determined from the graph.

2. Assay on Fibrinogen

Human or bovine fibrinogen, 0.2 ml, 0.4%, in 0.15 M Tris buffer pH 7.4, preheated during 2 min at 37° C, is mixed with 0.2 ml of either ancrod or batroxobin standard dilution and the time from the enzyme addition to the clot formation is recorded. A log-log graph is constructed and samples of unknown activity are read from the curve. Standard preparations should be diluted with a solution of the same composition as that of the samples to be tested (e. g., Arvin or Defibrase).

The original Twyford unit of ancrod was defined as the amount of enzyme which coagulates fibrinogen at the same velocity as 1 NIH unit of thrombin. Recent comparisons of thrombin and ancrod activity revealed that 1 ancrod unit corresponds to approximately one-third of one unit of thrombin (BARLOW and DEVINE, 1974).

The potency of batroxobin was originally assayed using citrated normal human plasma as a standard substrate and in a second step assayed against U.S. standard thrombin or fibrinogen. One batroxobin unit corresponds to approximately 0.17 NIH units, if assayed on human fibrinogen, and to approximately 0.43 NIH units, if assayed on bovine fibrinogen. The current batroxobin preparation, Defibrase, contains one BU in 50 µl.

3. In Vivo Activity Test on Mice

Batroxobin, 0.4 units, contained in 0.5 ml of physiologic saline are given by slow (2 min) i. v. injection to mice of 20 g body weight. After 1 h, 2 drops of blood from a tail vein are mixed with 50 µl of thrombin solution, 5 NIHU per ml, and clot formation is examined by means of a Pt hook. No firm clot should be detectable within 3 min, whereas blood of untreated mice coagulates in 20–40 s following thrombin addition.

C. Pharmacologic Properties of Ancrod and Batroxobin

I. Toxicity

1. Mice

The rapid i. v. administration of 10 batroxobin (BU) per kg body weight is tolerated without any visible signs of intoxication. At higher dose levels, an irregular pattern of mortality in each dosage group was observed. The mortality rate did not correlate with the administered amount of enzyme, suggesting that death was caused by thromboembolic processes, induced by too rapid intravenous injection. In animals being defibrinogenated by slow i.v. injection of 0.4 BU per kg, no mortality was observed upon administration of 450 BU per kg body weight, given in a concentration of 20 BU/ml by rapid i.v. injection. This statement is based on experiments carried out in our laboratory with seven different batches of batroxobin tested on 70 mice of 20–24 g.

2. Rat

Thirty units of ancrod per kg body weight were well tolerated, 90 U/kg caused respiratory failure followed by recovery of most of the animals, and 120 U/kg killed 80% of the rats. One hundred units of ancrod per kg administered i.v. to the anesthetized rat caused a fall in arterial blood pressure; respiration was slightly affected, and ECG was unaltered (ASHFORD et al., 1968).

Four sodium barbital–anesthetized rats of 250–300 g body weight, without previous defibrinogenation, tolerated administration of 36 600 BU dissolved in 20 ml, given by infusion during 2 h. (This corresponds to approx. 150 000 BU per kg body weight.)

3. Rabbit

According to ASHFORD et al. (1968), one out of 20 rabbits given 1 U of ancrod per kg died 1 h following i.v. injection; one other animal was in respiratory distress 6 min after the administration but recovered well; 3.5 U of ancrod per kg were always lethal.

As observed in our laboratory on 34 rabbits, 2 U of batroxobin per kg body weight i.v. are well tolerated. Death occurred 14 min following rapid i.v. injection of 20 BU per kg in one out of four animals.

The toxicity of anrod in the rabbit is considerably reduced if the enzyme is given by slow infusion (ASHFORD et al., 1968).

When ancrod and endotoxin or ancrod, aprotinin, and norepinephrine were given intravenously, glomerular microclots were found in the rabbit (MÜLLER-BERGHAUS and HOCKE, 1972; MÜLLER-BERGHAUS and MANN, 1973).

4. Cat

According to ASHFORD et al. (1968) the cat is less sensitive to the toxic effect of ancrod than the rabbit. One or 5 U/kg i.v. did not change arterial blood pressure, respiration, or ECG; 25 U/kg caused a fall in blood pressure, bradycardia, and fall in heart rate; recovery was slow. Severe reactions were observed at 30 and 50 U/kg i.v.: blood pressure rose steeply, followed by a sharp fall; respiration ceased. Necropsy on two cats after a lethal ancrod dose revealed a clot in the right ventricle and small thrombi in the coronary and pulmonary vessels as well as in the renal, hepatic, and splenic arteries.

5. Dog

Intravenous injection of 3.5 or 5.7 BU per kg, in unanesthetized dogs, did not cause changes exceeding the physiologic limits in red and white blood cell or platelet counts. The rapid i.v. injection of 5.7 BU per kg body weight did not produce any hemodynamic changes and did not affect the respiratory rate, depth, or pattern in four dogs.

In four sodium barbital–anesthetized dogs i.v. injection of 5.7 BU per kg did not reduce the renal blood flow.

6. Monkey (Yellow-Faced Baboon)

According to GINOCCHIO (1971, unpublished) batroxobin (Reptilase) was given i.v. at dose levels of 0.025, 0.25, and 2.5 BU per kg of body weight, per day, to groups of six animals each during a 3-month period. A control group of six baboons received daily injections of vehicle (containing 0.3% of phenol). None of the animals died, a lack of weight gain observed in some animals was not related to the treatment and the behavior of the animals was normal during the experiment. Hematologic studies revealed a moderate decrease in red cell parameters toward the middle of the dosing period but similar observations were made in the control group; this phenomenon should therefore rather be attributed to the effect of phenol than to batroxobin. Blood and urine analysis carried out periodically during the experiment did not show any alteration which could be related to a toxic effect of batroxobin. The macroscopic postmortem examination of brain, heart, liver, kidneys, spleen, adrenals, and gonads revealed no gross abnormalities other than slight mottling of the spleen in one female treated with 0.25 BU/kg/day and also in one male of the control group. Organ:brain weight ratio varied within the normal limits. The histologic examination of 33 tissue samples of each animal revealed in one control animal and in one animal of each dosage group lymphoid hyperplasia in the spleen and in the submucosa of the ileum and the colon.

7. Pigeon

Eighteen different batches of batroxobin (Defibrase) were tested for acute toxicity in our laboratory by injecting i.v. 20 BU per kg body weight into a total of 132 pigeons. No mortality was observed and no animals showed toxic symptoms.

II. Teratology

Teratogenicity of batroxobin has been studied in mice, rats, and rabbits on daily dose levels of 0.025, 0.25, 2.5, and 7 BU per kg body weight. No teratogenic or embryotoxic, nor any other adverse effects were observed. However, when batroxobin was given together with sodium salicylate, a compound with a known teratogenic action (LARSSON, 1970), increased embryo lethality and a potentiation of the teratogenic and the fetal damaging effect was observed in mice (GUTOVA and LARSSON, 1972).

III. Absorption and Metabolic Transformation of Ancrod and Batroxobin

Ancrod and batroxobin are absorbed from the intravenous, intramuscular (PITNEY et al., 1969b; STOCKER and BARLOW, 1975), the subcutaneous (GILLES et al., 1968; WYSS, 1975), and the intraperitoneal route (ASHBY et al., 1970; DONATI et al., 1975).

Moreover, ancrod was found to be absorbed from rectal compartments (BELL, 1974). Ancrod and batroxobin, administered to laboratory animals or man, progressively combine with α_2-macroglobulin (PITNEY and REGOECZI, 1970; EGBERG, 1974) and possibly with α_1-antitrypsin (MATSUDA et al., 1975) to form inactive complexes which are rapidly removed from the circulation and gradually metabolized, probably in the reticulo-endothelial system; enzyme degradation products are eliminated with the urine.

As demonstrated by REGOECZI and BELL (1969), the elimination of ^{131}I-labeled ancrod following i.v. administration into rabbits, is a multiexponential function, fast during the first few hours after the injection ($T^1/_2 = 3$–5 h) and gradually slower with increasing time ($T^1/_2 = 9$–12 days when only 6–10% of the initial dose remains in the plasma). Nephrectomy did not affect disappearance rate of the radio-labeled enzyme and rabbit leukocytes failed to phagocytose ancrod in vitro; the determination of nonprotein radioactivities as well as the characterization of urinary radioactive fractions, indicate a degradation of ancrod in vivo.

EGBERG (1974), by means of immunoelectrophoresis and autoradiography as well as by gel chromatography, was able to demonstrate the formation of a complex, when ^{125}I-labeled batroxobin was incubated in vitro with either dog plasma or purified α_2-macroglobulin. The complex had only a negligible clotting activity despite the fact that the amidolytic activity of the associated enzyme, as measured on Bz-Phe-Val-Arg-pNA, was almost intact. The complex was found to be stable during 24 h at 37° C, pH 7.4 at an ionic strength of 0.15; its dissociation was obtained by reduction of the ionic strength by means of dialysis. Intravenously given to the dog, ^{125}I-labeled batroxobin is to a large extent rapidly removed from the circulation but only slowly excreted by the urine. The half-life of the enzyme (3–10 h) was about the same when the radio-labeled batroxobin was injected into a dog with a normal fibrinogen level or into an animal defibrinogenated by the previous (24 h) injection of nonradioactive batroxobin, indicating that the capacity of α_2-macroglobulin to associate with new enzymes was unchanged or that the turnover rate for associated and nonassociated batroxobin was in the same range. No intact enzyme was found in the urine.

STRAUB et al. (1975) investigated the fate of ^{131}I-ancrod and of ^{131}I-batroxobin in the human organism following a single or repeated i.v. administration of either a low (nondefibrinogenating) or a high defibrinogenating dose (corresponding to 100 µCi) of the enzymes. Both ancrod and batroxobin behaved almost identically. The disappearance of the radiolabeled enzymes from the plasma was found to be faster than the drop in plasma fibrinogen level induced by their injection, and the excretion of radioactivity from the body was lagging behind the elimination of the enzymes from the circulation. A temporary sequestration, related to the complex formation with α_2-macroglobulin was admitted and confirmed by surface measurements on human beings following the i.v. administration of radio-labeled batroxobin; a transient accumulation of radioactivity in the liver, the spleen, and the lung was detected. Furthermore, a retention of radioactivity above a pre-existing as well as above a freshly formed thrombus was found, suggesting some fixation of radio-labeled batroxobin or of its α_2-macroglobulin complex to the thrombus. However, the velocity of elimination of ^{131}I-batroxobin was found to be equal in subjects with normal as well as with decreased fibrinogen level. A normal elimination rate of ^{131}I-ancrod was observed in one patient with a congenital afibrinogenemia.

IV. Effect of Ancrod and Batroxobin on Fibrinogen Metabolism

1. Fibrinogen Depletion

The dose of ancrod or batroxobin required for defibrinogenation varies considerably from one species to another; a refractoriness of the rat to ancrod and of the rabbit to batroxobin was observed (Table 8).

The fate of radio-labeled fibrinogen in the rabbit after i.v. application of crude *A. rhodostoma* venom was investigated by REGOECZI et al. (1966) and the metabolism of

Table 8. Defibrinogenating doses of ancrod and batroxobin for different laboratory animals

Enzyme	Species	Route of administration	Required dose per day, per kg		Authors
Ancrod	Rabbit	i.v.	1	U.	ASHFORD et al. (1968)
	Rabbit	i.m.	2–10	U.	ASHFORD et al. (1968)
	Dog	i.v.	1	U.	ASHFORD et al. (1968)
	Dog	i.m.	3.3	U.	ASHFORD et al. (1968)
	Cat	i.v.	60	U.	ASHFORD et al. (1968)
	Rat	i.v.	0.1–0.5	U.	ASHFORD et al. (1968)
	Mouse	i.p./i.v.	50	U.	HAGMAR (1972)
	Calf	i.v.	170	U.	SINGH et al. (1971)
	Monkey (M. nemestrina)	i.v.	25–30	U.	BARLOW et al. (1975)
Batroxobin	Rabbit	i.v.	>1000	B.U.	Unpublished
	Pig	i.v.	1060	B.U.	CHAMONE et al. (1974)
	Dog	i.v.	2	B.U.	OLSSON et al. (1973)
	Dog	s.c.	3.4	B.U.	WYSS (1975)
	Dog	i.m.	5.7	B.U.	STOCKER and BARLOW (1975)
	Rat	i.v.	200	B.U.	BLÜMEL ET AL. (1974)
	Mouse	i.v.	20	B.U.	Unpublished
	Mouse	i.p.	160	B.U.	DONATI et al. (1975)

^{125}I-labeled fibrinogen after administration of batroxobin was followed in a series of 34 dogs (EGBERG and NORDSTRÖM, 1969; EGBERG and LJUNGQVIST, 1973).

According to EGBERG (1973b) a total depletion of the circulating fibrinogen was accomplished in dogs within 2–6 h by i.v. infusion of batroxobin in doses ranging from 0.5 BU to 4.5 BU per kg body weight without provoking signs of vascular occlusion, bleeding, or toxic reactions. A minor decrease of the platelet count was observed. Pretreatment with heparin did not affect defibrinogenation. A secondary fibrinolytic process was observed during defibrinogenation. This fibrinolysis was not completely inhibited by administration of fibrinolytic inhibitors. Examination of sections from liver, kidney, lung, and spleen by autoradiography and immunofluorescent techniques revealed minor fibrin deposits in the lung capillaries in a few dogs. The glomerular filtration rate was not markedly affected by batroxobin, indicating that the defibrination did not produce circulatory disturbances. Only small amounts of fibrinogen-related material were demonstrated in the liver or the spleen, suggesting a minor importance of the reticuloendothelial system for the removal of the fibrin derivative formed under batroxobin. Eighty percent of the radioactivity administered by the injection of ^{125}I-fibrinogen was excreted with the urine within 8 days. The tested urine samples contained immunologically detectable fibrinogen degradation products.

The fate of ^{125}I-fibrinogen in five patients with venous thrombosis undergoing batroxobin-induced defibrinogenation was followed by STRAUB and HARDER (1971), by means of surface radioactivity measurements. A single i.v. dose of 1 BU per kg body weight led to a drop in plasma fibrinogen to 50 mg%, a fall in plasminogen, and to high amounts of circulating FDP. The radioactivity of the plasma decreased rapidly, while it increased in serum. A retention of radioactivity in the spleen and, less significantly also in the liver, but not in the lung, was observed.

The fibrinogen of platelets in dogs (JOHNSSON, 1975) and humans (LOPACIUK et al., 1975b) is not affected during treatment with batroxobin, while isolated platelet fibrinogen in vitro coagulates normally following the addition of the enzyme.

2. Fibrinogen Removal

As observed by REGOECZI et al. (1966) by means of autoradiography and histologic examination, i. v. injection of crude *A. rhodostoma* venom into rabbits caused formation of small fibrin aggregates which were found in various organs. This agrees with the fact that ancrod or batroxobin added in vitro to blood, causes clot formation at a velocity which is dependent upon the added enzyme quantity; a clot formed in vitro by ancrod or batroxobin is never dissolved spontaneously and no detectable fibrinolytic activity is generated in the blood itself. It was therefore believed that defibrinogenation consists of the formation of microclots which are subsequently removed by both fibrinolysis and phagocytosis. Fibrinolysis is most probably catalyzed by plasmin since the characteristic fibrin fragments X and Y as well as D and E, appear in the serum of ancrod-treated patients (PRENTICE et al., 1974). A fibrinolytic breakdown of soluble fibrin complexes should, however, be taken into consideration as an alternate pathway of fibrin removal; soluble fibrin seems to be a preferential substrate for plasmin.

COPLEY and LUCHINI (1964) demonstrated complex formation of fibrinogen with the particular type of fibrin monomer which is formed by the action of batroxobin. Fibrinogen was found to inhibit the polymerization of fibrinogen devoid of fibrinopeptide A (Des-Af-monomer). The soluble fibrin complex contained in human plasma previously incubated with 0.02 units of batroxobin per ml is much faster degraded by plasmin than native fibrinogen contained in untreated plasma (STOCKER and EGBERG, 1973). No D-dimer, a lysis product of γ-γ cross-linked fibrin, was detected in the plasma of ancrod-treated patients, indicating that lysis of soluble uncross-linked fibrin is the mechanism by which ancrod-produced fibrin derivatives are degraded (GAFFNEY and BRASHER, 1974; GAFFNEY, 1975).

The presence of soluble fibrin complexes in the plasma of human volunteers following a small dose of batroxobin has been detected by means of ultracentrifugation, cryoprecipitation, ethanol- as well as protaminsulphate gelation (HARDER and STRAUB, 1972). ASBECK et al. (1974, 1975), by means of gel chromatography, were able to demonstrate the simultaneous presence of soluble complexes with a higher molecular weight than fibrinogen and of fibrin(ogen) degradation products in the plasma of patients undergoing batroxobin treatment. MATHIAS et al. (1975), using insolubilized fibrinogen, detected the presence of soluble fibrin monomer in plasma of ancrod-treated patients, and PRENTICE et al. (1975) and MCKILLOP et al. (1975) separated, by means of agarose gel chromatography, high molecular soluble fibrin complexes from plasma of seven ancrod patients. MÜLLER-BERGHAUS and HOCKE (1972), and MÜLLER-BERGHAUS and MANN (1973) induced the formation of soluble fibrin complexes in the rabbit by ancrod infusion; no microthrombi were detected in the renal glomeruli. If, however, endotoxin was injected into ancrod-treated animals, fibrin-rich microthrombi were found in the glomerular capillaries, indicating endotoxin-induced polymerization of soluble fibrin monomer.

V. Effect of Ancrod and Batroxobin on the Plasminogen Metabolism

The plasminogen level in blood of animals and patients following ancrod or batroxobin administration, according to KWAAN and GRUMET (1975), decreases parallel with the fall of plasma fibrinogen. Although no activating effect of ancrod or batroxobin on plasminogen could be detected (PITNEY et al., 1970; HARDER and STRAUB, 1972), both enzymes may, by a proteolytic action on plasminogen, potentiate the effect of plasminogen activators (KWAAN and GRUMET, 1973).

EGBERG (1973a) reported from observations on 33 patients undergoing batroxobin treatment a fall of plasminogen in correlation with the decrease in fibrinogen. The plasminogen levels following batroxobin administration showed individual fluctuations and ranged from 28–94% of the initial values during the steady state of defibrinogenation. No increased fibrinolytic activity in the patient's plasma could be detected by fibrin plate techniques. The initial plasminogen concentration was regained within 4 days after the last batroxobin injection as determined in 5 out of 12 patients.

COLLEN and VERMYLEN (1973), COLLEN (1974), and COLLEN et al. (1975) examined, in five patients being defibrinogenated by batroxobin, the fate in the organism of ^{125}I-labeled plasminogen. The plasma radioactivity disappearance rate was accelerated from control value of ($T_{\frac{1}{2}}$) 2.24 ± 0.29 to 0.45–0.80 days; plasminogen half-life was as low as in patients undergoing thrombolytic therapy with streptokinase ($T_{\frac{1}{2}} = 0.50$–0.75 days) and corresponded to a daily plasminogen consumption of 10 mg/100 ml of plasma. Upon gel chromatography of serial plasma samples, collected on anti-batroxobin antiserum, besides a main peak corresponding to the plasminogen position, small amounts of radioactivity were eluted with an apparent molecular weight of 150000 to 200000—probably as plasmin-α_1-antiplasmin (P-AP) complex. As quantitatively estimated by means of a tanned red cell hemagglutination inhibition immunoassay, an elevated serum level of P-AP complex persisted during at least 48 h in three patients following the administration of 40 batroxobin units given as an i.v. infusion over 1 h. Unlike batroxobin, streptokinase causes a rapid but relatively short-lasting increase of P-AP level in the patient's serum. This indicates that plasminogen comsumption during batroxobin treatment is due, at least in part, to a secondary fibrinolytic response (COLLEN, 1975).

VI. Effect of Ancrod and Batroxobin on Hemostatic and Coagulation Parameters

1. The Hemostatic Function in the Defibrinogenated State

Bleeding tendency during defibrinogenation is, even at unmeasurably low fibrinogen levels, surprisingly low, except for the initial phase of fibrinogen depletion, when high amounts of FDP in the plasma inhibit platelet aggregation (KOWALSKI et al., 1964). According to KAKKAR et al. (1969) bleeding complications in patients under ancrod therapy are less common than with heparin; normal bleeding times were found in 9 ancrod-treated patients (BELL et al., 1968b; OLSSON, 1975), summarizing the experience collected during venous surgery in 16 patients defibrinogenated with batroxobin. Only minor bleeding in all cases was reported and no blood had to be transfused. However, in 7 out of 9 cases undergoing arterial surgery, defibrinogenation had to be discontinued because of excessive bleeding, probably caused by FDP formed during the continuous defibrinogenation of transfused blood.

OLSSON et al. (1971) and OLSSON and JOHNSSON (1972) quantitatively measured the blood loss from standardized skin wounds in dogs kept defibrinogenated for 3 days before and during the experiment. The wounds on the chest of the anesthetized animals were obtained by cutting two skin flaps of 5×5 cm. Small arteries were coagulated with electrocautery and the wound was roughed with sandpaper to obtain capillary bleeding. The mean blood loss was 1.8 g per 5 min per 50 cm^2 of wound surface in the defibrinogenated dogs. When acetylsalicylic acid was given in addition to batroxobin, the blood loss increased to 680%, when heparin was additionally given, to 215%, and when FDP were injected into the defibrinogenated animals, the blood loss increased to 170%. Chlorpromazine, despite its in vitro inhibitory effect on platelet aggregation, did not increase bleeding in defibrinogenated dogs, as measured by the above method (JOHNSSON and NIKLASSON, 1974). BROWSE (1975), during experimental venous surgery on batroxobin defibrinogenated dogs, observed no excessive bleeding by comparison with control animals. BLÜMEL et al. (1975), during experimental skin transplatation in the batroxobin defibrinogenated rat, did not encounter any significant bleeding tendency.

BERGLIN et al. (1975a, b, 1976) measured the blood loss according to the technique of OLSSON and JOHNSSON (1972) in dogs undergoing 6 h extracorporeal circulation and oxygenation, being anticoagulated with a) heparin or b) batroxobin. The blood loss was 155–455 ml in the heparin group and 43–133 ml in the batroxobin group.

2. Effects of Ancrod and Batroxobin on Platelets

Ancrod (PRENTICE et al., 1969; BROWN et al., 1972) and batroxobin (NIEWIAROWSKI et al., 1972) do not induce platelet aggregation and release reactions in vitro. Neither enzyme activates the contractile system of platelets and forms therefore with platelet-rich plasma nonretracting clots (BOUNAMEAUX, 1970). Platelets incubated with batroxobin do not undergo any change in ultrastructure nor do they lose their ability to aggregate upon addition of ADP, adrenalin, collagen, or thrombin (NIEWIAROWSKI et al., 1975). Platelet survival in dogs (MARTIN et al., 1971) and rabbits (BROWN et al., 1972) during ancrod treatment remained normal.

According to BELL et al. (1968b) based on observations on nine patients, defibrination with ancrod did not change the platelet number nor its ability to aggregate and adhere to glass. VINAZZER (1975) reports from an investigation on 82 Arvin-treated patients a moderate drop in platelet count and a diminution of platelet factors III and IV during the initial ancrod infusion, which was attributed to platelet damage by trapping into microclots.

A moderate and transient fall in platelet count during batroxobin-induced defibrinogenation in dogs has been reported by OLSSON et al. (1971, 1973) and by EGBERG (1973b) and a similar phenomenon was noticed in man (EGBERG, 1973a, b; STRAUB and HARDER, 1971).

LATALLO and LOPACIUK (1973), in order to investigate the mechanism of the moderate drop and the surprisingly rapid restitution of the platelet count, labeled the patient's own platelets with ^{51}Cr, reinfused them before starting batroxobin treatment and followed the changes in platelet count and radioactivity at various time intervals. It was found that some of the platelets were removed from the circulation for a short time period (max. 8 h) but reappeared; their survival was found to be within the normal range during 7 days of defibrinogenation.

FOLLANA et al. (1975) noted a significant but transient decrease in platelet count in two patients following the rapid (15 min) infusion of 1 batroxobin unit per kg body weight, diluted in 50 ml of physiologic saline. The initial platelet count was restored within 6 h after the infusion. It was noticed that the maximum drop in platelets coincides with the highest level of soluble fibrin complexes in the plasma, an observation which confirmed previous findings (HARDER et al., 1972; LATALLO and LOPACIUK, 1973).

Platelet aggregation in plasma of dogs treated with batroxobin was found to be impaired when the fibrinogen level was below the critical value of 50 mg-% (EGBERG et al., 1975). A complete restitution of ADP-induced aggregation was observed, when the fibrinogen level of the plasma was reconstituted artificially to 180 mg-%. FDP added to such plasma did not affect ADP-induced platelet aggregation; thrombin-induced aggregation occurred irrespective of the fibrinogen concentration. The bleeding time, as measured by the Ivy method, was prolonged by FDP at fibrinogen levels of more than the critical 50 mg-%, when ADP-induced aggregation was still normal. These findings are in agreement with the observations of PRENTICE et al. (1969) on patients who showed impaired ADP-induced platelet aggregation following ancrod infusion.

Platelet adhesiveness to glass, according to MARTIN and MARTIN (1975) was found to be virtually unaffected in patients under batroxobin treatment, at fibrinogen levels around 90 mg-%, irrespective, of the presence of FDP. Platelet fibrinogen in dogs following batroxobin infusion, remains unaffected (JOHNSSON, 1975), it is also unaffected in batroxobin-treated patients (LOPACIUK et al. 1975b).

3. Effect of Ancrod and Batroxobin on Plasma Coagulation Factors

No significant reduction in the plasma levels of factors II, V, VIII, IX, and X has been observed during ancrod and batroxobin treatment of laboratory animals or human beings. Respective investigations in man are listed in Table 9.

LOPACIUK and LATALLO (1973) showed that incubation of human factor VIII with batroxo-bin neither reduces the activity nor alters the immunologic properties of factor VIII.

EGBERG (1973a), as measured by the fluorescent amine incorporation method, observed in three patients under batroxobin treatment a significant decrease in factor XIII in the plasma.

Factor VII, according to BELL et al. (1968a) is markedly decreased in plasma samples defibrinogenated by ancrod in vitro, however no significant decrease in factor VII was found in plasma of patients undergoing defibrinogenating therapy with either ancrod or batroxobin.

VII. Effect of Ancrod and Batroxobin on Wound Healing

Impaired tissue repair in laboratory animals defibrinogenated by ancrod has been reported by HOLT et al. (1970) as well as by SILBERMANN and KWAAN (1971). According to WYSS (1975) the tearing resistance, measured on standardized skin wounds in the anesthetized dog, was significantly reduced in batroxobin-defibrinogenated animals as compared with a control group, but during the first 4 postoperative days only. From the 5th to the 12th postoperative day, due to fibroplasia, the wound tearing resistance in both groups became equal.

BLÜMEL et al. (1974) reported no difference in wound tearing resistance measured in normal and batroxobin defibrinogenated rats.

BROWSE (1975) observed minor skin dehiscence in dogs following venous surgery under batroxobin anticoagulation.

BARLOW et al. (1975) demonstrated that ancrod defibrinogenation does not impair the healing process of the myocardium in experimental myocardial infarction in the pigtail monkey.

VIII. Effect of Ancrod and Batroxobin on Hemorheology

In agreement with WELLS et al. (1964) who demonstrated a correlation between the fibrinogen level and the viscosity of the blood, therapeutic reduction of the plasma fibrinogen concentration either by ancrod (PITNEY et al., 1970; EHRINGER et al., 1971; VINAZZER, 1971; EHRLY, 1973a, b), or by batroxobin (VÖLKER and MARTIN, 1973; VÖLKER, 1975) results in a significant decrease of whole blood viscosity and a less pronounced decrease of plasma viscosity.

EHRLY (1973b) observed a decrease of the relative whole blood viscosity from 4.74 to 4.41 ($H_2O = 1$) and of the plasma viscosity from 1.68 to 1.57 in 12 patients undergoing ancrod therapy. Whole blood viscosity was measured by means of an Ostwald capillary viscosimeter as well as a Brookfield viscosimeter, plasma viscosity was measured with the Ostwald instrument only. The pathologically increased red cell aggregation in some patients was normalized under ancrod therapy. As estimated by the filtration technique of EHRLY and ROSSBACH (1973), the flexibility of erythrocytes remained normal during ancrod treatment. EHRINGER et al. (1974), in a study on 10 ancrod-treated patients, noticed a reduction in whole blood viscosity by a maximum of 35% as measured with the Wells-Brookfield viscosimeter at a shear rate of $11.5 \, s^{-1}$. Similar results have been reported by VÖLKER (1975) from a study on 11 batroxobin patients. The relative whole blood viscosity, measured with a Wells-Brookfield viscosimeter at a shear rate of $11.5 \, s^{-1}$, reached a minimum of 62% of the initial value at fibrinogen levels of approximately 100 mg-%. Further reduction of the plasma fibrinogen content did not cause any additional decrease in viscosity. The plasma viscosity fell to about 90% of the initial value. Red cell aggregation and desaggregation was followed by means of a rheoscope according to SCHMID-SCHÖNBEIN et al. (1969); a strong reduction of aggregability of erythrocytes was observed in all the batroxobin-treated patients.

Since, according to HARDER and STRAUB (1972), the initial phase of defibrinogenation, or the state following the administration of a low dose of the defibrinogenating agent, is characterized by reduced blood coagulation and bleeding times and by the presence of soluble fibrin complexes, BLÄTTLER et al. (1974) measured the whole blood viscosity and the suspension stability of red cells in 15 healthy volunteers following the i.v. application of 0.13 batroxobin units per kg of body weight, as a low, nondefibrinogenating dose. The presence of soluble fibrin complexes was confirmed by ethanol gelation, by the formation of cryofibrinogen, and by gel filtration; the plasma fibrinogen level decreased to about 80% of its initial value within 24 h. Comparing the measurements on four control persons, the whole blood viscosity was unchanged at 37° C but drastically increased at 22° C. Erythrocyte suspension stability, measured at both temperatures, was increased. In all cases microscopic inspection of blood revealed a decrease in number and size of red cell aggregates and their rate of formation was slower in the subjects receiving batroxobin.

KÖHLER et al. (1973) and KÖHLER (1975) founds, as a consequence of the reduced blood viscosity, in ten patients with unilateral femoral occlusion stage II (according to Fontaine), a significantly increased blood oxygenation in the femoral vein.

D. Preclinical Trials

I. Antithrombotic Effect of Ancrod and Batroxobin

Specific fibrinogen removal, discontinuation of fibrin accretion in an established thrombus, a potential moderate thrombolytic action as well as reduction of blood viscosity by ancrod and batroxobin have been applied in numerous animal trials to prevent and/or to treat experimental and arterial thrombosis and to investigate the role of fibrinogen in thrombogenesis.

MARSTEN et al. (1966) prevented, by postoperative infusion of crude *A. rhodostoma* venom, the formation of thrombi induced by introduction of umbilical tape into the inferior vena cava of dogs. CHAN (1968), by i.v. administration of 500 µg of crude *A. rhodostoma* venom per rat (180–250 g of body weight), achieved a statistically significant reduction of thrombus formation induced by incorporation of a polyethylene tube into the left carotid artery.

According to OLSEN and PITNEY (1969) ancrod treatment produced alterations in the histologic structure of experimental pulmonary emboli in the rabbit. Early and extensive necrosis was observed in emboli produced by injection of autogenous thrombi into a marginal ear vein of those animals who received 1 ancrod unit per kg body weight twice daily, beginning 1–2 h following the experimental embolism. The emboli disappeared more rapidly from the pulmonary vessels of the treated than the nontreated animals. SHARMA et al. (1973) induced experimental pulmonary emboli in dogs by isolating short segments of jugular and femoral veins, allowing the clots formed by this procedure to consolidate for 72 h, and releasing them into circulation to produce pulmonary emboli. Twenty-two dogs were subdivided into a control group, a group receiving heparin therapy and a group undergoing ancrod therapy. Production of embolism and success of treatment were controlled by four-view perfusion lung scan and pulmonary angiographic studies. Autopsy was carried out in all animals at the end of the 5-day treatment. As compared with the control and the heparin group, the ancrod-treated animals showed the highest rate of emboli resolution.

SINGH et al. (1970, 1971), in a series of calves, replaced the tricuspid valve by polypropylene prosthetic heart valves under heparin anticoagulation and total cardiopulmonary bypass. In nontreated animals thrombus deposition on the prostheses were found within 72 h whereas no thrombus formation occurred in the calves defibrinogenated with ancrod in a daily dose of 24–26 ancrod units per kg body weight. VAN DER ZIEL et al. (1970) prevented occlusion of venous shunts in the dogs and BELL (1974) reported the successful application of ancrod in preventing thrombus formation on fiberoptic catheters.

OLSON et al. (1972) and OLSON (1975) were able to prevent thrombus formation in steel tubes implanted into carotid arteries and external jugular veins of anesthetized dogs, when the fibrinogen level was reduced by previous batroxobin administration to unmeasurable values. With increasing plasma fibrinogen concentration, there was an almost linear increase of thrombus weight up to a fibrinogen concentration of 60 mg%. When in the same model the platelet count was reduced below $10000/mm^3$ by means of antiplatelet serum, hardly any thrombi were found in the arterial steel tubes whereas deposits still formed in the venous tubes. Thus platelets play a dominant role in thrombus formation but fibrinogen also seems to be a necessary factor in thrombus development both in the arterial and the venous circulation.

BUSCH et al. (1973) and BUSCH (1973) prevented, by defibrinogenation with batroxobin, respiratory insufficiency induced by i.v. infusion of thrombin and tranexamic acid in the dog. Pulmonary uptake of ^{51}Cr-platelets and ^{125}I-fibrin was followed up by surface measurements and these results have been confirmed by LINDQUIST (1975) on the same animal model. Elimination of platelets by anti-platelet serum and of platelets and leukocytes by Alkeran, did not prevent thrombin- and AMCA-induced pulmonary insufficiency, demonstrating that the presence of fibrin is a prerequisite for this damage.

OLSSON et al. (1973) prevented, by the use of batroxobin, the thrombotic obstruction of dacron grafts inserted into the inferior vena cava of dogs. When the operation was carried out on previously defibrinogenated animals, all the prostheses remained patent and none of the animals died. BROWSE (1975) substituted 3 cm segments of the femoral veins of dogs by woven dacron prostheses. This operation carried out in untreated animals, led within 7 days to the complete blockade of the grafts in 3, and to an 80% occlusion in 2 out of 5 animals. In the operated dogs, however, on the 2nd day of batroxobin defibrinogenation, three grafts were found fully patent and one was found 70% occluded. BROWSE (1975), in a further experiment, studied the incidence of rethrombosis in dogs following the removal, by means of phlebotomy, of a polyethylene-induced thrombus from the femoral vein. Rethrombosis was observed in 4 out of 10 untreated control animals, whereas in the defibrinogenated dogs, no signs of rethrombosis were found at autopsy carried out 7 days after thrombectomy.

BOURGAIN and SIX (1975a, b) and BOURGAIN (1975) studied the antithrombotic effect of batroxobin in the rat. A white platelet thrombus was induced by means of electrostimulation and subsequent ADP perfusion in a mesenteric artery. Formation, structural behavior and disappearance of the thrombus were continuously followed by measuring variations in light reflection on the arterial segment by means of a set of 30 light-depending resistances and continuously registered as analog signals on magnetic tape. The registered signals were analyzed by computer. As shown in a group of 15 rats defibrinogenated by the rapid injection of 1 ml of Defibrase (20 batroxobin units) per animal, the total thrombus value, its duration and the thrombus surface were strongly reduced as compared with the pretreatment values. The mobility of the maximum intensity value of a thrombus formed in defibrinogenated animals was increased, indicating the instability of its structure. Electron-microscopic studies revealed also a particular type of thrombus after batroxobin. The distance between individual platelets in the thrombus was found to be approx. 25000 Å, whereas in a normal thrombus, platelets were found to be closely packed with interspaces of approx. 500 Å only.

BERGLIN et al. (1975a, b, 1976) compared the effect of batroxobin with that of heparin during 6 h partial extracorporeal circulation in dogs, using a membrane oxygenator in the perfusion circuit. Blood loss in the heparin group, as measured by the skin-flap technique of OLSSON and JOHNSSON (1972), was significantly higher than in the batroxobin-treated animals. The flow through the perfusion unit was 22–40 ml per min and kg body weight in the heparin and 38–63 ml in the batroxobin group. Platelet deposition on the oxygenator membranes and in the lung, as measured by means of ^{51}Cr-labeled platelets, was higher in heparinized dogs than in the defibrinogenated animals. As revealed by scanning electron microscopy, platelet deposits covered 78% of the oxygenator membrane surface in the heparin group, whereas 31% of the membrane surface was found to be covered in the batroxobin group. Immunoelectrophoresis showed no difference in fibrin deposition in the membranes from the two groups. No difference between the two groups was found in gas exchange across the oxygenator membranes. Batroxobin appeared to be a superior alternative to heparin in extracorporeal circulation. A similar statement was made for ancrod (SHARP, 1975).

CHAMONE et al. (1974) diminished platelet sequestration and fibrin deposition in the isolated pig liver perfused with human blood, when the donor pig was defibrinogenated in vivo and when fibrinogen was removed from the human blood by in vitro addition of batroxobin.

II. Defibrinogenation and Transplant Rejection

Since fibrin formation has been suspected to play a key role in acute transplant rejection, experimental transplantation was carried out on defibrinogenated animals. Removal of fibrinogen from recipient dogs did not prevent or retard rejection of renal allografts and of sheep-to-dog xenografts as compared to control animals (MacDonald et al., 1972; Bell, 1974).

A decrease in transplant rejection rate and an improved capillary blood flow in tubed pedicle autografts of the rat, kept defibrinogenated by batroxobin, had to be attributed to thrombosis prevention and especially to a decrease of blood viscosity since similar results were obtained when instead of batroxobin, low molecular dextran was given (Blümel et al., 1975).

III. Defibrinogenation and Tumor Growth

A single dose of ancrod increased the metastasis formation in the liver and other extrapulmonary organs of mice following intravenous tumor cell injection (Hagmar, 1972). As demonstrated by Ivarsson (1975) a single dose of batroxobin decreased the number of pulmonary metastases following intravenous tumor cell injection in the rat. Donati et al. (1975) studied the effect of defibrinogenation by daily i.p. injection of 80 batroxobin units per kg body weight on tumor growth and metastasis formation in mice with Lewis lung carcinoma (3 LL). As compared with untreated, tumor-bearing animals, the survival time and the primary tumor weight (in those animals who received daily batroxobin injections beginning 1 day before tumor transplantation and continued till the death of the animals) were unchanged. However, the lung weight, the metastasis number, and the total metastasis weight were increased.

E. Clinical Experience

I. Dose-Response Studies

Observations of the effect on patients of the bite of *A. rhodostoma* or *B. atrox* together with clinical experience with batroxobin-containing drugs used as hemostatic agents (Klobusitzky, 1951; Berger et al., 1968) and pharmacologic and preclinical trials with ancrod and batroxobin on laboratory animals, proved a high degree of safety in the application of these drugs. Dose-response studies in patients requiring anticoagulant treatment were then carried out with ancrod and batroxobin (Table 9).

As a result of these dose-response trials the following guide-lines for the dosage of ancrod and batroxobin are being recommended by the manufactures of these drugs:

Ancrod, intravenous route. Induction: 2–5 ancrod units per kg body weight, in 50–500 ml saline, by intravenous infusion over 4–12 h (usually 6–8 h). Maintenance: 1–2 ancrod units per kg body weight, in 10–20 ml saline every 12 h by slow i.v. injection (about 5 min). This dose can also be given by continuous slow infusion. The dose should be adjusted according to plasma fibrinogen concentration. *Ancrod, subcutaneous route*: 1 ancrod unit per kg body weight daily until plasma fibrinogen level decreases to 70–100 mg-% (usually 4 days), followed by maintenance doses of 4 ancrod units per kg body weight, given every 3–4 days as a single subcutaneous injection. *Batroxobin, intravenous route.* Induction: 1–2 batroxobin units per kg body weight, diluted in 100 ml saline, by intravenous infusion over at least 1 h. If immediate anticoagulation is required, 12 500 IU of heparin may be added to the batroxobin infusion. Maintenance: 1–3 BU per kg

Table 9. Dose-response trials with ancrod and batroxobin

Author	No. of patients	Route	Laboratory control
Ancrod			
BELL et al. (1968a)	15	i.v.	Factors I, II, V, VII, VIII, IX, X, XI and XII, thrombotest
BELL et al. (1968b)	9	i.v.	Bleeding time, platelet count, adhesivity and aggregation (ADP), F.I, fibrin plate, FDP, plasminogen, thrombin clotting time
DONAHOE et al. (1972)	10	i.v.	Fibrinogen, FDP, plasma clotting factors
EHRLY (1973b)	11	s.c.	Fibrinogen, erythrocyte sedimentation rate
EHRLY and BREDDIN (1972)	12	i.v.	Blood and plasma viscosity, red cell aggregation and flexibility, fibrinogen
EHRLY and JUNG (1973)	10	s.c.	Blood and plasma viscosity, red cell aggregation, fibrinogen
PAAR and KLÜKEN (1975)	38	s.c.	Fibrinogen, Quick time, thrombin time, reptilase time
SHARP et al. (1968)	19	i.v.	Coagulation and bleeding times, F. I, II, V, VII, VIII, IX and X, thrombin time, euglobulin lysis time, platelet adhesiveness, FDP
VINAZZER (1975)	82	i.v./s.c.	Fibrinogen, FDP, platelet functions, antibodies
Batroxobin			
BLÄTTLER et al. (1974)	15	i.v.	Fibrinogen, FDP, EtOH gelation, PTT, blood viscosity, red cell sedimentation
BLOMBÄCK et al. (1970)	7	i.v.	F. I, II, V, VIII, X, normotest, platelet count, fibrin plate, FDP, plasminogen, $\alpha 2$-macroglobulin
EGBERG (1973)	33	i.v.	F. I, II, V, VIII, X, XII, XIII, Normotest, Thrombotest, ethanol gelation, FDP, euglobulin lysis time, plasminogen, antithrombin III, α_2-macroglobulin
EGBERG et al. (1971)	13	i.v.	F. I, II, VII, X, XIII, FDP, plasminogen, antithrombin III, α_2-macroglobulin, thrombin time, reptilase time
HARDER et al. (1972)	10	i.v.	Clotting time, bleeding time, recalc. time, prothrombin complex, F. I, II, VIII, thrombin time, reptilase-time, FDP, euglobulin lysis, fibrin plate, platelet count
MARTIN et al. (1973)	33	i.v.	Fibrinogen, PTT, reptilase time
MARTIN and AUEL (1975)	10	s.c.	Fibrinogen, antibodies
STRAUB and HARDER (1971)	5	i.v.	Fibrinogen, plasminogen, thrombin time, Quicktime, platelet count, euglobulin lysis time, protamine sulphate test, FDP
VÖLKER and MARTIN (1973)	18	i.v.	Blood and plasma viscosity, red cell aggregation

body weight, every 24 h either by infusion or by slow intravenous injection. The dose should be adjusted according to plasma fibrinogen concentration. *Batroxobin, subcutaneous route*: 0.5–1 batroxobin units per kg body weight daily until plasma fibrinogen level reaches 50–100 mg-%, followed by maintenance dose of daily 0.5–1 BU or every 3–4 days 2–4 BU, according to the plasma fibrinogen level.

Table 10. Indications for ancrod and batroxobin currently under investigation

---

Deep-vein thrombosis with or without pulmonary embolism
Central retinal vein thrombosis
Myocardial infarction
Embolism from prosthetic valves
Priapism
Sickle cell anemia
Rheumatoid arthritis
Transplant rejection
Prevention of rethrombosis following surgical or fibrinolytic therapy
Anticoagulation and thrombosis prevention in venous surgery
Extracorporeal hemodialysis
Artificial heart-lung life support
Peripheral arterial occlusions
Coronary arterial stenoses

Should ancrod or batroxobin therapy be rapidly interrupted and plasma fibrinogen level be restored to normal values within a minimum delay, antiancrod (LEWIS et al., 1971) or antibatroxobin preparations (ENGELKEN, 1974) should be given, eventually followed by infusion of washed red cells. Following neutralization of ancrod or batroxobin by antivenin, replacement therapy with whole blood, plasma or fibrinogen is safe and efficient.

II. Laboratory Monitoring

Plasma fibrinogen concentration is the most important indicator of the adequacy of treatment. The rapid method for fibrinogen determination according to CLAUSS (1957) furnishes accurate results 24 h after starting defibrinogenating therapy by intravenous infusion, when FDP level returns to low values (MARTIN and KNOLLMANN, 1975). The occasional measurement of hematocrit, white blood cell count, platelet count as well as urine and stool control (for occult blood) have been suggested (BELL, 1974). The determination of blood viscosity, oxygen concentration in tissue, and FDP are of interest but not essential.

III. Exploratory Clinical Trials

Speculating upon the anticoagulant, thrombosis-preventing thrombolytic or rheologic effects of ancrod and batroxobin, many workers carried out preliminary experiments in order to establish a pattern for organized clinical trials. Categories of potential indications being actually investigated are listed in Table 10. The results of exploratory clinical trials are given in Table 11.

IV. Comparative Clinical Trials

Ancrod, heparin, and streptokinase in deep vein thrombosis (KAKKAR et al., 1969). Thirty patients with deep vein thrombosis of the legs of less than 4 days duration were allocated at random to treatment with ancrod, heparin or streptokinase. Assessment of progress by radiography and by means of an isotope method as well as clinical examination showed the highest incidence of complete thrombolysis in the streptokinase group. Bleeding complications were least in the

Table 11. Results of exploratory clinical trials with ancrod and batroxobin

Author	Disease/Indication	No. of patients	Criteria	Response[a]		
				C	P	N
Ancrod						
BELL et al. (1968b)	DVT	7	Clinical	6	1	—
SHARP et al. (1968)	DVT	9	Clinical	9	—	—
KAKKAR et al. (1969)	DVT	10	a) Clinical	10		
			b) Radiological/isotope	1	3	6
PITNEY (1969)	DVT	18	Clinical	11	—	7
BELL and PITNEY (1969)	Priapism	2	Clinical	2	—	—
PITNEY (1969)	Priapism	1	Clinical	—	—	1
SHARP et al. (1968)	Arterial thrombosis	5	Combined surg.	4	—	1
GILLES et al. (1968)	Sickle cell crisis	11	Clinical	9	2	—
REID and CHAN (1968)	Sickle cell crisis	8	Clinical	5	3	1
BOWELL et al. (1970)	Central retinal vein thrombosis	8	Ret. photogr.	6	1	1
PITNEY (1969)	Prosthetic valve with embolism	8	Clinical	—	—	8
PITNEY (1969)	Chronic pulmonary hypertension	7	Clinical	—	—	7
LEUBE et al. (1972)	Venous thrombosis	9	Clinical	6	—	3
LEUBE et al. (1972)	Arterial thrombosis	2	Oscillographic/radiological	—	—	2
LEUBE et al. (1972)	Pulmonary embolism	3	Clinical	2	—	1
EHRINGER et al. (1973)	Arterial thrombosis	9	Clinical	5	2	2
HALL et al. (1970)	Anticoagulation in hemodialysis	4	Clinical/urea clearance	—	4	—
EHRINGER et al (1972)	Thrombosis prevention following SK therapy	14	Plethysmographic/ultra sonic flow meter	11	—	3
EHRLY and BREDDIN (1972)	Arterial thrombosis	12	Blood viscosity	12	—	—
Batroxobin						
BLOMBÄCK et al. (1970)	DVT	5	Radiological	1	1	3
EGBERG et al. (1971)	DVT	8	Radiological	3	—	5
BLOMBÄCK et al. (1970)	Central retinal vein thrombosis	3	Retinal circulation time	1	—	1
EGBERG and NILSSON (1975)	Cehtral retinal vein thrombosis	5	a) Retinal circulation time	5	—	—
			b) Visual acuity	3	—	2
KÖHLER (1975)	Arterial thrombosis	10	Oxygen determination	10	—	—
Völker (1975)	Arterial thrombosis	29	Blood viscosity	29	—	—
ENGELKEN (1974)	Arterial thrombosis	10	Clinical		5	5
LATALLO and LOPACIUK (1973)	Thrombosis prevention following SK therapy	7	Clinical	6	1	—
LOPACIUK et al. (1975)	Thrombosis prevention following SK therapy	7	Clinical, radiological	3	3	1
OLSSON et al. (1971)	Thrombosis prevention in venous surgery	1	radiological	1	—	—
OLSSON (1975)	Thrombosis prevention in venous surgery	6		2		
OLSSON (1975)	Thrombosis prevention in arterial surgery	9		1	—	8

[a] C=complete, P=partial, N=none.

ancrod group and highest in the streptokinase group. *Ancrod versus heparin in hemodialysis* (HALL et al., 1970). The effect of ancrod and heparin was compared in four patients during intermittent hemodialysis. As compared with the heparin-treated patients, deposition of fibrin and leukocytes on the membrane was less during anticoagulation with ancrod, however the urea dialysis rate was decreased during ancrod therapy. *Ancrod, heparin, and streptokinase in myocardial infarction* (LEUBE et al., 1972). Sixty patients with acute myocardial infarction, qualified for anticoagulant therapy, were allocated at random into two groups. Twenty-seven patients received ancrod, 33 patients received heparin. Those patients of both groups who were accepted for treatment not later than 12 h following the initial manifestation of angina pectoris, were submitted to 20 h fibrinolytic treatment with streptokinase, prior to anticoagulation with either heparin or ancrod. The mortality rate in both groups examined during 40 days was equal (18.2 and 18.5%). *Prevention of rethrombosis by ancrod or batroxobin following SK-therapy* (EHRINGER et al., 1974). Heparin and ancrod were compared in the change-over phase from streptokinase to peroral anticoagulation in 46 patients with peripheral arterial occlusions. In the heparin group, a final rate of thrombolysis of only 55% (17 out of 31 cases, 1 week after SK) was achieved, whereas in the ancrod group a rate of 80% thrombolysis (12 out of 15 patients) was obtained. *Treatment of peripheral arterial occlusions with ancrod or heparin* (TILSNER, 1975). Patients with peripheral arterial occlusions stage 3–4 according to FONTAINE, in whom it was not possible to perform surgical or thrombolytic therapy, were submitted to subcutaneously administered heparin or ancrod therapy. The efficacy of treatment was estimated following the disappearance rate of rest pain. Treatment was successful in 29 out of 41 ancrod cases and in 2 out of 25 heparin-treated patients. *Double-blind clinical trial with batroxobin in patients suffering from intermittent claudication* (MARTIN et al., 1975). Twenty patients were allocated at random to either batroxobin or placebo treatment during 3 weeks. No significant difference between the two groups was found with respect to both the walking distance and the poststenotic pressure.

V. Immunologic Resistance to Ancrod and Batroxobin

Acquired resistance to ancrod during repeated treatment has been described by PITNEY et al. (1969 b). Two patients who underwent defibrination with ancrod were found to be refractory to a second course of treatment. Plasma from both neutralized the clotting activity of ancrod, in vitro, and hypofibrinogenemia, as a response to the administered ancrod dose, was poor. A similar resistance was observed in 2 out of 14 patients treated intravenously and in 3 out of 4 treated intramuscularly with ancrod. VINAZZER (1973), by measuring quantitatively the ancrod-neutralizing potency of the patients'serum in a plasma-clotting system, detected resistance to ancrod in 4 out of 19 patients who underwent ancrod treatment.

LATALLO and LOPACIUK (1973) observed an unsatisfactory dose-response in one patient undergoing a second treatment with batroxobin, the fibrinogen level in the plasma promptly decreased when batroxobin was substituted by ancrod. Based on these and similar, unpublished clinical observations who implied immunologic nonidentity of ancrod and batroxobin, BARLOW et al. (1973) and STOCKER and BARLOW (1975) demonstrated, by means of gel diffusion studies carried out with the pure enzymes versus specific antiancrod and antibatroxobin, that no cross-reaction between the enzymes occurs. The nonidentity of ancrod and batroxobin was further confirmed by making dogs resistant to each enzyme respectively; in both cases, the alternate enzyme could bring about defibrination.

VINAZZER (1975) demonstrated the development of resistance in patients following 4–6 weeks of ancrod treatment. The half-life of the antibody was established at 97 days. Patients resistant to ancrod were defibrinogenated by batroxobin and vice versa.

MARTIN and AUEL (1975) detected resistance to batroxobin in 4 out of 10 patients, 2–4 weeks after starting therapy by subcutaneous injections of the drug. After replacing batroxobin by ancrod, a prompt fibrinogen depression was observed. Quantitation of batroxobin-neutralizing capacity of patient serum, determined according to STOCKER and YEH (1975), correlated with the respective rate of fibrinogen depression.

VI. Side-Effects

The most commonly encountered complication with ancrod was bleeding, which, however seems to occur less frequently than with heparin or with streptokinase. According to SHARP (1971), 14 out of 104 patients treated with ancrod showed bleeding episodes of which 10 were severe enough to warrant discontinuation of therapy. EHRINGER (1975) observed two severe bleeding accidents in patients on ancrod treatment following thrombolytic therapy with SK. In one case, hematoma and rupture of the liver led to death, the other patient with hematoma and rupture of the spleen was saved by splenectomy. BELL (1974) reports headache in approximately 1% of the ancrod-treated patients.

Whereas in general a particularly low bleeding tendency during batroxobin treatment has been reported, OLSSON (1975) encountered a high bleeding tendency during arterial surgery, which might be explained by continuous FDP formation due to frequent blood transfusions. MARTIN (1975) observed a nonlethal subarachnoidal bleeding in a patient under combined streptokinase and batroxobin therapy. A pneumoencephalogram carried out 3 weeks following this episode showed a left-temporal cyst; it was not clear whether this lesion existed already before the treatment or whether it was caused by the latter. EGBERG (1973b) encountered a sensitivity reaction manifested as headache and vomiting in 1 out of 33 patients treated with batroxobin.

References

Andersson, L.: A study of the coagulant action of some snake venoms. Haemostasis **1**, 31 (1972)

Asbeck, F., Lechler, E., Martin, M., Loo, J., van de: Derivatives of fibrinogen and fibrin during Defibrase therapy. Haemostasis **3**, 340—347 (1974)

Asbeck, F., Loo, J., van de: Fibrinogen-Fibrin-Derivate unter Defibrasebehandlung. In: Martin, M., Schoop, W. (Eds.): Defibrinierung mit thrombin-ähnlichen Schlangengiftenzymen, pp. 79—83. Bern-Stuttgart-Vienna: Huber 1975

Ashby, E. C., James, D. C. O., Ellis, H.: The effect of intraperitoneal Malayan pit-viper venom on adhesion and peritoneal healing. Brit. J. Surg. **57**, 863 (1970)

Ashford, A., Ross, J. W., Southgate, P.: Pharmacology and toxicology of a defibrinating substance from Malayan pitviper venom. Lancet **1968 I**, 486—489

Barlow, G. H., Devine, E. M.: A study on the relationship between ancrod and thrombin clotting units. Thrombos. Res. **5**, 695—698 (1974)

Barlow, G. H., Lewis, L. J., Finley, R., Martin, D., Stocker, K.: Immunochemical identification of Ancrod (A 38414) and Reptilase (Defibrase). Thrombos. Res. **2**, 17—22 (1973)

Barlow, G. H., Martin, D. L., Tekeli, S., Donahoe, J., Somani, P.: Effect of treatment with ancrod (Venacil) on healing of myocardial infarction in the pigtail monkey. Abstr. Symp. on thrombin-like enzymes. July 15—17, Trier (1975)

Bell, W. R.: Defibrinogenation with Arvin in thrombotic disorders. In: Sherry, S., Scriabine, A. (Eds.): Platelets and Thrombosis, pp. 274—298. Munich-Berlin-Vienna: Urban and Schwarzenberg 1974

Bell, W. R., Bolton, G., Pitney, W. R.: The effect of Arvin on blood coagulation factors. Brit. J. Haemat. **15**, 589—602 (1968 a)

Bell, W. R., Pitney, W. R.: Management of priapism by therapeutic defibrination. New Engl. J. Med. **280**, 649—650 (1969)

Bell, W. R., Pitney, W. R., Goodwin, J. F.: Therapeutic defibrination in the treatment of thrombotic disease. Lancet **(1968 b)** 490—493

Berger, E., Laurent, A. J., Stocker, K. F.: The prophylatic and therapeutic use of Reptilase. Praxis **57**, 611—616 (1968)

Berglin, E., Hansson, H. A., Teger-Nilsson, A. C., William-Olsson, G.: Six hours extracorporeal perfusion. A comparison between heparinisation. Abstr. Symp. on thrombin-like enzymes. July 15—17, Trier (1975b)

Berglin, E., Svalander, Ch., Teger-Nilsson, A. C., William-Olsson, G.: Anticoagulation with Defibrase during prolonged extracorporeal circulation in the dog. Scand. J. thorac. cardiovasc. Surg. **10**, 225, (1976)

Berglin, E., Teger-Nilsson, A. C., William-Olsson, G.: Anticoagulation during six hours of extracorporeal perfusion. A comparison between heparinisation and defibrinogenation. Abstr. X. Congr. Europ. Soc. exp. Surg. April 6—9, Paris (1975a)

Blättler, W., Straub, P. W., Peyer, A.: Effect of in vivo produced fibrinogen-fibrin intermediates on viscosity of human blood. Thrombos. Res. **4**, 787—801 (1974)

Blombäck, B.: Report of the Subcommittee on Nomenclature. Thrombos. Diathes. haemorrh. Suppl. **54**, 425 (1973)

Blombäck, B., Blombäck, M., Gröndahl, N. J., Holenberg, E.: Structure of fibrinopeptides—its relation to enzyme specificity and phylogeny and classification of species. Ark. Kemi **25**, 411 (1966).

Blombäck, B., Blombäck, M., Nilsson, I. M.: Coagulation studies on Reptilase, an extract of the venom from *Bothrops jararaca*. Thrombos. Diathes. haemorrh. **1**, 1—13 (1957)

Blombäck, M., Egberg, N., Gruder, E., Johansson, S. A., Johnsson, H., Nilsson, S. E. G., Blombäck, B.: Treatment of thrombotic disorders with Reptilase. Thrombos. Diathes. haemorrh. Suppl. **45**, 51 (1970)

Blümel, J., Köhnlein, H. E., Härtwig, J., Seidel, B.: Transplantationschirurgie an der Ratte unter Einfluß von Defibrase. In: Martin, M., Schoop, W. (Eds.): Defibrinierung mit thrombinähnlichen Schlangengiftenzymen, pp. 157—163. Bern-Stuttgart-Wien: Huber 1975

Blümel, J., Köhnlein, H. E., Krieg, G., Kutschera, H.: Einfluß der therapeutischen Defibrinierung und Faktor XIII-Substitution auf die Wundreißfestigkeit im Tierversuch. Langenbecks Arch. klin. Chir. Suppl. Chir. Forum. 245—248 (1974)

Bonilla, A. C.: Defibrinating enzyme from timber rattlesnake *(Crotalus H. Horridus)* venom: a potential agent for therapeutic defibrination. I. Purification and properties. Thrombos. Res. **6**, 151—169 (1975)

Bounameaux, Y.: Exploration fonctionelle des plaquettes. Description d'un test original. In: Hormones, Lipids and Miscellaneous, Vol. 3, 374. Basel-München-New York: Karger 1970

Bourgain, R. H.: The action of Defibrase on the arterial thrombus. Abstr. Symp. on thrombin-like enzymes. July 15—17, Trier (1975)

Bourgain, R. H., Six, F.: The effect of Defibrase on arterial thrombus formation. Thrombos. Res. **6**, 195—200 (1975a)

Bourgain, R. H., Six, F.: Effet d'une enzyme du type thrombique, la Défibrase sur la formation du thrombus blanc intra-artériel. C. R. Soc. Biol. (Paris) **169**, 709—712 (1975b)

Bowell, E., Marmion, V. E., McCarthy, C. F.: Treatment of central retinal vein thrombosis with ancrod. Lancet **1970I**, 173

Brown, C. H., Bell, W. R., Shreiner, D. P., Jackson, D. P.: Effects of Arvin on blood platelets. In vitro and in vivo studies. J. Lab. clin. Med. **79**, 758—769 (1972)

Browse, N. C.: Vein surgery during defibrination. In: Martin, M., Shoop, W. (Eds.): Defibrinierung mit thrombin-ähnlichen Schlangengiftenzymen, pp. 152—155. Bern-Stuttgart-Wien: Huber 1975

Busch, Ch.: Kinetics of thrombin induced microembolism. Acta Univ. Upsaliensis **173**, 1—46 (1973)

Busch, Ch., Lindquist, O., Saldeen, T.: Effect of Reptilase on respiratory insufficiency induced by intravenous infusion of thrombin and AMCA (Tranexamic acid) in the dog. Bibl. anat. (Basel) **12**, 254—259 (1973)

Chamone, D. F., Raia, S., Mies, S., Jamra, M.: Isolated perfusion of pig liver. Effects of Reptilase in hemostasis. Rev. bras. Pesqui. med. biol. **7**, 427—433 (1974)

Chan, K. E.: The modification of experimental occlusive arterial thrombosis in the rat by Malayan pit-viper venom. Thrombos. Diathes. haemorrh. **19**, 242—243 (1968)

Chen, K. H., Simpson, I., Buner-Lorand, J., Lorand, L.: Kinetics of Arvin, Reptilase, thrombin and trypsin. Abstr. FASEB-Meeting (1972)

Clauss, A. V.: Gerinnungsphysiologische Schnellmethode zur Bestimmung des Fibrinogens. Acta haemat. **17**, 237 (1957)

Collen, D.: Plasminogen and prothrombin metabolism in man (Thesis) ACCO. Leuven (1974)

Collen, D.: Quantitative estimation of thrombin-antithrombin III and plasmin -α_l-antiplasmin complexes in human plasma. Abstr. V. Cong. Int. Soc. Thrombos. and Haemostasis. July 21—26, Paris (1975)

Collen, D., De Cock, F., Verstraete, M.: Plasminogen consumption and plasmin-antiplasmin complex formation during Defibrase therapy in man. Abstr. Symp. on thrombin-like enzymes. July 15—17, Trier (1975)

Collen, D., Vermylen, J.: Metabolism of iodine-labeled plasminogen during streptokinase and Reptilase in man. Thrombos. Res. **2**, 239—250 (1973)

Collins, J. P., Jones, J. G.: Studies on the active site of IRC- 50 Arvin the purified coagulant enzyme from *Agk. rh.* venom. Europ. J. Biochem. **26**, 510—517 (1972)

Copley, A. L., Banerjee, S., Davi, A.: Studies of snake venoms on blood coagulation I. The thromboserpentin (thrombin-like) enzyme in the venoms. Thrombos. Res. **2**, 487—508 (1973)

Copley, A. L., Luchini, B. W.: The binding of human fibrinogen to native and fraction fibrins and the inhibition of polymerization of a new human fibrin monomer by fibrinogen. Life Sci. **3**, 1293—1305 (1964)

Csako, G., Gazdy, E., Csernyanszky, H., Szilagyi, T.: Specificity of bovine thrombin and Reptilase for mammalian plasmas. Blut **30**, 283—288 (1975)

Denson, K. V. E.: Coagulant and anticoagulant action of snake venoms. Toxicon **7**, 5—11 (1969)

Denson, K. V. E., Russell, F. E., Almagro, D., Bishop, R.: Characterization of the coagulant activity of some snake venoms. Toxicon **10**, 557 (1972)

Devi, A., Banerjee, S., Copley, A. L.: Coagulant and esterase activities of thrombin and *Bothrops atrox* venom. Toxicon **10**, 563—573 (1972)

De Vries, A., Cohen, I.: Hemorrhagic and blood coagulation disturbing action of snake venoms. In: Poller, L. (Ed.): Recent Adv. in Blood Coagulation, pp. 277. Boston: Little, Brown & Co. 1969

Didisheim. P., Lewis, J. H.: Fibrinolytic and coagulant activities of certain snake venoms and proteases. Proc. Soc. expl. Biol. (N. Y.) **93**, 10 (1956)

Donahoe, J. F., Barlow, G. H., McMabon, F. G., Ryan, J. R., Kwaan, H. C.: A study of Abbott-38414 (ancrod) in the normal adult human. Abstr. 3. Cong. Int. Soc. Thrombos. and Haem. Washington (1972)

Donati, M. B., Poggi, A., Mussoni, L., de Gaetano, G., Garattini, S.: The role of fibrin formation in experimental tumor growth and metastases: A pharmacological approach with a defibrinogenating enzyme (Defibrase). Symp. on thrombinlike-enzymes. July 15—17, Trier (1975)

Edgar, W., Prentice, C. R. M.: The proteolytic action of ancrod on human fibrinogen and its polypeptide chains. Thrombos. Res. **2**, 85—96 (1973)

Egberg, N.: Coagulation studies in patients treated with Defibrase. Acta med. scand. **194**, (1973a)

Egberg, N.: Experimental and clinical studies on the thrombin-like enzyme from the venom of Bothrops atrox. On the primary structure of fragment E. Acta phys. scand. Suppl. **400**, (1973b)

Egberg, N.: On the metabolism of the thrombin-like enzyme from the venom of Bothrops atrox. Thrombos., Res., **4**, 35—53 (1974)

Egberg, N., Blombäck, M., Johnsson, H., Abildgaard, U., Blombäck, B., Diener, G., Ekestroem, S., Göransson, L., Johansson, S. A., McDonagh, J., McDonagh, R., Nilsson, S. E., Nordström, S., Olsson, P., Wiman, B.: Clinical and experimental studies on Reptilase. Thrombos. Diathes. haemorrh. Suppl. **47**, 379—387 (1971)

Egberg, N., Ljungqvist, A.: On fibrin distribution in organs of dogs during defibrination with the thrombin-like enzymes from *Bothrops atrox*. Thrombos. Res. **3**, 191—207 (1973)

Egberg, N., Nilsson, S. E. G.: Treatment of central retinal vein thrombosis with Defibrase induced defibrination. In: Martin, M., Schoop, W. (Eds.): Defibrinierung mit thrombin-ähnlichen Schlangengiftenzymen, pp. 231—232. Bern-Stuttgart-Wien: Huber 1975

Egberg, N., Nordström, S.: In vivo effect of Reptilase on fibrinogen metabolism in dogs. Scand. J. clin. Lab. Invest. **24**, 383—385 (1969)

Egberg, N., Nordström, S.: Effects of Reptilase induced intravascular coagulation in dogs. Acta physiol. scand. **79**, 493—505 (1970)

Egberg,N., Olsson,P., Johnsson,H.: Studies on the influence of FDP and hypofibrinogenaemia on platelet aggregation and bleeding tendency on dogs. In: Martin,M., Schoop,W. (Eds.): Defibrinierung mit thrombin-ähnlichen Schlangengiftenzymen, pp. 96—101. Bern-Stuttgart-Wien: Huber 1975

Ehringer,H.R.: Side-effects, discussion. In: Martin,M., Schoop,W. (Eds.): Defibrinierung mit thrombinähnlichen Schlangengiftenzymen, p. 242. Bern-Stuttgart-Wien: Huber 1975

Ehringer,H.R., Dudczak,G., Kleinberger,R., Lechner,K., Reiterer,W.: Arvin: Schlangengift als neue Therapiemöglichkeit bei Durchblutungsstörungen. Wien klin. Wschr. **83**, 411 (1971)

Ehringer,H.R., Dudczak,R., Lechner,K.: Therapeutische Defibrinierung mit Ancrod. Dtsch. med. Wschr. **98**, 2298—2304 (1973)

Ehringer,H.R., Dudczak,R., Lechner,K.: A new approach in the treatment of peripheral arterial occlusions: Defibrination with arvin. Angiology **25**, 279—289 (1974)

Ehringer,H.R., Dudczak,R., Lechner,K., Wildhalm,F.: Therapeutische Defibrinierung mit Schlangengift (Arwin) bei arteriellen Durchblutungsstörungen. Verh. dtsch. Ges. inn. Med. **78**, 624—627 (1972)

Ehrly,M.: Dosis-Wirkungsbeziehungen von subkutan appliziertem Arwin bei Patienten mit chronischen arteriellen Durchblutungsstörungen. Vasa **4**, 161—167 (1975)

Ehrly,M.: Verbesserung der Fließeigenschaften des Blutes: ein neues Prinzip zur medikamentösen Therapie chronischer peripherer arterieller Durchblutungsstörungen. Vasa Suppl. **1**, 1—18 (1973a)

Ehrly,M.: Zur Wirkung von Arwin auf die Fließeigenschaften des Blutes. Herz Kreisl. **5**, 135 (1973b)

Ehrly,M., Breddin,K.: Verbesserung der Fließeigenschaften des Blutes durch Arwin. Verh. dtsch. Ges. inn. Med. **78**, 620—624 (1972)

Ehrly,M., Jung,H.J.: Verbesserung der Fließeigenschaften menschlichen Blutes durch subcutane Applikation von Arvin. Verh. dtsch. Ges. inn. Med. **79**, 1397—1400 (1973)

Ehrly,M., Köhler,H.J., Schröder,W., Müller,R.: Sauerstoffdruckwerte im ischämischen Muskelgewebe von Patienten mit chronischen peripheren arteriellen Verschlußkrankheiten. Klin. Wschr. **53**, 687—688 (1975)

Ehrly,M., Rossbach,P.: The detection of changes in erythrocyte shape by a filtration method using 8 µm filters. In: Erythrocytes, Thrombocytes, Leukocytes. Gerlach,E., Moser,K., Deutsch,E., Wilmans,W. (Eds.)., p. 52, Stuttgart: Thieme 1973

Engelken,H.J.: Gerinnungsphysiologische Untersuchungen und klinische Beobachtungen bei der Behandlung mit dem thrombinähnlichen Schlangengiftenzym Defibrase. Dissertation, Bonn (1974)

Esnouf,M.P., Tunnah,G.W.: The isolation and properties of the thrombin-like activity from *Agkistrodon rhodostoma* venom. Brit. J. Haemat. **13**, 581—590 (1967)

Ewart,M.R., Hatton,M.W.C., Basford,J.M., Dogson,K.S.: The proteolytic action of arvin on human fibrinogen. Biochem. J. **118**, 603—609 (1970)

Exner,T., Koppel,J.C.: Observations concerning the substrate specificity of Arvin. Biochim. biophys. Acta (Amst.) **258**, 825—829 (1972)

Follana,R., Sampol,J., Salvadori,J.M., Olmer,M.: The use of Defibrase against hyperfibrinogenemia in patients with nephrotic syndrome. In: Martin,M., Schoop,W. (Eds.): Defibrinierung mit thrombin-ähnlichen Schlangengiftenzymen, pp. 233—240. Bern-Stuttgart-Wien: Huber 1975

Fumarola,D., Pasquetto,T., Telesforo,P., Donati,M.B.: Studies on the clotting mechanism of *Limulus polyphemus*. Thrombos. Res. **7**, 401—408 (1975)

Gaffney,P.J.: Defibrination with ancrod. A proposed mechanism of action. Abstr. Symp. on thrombin-like enzymes. July 15—17, Trier (1975)

Gaffney,P.I., Brasher,M.: Mode of action of ancrod as a defibrinating agent. Nature (Lond.) **251**, 53—54 (1974)

Ghitis,J., Bonelli,V.: Fibrinogenemia in snake bite. Ann. intern. Med. **59**, 737 (1963)

Gilles,H.M., Reid,H.A., Odutola,A., Ransome-Kuti,O., Ransome-Kuti,S.: Arvin treatment for sickle-cell crisis. Lancet **1968 II**, 542

Ginocchio,A.V.: Reptilase, three month toxicity study in yellow-faced baboons, Personal communications (1971)

Gutova,M., Larsson,K.S.: Teratogenic interaction of two substances: Effect of sodium salicylate and Defibrase upon pregnant mice. Thrombos. Res. **1**, 127—134 (1972)

Hagmar, B.: Defibrination and metastasis formation: Effect of Arvin on experimental metastasis in mice. Europ. J. Cancer **8**, 17 (1972)

Hall, R. J. C., Young, C., Sutton, G. C., Campbell, S.: Anticoagulation by ancrod for haemodialysis. Brit. med. J. **4**, 591 (1970)

Harder, A. J., Stadelmann, H., Straub, P. W.: Reptilase-induced shortening of coagulation times in normal and haemophilic individuals. Thrombos. Diathes. haemorrh. **27**, 349—360 (1972)

Harder, A. J., Straub, P. W.: In vitro and in vivo induction of cryofibrinogen and "paracoagulation" by Reptilase. Thrombos. Diathes. haemorrh. **27**, 337—348 (1972)

Hatton, M. W. C.: Studies on the coagulant enzyme from *Agkistrodon rhodostoma* venom. Biochem. J. **131**, 799—807 (1973)

Herzig, R. H., Ratnoff, O. D., Shainoff, J. R.: Studies on a procoagulant fraction of southern copperhead snake venom: The preferential release of fibrinopeptide B. J. Lab. clin. Med. **76**, 451—465 (1970)

Hessel, B.: Personal communication (1975)

Hessel, B., Blombäck, M.: The proteolytic action of the snake venom enzymes Arvin and Reptilase on N-terminal chain-fragments of human fibrinogen. FEBS-Letters **18**, 318—320 (1971)

Hoge, A. R.: Preliminary account on neotropical crotalinae. Mem. Inst. Butantan **32**, 109—184 (1965)

Hohnen, H. W.: Experimentelle Studien zur Frage der Beeinflussung der Blutgerinnung durch Reptilase. Z. ges. exp. Med. **128**, 427—436 (1957)

Holt, P. J. L., Holloway, V., Raghnpati, N., Calnan, J. S.: Effect of a fibrinolytic agent (Arvin) on wound healing and collagen formation. Clin. Sci. **38**, (1970)

Ivarsson, L.: Personal communication (1975)

Jansky, B.: The relation between the proteolytic and blood clotting activity of snake venoms. Arch. Biochem. **28**, 139 (1950)

Johnsson, H.: On platelet fibrinogen in plasma defibrinogenated dogs and in uremic patients before and after hemodialysis. Thrombos. Res. **7**, 161—174 (1975)

Johnsson, H., Niklasson, P. M.: The effect of moderate doses of chlorpromazine on the hemostasis in dogs defibrinogenated with Defibrase. Thrombos. Res. **4**, 229—236 (1974)

Jorpes, E., Vrethammar, T., Oehman, B., Blombäck, B.: On the assay of thrombin preparations J. Pharm. (Lond.) **10**, 561—573 (1958)

Kakkar, V. V., Flanc, C., Howe, C. T., O'Shea, M., Flute, P. T.: Treatment of deep vein thrombosis. A trial of heparin, streptokinase and Arvin. Brit. med. J. **1**, 806—810 (1969)

Karpatkin, S., Karpatkin, M.: Inhibition of the enzymatic activity of thrombin by concanavalin A. Biochem. biophys. Res. Commun. **57**, 1111—1118 (1974)

Klobusitzky, D., von: Gerinnungsfördernde Wirkung hämostatischer Bothrops-Gift-Präparate. Naunyn-Schmiedeberg's Arch. exp. Path. Pharmak. **213**, 361—364 (1951)

Klobusitzky, D., von, Koenig, P.: Biochemische Studien über die Gifte der Schlangengattung Bothrops. Naunyn-Schmiedeberg's Arch. exp. Path. Pharmak. **181**, 387—398 (1936)

Köhler, M.: Untersuchungen zur Wirkung einer Defibrinierung mittels Schlangengiftenzym auf den Stoffwechsel bei chronischer peripherer Arteriopathie. In: Martin, M., Schoop, W. (Eds.): Defibrinierung mit thrombin-ähnlichen Schlangengiftenzymen, pp. 132—138. Bern-Stuttgart-Wien: Huber 1975

Köhler, M., Martin, M., Krüpe, M.: Therapeutische Effekte auf den Sauerstoffwechsel durch Verminderung der Blutviskosität (Defibrase). Verh. dtsch. Ges. inn. Med. **79**, 1400—1402 (1973)

Kornalik, F., Hladovec, J.: The effect of Ecarin-defibrinating enzyme isolated from *Echis carinatus*—on experimental arterial thrombosis. Thrombos. Res. **7**, 611—622 (1975)

Kowalski, E., Kopec, M., Wegrzynowicz, Z.: Influence of fibrinogen degradation products (FDP) on platelet aggregation, adhesiveness and viscous metamorphosis. Thrombos. Diathes. haemorrh. **12**, 69 (1964)

Krause, W., Zimmermann, P.: Quantitative elektronenmikroskopische Untersuchungen zur Fibrinstruktur bei Dysfibrinogenämie. Klin. Wschr. **50**, 557—561 (1972)

Kwaan, H. C., Barlow, G. H.: The mechanism of action of Arvin and Reptilase, Thrombos. Diathes. haemorrh. Suppl. **47**, 361—369 (1971)

Kwaan, H. C., Barlow, G. H., Suwanwela, N.: Fibrinogen and its derivatives in relationship to Ancrod and Reptilase. Thrombos. Res. **2**, 123 (1973)

Kwaan,H.C., Grumet,G.N.: Potentiation of plasminogen activation by Ancrod and Reptilase. Fed. Proc. **32**, 427 (1973)

Kwaan,H.,C., Grumet,G.N.: The place of thrombolytic and defibrinating agents in the treatment of venous thromboembolism. In: Nicolaides,A.N. (Ed.): Thromboembolism, pp. 251—267. Lancaster: Med. and Tech. Publ. Co. 1975

Larrieu,M.J., Rigollot,C., Marder,V.J.: Comparative effects of fibrinogen degradation fragments D and E on coagulation. Brit. J. Haemat. **22**, 719—733 (1972)

Larsson,K.S.: Action of salicylates on prenatal development. In: Tuchmann-Duplessis,H. (Ed.): Congenital Malformation of Mammalia, p. 171, Paris: Masson & Cie. 1970

Latallo,Z.S., Lopaciuk,S.: New approach to thrombolytic therapy. The use of Defibrase in connection with streptokinase. Thrombos. Diathes. haemorrh. Suppl. **56**, 253—255 (1973)

Leloup,P.: Essais de rationalisation dans le maintien d'un serpentarium à but industriel. Acta trop. (Basel) **30**, 281—311 (1973)

Leloup,P.: Observations sur la reproduction de *Bothrops moojeni* Hoge en captivité, Acta zool. path. Antverp **62**, 173—201 (1975)

Leube,G., Kühn,J.J., Hartert,H.: Erste Erfahrungen mit Arvin, der gerinnungsfördernden Fraktion eines Schlangengiftes. Med. Welt **23**, 601—605 (1972)

Lewis,L.J., Martin,D.L., Buckner,S., Finley,R., Lazer,L., Fedor,E.J.: Studies on the type specific immunity to the whole venom and a fraction of *Agkistrodon rhodostoma*. Res. Commun. Path. Pharmacol. **2**, 649 (1971)

Lindquist,O.: Pulmonary microembolism, fibrinolysis inhibition and pulmonary insufficiency. Thesis, Uppsala Dissertations Abstr. Uppsala (1975)

Lopaciuk,S., Latallo,Z.S.: Separation of human antihaemophilic factor (AHF, factor VIII) from fibrinogen by means of Defibrase (Reptilase). Abstr. Lecture presented at IV Int. Congr. on Thromb. and Haem. June 19—22, Vienna (1973)

Lopaciuk,S., Meissner,J., Ziemski,J.M., Latallo,Z.S.: Defibrination as a follow-up of thrombolytic therapy. In: Martin,M., Schoop,W. (Eds.): Defibrinierung mit thrombin-ähnlichen Schlangengiftenzymen, pp. 191—199. Bern-Stuttgart-Wien: Huber 1975a

Lopaciuk,S., Sulek,K., Latallo,Z.S.: Platelet fibrinogen during Defibrase therapy. Abstr. Symp. on thrombin-like enzymes. July 15—17, Trier (1975b)

MacDonald,A.S., Bell,W.R., Busch,G.J., Ghose,T., Chan,C.C., Falvey,C.F., Merill,I.: A comparison of hyperacute canine renal allograft and sheep-to-dog xenograft rejection. Transplantation **13**, 146 (1972)

Markland,F.S., Damus,P.S.: Purification and properties of a thrombinlike enzyme from the venom of *Crotalus adamanteus* (Eastern Diamondback Rattlesnake). J. biol. Chem. **246**, 6460—6473 (1971)

Markwardt,F., Landmann,H., Walsmann,P.: Comparative studies on the inhibition of trypsin, plasmin and thrombin by derivatives of benzylamine and benzamidine. Europ. J. Biochem. **6**, 502 (1968)

Marsh,N.A., Whaler,B.C.: Separation and partial characterization of a coagulant enzyme from *Bitis gabonica* venom. Brit. J. Haemat. **26**, 295—306 (1974)

Marsten,J.L., Chan,K.E., Ankeney,J.L., Botti,R.E.: Antithrombotic effect of Malayan pit viper venom on experimental thrombosis of the inferior vena cava produced by a new method. Circulat. Res. **19**, 514—519 (1966)

Martin,D.L., Hirdes,E., Mann,S., Auel,H.: Defibrinogenating treatment in patients suffering from severe intermittent claudication. Abstr. Symp. on thrombin-like enzymes. July 15—17, Trier (1975)

Martin,D.L., Hollinger,R.E., Suwanwela,N., Fedor,E.J.: Experimental defibrination produced by Abbott 38414 (Ancrod) and associated effects on some other factors of the hemostatic system. Fed. Proc. **30**, 424 (1971)

Martin,D.L., Knollmann,G.: Kontrolle der Fibrinogenbestimmung unter defibrinierender Behandlung. In: Martin,M., Schoop,W. (Eds.): Defibrinierung mit thrombin-ähnlichen Schlangengiftenzymen, pp. 166—170. Bern-Stuttgart-Wien: Huber 1975

Martin,D.L., Martin U.: Verhalten der Thrombozytenadhäsivität unter Defibrase®-Therapie. In: Martin,M., Schoop,W. (Eds.): Defibrinierung mit thrombinähnlichen Schlangengiftenzymen, pp. 102—107. Bern-Stuttgart-Wien: Huber 1975

Martin,D.L., Auel,H.: The technique and laboratory control of subcutaneously administered Defibrase. Abstr. Symp. on thrombin like enzymes. July 15—17, Trier (1975)

Martin, D. L., Engelken, H. J., Tambert, F.: Senkung der Fibrinogenkonzentration im Blut durch Defibrase: Möglichkeiten und Grenzen. Verh. dtsch. Ges. inn. Med. **79**, 1336—1338 (1973)

Martin, M.: Side effects. Discussion, In: Martin, M., Schoop, W. (Eds.): Defibrinierung mit thrombinähnlichen Schlangengiftenzymen, p. 242. Bern-Stuttgart-Wien: Huber 1975

Marx, R.: Discussion. Thrombos. Diathes. haemorrh. Suppl. **19**, 179 (1966)

Mathias, F. R., Reinicke, R., Müller, W.: Detection of soluble fibrin monomer in plasma of patients after arvin-treatment by means of insolubilized fibrinogen (FG-ag). Abstr. Symp. on thrombin-like enzymes. July 15—17, Trier (1975)

Matsuda, T., Hideno, K., Ogawara, M., Kodama, N., Murakami, M.: Therapeutic defibrination by *Bothrops marajoensis* venom. Acta haemat. jap. **38**, 299—305 (1975)

Mattock, P., Esnouf, M. P.: Differences in the subunit structure of human fibrin formed by the action of Arvin, Reptilase and thrombin. Nature (Lond.) New Biol. **233**, 277—279 (1971)

McDonagh, J., McDonagh, R. P.: Alternative pathways for the activation of F. XIII. Brit. J. Haemat. **30**, 465—477 (1975)

McDonagh, J., McDonagh, R. P., Duckert, F.: The influence of fibrin crosslinking on the kinetics of urokinase-induced clot lysis. Brit. J. Haemat. **21**, 323 (1971)

McDonagh, J., Messel, H., McDonagh, R. P., Murano, G., Blombäck, B.: Molecular weight analysis of fibrinogen and fibrin chains by an improved sodium-dodecyl-sulphate gel electrophoresis method. Biochim. biophys. Acta (Amst.) **257**, 135—142 (1972)

McKillop, C., Edgar, W., Forbes, C. D., Prentice, C. R. M.: In vivo production of soluble complexes containing fibrinogen-fibrin related antigen during ancrod therapy. Thrombos. Res. **7**, 361—372 (1975)

Mitrakul, Ch.: Effects of green pit-viper (*Trimesurus erythurus* and *Trimesurus popeorum*) venoms and blood coagulation, platelets and the fibrinolytic enzyme systems. Amer. J. clin. Path. **60**, 654—662 (1973)

Mugneret, P.: A propos d'une observation de morsure de Crotale viridis viridis. Etude clinique et expérimentale de l'incidence des venins de crotalidae sur la coagulabilité sanguine, déductions thérapeutiques. Thesis. Dijon (1973)

Müller-Berghaus, G., Hocke, M.: Effect of endotoxin on the formation of microthrombi from circulating fibrin monomers complexes in the absence of thrombin generation. Thrombos. Res. **1**, 541—548 (1972)

Müller-Berghaus, G., Mann, B.: Precipitation of ancrod-induced soluble fibrin by Aprotinin and Norepinphrine. Thrombos. Res. **2**, 305—322 (1973)

Niewiarowski, S., Regoeczi, E., Stewart, G. J., Senyi, A. F., Mustard, J. F.: Platelet interaction with polymerizing fibrin. J. Lab. clin. Invest. **51**, 685—700 (1972)

Niewiarowski, S., Stewart, G. J., Nath, N., Sha, A. T., Liebermann, G. E.: ADP, Thrombin and *Bothrops atrox* enzymes in platelet dependent fibrin retraction. Amer. J. Physiol. **229**, 737 (1975)

Okamoto, S., Hijikata, A., Kinjo, K., Kikumoto, R., Ohkubo, K., Tonomura, Sh., Tamao, Y.: A novel series of synthetic thrombin-inhibitors having extremely potent and highly selective action. Kobe J. med. Sci. **21**, 43—51 (1975)

Olsen, E. G. J., Pitney, W. R.: The effect of arvin on experimental pulmonary embolism in the rabbit. Brit. J. Haemat. **17**, 425—429 (1969)

Olson, P. S.: The contribution of platelets and fibrinogen in the early development of experimental arterial and venous thrombi. In: Martin, M., Schoop, W. (Eds.): Defibrinierung mit thrombinähnlichen Schlangengiftenzymen, pp. 108—113. Bern-Stuttgart-Wien: Huber 1975

Olson, S., Ljungqvist, U., Bergentz, S. E.: The effect of Reptilase on the formation of experimental thrombi. Abstr. 7, Congr. Europ. Soc. exp. Surg. Amsterdam (1972)

Olsson, P.: Discussion. In: Martin, M., Schoop, W. (Eds.): Defibrinierung mit thrombin-ähnlichen Schlangengiftenzymen, 179—180. Bern-Stuttgart-Wien: Huber 1975

Olsson, P., Blombäck, M., Egberg, N., Ekeström, S., Göransson, L., Johnsson, H.: Studies on the bleeding tendency and on the possibility of surgery in states of Reptilase-induced defibrinogenation. Thrombos. Diathes. haemorrh. Suppl. **47**, 389—396 (1971)

Olsson, P., Johnsson, H.: Interference of acetyl salicylic acid, heparin and fibrinogen degradation products in haemostasis of Reptilase-defibrinogenated dogs. Thrombos. Res. **1**, 135—146 (1972)

Olsson, P., Ljungquist, A., Göransson, L.: Vein graft surgery in Defibrase defibrinogenated dogs. Thrombos. Res. **3**, 161—172 (1973)

Ouyang, C., Hong, I. S., Teng, Ch. M.: Purification and properties of the thrombin-like principle of *Agkistrodon acutus* and its comparison to bovine thrombin. Thrombos. Diathes. haemorrh., **26**, 224—234 (1971)

Ouyang, C., Yang, F. Y.: Purification and properties of the thrombinlike enzymes from *Trimesurus gramineus* venom. Biochim. biophys. Acta (Amst.) **351**, 354—363 (1974)

Paar, D., Klüken, N.: Beziehungen zwischen der Fibrinogenkonzentration, der Thromboplastinzeit, Thrombin- und Reptilasezeit bei Patienten unter Arwin-Therapie. Med. Welt **26**, 1700—1701 (1975)

Pitney, W. R.: Clinical experience with Arvin. Thrombos. Diathes. haemorrh. Suppl. **38**, 81 (1969 c)

Pitney, W. R., Bell, W. R., Bolton, G.: Blood fibrinolytic activity during Arvin therapy. Brit. J. Haemat. **16**, 165—171 (1969 a)

Pitney, W. R., Bray, C., Holt, P. J. L., Bolton, G.: Acquired resistance to treatment with Arvin. Lancet **1969 b I**, 79—81

Pitney, W. R., Oakley, C. M., Goodwin, J. F.: Therapeutic defibrination with Arvin. Amer. Heart J. **80**, 144—146 (1970)

Pitney, W. R., Regoeczi, E.: Inactivation of Arvin by plasma proteins. Brit. J. Haemat. **19**, 67—81 (1970)

Pizzo, S. V., Schwartz, M. L., Hill, R. L., McKee, P. A.: Mechanism of ancrod. A direct proteolytic effect on fibrin. J. clin. Invest. **51**, 2841 (1972)

Prentice, C. R. M., Edgar, W., McNicol, G. P.: Characterization of fibrin degradation products in patients on ancrod therapy: Comparison with fibrinogen derivatives produced by plasmin. Brit. J. Haemat. **27**, 77—87 (1974)

Prentice, C. R. M., Hassanein, A. A., Turpie, A. G. G., McNicol, G. P., Douglas, A. S.: Changes in platelet behaviour during Arvin therapy. Lancet **1969 I**, 644—647

Prentice, C. R. M., McKillop, C. A., Edgar, W., Forbes, C. D.: Soluble complexes production during defibrination with ancrod infusion. Abstr. Symp. on thrombin-like enzymes. July 15—17, Trier (1975)

Regoeczi, E., Bell, W. R.: In vivo behaviour of the coagulant enzyme from *Agkistrodon rhodostoma* venom: Studies using 131$_I$-Arvin. Brit. J. Haemat. **16**, 573—587 (1969)

Regoeczi, E., Gergely, J., McFarlane, A. S.: In vivo effects of *Agkistrodon rhodostoma* venom: Studies with fibrinogen—^{131}I. J. clin. Invest. **115**, 1202—1212 (1966)

Reid, H. A., Chan, K. E.: The paradox in therapeutic defibrination Lancet **1968 I**, 485—486

Reid, H. A., Thean, P. C.: Prolonged coagulation defect (defibrination syndrome) in Malayan viper bite. Lancet **1963 I**, 621

Sato, T., Iwanaga, S., Mizushima, Y., Suzuki, T.: Studies on snake venoms. J. Biochem. **57**, 380—391 (1965)

Schmid-Schönbein, H., Wells, R., Schildkraut, R.: Microscopy and viscometry of blood under uniform shear rate (rheoscopy). J. appl. Physiol. **26**, 674 (1969)

Sharma, G. V. R. K., Godin, P. F., Belko, J. S., Bell, W. R., Sasahara, A. A.: Arvin therapy in experimental pulmonary embolism. Amer. Heart J. **85**, 72—77 (1973)

Sharp, A. A.: Clinical use of Arvin. Thrombos. Diathes. haemorrh. Suppl. **45**, 69 (1971)

Sharp, A. A.: Clinical experience with Arvin. Abstr. Symp. on thrombinlike enzymes. July 15—17, Trier (1975)

Sharp, A. A., Warren, B. A., Paxton, A. M., Allington, M. J.: Anticoagulant therapy with a purified fraction from Malayan pit viper venom. Lancet **1968 I**, 493—499

Silbermann, S., Kwaan, H. C.: The effect of "Arvin" on wound healing in the rat. Fed. Proc. **30**, 424 (1971)

Singh, M. P., Pentall, H. H., Bell, W. R., Olsen, E. G. J., Allwork, S. P.: The use of ancrod to prevent thrombosis on prosthetic heart valves. Thorax **25**, 472 (1970)

Singh, M. P., Pitney, W. R., Melrose, D. G.: Further experience in the use of ancrod (Arvin) to prevent thrombosis on prosthetic heart valves. Thorax **26**, 167—171 (1971)

Soria, J., Soria, C., Yver, J., Samama, M.: Temps de Reptilase. Etude de la polymérisation de la fibrine en présence de Reptilase. Coagulation **2**, 173—175 (1969)

Stocker, K., Barlow, G. H.: Characterization of Defibrase. In: Martin, M., Schoop, W. (Eds.): Defibrinierung mit thrombin-ähnlichen Schlangengiftenzymen, pp. 45—62. Bern-Stuttgart-Wien: Huber 1975

Stocker, K., Christ, W., Leloup, P.: Characterization of the venoms of various *Bothrops* species by immunoelectrophoresis and reaction with fibrinogen agarose. Toxicon **12**, 415—417 (1974)

Stocker, K., Egberg, N.: Reptilase as a defibrinogenating agent. Thrombos. Diathes. haemorrh. Suppl. **54**, 361—370 (1973)

Stocker, K., Straub, P. W.: Rapid detection of fibrinopeptides by bidimensional paper electrophoresis. Thrombos. Diathes. haemorrh. **24**, 248—255 (1970)

Stocker, K., Yeh, H.: A simple and sensitive test for the detection of inhibitors of Defibrase and Arwin in serum. Brief Commun. Thrombos. Res. **6**, 189—194 (1975)

Straub, P. W.: Personal communication (Cerastes cerastes) (1971)

Straub, P. W., Bollinger, A., Blättler, W.: Metabolism of labeled thrombin-like snake venom enzymes. In: Martin, M., Schoop, W. (Eds.): Defibrinierung mit thrombin-ähnlichen Schlangengiftenzymen, pp. 72—78. Bern-Stuttgart-Wien: Huber 1975

Straub, P. W., Harder, A.: Verhalten von ^{125}I-Fibrinogen bei therapeutischer Defibrinierung mit hochgereinigter Reptilase (Defibrase). Schweiz. med. Wschr. **101**, 1802—1804 (1971)

Svendsen, L., Blombäck, B., Blombäck, M., Olsson, P.: Synthetic chromogenic substrates for determination of trypsin, thrombin and thrombin-like enzymes. Thrombos. Res. **1**, 267—278 (1972)

Tilsner, V.: Vorläufige Mitteilung über die Ergebnisse einer Gemeinschaftsstudie mit Arwin. In: Martin, M., Schoop, W. (Eds.): Defibrinierung mit thrombinähnlichen Schlangengiftenzymen, pp. 225—230. Bern-Stuttgart-Wien: Huber 1975

Turpie, A. G. G., Prentice, C. R. M., McNicol, G. P., Douglas, A. S.: In vitro studies with ancrod (Arvin). Brit. J. Haemat. **20**, 217—224 (1971)

Vaz, E., Pereira, A.: Agao hemocoagulante de veneno botropico, An. Inst. Pinheiros **3**, 5 (1940)

Vellard, J.: Une Lachesis peu connue du Nord-Est du Brésil, L. erythromelas. C. R. Soc. Biol. (Paris) **127**, 38 (1938)

Vinazzer, H.: Zur Wirkung von Arvin auf die Blutgerinnung. Wien. Z. inn. Med, **52**, 378—392 (1971)

Vinazzer, H.: Acquired resistance to ancrod. Its evaluation and clinical occurrence. Thrombos. Diathes. haemorrh. **29**, 339—346 (1973)

Vinazzer, H.: Coagulation studies during therapeutic application of Arvin. Abstr. Symp. on thromin-like enzymes. July 15—17, Trier (1975)

Völker, D.: Rheologische Veränderungen unter der Therapie mit Defibrase. In: Martin, M., Schoop, W. (Eds.): Defibrinierung mit thrombin-ähnlichen Schlangengiftenzymen, pp. 171—178. Bern-Stuttgart-Wien: Huber 1975

Völker, D., Martin, M.: Verhalten der Blutviskosität unter Defibrase und kombinierter Defibrase-Streptokinasetherapie, Verh. dtsch. Ges. inn. Med. **79**, 1338—1340 (1973)

Walter, M., Nyman, D., Duckert, F.: Ancrod, batroxobin and F. XIII. Abstr. Symp. on thrombin-like enzymes. July 15—17, Trier (1975)

Weiss, H. J., Allen, S., Davidson, E., Kochwa, S.: Afibrinogenemia in man following the bite of a rattle snake (*Crotalus adamanteus*) Amer. J. Med. **47**, 625—634 (1969)

Weiss, H. J., Phillips, L. L., Hopenwell, W. S., Phillips, G., Christy, N. P., Nitti, J. F.: Heparin therapy in a patient bitten by a saw-scaled viper (*Echis carinatus*), a snake whose venom activates prothrombin. Amer. J. Med. **54**, 654 (1973)

Wells, R. E., Gaweonski, T. H., Cox, P. J., Perera, R. D.: Influence of fibrinogen on flow properties of erythrocyte suspensions. Amer. J. Physiol. **207**, 1035 (1964)

Wik, K. O., Tangen, O., McKenzie, N.: Blood-clotting activity of Reptilase and bovine thrombin in vitro: A comparative study on seven different species. Brit. J. Haemat. **23**, 37—45 (1972)

Wyss, W.: Wundheilung bei experimenteller Defibrinogenierung. Thesis. Zürich (1975)

Zajdel, M., Wegrzynowicz, Z., Sawecka, J., Kopeč, M.: Subunits and susceptibility of fibrins formed from bovine fibrinogen by Arvin, reptilase, thrombin and staphylothrombin. Thrombos. Res. **6**, 337—344 (1975)

Ziel, C., van der, Joison, J., Siso, H., Saravis, C., Slapak, M.: The effect of Arvin on blood coagulation and patency of venovenous shunts in the dog. Abstr. Brit. J. Surg. **57**, 856 (1970)

Antifibrinolytics

Naturally Occurring Inhibitors of Fibrinolysis

F. Markwardt

Disturbances of hemostasis play an important role in clinical practice. To prevent fatal bleedings their judicious treatment with appropriate drugs is an absolute necessity.

In the past several years new hemostyptics have been developed which have led to an improved therapy of disturbances in the formation and consumption of clotting factors. Congenital abnormalities in the formation of clotting factors require substitution therapy. Improved methods of plasma fractionation allow us to obtain sufficient quantities of clotting factors with high activity. Localized and generalized hyperfibrinolytic states belong to the acquired disturbances of consumption. When activators of fibrinolysis are rapidly released into the circulation, the activation of plasminogen occurs more rapidly than the inactivation of plasmin by inhibitors in blood, so that the enzyme may appear in the blood in an active form. Moreover, the hyperplasminemia may be caused by a pathologically decreased antiplasmin content of the blood.

The appearance of free plasmin in the blood represents a particular danger to the organism. Because of the general proteolytic activity of this enzyme, not only fibrin is digested but also plasma proteins, particularly fibrinogen and other clotting factors. Besides, the resulting fibrin(ogen) degradation products inhibit blood coagulation. This causes a disturbance of hemostasis which may produce a clinically relevant hemorrhagic diathesis. For its treatment an interference in this pathophysiologic process is required. Therefore, endogenous inhibitors of fibrinolysis, and those which are obtained from animals and plants, have stimulated growing interest.

A. Endogenous Inhibitors

Naturally occurring inhibitors of fibrinolysis are divided into two groups, one inhibiting the activation of plasminogen, the other acting against plasmin directly.

I. Inhibitors from Plasma

In blood plasma, inhibitors of plasminogen activation and of active plasmin are present. The existence of an inhibitor of plasminogen activation was suggested as early as 1937 by Schmitz and subsequently by Hultin and Lundblad (1949) and Lewis and Ferguson (1951). The presence of this antiactivator was proved indirectly by use of clot lysis methods (Gormsen, 1962; Dudok de Wit, 1964). Although Paraskevas et al. (1962) and Bennett (1967) pointed out that the clot lysis system used by them measured predominantly the antiactivator level in serum, it is likely

Table 1. Plasmin inhibitors in human serum

Inhibitor	Type of inhibition	Mol wt.	Mean concentration (mg/ 100 ml)	References
α_1-Antitrypsin	Progressive	54000	290	SHULMAN (1952), JACOBSSON (1955), MOLL et al. (1958), NORMAN (1958), BUNDY and MEHL (1959), SCHULTZE et al. (1962), HEIMBURGER and HAUPT (1966), RIMON et al. (1966), CRAWFORD (1973), CRAWFORD and OGSTON (1974)
α_2-Macroglobulin	Immediate	820000	260	SHULMAN (1952), BROWN et al. (1954), JACOBSSON (1955), NORMAN and HILL (1958), SCHULTZE et al. (1963), MEHL et al. (1964), STEINBUCH et al. (1965, 1972), GANROT (1967), GANROT and SCHERSTEN (1967)
Inter-α-inhibitor	Immediate	160000	50	STEINBUCH and LOEB (1961), HEIDE et al. (1965), HEIMBURGER and HAUPT (1965), SCHWICK et al. (1966), STEINBUCH et al. (1966)
CĪ-inactivator	Immediate	104000	24	HAUPT et al. (1970), HEIMBURGER et al. (1971)
Antithrombin III	Progressive	65000	40	HEIMBURGER (1967), TELESFORO et al. (1975)

that none of these methods completely exclude inhibitory effects of antiplasmin substances. An activator inhibitor in normal serum has repeatedly been demonstrated by means of clot lysis methods (NILSSON et al., 1961; HAWKEY and STAFFORD, 1964; BENNETT, 1967, 1970; DEN OTTOLANDER et al., 1967, 1969a, b). The activator inhibitor level varies independently of those of α_2-macroglobulin or α_1-antiplasmin (PARASKEVAS et al., 1962; BENNETT, 1967).

Thus, there is good evidence for the existence of an inhibitor of plasminogen activation in human serum, but little is known about its chemical nature and properties.

The activator inhibitor of human serum is an α_2-globulin (NILSSON et al., 1961). It is destroyed by heating at 56° C for 30 min. The activity decreases markedly also after storage at room temperature or at 4° C for more than 24 h. Acidification to pH 2.0 destroys the activity (NILSSON et al., 1961; BENNETT, 1967). The inhibitor is not dialyzable and not adsorbed on $BaSO_4$ (NILSSON et al., 1961).

Plasmin inhibitors of human plasma have been purified and well characterized as proteins (SCHULTZE et al., 1962; SHAMASH and RIMON, 1964; HEIMBURGER and HAUPT, 1966) (Table 1). They are able to inhibit other proteolytic enzymes besides plasmin, such as trypsin, thrombin, and chymotrypsin.

In the α_1-globulin fraction of human plasma an inhibitor is present which inactivates plasmin in a time-dependent reaction (progressive antiplasmin) (ROWLEY and

OETTE, 1973; HERCZ, 1974). This inhibitor, also termed α_1-antitrypsin, constitutes 90% of the antiplasmin activity of plasma. Its concentration in plasma is 2–5 mg/ml (SCHWICK, 1967). A further plasmin inhibitor which causes a rapid plasmin inactivation is present in the α_2-globulin fraction (immediate antiplasmin). The inhibitor possesses the characteristics of a macroglobulin and is present in plasma in a concentration of 2.2–3.8 mg/ml (STEINBUCH and BLATRIX, 1968; IWAMOTO and ABIKO, 1970). The plasmin binding to α_2-macroglobulin is reversible. Thus, the inhibitor possibly possesses a transport function for plasmin. Further human plasma inhibitors which cause an inhibition of plasmin are: the inter-α-trypsin inhibitor which is presumably identical with protein II described by STEINBUCH et al. (1966), and the C1-inactivator which combines immediately with plasmin (HEIMBURGER et al., 1971; HARPEL and COOPER, 1975). Antithrombin III, which is mainly responsible for the physiologic thrombin inactivation in plasma, is also able to inhibit plasmin (HEIMBURGER and HAUPT, 1966). How far it participates in the physiologic plasmin inactivation has remained unclear.

Plasmin inhibitors are present in the blood in excess of requirements. While a maximum amount of 3–4 caseinolytic units of plasmin is produced in 1 ml of human plasma, the quantity of inhibitor of this volume is sufficient to neutralize 5 caseinolytic units of plasmin (FEARNLEY, 1965). According to other authors (NORMAN and HILL, 1958; SHAMASH and RIMON, 1964; SCHWICK, 1967), the antiplasmin activity of plasma is even 10–30 times higher than required for the neutralization of the maximum amount of plasmin formed. A comparative study on the inhibitors of fibrinolysis in human, dog, and rabbit blood was performed by GALLIMORE et al. (1965).

II. Inhibitors from Blood Platelets

In blood platelets a highly effective antiplasmin exists which may be obtained by repeated freezing and thawing (JOHNSON and SCHNEIDER, 1953; STEFANINI, 1956; ALKJAERSIG, 1961; GANGULY, 1972). The antiplasmin activity of blood platelets amounts only to 3% of the total plasma activity. This is in agreement with the finding that blood platelets have a low antitrypsin content (LANDMANN et al., 1969). They are, however, supposed to have a higher antiactivator content (DEN OTTOLANDER et al., 1967, 1969a, b).

III. Inhibitors from Other Body Fluids and Tissues

Endogenous inhibitors of fibrinolysis have been found in other body fluids and tissues besides blood (STAMM, 1962). Inhibitors from tissues are thought to be mainly protein-like substances localized in several cells and effective against many proteolytic enzymes. Furthermore, specific inhibitors of fibrinolysis have been detected in human tissues, e.g., a urokinase inhibitor of human placenta (KAWANO et al., 1968; USZYNSKI and ABILDGAARD, 1971; ÅSTEDT et al., 1972) and of amniotic fluid (USZYNSKI and USZYNSKI-FOLEJEWSKA, 1969). The urokinase inhibitor of placenta has been purified and separated by gel filtration into two fractions with molecular weights of 70000 and 43000 (KAWANO et al., 1970). An inhibitor of plasminogen activation from the walls of human blood vessels was described by AOKI and VON KAULLA (1971). The antiplasmin action of the inhibitor mingin present in human urine was investigated in great detail (ASTRUP and STERNDORF, 1955; ASTRUP and ALBRECHTSEN, 1957; EGEBLAD and ASTRUP, 1963). An inhibitor of fibrinolysis has recently been demonstrated in the wall of human arteries (NOORDHOEK HEGT and BRAKMAN, 1974).

B. Animal Inhibitors

Naturally occurring inhibitors of proteolytic enzymes were first demonstrated in intestinal parasites which produce antipeptically and antitryptically active substances in order to protect themselves from an attack of digestive enzymes of the host organism (WEINLAND, 1903; MENDEL and BLOOD, 1910). Subsequently, such inhibitors were isolated from several animal organs (for review see GREEN and NEURATH, 1954; LASKOWSKI and LASKOWSKI, 1954; LASKOWSKI, 1955; LASKOWSKI et al., 1966; KASSELL, 1970; VOGEL and WERLE, 1970; WERLE and ZICKGRAF-RÜDEL, 1972; TSCHESCHE, 1974). These are high molecular weight polypeptides which form complexes with several proteases, whereby the activity of the enzymes is blocked. The general characteristics of this reaction are: definite molar ratio of the complex formed, rapid equilibrium of the reaction, complete recovery of activity of the enzyme after splitting of the complex, and blockade of the active centers of the enzymes. These substances took on practical therapeutic importance after it was shown that they are able to inhibit the serine proteases trypsin and chymotrypsin as well as the specific proteolytic enzyme kallikrein, whereby the formation of the plasma kinins bradykinin and kallidin is prevented. They are used in the therapy of diseases in whose pathogenesis these proteolytic enzymes play a role.

Since plasmin is also a serine protease, it was reasonable to use these inhibitors for its inhibition. It has been shown that some of them act as antiplasmins (FEENEY et al., 1969). With the developments in the field of fibrinolysis research, they have, therefore, become very important.

In the following, the inhibitor isolated from bovine organs, aprotinin, which has therapeutic importance as an antifibrinolytic, is reported in detail, whereas other animal inhibitors of proteases with antiplasmin activity are only briefly described.

I. Aprotinin

As early as 1936, a protease inhibitor was isolated from bovine pancreas by KUNITZ and NORTHROP. It was found to be a basic protein with a molecular weight of 9000 (GREEN and WORK, 1953). Subsequently, inhibitors with similar properties were isolated from bovine parotid glands and lungs (ASTRUP, 1952; ASTRUP and STAGE, 1956; KRAUT and KÖRBEL-ENKHARDT, 1958; FREY et al., 1959). These inhibitors were characterized in detail. Each of them was found to possess antifibrinolytic activity (ASTRUP and STAGE, 1956; MARX et al., 1959, 1963; HLADOVEC and MANS-FELD 1960; MANSFELD et al., 1960; VAIREL and CHOAY, 1960; VAIREL and THELY, 1960; STEICHELE and HERSCHLEIN, 1961; SCHMUTZLER and BECK, 1962; GODAL and THEODOR, 1965). They are used therapeutically and are registered as Iniprol (inhibitor from pancreas), Trasylol (inhibitor from parotid glands) and Contrykal (inhibitor from lungs).

Studies on highly purified inhibitor preparations revealed conspicuous similarities between these inhibitors, so that they were assumed to be identical (KASSELL et al., 1963; KRAUT et al., 1963; KRAUT and BHARGAVA, 1964; ANDERER and HÖRNLE, 1965 c). This assumption was confirmed after the structure of these inhibitor proteins had been elucidated (CHAUVET et al., 1964; ANDERER and HÖRNLE, 1965 a b; DLOUHA et al., 1965; KASSELL and LASKOWSKI, 1965; KASSELL et al., 1965). Presumably, the inhibitors isolated from bovine liver and from other bovine organs are also identical (FRITZ et al., 1967; WERLE et al., 1967). The inhibitor from bovine organs was named aprotinin.

A further inhibitor localized in bovine pancreas, which was first purified and tested by KAZAL in 1948, has to be distinguished from aprotinin. It is an acidic protein delivered into the pancreatic juice which acts specifically against trypsin. It does not influence the fibrinolytic system (GREENE et al., 1966; BURCK, 1970).

1. Chemistry

The inhibitor from bovine organs, aprotinin, was the first naturally occurring inhibitor of proteases to be isolated in purified form, and the first substance of this nature whose structure has been elucidated. Several research groups independently devoloped methods for the isolation of the inhibitor (for review, see VOGEL and WERLE, 1970). The molecule consists of 58 amino acids and possesses a molecular weight of 6500 (Fig. 1). Earlier reports of higher molecular weights can be explained by dimerization. The isoelectric point was found at pH 10–10.5. The molecule possesses a compact tertiary structure which provides a high stability against acids, heating, and proteolytic degradation (SCHOLTAN and LIE, 1966; SCHOLTAN and ROSENKRANZ, 1966; CHAUVET and ACHER, 1967 a). Its stability decreases with increasing pH values. Proteolytic degradation occurs only after cleavage of disulfide bonds (KASSELL and LASKOWSKI, 1966; SCHULTZ, 1967).

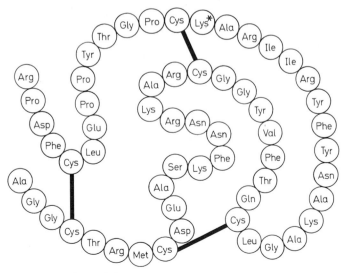

Fig. 1. Primary structure of aprotinin

2. Mechanism of Action

Aprotinin forms complexes with several esteroproteolytic enzymes belonging to the serine proteases. Detailed studies exist on the kinetics and molecular mechanism of the inhibition of trypsin and kallikrein (GREEN, 1957, 1963; TRAUTSCHOLD and WERLE, 1961; VOGEL and TRAUTSCHOLD, 1966; PÜTTER, 1967; VOGEL and WERLE, 1970). In both cases, the reaction proceeds at high velocity; it is, however, clearly time-dependent. The second order rate constant amounts to $3 \times 10^5 \, l \times mol^{-1} \times s^{-1}$ at optimal ionic strength and neutral pH. The reaction is reversible. The dissociation of the complex depends on the pH value. At pH values below 3—4 no noteworthy complex formation is observed. In case of neutral reaction, the dissociation constant for the trypsin-inhibitor complex amounts to 10^{-11} M, and for the kallikrein-inhibitor complex 10^{-8} M. The reaction of the inhibitor with kallikrein is not impaired in the presence of substrate. However, the trypsin-inhibitor reaction is retarded by substrates of the enzyme.

Many investigators examined the active center of the inhibitor. Changes in the molecule concerning methionine, tyrosine, serine, and four lysines are without effect on the inhibitor activity. Only the lysine residue at 15 position (in Fig. 1 with asterisk) participates in complex binding (CHAUVET and ACHER, 1967b). Acetylation and methylation of the inhibitor lead to a loss of inhibiting capacity, pointing to the rate of carboxyl and primary amino groups. Studies on the structure of the complex formed by bovine trypsin and aprotinin have recently been reported (HUBER et al., 1974, 1975).

The reaction of the inhibitor with plasmin, i.e., its antifibrinolytic effect, follows the same mechanism as the inhibition of trypsin (MARKWARDT and LANDMANN, 1967). After addition of increasing amounts of inhibitor to a plasmin solution, the determination of the remaining plasmin activity revealed that a defined amount of inhibitor always blocks an equivalent amount of enzyme (Fig. 2). Thus, the reaction between plasmin and inhibitor proceeds stoichiometrically according to the following simple scheme:

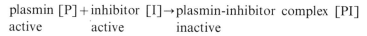

plasmin [P] + inhibitor [I] → plasmin-inhibitor complex [PI]
active   active   inactive

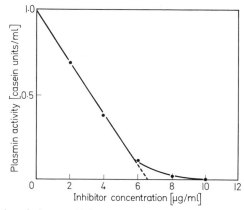

Fig. 2. Inhibition of plasmin by aprotinin

The deviation from the stoichiometric reaction near the equivalence point indicates the dissociation of the plasmin-inhibitor complex under present test conditions. From the remaining plasmin activity in the presence of an equivalent amount of inhibitor the dissociation constant for the equilibrium $[P] + [I] = [PI]$ can be determined as 1.8×10^{-9} M. Accordingly, the dissociation of the plasmin-inhibitor complex is very small, so that the complex is practically undissociated. One μg inhibitor inhibits 38.4 μg plasmin Novo (VOGEL et al., 1966). Inhibition of the fibrinolytic action of streptokinase-activated plasmin has been reported (HLADOVEC et al., 1958; MARX et al., 1959; MANSFELD et al., 1960; SOULIER et al., 1960; SCHMUTZLER and BECK, 1962; BERGHOFF and GLATZEL, 1963; GODAL and THEODOR, 1965; MAXWELL et al., 1965; MAKI and BELLER, 1966).

In addition to its antiplasmin effect, aprotinin is said to possess inhibitory activity on plasminogen activation (SCHMUTZLER, 1963; BERGHOFF and GLATZEL, 1964; DE BARBIERI, 1965; MAKI and BELLER, 1966). From a critical point of view, however, the experimental approach to this problem is not convincing. The measurement of inhibition of activation must lead to misinterpretations, since it is based on the determination of the plasmin formed which itself is blocked by the inhibitor. Besides the endogenous antiactivators, no protein-like inhibitor able to inhibit a plasminogen-activating enzyme under biochemically well-defined conditions is presently known. Thus, the inhibitors from bovine organs as well as from soybeans and human urine (mingin) do not inhibit urokinase (LORAND and CONDIT, 1965; WALTON, 1967; DUCKERT, 1968). The streptokinase-induced kinase activity also is not inhibited by soybean inhibitors (KLINE and FISHMAN, 1957, 1961; SPRITZ and CAMERON, 1962; TS'AO and KLINE, 1969).

3. Determination of Activity, Standardization

Because of its polypeptide nature the chemical proof of the inhibitor is difficult. Therefore, only test methods based on the biological activity of the inhibitor are used (RICHTER, 1967). For methods of testing naturally occurring protease inhibitors, see VOGEL and WERLE (1970). To determine the inhibitor, its ability to form stoichiometrically defined complexes with the enzymes plasmin, trypsin, or kallikrein is utilized and its activity is expressed in units. Generally, one inhibitor unit is defined as that quantity which inhibits one unit of the particular enzyme used. The activities obtained, however, show marked differences because they refer to different enzymes and different definitions of enzyme activity (MARKWARDT and RICHTER, 1969). These differences become evident when the various preparations from bovine organs are compared. For example, the activity of Contrykal is expressed in antitrypsin units (ATrU). One trypsin unit (TrU) is equal to that amount of enzyme able to cleave 1 μmol N^α-tosyl-L-arginine methyl ester (TAME) at 25° C under optimal conditions. The activity of Iniprol is measured in Unités Inhibitrice des Peptidases (U.I.P.). Here the activity of trypsin is determined by means of cleavage of N^α-benzoyl-L-arginine ethyl ester (BAEE) according to the method of Schwert and Takenaka. One Schwert-Takenaka unit (STU) is that quantity of trypsin which causes an increase in the optical density by 0.001 per min at 253 nm. The activity of Trasylol is expressed in kallikrein-inactivator units (KIU). One kallikrein unit (KU) is equal to that quantity of kallikrein which after i.v. injection into dogs causes the same effect on blood pressure as 5 ml human urine of healthy subjects (taken from samples containing at least 50 l and dialyzed for 24 h through a cellophane membrane against flowing water). The standardization by biological determination of the kallikrein activity is rather difficult. Therefore, to measure the enzyme activity and its inhibition by protease inhibitors, the synthetic substrates N^α-benzoyl-L-arginine ethyl ester or N^α-benzoyl-DL-arginine-p-nitroanilide (BAEE, BAPNA) are used.

Because of the different procedures of standardization the activities of various preparations of protease inhibitors can hardly be compared. Further difficulties arise because a valid standardization requires optimal test methods, the same substrate, the same kind of enzymes, and even the same enzyme preparation. According to the results obtained by other authors (TRAUTSCHOLD and WERLE, 1961), trypsin preparations of various provenance vary in their susceptibility to the protease inhibitor aprotinin, although they all had the same enzyme activity. Therefore, a standard trypsin preparation from bovine pancreas is recommended for the determination of inhibitor activity. A practical way of comparison was found by determining the activities of pure inhibitor and of commercial preparations by the same method, and comparing the measured activity with that stated by the manufacturer in declared units (MARKWARDT and RICHTER, 1969). After purification and analysis of the polypeptide the preparations are best defined according to their inhibitor protein content. Thus, the standardization of the pure inhibitor activity would be independent of the test method used.

The following data on specific activity of the pure inhibitor are given: 1 mg aprotinin = 7150 KIU (TRAUTSCHOLD et al., 1966) = 50 000 U.I.P. (CHAUVET et al., 1964) = 1180 ATrU (MARKWARDT and WALSMANN, 1964). Knowing these ratios, the conversion of inhibitor units into inhibitor content is possible: 1 ATrU = 0.85 µg aprotinin, 1 KIU = 0.14 µg aprotinin, 1 U.I.P. = 0.02 µg aprotinin.

The antifibrinolytic activity of the inhibitor can be followed in the blood by means of the plasma lysis test (MARKWARDT and LANDMANN, 1967): in test tubes of 6–7 mm diameter, 0.2 ml human-citrated plasma is mixed with 0.1 ml Tris buffer (pH 7.5), 0.1 ml streptokinase (500 U/ml) and 0.1 ml thrombin (50 NIH U/ml), are incubated at 37° C. After coagulation has occurred, a glass bead (4 mm diameter) is placed on the surface of the clot and the time from the addition of thrombin until the bead falls freely to the bottom of the test tube is measured (Fig. 3).

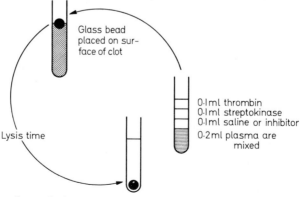

Fig. 3. Scheme of the plasma lysis test

4. Experimental Pharmacology

a) Toxicity

Aprotinin is well tolerated, even in relatively high doses. In rats and dogs, intravenous application of doses up to 100 mg/kg did not produce toxic side-effects (MARKWARDT et al., 1972). Further studies on the toxicity of therapeutically used protease inhibitors were done by the manufacturers of the various preparations. The determination of acute toxicity of i.v. administered Trasylol revealed an LD_{50} of 2.5 million KIU/kg mouse and 1.25–2.5 million KIU/kg rat (BEUCHELT, 1963). After application of lethal doses the animals died of acute cardiac and circulatory failure.

Studies on the chronic toxicity revealed that i.p. or i.v. application of 10000–300000 KIU/kg per day in rats and 5000–25000 KIU/kg per day in dogs over a period of 13 weeks did not cause gross pathologic changes. Histologic examinations in animals treated with the high dose showed reversible alterations in kidney tissue, and the weight gain of the animals was less than normal.

Up to 80000 KIU/kg were injected into pregnant rats for 5 days during the first trimester of pregnancy. Neither the dam nor the developing fetus were affected.

b) Pharmacokinetics

Determination of aprotinin in the blood was performed according to the plasma lysis test (Fig. 3), which has been used also for the quantitative determination of synthetic inhibitors of fibrinolysis in plasma and urine (MARKWARDT et al., 1964, 1966; MARKWARDT and KLÖCKING, 1965). The inhibitor concentrations were determined from the lysis times of clots from plasma samples with the aid of a calibration curve obtained by addition of increasing inhibitor amounts to the same plasma. When the lysis time was higher than the maximum value of the calibration curve, the samples were diluted by addition of normal plasma until the measured values fell within the range of the calibration curve. To determine the inhibitor content in urine or other body fluids, human-citrated plasma was used as substrate and the solution to be tested was added. The lysis test was performed as described above.

To study the pharmacokinetics, the inhibitor concentration in the blood of experimental animals was followed and the excretion in the urine was determined (KLÖCKING, 1967). The inhibitor is not absorbed from oral administration and can only be given parenterally. After subcutaneous, intramuscular or intraperitoneal application, a maximum blood level is reached after 1–2 h. Figure 4 shows the blood level after intravenous injection of inhibitor into rabbits. Owing to rapid elimination, the inhibitor level dropped sharply and was no longer detectable after 4 h. Within the first hours after injection 10–15% of the inhibitor was excreted in the urine in active form. Thereafter, no further excretion of active inhibitor was measured and the quantity of inhibitor in the 24-h urine did not increase. After the distribution equilibrium was reached (30 min p.i.) the semilogarithmic plot of the plasma level revealed a half-life of 75 min. After intravenous application in rats the half-life was 70 min (WERLE, 1969). Investigations in dogs (TRAUTSCHOLD et al., 1964) and mice (KALLER, 1963) showed a similar behavior of the inhibitor. Thus, the inhibitor disappeared relatively rapidly from the blood.

Using biological test methods, only the antifibrinolytically effective inhibitor portion is detectable, whereas the inactivated portion cannot be estimated. There-

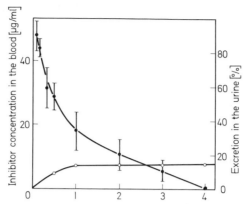

Fig. 4. Elimination of aprotinin after i.v. injection of 5 mg/kg into rabbits

fore, these studies did not reveal the fate of the remaining portion, whether excreted in inactive form or eliminated by other routes.

Studies in nephrectomized animals showed that elimination occurs mainly through the kidneys (KALLER, 1964). TRAUTSCHOLD et al. (1964) proposed that the inhibitor is fixed and slowly inactivated in the kidneys and that only a small amount of the administered inhibitor is excreted in the urine in active form. After application of a tritium-labeled inhibitor preparation, an accumulation of tritium activity was first observed in the liver and then in the kidneys. The inhibitor is thought to be chemically changed in the liver, bound to a higher molecular substance, and stored in the kidneys (REICHENBACH-KLINKE et al., 1969). It is evenly distributed to other organs. Studies in mice showed that the inhibitor is distributed mainly in the extracellular space; it does not penetrate into cells and does not pass the blood-brain barrier (KALLER, 1968).

c) Antifibrinolytic Action

Fibrinolysis is inhibited by aprotinin not only in vitro but also in vivo (MARX et al., 1959; STEICHELE and HERSCHLEIN, 1961; ENKE et al., 1966; MARKWARDT et al., 1966; AMBRUS et al., 1968). To demonstrate the antifibrinolytic action of the inhibitor in vivo, the antifibrinolytic activity was followed in the blood (MARKWARDT et al., 1966; KLÖCKING, 1967). It has been shown that prior inhibitor application prevents experimental fibrinolysis, and that fibrinolysis is interrupted by subsequent application. For experimental studies of the antifibrinolytic action rabbits and dogs are particularly well-suited. In these species intravascular fibrinolysis can be induced with streptokinase.

To demonstrate the antifibrinolytic action of the inhibitor, fibrinolysis was induced by i.v. injection of 2500 U streptokinase/kg into rabbits. Blood for thrombelastograms was taken by venipuncture with the aid of a polished coneless stainless steel cannula. Fibrinolysis was completely prevented by injection of 1 mg aprotinin/kg 10 min before streptokinase application, so that, in contrast to the streptokinase control, the thrombelastogram did not show any deviation.

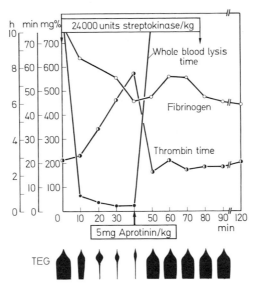

Fig. 5. Influence of aprotinin (5 mg/kg i.v.) on streptokinase-induced fibrinolysis in rabbits. Lysis time [h]; thrombin time [min]; fibrinogen [mg%]

The influence of the inhibitor on established intravascular hyperfibrinolysis was studied (KLÖCKING and MARKWARDT, 1969). Intravascular fibrinolysis was induced and maintained over a period of 1 h in rabbits by infusion of streptokinase. To demonstrate the increase in fibrinolysis, the lysis of whole blood clots was determined. Furthermore, fibrinogen degradation as well as formation of degradation products which inhibit the coagulation were estimated by measurements of the fibrinogen level and thrombin time. The results in Figure 5 show that extensive fibrinolysis was caused by continuous i.v. infusion of 400 U streptokinase/kg/min over 60 min. Lysis time shortened, the fibrinogen level decreased, and thrombin times were prolonged. The hyperfibrinolytic state was demonstrated also in the thrombelastogram of whole blood. Forty min after the start of streptokinase infusion, fibrinolysis was terminated immediately by i.v. injection of 5 mg aprotinin/kg, and all parameters returned to normal.

5. Clinical Pharmacology

a) Pharmacokinetics

Studies on the fate of the inhibitor in the human organism confirmed the results obtained in animal experiments, which revealed that the inhibitor is rapidly eliminated from the circulation. After i.v. injection of inhibitor the plasma concentration decreased markedly, as is shown by the time course of the inhibition of fibrinolysis in plasma (Fig. 6). The analysis of pharmacokinetic data revealed an elimination constant of $0.29 \, \text{h}^{-1}$ and a half-life of 140 min, which was also observed by other investigators (BELLER et al., 1966; KALLER, 1968). The volume of distribution amounted to about 60% of body weight. In the urine, the inhibitor was not excreted in an active

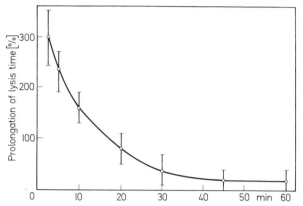

Fig. 6. Inhibition of streptokinase-induced lysis time in human plasma after injection of 1 mg aprotinin/kg

form. Because of the relatively rapid rate of elimination, the maintenance of a high inhibitor level over a longer period of time is possible only by continuous infusion. From the half-life and the distribution volume of the inhibitor, the amounts necessary to obtain a certain blood level by intravenous injection, and for its maintenance by subsequent infusion, can be calculated.

Different opinions prevail on the placental transfer of the inhibitor. While BELLER et al. (1966) found that the inhibitor does not cross the placental barrier, LUDWIG (1968) as well as HOFBAUER and DOBBECK (1970) believe to have provided evidence for a placental transfer, since they have observed an inhibition of fibrinolysis in fetal blood.

b) Therapeutic Use

α) Indications

The use of the inhibitor is indicated in pathologic fibrinolytic states in which there is a high incidence of bleeding. For reports on the clinical use of the protease inhibitor as an antifibrinolytic agent, see MARKWARDT et al. (1972). At first, the protease inhibitor was expected to be useful for the arrest of generalized fibrinolysis. However, such hyperfibrinolytic states develop mainly as the consequence of diffuse intravascular coagulation. If primary fibrinolysis cannot be definitively assured by differential diagnosis, the use of an antifibrinolytic is contraindicated. Reactive secondary fibrinolysis must be considered as a rational biological control mechanism which eliminates fibrin deposits. The inhibition of this process would allow the continued formation of microthrombi and thus increase further the risk of organ damage.

Antifibrinolytics are mainly applied in bleedings caused by a localized increase in fibrinolysis. Compared to the use of synthetic antifibrinolytics, that of aprotinin is limited because of its pharmacokinetics. Since the inhibitor is a protein, it is destroyed after oral administration. Therefore, it can only be used parenterally. Furthermore, it has to be kept in mind that the inhibitor is not excreted in the urine in active form, so that no antifibrinolytic effect can be expected in fibrinolytic bleeding from the urinary tract. Bleeding after operations on the thorax, abdomen, and prostate as well as cerebral hemorrhages are very rarely observed following prior administration of inhibitor. Hyperfibrinolytic bleeding as a consequence of obstetric and gynecologic operations can also be controlled with the aid of the inhibitor.

Because of the supposed anticoagulant effect of the protease inhibitor, the use of extremely high inhibitor doses has been recommended for the simultaneous inhibition of coagulation (AMRIS, 1966; NORDSTRÖM et al., 1966; MARX, 1968; MATIS and MÖRL, 1968). This anticoagulant activity of the inhibitor, which could not be confirmed by GORMSEN and JOSEPHSEN (1967), does not seem to be sufficient for an effective interruption of intravascular coagulation, so that in these cases the use of a direct anticoagulant, such as heparin, is recommended.

β) Side-Effects

The inhibitor is relatively well-tolerated (BECK et al., 1963). A single dose of 1–1.5 million KIU of Trasylol, when slowly injected i.v., was tolerated without any reaction (MÖRL, 1968). When extremely slowly injected, nausea and vomiting were reported in about 5% of cases. Because of the low molecular weight, sensitization against the inhibitor was not commonly observed. The frequency of side-effects during therapeutic use amounted to about 0.1% (HABERLAND and MATIS, 1967).

γ) Doses

Because of the rapid elimination of aprotinin from the blood, the inhibitor should be administered by intravenous drip or repeated injection. For this therapy the following doses are recommended.

	Initial dose	Maintenance dose	
Iniprol	5×10^6 antipeptidase units (U.I.P.)	1×10^6 U.I.P. every h	Until
Trasylol	500000 kallikrein inactivator units (KIU)	200000 KIU every 4–6 h	bleeding
Contrykal	100000 antitrypsin units (ATrU)	40000 ATrU every 4–6 h	is arrested

The difference in doses of the several preparations is the result of the different definitions of units used for standardization (see above). The listed doses correspond to 70–100 mg pure aprotinin per day. In general, the therapy of hyperfibrinolytic bleeding was initiated with an i.v. injection of 10–20% of the total dose of inhibitor and was continued by i.v. drip until bleeding stopped. For prophylaxis, 10–20% of the therapeutic dose was commonly applied, preferably as an infusion.

II. Miscellaneous Inhibitors

Besides the inhibitor from bovine organs, only a few animal inhibitors able to inhibit the fibrinolytic enzyme plasmin have been detected (Table 2). With the other not-so-well-characterized inhibitors, such as the trypsin-kallikrein inhibitor from seminal vesicles and sperm of mammals, only qualitative investigations of the inhibitory effect on plasmin were performed. Plasmin is also inhibited by a protease inhibitor from the submandibular glands of dogs, but much more weakly than other proteases,

Table 2. Plasmin inhibitors of animal origin

Source of inhibitor	Mol wt. approx.	References
Bovine organs (aprotinin)	6 500	KUNITZ and NORTHROP (1936), TRAUTSCHOLD et al. (1966, 1967)
Bovine colostrum	10 500	FEENEY and ALLISON (1969), FEENEY et al. (1969)
Guinea-pig (seminal vesicles)	6 000	HAENDLE et al. (1965), VOGEL et al. (1966), FRITZ et al. (1972)
Dog (submandibular glands)	13 000	VOGEL et al. (1968), FRITZ et al. (1971)
LEECHES (*Hirudo medicinalis*)	6 000	FRITZ et al. (1969, 1971)
Snails (*Helix pomatia*)	6 500	TSCHESCHE and DIETL (1972), TSCHESCHE et al. (1972)

such as trypsin and chymotrypsin. Recently, proteins obtained from medicinal leeches, termed bdelline, have been shown to possess an inhibitory action on trypsin and plasmin. The possible use of these inhibitors in medical therapy for the purpose of plasmin inhibition is under investigation. Broad-spectrum protease inhibitors which are also able to inhibit plasmin were isolated from snails *(Helix pomatia)* and sea anemones *(Anemonia sulcata)*.

C. Plant Inhibitors

Certain storage organs of plants, such as seeds from the *Leguminosae* and *gramineae* families, and tubers from the *Solanaceae* family, are excellent sources of protease inhibitors (VOGEL et al., 1968). These inhibitors are quite diverse in number and in specificity toward various enzymes. The activities of these inhibitors against human plasmin were generally similar to those against human trypsin. For inhibitors known to inhibit the fibrinolytic enzyme plasmin, see Table 3.

Among the plant inhibitors the trypsin inhibitor from soybeans (KUNITZ and NORTHROP, 1947) provoked early interest as an inhibitor of fibrinolysis. Its effect is exerted through the inhibition of plasmin. The dissociation of the complex between plasmin and the soybean inhibitor is very low (KUNITZ, 1947a); NANNINGA and GUEST (1964) ascertained a dissociation constant of 2×10^{-10} M. The antifibrinolytic

Table 3. Plant inhibitors of plasmin

Source of inhibitor	Mol wt. approx.	References
Soybeans	22 000	KUNITZ (1947a, b, c), KUNITZ and NORTHROP (1947)
Potatoes	24 000	WERLE and MAIER (1952), MANSFELD et al. (1959), HOCHSTRASSER and WERLE (1969), HOJIMA et al. (1971)
Peanuts	18 000	HOCHSTRASSER et al. (1969)
Lima beans	9 000	FRAENKEL-CONRAT et al. (1952), JONES et al. (1963), HAYNES and FEENEY (1967), FRICKE et al. (1969)

effect of this substance, in vitro and in vivo, was reported in a great number of publications (TAGNON and SOULIER, 1948; LEWIS and FERGUSON, 1950; RUSH and CLIFFTON, 1951; NANNINGA and GUEST, 1964; EGEBLAD, 1966).

Studies on the toxicity of the inhibitor were done by LIENER (1951). Single doses of the crude inhibitor have been found to produce death in rats and chicks when administered by intraperitoneal injection. The LD_{50} in rats and chicks was 200 and 2000 mg/kg respectively. Until now, the inhibitor did not prove useful in the therapy of hyperfibrinolysis. Furthermore, it is of interest that the inhibitor possesses an anticoagulant effect by inhibiting prothrombin activation (MACFARLANE and PILLING, 1946; TAGNON and SOULIER, 1946; GLENDENING and PAGE, 1951; LANCHANTIN et al., 1969; MARKWARDT and LANDMANN, 1971).

Besides the trypsin inhibitor from soybeans, other vegetable protease inhibitors with antifibrinolytic activity have been identified, such as the inhibitor from peanut shells (ČEPELÁK et al., 1963; EGEBLAD, 1967). This is assumed to possess a specific hemostatic effect in hemophilia (BOUDREAUX et al., 1960; BOUDREAUX and FRAMPTON, 1960). According to ASTRUP et al. (1960, 1962) and BRAKMAN et al. (1962) this effect is ascribed to an inhibition of fibrinolysis. A further protease inhibitor with antifibrinolytic activity was found in Lima beans (LEWIS and FERGUSON, 1953; MAXWELL et al., 1965) and in potatoes (HLADOVEC et al., 1958; MANSFELD et al., 1960, RABEK and MANSFELD, 1963). Pharmacologic observations on the inhibitor from potatoes were made by HLADOVEC et al. (1961) and DEEDS et al. (1964), but experiences in the therapeutic use of these inhibitors are lacking.

References

Alkjaersig, N.: The antifibrinolytic activity of platelets. In: Internat. Symp. on Blood Platelets, p. 329. Boston: Little, Brown 1961

Ambrus, C. M., Ambrus, J. L., Lassman, H. B., Mink, I. B.: Studies on the mechanism of action of inhibitors of the fibrinolysin system. Ann. N.Y. Acad. Sci. **146**, 430 (1968)

Amris, C. J.: Inhibition of thromboplastic activity by Trasylol. In: Gross, R., Kroneberg, G. (Eds.): Neue Aspekte der Trasylol-Therapie, p. 52. Stuttgart: Schattauer 1966

Anderer, F. A., Hörnle, S.: Strukturuntersuchungen am Kallikrein-Inaktivator aus Rinderlunge. I. Molekulargewicht, Endgruppenanalyse und Aminosäure-Zusammensetzung. Z. Naturforsch. B **20**, 457 (1965a)

Anderer, F. A., Hörnle, S.: Strukturuntersuchungen am Kallikrein-Inaktivator aus Rinderlunge. II. Bestimmung der Aminosäuresequenz. Z. Naturforsch. B **20**, 462 (1965b)

Anderer, F. A., Hörnle, S.: Zur Identität des Kallikrein-Inaktivators aus Rinderlunge und Rinderparotis. Z. Naturforsch. B **20**, 499 (1965c)

Aoki, N., Kaulla, K. N., von: Human serum plasminogen antiactivator: its distinction from antiplasmin. Amer. J. Physiol. **220**, 1137 (1971)

Åstedt, B., Pandolfi, M., Nilsson, I. M.: Inhibitory effect of placenta on plasminogen activation in human organ culture. Proc. Soc. exp. Biol. (N.Y.) **139**, 1421 (1972)

Astrup, T.: Fibrinolysis. Acta haemat. (Basel) **7**, 271 (1952)

Astrup, T., Albrechtsen, O. K.: Estimation of the plasminogen activator and the trypsin inhibitor in animal and human tissue. Scand. J. clin. Lab. Invest. **9**, 233 (1957)

Astrup, T., Brakman, P., Ollendorff, P., Rasmussen, J.: Haemostasis in haemophilia in relation on the haemostatic balance in the normal organism and the effect of peanuts. Thrombos. Diathes. haemorrh. (Stuttg.) **5**, 329 (1960)

Astrup, T., Brakman, P., Sjölin, K. E.: Haemophilia and the protease inhibitor in peanuts. Nature (Lond.) **194**, 980 (1962)

502   F. Markwardt

Astrup, T., Stage, A.: A protease inhibitor in ox lung tissue. Acta med. chem. scand. **10**, 617 (1956)
Astrup, T., Sterndorff, I.: The plasminogen activator in urine and the urinary trypsin inhibitor. Scand. J. clin. Lab. Invest. **7**, 239 (1955)
Barbieri, A. de: Enzymology of the fibrinolytic system and its clinical significance. In: Ruyssen, R., Vandendriesche, L. (Eds.): Enzymes in Clinical Chemistry, p. 32. Amsterdam-London-New York: Elsevier 1962
Beck, E., Schmutzler, R., Duckert, F.: Inhibition of fibrinolysis and fibrinogenolysis in man: comparison of ε-aminocaproic acid and kallikrein inhibitor. Thrombos. Diathes. haemorrh. (Stuttg.) **10**, 106 (1963)
Beller, F. K., Epstein, M. D., Kaller, H.: Distribution, half life time and placental transfer of the protease inhibitor Trasylol. Thrombos. Diathes. haemorrh. (Stuttg.) **16**, 302 (1966)
Bennett, N. B.: A method for the quantitative assay of inhibitor of plasminogen activation in human serum. Thrombos. Diathes. haemorrh. (Stuttg.) **17**, 12 (1967)
Bennett, N. B.: Further studies on an inhibitor of plasminogen activation in human serum. Thrombos. Diathes. haemorrh. (Stuttg.) **23**, 553 (1970)
Berghoff, A., Glatzel, H.: Untersuchungen in einem Plasmin-Präparat unter Verwendung des Kaseinspaltungstestes: Die Aktivität von Plasmin-Novo und seine Hemmbarkeit durch Epsilon-Aminocapronsäure und Trasylol. Thrombos. Diathes. haemorrh. (Stuttg.) **12**, 418 (1964)
Beuchelt, H.: Trasylol, ein Proteinasen-Inhibitor, in Experiment und klinischer Anwendung. Med. Chem. **7**, 763 (1963)
Boudreaux, H. B., Boudreaux, R. M., Brandon, M., Frampton, V. L., Lee, L. S.: Biologische Prüfung eines hämostatischen Faktors aus Erdnüssen. Arch. Biochem. **89**, 276 (1960)
Boudreaux, H. B., Frampton, V. L.: A peanut factor for haemostasis in haemophilia. Nature (Lond.) **185**, 570 (1960)
Brakman, P., Sjølin, K. E., Astrup, T.: Is there a hemostatic effect of peanuts in hemophiloid disorders? Thrombos. Diathes. haemorrh. (Stuttg.) **8**, 442 (1962)
Brown, R. K., Baker, W. H., Peterkofsky, A., Kauffman, D. L.: Crystallization and properties of a glycoprotein from human plasma. J. Amer. chem. Soc. **76**, 4244 (1954)
Bundy, H. F., Mehl, J. W.: Trypsin inhibitor of human serum. II. Isolation of the α_1-inhibitor and its partial characterization. J. biol. Chem. **234**, 1124 (1959)
Burck, P. J.: Pancreatic secretory trypsin inhibitors. In: Colowick, S. P., Kaplan, N. O. (Eds.): Methods in Enzymology, Vol. XIX. Perlman, G. E., Lorand, L. (Eds.): Proteolytic Enzymes, p. 906. New York-London: Academic Press 1970
Čepelák, V., Horáková, Z., Pádr, Z.: Protease inhibitor from groundnut skins. Nature (Lond.) **198**, 295 (1963)
Chauvet, J., Acher, R.: La structure covalente d'un inhibiteur polypeptidique de la trypsine (inhibiteur de Kunitz et de Northrop). Bull. Soc. Chim. biol. (Paris) **49**, 985 (1967 a)
Chauvet, J., Acher, R.: The reactive site of basic trypsin inhibitor of pancreas. Role of lysine 15. J. biol. Chem. **242**, 4274 (1967 b)
Chauvet, J., Nouvel, G., Acher, R.: Structure primaire d'un inhibiteur pancréatique de la trypsine (inhibiteur de Kunitz et Northrop). Biochim. biophys. Acta (Amst.) **92**, 200 (1964)
Crawford, G. P. M., Ogston, D.: The influence of α-1-antitrypsin on plasmin, urokinase and Hageman factor cofactor. Biochim. biophys. Acta (Amst.) **354**, 107 (1974)
Crawford, I. P.: Purification and properties of normal human α_1-antitrypsin. Arch. Biochem. **156**, 215 (1973)
DeEds, F., Ryan, C. A., Balis, A. K.: Pharmacological observations on a chymotryptic inhibitor from potatoes. Proc. Soc. exp. Biol. (N.Y.) **115**, 772 (1964)
Dlouha, V., Popišilová, D., Meloun, B., Šorm, F.: On proteins. XCIV. Primary structure of basic trypsin inhibitor from beef pancreas. Coll. Csl. chem. Commun. **30**, 1311 (1965)
Duckert, F.: Urokinase. In: Aebi, H., Mattenheimer, H., Schmidt, F. W. (Eds.): Current Problems in Clinical Biochemistry, Vol. II. Dubach, U. C. (Ed.): Enzymes in Urine and Kidney, p. 237. Bern-Stuttgart: Huber 1968
Dudok de Wit, C.: Investigation on the inhibitors of the fibrinolytic system. Thrombos. Diathes. haemorrh. (Stuttg.) **12**, 105 (1964)
Egeblad, K.: Effects of soybean trypsin inhibitor on fibrin clot lysis. Thrombos. Diathes. haemorrh. (Stuttg.) **15**, 542 (1966)

Egeblad,K.: Effects on fibrin clot lysis of a trypsin inhibitor in peanuts *(Arachis hypogaea)*. Thrombos. Diathes. haemorrh. (Stuttg.) **17**, 31 (1967)

Egeblad,K., Astrup,T.: ε-Aminocaproic acid and urinary trypsin inhibitor: Potentiated inhibition of urokinase induced fibrinolysis. Proc. Soc. exp. Biol. (N.Y.) **112**, 1020 (1963)

Encke,A., Schimpf,K., Kommerell,B., Grözinger,K.H., Gilsdorf,H., Wanke,M., Lasch,H.G.: Veränderungen der Blutgerinnung bei der akuten experimentellen Pankreatitis des Hundes. Klin. Wschr. **44**, 90 (1966)

Fearnley,G.R.: Fibrinolysis. London: Edward Arnold 1965

Feeney,R.E., Allison,R.G.: The Evolutionary Biochemistry of Proteins. New York: Wiley 1969

Feeney,R.E., Means,G.E., Bigler,J.C.: Inhibition of human trypsin, plasmin and thrombin by naturally occurring inhibitors of proteolytic enzymes. J. biol. Chem. **244**, 1957 (1969)

Fraenkel-Conrat,H., Bean,R.C., Ducey,E.D., Olcott,H.S.: Isolation and characterization of a trypsin inhibitor from Lima beans. Arch. Biochem. **37**, 393 (1952)

Frey,E.K., Kraut,H., Werle,E.: Kallikrein. Stuttgart: Enke, 1959

Fritz,H., Brey,B., Beress,L.: Polyvalente Isoinhibitoren für Trypsin, Chymotrypsin, Plasmin und Kallikreine aus Seeanemonen (Anemonia sulcata), Isolierung, Hemmverhalten und Aminosäurezusammensetzung. Hoppe-Seylers Z. physiol. Chem. **353**, 19 (1972)

Fritz,H., Fink,E., Gebhardt,M., Hochstrasser,K., Werle,E.: Identifizierung von Lysin- und Argininresten als Hemmzentren von Proteaseninhibitoren mit Hilfe von Maleinsäureanhydrid und Butandion-(2.3). Hoppe-Seylers Z. physiol. Chem. **350**, 933 (1969)

Fritz,H., Fink,E., Meister,R., Klein,G.: The isolation of trypsin inhibitors and trypsin-plasmin inhibitors from the seminal vesicles of guinea pig. Hoppe-Seylers Z. physiol. Chem. **353**, 19 (1972)

Fritz,H., Gebhardt,M., Meister,R., Fink,E.: Trypsin-plasmin inhibitors from leeches. Isolation, amino acid composition, inhibitory characteristics. In: Fritz,H., Tschesche,E. (Eds.): Proc. Int. Res. Conf. on Proteinase Inhibitors, p. 271. Berlin-New York: De Gruyter 1971

Fritz,H., Hutzel,M., Werle,E.: Über Proteinaseninhibitoren. VI. Zur Identität des Proteinaseninhibitors aus Rinderleber mit dem Trypsin-Kallikrein-Inhibitor (Trasylol). Hoppe-Seylers Z. physiol. Chem. **348**, 950 (1967)

Fritz,H., Oppitz,K.-H., Gebhardt,M., Oppitz,I., Werle,E., Marx,R.: Über das Vorkommen eines Trypsin-Plasmin-Inhibitors in Hirudin. Hoppe-Seylers Z. physiol. Chem. **350**, 91 (1969)

Gallimore,M.J., Nulkar,M.V., Shaw,J.T.B.: A comparative study of the inhibitors of fibrinolysis in human, dog and rabbit blood. Thrombos. Diathes. haemorrh. (Stuttg.) **14**, 145 (1965)

Ganguly,P.: A low molecular weight antiplasmin of human blood platelets. Clin. chim. Acta **39**, 466 (1972)

Ganrot,P.O.: Inhibition of plasmin activity by α_2-macroglobulin. Clin. chim. Acta **16** 328 (1967)

Ganrot,P.O., Scherstén,B.: Serum α_2-macroglobulin concentration and its variation with age and sex. Clin. chim. Acta **15**, 113 (1967)

Glendening,H.B., Page,E.W.: The site of inhibition of blood clotting by soy bean trypsin inhibitor. J. clin. Invest. **30**, 1298 (1951)

Godal,H.C., Theodor,I.: In vitro inhibition of streptokinase-induced proteolysis by trasylol and epsilon aminocaproic acid. Scand. J. clin. Lab. Invest. **17**, Suppl. 84, 199 (1965)

Gormsen,J.: Fibrinolytic activity. Inhibition of plasminogen activation. Acta med. scand. **172**, 657 (1962)

Gormsen,J., Josephsen,P.: The effect of trasylol on blood coagulation after intravenous injection. Thrombos. Diathes. haemorrh. (Stuttg.) **17**, 51 (1967)

Green,N.M.: Kinetics of the reaction between trypsin and the pancreatic trypsin inhibitor. Biochem. J. **66**, 407 (1957)

Green,N.M.: Competition between trypsin inhibitors. J. biol. Chem. **205**, 535 (1963)

Green,N.M., Neurath,H.: Proteolytic enzymes. In: Neurath,H., Bailey,K. (Eds.): The Proteins, Vol. II, Part 25. New York: Academic Press 1954

Green,N.M., Work,E.: Pancreatic trypsin inhibitor, II. Reaction with trypsin. Biochem. J. **54**, 347 (1953)

Greene,L.J., Rickbi,M., Fackre,D.S.: Trypsin inhibitors from bovine pancreatic juice. J. biol. Chem. **241**, 5610 (1966)

Haberland,G.L., Matis,P.: Trasylol, ein Proteinaseninhibitor bei chirurgischen und internen Indikationen. Med. Welt (Stuttg.) **1967**, I, 1367

Haendle, H., Fritz, H., Trautschold, I., Werle, E.: Über einen hormonabhängigen Inhibitor für proteolytische Enzyme in männlichen accessorischen Geschlechtsdrüsen und im Sperma. Hoppe-Seylers Z. physiol. Chem. **343**, 185 (1965)

Harpel, P. C., Cooper, N. R.: Studies on human plasma C1-inactivator-enzyme interactions. I. Mechanisms of interaction with C1s, plasmin, and trypsin. J. clin. Invest. **55**, 593 (1975)

Haupt, H., Heimburger, N., Kranz, T., Schwick, H. G.: Ein Beitrag zur Isolierung und Charakterisierung des C 1-Inaktivators aus Humanplasma. Europ. J. Biochem. **17**, 254 (1970)

Hawkey, Ch. M., Stafford, J. L.: A standard clot method for the assay of plasminogen activators, antiactivators, and plasmin. J. clin. Path. **17**, 175 (1964)

Haynes, R., Feeney, R. E.: Fractionation and properties of trypsin and chymotrypsin inhibitors from Lima beans. J. biol. Chem. **242**, 5378 (1967)

Heide, K., Heimburger, N., Haupt, H.: An inter-alpha trypsin inhibitor of human serum. Clin. chim. Acta **11**, 82 (1965)

Heimburger, N.: On the protease inhibitors of human plasma with especial reference to antithrombin, p. 353. Marburg/Lahn: Behringwerke A.G., 1967

Heimburger, N., Haupt, H.: Charakterisierung von α_1X-Glykoprotein als Chymotrypsin-Inhibitor des Humanplasmas. Clin. chim. Acta **12**, 116 (1965)

Heimburger, N., Haupt, H.: Zur Spezifität der Antiproteinasen des Humanplasmas für Elastase. Klin. Wschr. **44**, 1196 (1966)

Heimburger, N., Haupt, H., Schwick, H. G.: Proteinase inhibitors of human plasma. In: Fritz, H., Tschesche, H. (Eds.): Proc. Int. Res. Conf. on Proteinase Inhibitors, p. 1. Berlin-New York: de Gruyter 1971

Hercz, A.: The inhibition of proteinases by human α_1-antitrypsin. Europ. J. Biochem. **49**, 287 (1974)

Hladovec, J., Horáková, Z., Mansfeld, V.: Die entzündungshemmende Wirkung des Proteasen-Inhibitors aus Kartoffeln bei experimentellen Verbrennungen. Arzneimittel-Forsch. **11**, 104 (1961)

Hladovec, J., Mansfeld, V.: Antifibrinolytische Aktivität des Proteasen-Inhibitors aus Pankreas. Z. ges. inn. Med. **15**, 312 (1960)

Hladovec, J., Mansfeld, V., Horáková, Z.: Antifibrinolytische Aktivität einiger Trypsininhibitoren. Naturwissenschaften **45**, 575 (1958)

Hochstrasser, K., Illchmann, K., Werle, E.: Über pflanzliche Proteaseninhibitoren. VI. Reindarstellung der polyvalenten Proteaseninhibitoren aus Arachis hypogaea. Hoppe-Seylers Z. physiol. Chem. **350**, 929 (1969)

Hochstrasser, K., Werle, E.: Über pflanzliche Proteaseninhibitoren. V. Isolierung und Charakterisierung einiger polyvalenter Proteaseninhibitoren aus Solanum tuberosum. Hoppe-Seylers Z. physiol. Chem. **350**, 897 (1969)

Hoffbauer, H., Dobbeck, P.: Untersuchungen über die Placentapassage des Kallikrein-Inhibitors. Klin. Wschr. **48**, 183 (1970)

Hojima, Y., Moriya, H., Moriwaki, C.: Studies of kallikrein inhibitors in potatoes, partial purification and some properties. J. Biochem. **69**, 1019 (1971)

Huber, R., Bode, W., Kukla, D., Kohl, U.: The structure of the complex formed by bovine trypsin and bovine pancreatic trypsin inhibitor. III. Structure of the anhydro-trypsin-inhibitor complex. Biophys. Struct. Mechanism **1**, 189 (1975)

Huber, R., Kukla, D., Bode, W., Schwager, P., Bartels, K., Deisenhofer, J., Steigemann, W.: Structure of the complex formed by bovine trypsin and bovine pancreatic trypsin inhibitor. II. Crystallographic refinement at 1.9 Å resolution. J. molec. Biol. **89**, 73 (1974)

Hultin, E., Lundblad, G.: Investigations on plasmin. III. On the formation of plasmin from plasminogen. Acta chem. scand. **3**, 620 (1949)

Iwamoto, M., Abiko, Y.: Plasminogen-plasmin system. IV. Preparation of α_2-macroglobulin antiplasmin from human plasma. Biochim. biophys. Acta (Amst.) **214**, 402 (1970)

Jacobsson, K.: Studies on the trypsin and plasmin inhibitors in human blood serum. Scand. J. clin. Lab. Invest. Suppl. **14**, 55 (1955)

Johnson, S. A., Schneider, C. L.: Existence of antifibrinolysin activity in platelets. Science **117**, 229 (1953)

Jones, G., Moore, S., Stein, W.: Properties of chromatographically purified trypsin inhibitors from Lima beans. Biochemistry **2**, 66 (1963)

Kaller, H.: Tierexperimentelle Untersuchungen über die Wirkungsdauer und Elimination von Trasylol. Naunyn-Schmiedeberg's Arch. exp. Path. Pharmak. **246**, 92 (1963)

Kaller, H.: Tierexperimentelle Untersuchungen über die Wirkungsdauer und Elimination von Trasylol. In: Heinkel, K., Schön, H. (Eds.): Pathogenese, Diagnostik, Klinik und Therapie der Erkrankungen des exokrinen Pankreas, p. 307. Stuttgart: Schattauer 1964

Kaller, H.: Pharmakologie des Trasylols. In: Marx, R., Imdahl, H., Haberland, G. L. (Eds.): Neue Aspekte der Trasylol-Therapie, p. 11. Stuttgart-New York: Schattauer, 1968

Kassell, B.: Naturally occurring inhibitors of proteolytic enzymes. In: Colowick, S. P., Kaplan, N. O. (Eds.): Methods in Enzymology, Vol. XIX. Perlmann, G. E., Lorand, L. (Eds.): Proteolytic Enzymes, p. 839. New York-London: Academic Press 1970

Kassell, B., Laskowski, M.: The basic trypsin inhibitor of bovine pancreas. V. The disulfide linkages. Biochem. biophys. Res. Commun. **20**, 463 (1965)

Kassell, B., Laskowski, M.: The basic trypsin inhibitor of bovine pancreas. VI. Sequence studies and disulphide linkages. Acta biochim. polon. **13**, 287 (1966)

Kassell, B., Radicevic, M., Ansfield, M. J., Laskowski, M.: The basic trypsin inhibitor of bovine pancreas. IV. The linear sequence of the 58 amino acids. Biochem. biophys. Res. Commun. **18**, 255 (1965)

Kassell, B., Radicevic, M., Berlow, S., Peanasky, R. I., Laskowski, M.: The basic trypsin inhibitor of bovine pancreas. I. An improved method of preparation and amino acid composition. J. biol. Chem. **238**, 3274 (1963)

Kawano, T., Morimoto, K., Uemura, Y.: Urokinase inhibitor in human placenta. Nature (Lond.) **217**, 253 (1968)

Kawano, T., Morimoto, K., Uemura, Y.: Partial purification and properties of urokinase inhibitor from human placenta. J. Biochem. (Tokyo) **67**, 333 (1970)

Kazal, L. A., Spicer, D. S., Brahinsky, R. A.: Isolation of a crystalline trypsin inhibitor-anticoagulant protein from pancreas. J. Amer. chem. Soc. **70**, 304 (1948)

Kline, D. L., Fishman, J. B.: Plasmin: the humoral protease. Ann. N.Y. Acad, Sci. **68**, 25 (1957)

Kline, D. L., Fishman, J. B.: Proactivator function of human plasmin as shown by lysine esterase assay. J. biol. Chem. **236**, 2807 (1961)

Klöcking, H.-P.: Zum Nachweis der antifibrinolytischen Wirkung des Proteaseninhibitors Contrykal in vivo. Folia haemat. (Lpz.) **88**, 136 (1967)

Klöcking, H.-P., Markwardt, F.: Tierexperimentelle Verfahren zur Testung von Fibrinolytika und Antifibrinolytika. Folia haemat. (Lpz.) **92**, 84 (1969)

Kraut, H., Bhargava, N.: Versuche zur Isolierung des Kallikrein-Inaktivators. V. Isolierung eines Kallikrein-Inaktivators aus Rinderlunge und seine Identifizierung mit dem Inaktivator aus Rinderparotis. Hoppe-Seylers Z. physiol. Chem. **338**, 231 (1964)

Kraut, H., Bhargava, N., Schultz, F., Zimmermann, H.: Versuche zur Isolierung des Kallikrein-Inaktivators. IV. Kristallisation und Aminosäurezusammensetzung. Vergleich mit dem Trypsin-Inhibitor von Kunitz und Northrop. Hoppe-Seylers Z. physiol. Chem. **334**, 230 (1963)

Kraut, H., Körbel-Enkhardt, R.: Versuche zur Isolierung des Kallikrein-Inaktivators. Hoppe-Seylers Z. physiol. Chem. **309**, 243 (1957); **312**, 161 (1958)

Kunitz, M.: Crystalline soybean trypsin inhibitor. J. gen. Physiol. **29**, 149 (1947a)

Kunitz, M.: Crystalline soybean trypsin inhibitor. II. General properties. J. gen. Physiol. **30**, 291 (1947b)

Kunitz, M.: Isolation of a crystalline protein compound of trypsin and of soybean trypsin inhibitor. J. gen. Physiol. **30**, 311 (1947c)

Kunitz, M., Northrop, J. H.: Isolation from beef pancreas of crystalline trypsinogen, trypsin and an inhibitor trypsin compound. J. gen. Physiol. **19**, 991 (1936)

Kunitz, M., Northrop, J. H.: Crystalline soybean trypsin inhibitor. II. General properties. J. gen. Physiol. **30**, 291 (1947)

Lanchantin, G. F., Friedmann, J. A., Hart, D. W.: Interaction of soybean trypsin inhibitor with thrombin and its effect on prothrombin activation. J. biol. Chem. **244**, 865 (1969)

Landmann, H., Markwardt, F., Perlewitz, J.: Die Beeinflussung der Wirkung des Trypsins auf die Blutgerinnung durch natürliche und synthetische Trypsin- und Thrombininhibitoren. Thrombos. Diathes. haemorrh. (Stuttg.) **22**, 552 (1969)

Laskowski, M.: Naturally occurring trypsin inhibitors. In: Colowick, S. P., Kaplan, N. O. (Eds.): Methods in Enzymology. Vol. II. Preparation and Assay of Enzymes, p. 36. New York: Academic Press 1955

Laskowski, M., Kassell, B., Peanasky, R. J., Laskowski, M.: Endopeptidases. In: Lang, K., Lehnartz, E. (Eds.): Hoppe-Seyler/Thierfelder Handbuch der physiologisch- und pathologisch-chemischen Analyse. 10th Ed. Vol. VI C, p. 256. Berlin-Heidelberg-New York: Springer, 1966

Laskowski, M., Laskowski, M. Jr.: Naturally occurring trypsin inhibitors. Advanc. Protein Chem. **9**, 203 (1954)

Lewis, J. H., Ferguson, J. H.: Studies on a proteolytic enzyme system of the blood. I. Inhibition of fibrinolysis. J. clin. Invest. **29**, 486 (1950)

Lewis, J. H., Ferguson, J. H.: Studies on a proteolytic enzyme system of the blood. IV. Activation of profibrinolysin by serum fibrinolysokinase. Proc. Soc. exp. Biol. (N.Y.) **78**, 184 (1951)

Lewis, J. H., Ferguson, J. H.: The inhibition of fibrinolysin by Lima bean inhibitor. J. biol. Chem. **204**, 503 (1953)

Liener, E.: The intraperitoneal toxicity of concentrates of the soybean trypsin inhibitor. J. biol. Chem. **193**, 189 (1951)

Lorand, L., Condit, E. V.: Ester hydrolysis by urokinase. Biochemistry **4**, 265 (1965)

Ludwig, H.: Mikrozirkulationsstörungen und Diapedeseblutungen im fetalen Gehirn bei Hypoxie. Bibl. gynaec. (Basel) **46**, 1 (1968)

MacFarlane, R. G., Pilling, J.: Anticoagulant action of soya-bean trypsin inhibitor. Lancet **1946 II**, 888

Maki, M., Beller, F. K.: Comparative studies of fibrinolytic inhibitors in vitro. Thrombos. Diathes. haemorrh. (Stuttg.) **16**, 668 (1966)

Mansfeld, V., Rybak, M., Horáková, Z., Hladovec, J.: Die antitryptische, antifibrinolytische und antiphlogistische Aktivität natürlicher Proteasen-Inhibitoren. Hoppe-Seylers Z. physiol. Chem. **318**, 6 (1960)

Mansfeld, V., Ziegelhöfer, A., Horáková, Z., Hladovec, J.: Isolierung der Trypsin-Inhibitoren aus einigen Hülsenfrüchten. Naturwissenschaften **46**, 172 (1959)

Markwardt, F., Haustein, K.-O., Klöcking, H.-P.: Die pharmakologische Charakterisierung des neuen Antifibrinolytikums p-Aminomethylbenzoesäure (PAMBA). Arch. int. Pharmacodyn. **152**, 223 (1964)

Markwardt, F., Klöcking, H.-P.: Über das Stoffwechselschicksal der p-Aminomethylbenzoesäure (PAMBA) beim Menschen. Acta biol. med. germ. **14**, 519 (1965)

Markwardt, F., Klöcking, H.-P., Haustein, K.-O., Perlewitz, J.: Tierexperimentelle Untersuchungen über die Wirkung eines Proteaseninhibitors aus Rinderlunge. Acta biol. med. germ. **16**, 15 (1966)

Markwardt, F., Landmann, H.: Blutgerinnungshemmende Proteine, Peptide und Aminosäurederivate. In: Heffter, A., Heubner, W. (Eds.): Handbuch der experimentellen Pharmakologie, Vol. 27, p. 76. Markwardt, F. (Ed.): Anticoagulantien. Berlin-Heidelberg-New York: Springer, 1971

Markwardt, F., Landmann, H., Klöcking, H.-P.: Fibrinolytika und Antifibrinolytika. Jena: Fischer, 1972

Markwardt, F., Richter, M.: Zur Standardisierung des Proteaseninhibitors aus Rinderorganen. Pharmazie **24**, 620 (1969)

Markwardt, F., Walsmann, P.: Zur quantitativen Bestimmung von Proteaseninhibitoren. Pharmazie **19**, 453 (1964)

Marx, R.: Kallikreininhibitoren als Gerinnungshemmstoffe. In: Marx, R., Imdahl, H., Haberland, G. L. (Eds.): Neue Aspekte der Trasylol-Therapie, p. 89. Stuttgart-New York: Schattauer 1968

Marx, R., Clemente, P., Werle, E., Appel, W.: Zum Problem eines Antidots in der internen Therapie mit Fibrinolytika. Blut **5**, 367 (1959)

Marx, R., Clemente, P., Werle, E., Appel, W.: Über die Wirkung von Proteaseninhibitor-Präparaten (Leber- und Parotisinhibitor) auf die extravasale Fibrinolyse und Blutgerinnungskonstanten im Menschenblut. Blut **9**, 164 (1963)

Matis, P., Mörl, F. K.: Effect of proteinase inhibition on blood coagulation, fibrinolysis and wound healing in patients during and after surgery. Ann. N.Y. Acad. Sci. **146**, 715 (1968)

Maxwell, R. E., Lewandowski, V., Nickel, V. S.: Enhancement of fibrinolysis and antagonism of antiplasmin by reversible plasmin inhibitors. Life Sci. **4**, 45 (1965)

Mehl, J. W., O'Connell, W., de Grott, J.: Macroglobulin from human plasma which forms an enzymatically active component with trypsin. Science **145**, 821 (1964)

Mendel, L. D., Blood, A. F.: Trypsin inhibitors. J. biol. Chem. **8**, 177 (1910)

Moll, F. C., Sunden, S. F., Brown, J. R.: Partial purification of the serum trypsin inhibitor. J. biol. Chem. **233**, 121 (1958)

Mörl, F. K.: Klinik der Proteaseninhibitoren in der Chirurgie. Ergebnisse einer alternierenden Applikation des Proteinaseninhibitors Trasylol. Thrombos. Diathes. haemorrh. (Stuttg.) Suppl. **31** (1968)

Nanninga, L. B., Guest, M. M.: On the interaction of fibrinolysin (plasmin) with the inhibitors antifibrinolysin and soybean trypsin inhibitor. Arch. Biochem. **108**, 542 (1964)

Nilsson, I. M., Krook, H., Sternby, N. H., Söderberg, E., Söderstrom, N.: Severe thrombotic disease in a young man with bone marrow and sceletal changes and with a high content of an inhibitor of the fibrinolytic system. Acta med. scand. **169**, 323 (1961)

Noordhoek Hegt, V., Brakman, P.: Inhibition of fibrinolysis by the human vascular wall related to the presence of smooth muscle cells. Haemostasis **3**, 118 (1974)

Nordström, S., Olsson, P., Blombäck, M.: On the antithromboplastic activity of Trasylol. In: Gross, R., Kroneberg, G. (Eds.): Neue Aspekte der Trasylol-Therapie. Stuttgart: Schattauer 1966, p. 44

Norman, P. S.: Studies of the plasmin system. II. Inhibition of plasmin by serum or plasma. J. exp. Med. **108**, 53 (1958)

Norman, P. S., Hill, B. M.: Studies of the plasmin system. III. Physical properties of the two plasmin inhibitors in plasma. J. exp. Med. **108**, 639 (1958)

Ottolander, G. J. H. den, Leijnse, B., Cremer-Elfrink, H. M. J.: Plasmatic and platelet anti-plasmins and anti-activators. Thrombos. Diathes. haemorrh. (Stuttg.) **18**, 404 (1967)

Ottolander, G. J. H. den, Leijnse, B., Cremer-Elfrink, H. M. J.: Plasmatic and thrombocytic antiplasmins and anti-activators. II. Thrombos. Diathes. haemorrh. (Stuttg.) **21**, 26 (1969a)

Ottolander, G. J. H. den, Leijnse, B., Cremer-Elfrink, H. M. J.: Plasmatic and platelet anti-plasmins and anti-activators. III. Results in normal people, in patients and in those with venous thrombosis. Thrombos. Diathes. haemorrh. (Stuttg.) **21**, 35 (1969b)

Paraskevas, M., Nilsson, I. M., Martinsson, G.: A method for determining serum inhibitors of plasminogen activation. Scand. J. clin. Lab. Invest. **14**, 138 (1962)

Pütter, J.: Zur Kinetik der Reaktion zwischen dem Kallikrein-Inaktivator und Trypsin. Hoppe-Seylers Z. physiol. Chem. **348**, 1197 (1967)

Rabek, V., Mansfeld, V.: Gefiltration von Protease-Inhibitoren der Kartoffel. Experientia (Basel) **19**, 151 (1963)

Reichenbach-Klinke, K. E., Meckl, D., Kemkes, B., Hochstrasser, K., Fritz, H., Werle, E.: Die Fixierung und Veränderung eines Proteinasenhemmstoffes in der Niere. Arzneimittel-Forsch. **19**, 1025 (1969)

Richter, M.: Die Bestimmung natürlicher Proteaseninhibitoren im biologischen Material. Folia haemat. (Lpz.) **88**, 130 (1967)

Rimon, A., Shamash, J., Shapiro, B.: The plasmin inhibitor of human plasma. IV. Its action on plasmin, trypsin, chymotrypsin, and thrombin. J. biol. Chem. **241**, 5102 (1966)

Rowley, P. T., Oette, D.: Characteristics of the antitrypsin activity of human serum. J. clin. Path. **26**, 48 (1973)

Rush, B., Cliffton, E. E.: Control of proteolytic activity in serum: effect of soybean inhibitor in vivo in the mouse. Amer. J. Physiol. **166**, 485 (1951)

Schmitz, A.: Über die Freilegung von aktivem Trypsin aus Blutplasma. Zweite Mitteilung zur Kenntnis des Plasmatrypsinsystems. Hoppe-Seylers Z. physiol. Chem. **250**, 37 (1937)

Schmutzler, R.: Spontanfibrinolysen und Hemmwirkung von Epsilon-Amino-Capronsäure und Trasylol. Folia haemat. (Frankf.) **8**, 33 (1963)

Schmutzler, R., Beck, E.: Die Wirkung von ε-Aminocapronsäure und Trasylol auf die Fibrinolyse. Schweiz. med. Wschr. **92**, 1368 (1962)

Scholtan, W., Lie, S. Y.: Molekulargewichtsbestimmung des Kallikrein-Inaktivators mittels der Ultrazentrifuge. Makromolek. Chem. **98**, 204 (1966)

Scholtan, W., Rosenkranz, H.: Optisches Drehungsvermögen. Circulardichroismus und Ultraviolett-Spektrum des Kallikrein-Inaktivators. Makromolek. Chem. **99**, 254 (1966)

Schultz, F.: Kristallisation des Kallikrein-Trypsin-Inhibitors als freies basisches Polypeptid. Naturwissenschaften **54**, 338 (1967)

Schultze, H. E., Heide, K., Haupt, H.: α_1-Antitrypsin aus Humanserum. Klin. Wschr. **40**, 427 (1962)

Schultze, H. E., Heimburger, N., Heide, K., Haupt, H., Störiko, K., Schwick, H. G.: Preparation and characterization of α_1-trypsin inhibitor and α_2-plasmin inhibitor of human serum. In: Proc. IXth Congr. Europ. Soc. Haemat., p. 1315. Basel-New York: Karger 1963

Schwick, H. G.: Biochemie der Fibrinolyse. Thrombos. Diathes. haemorrh. (Stuttg.) Suppl. **22**, 7 (1967)

Schwick, H. G., Heimburger, N., Haupt, H.: Antiproteinasen des Humanserums. Z. ges. inn. Med. **21**, 193 (1966)

Shamash, Y., Rimon, A.: The plasmin inhibitors of plasma. I. A method for their estimation. Thrombos. Diathes. haemorrh. (Stuttg.) **12**, 119 (1964)

Shulman, N. R.: Studies on the inhibition of proteolytic enzymes by serum. III. Physiological aspects of variation in proteolytic inhibition. The concurrence of changes in fibrinogen concentration with changes in trypsin inhibition. J. exp. Med. **95**, 605 (1952)

Soulier, J. P., Prou-Wartelle, O., Dormont, J.: Etude de divers inhibiteurs d'enzymes protéolytiques sur la coagulation et la fibrinolyse. Rev. Hémat. **15**, 431 (1960)

Spritz, N., Cameron, D. J.: Streptokinase induced lysine-methyl-esterase activity of human euglobulin. Proc. Soc. exp. Biol. (N.Y.) **109**, 848 (1962)

Stamm, H.: Einführung in die Klinik der Fibrinolyse. Basel-New York: Karger, 1962

Stefanini, M., Murphy, I. S.: Human platelets as source of antifibrinolysin. J. clin. Invest. **35**, 355 (1956)

Steichele, D. F., Herschlein, H. J.: Zur antifibrinolytischen Wirkung des Trypsin-Kallikrein Inaktivators. Med. Welt (Stuttg.) **1961**, II, 2170

Steinbuch, M., Audran, R., Reuge, C., Blatrix, Ch.: Etude d'une α-globuline contenant du zinc: la protéine Π. Prot. Biol. Fluids **14**, 185 (1966)

Steinbuch, M., Blatrix, C.: Action anti-protéase de l'α_2-macroglobuline. I. Activités antiplasmine et antitrypsine. Rev. franç. Et. clin. biol. **13**, 142 (1968)

Steinbuch, M., Blatrix, C., Drouet, J., Amouch, P.: Study of the α_2-macroglobulin/plasmin interaction mechanism. Path. Biol. Suppl. **20**, 50 (1972)

Steinbuch, M., Loeb, J.: Isolation of an α_2-globulin from human plasma. Nature (Lond.) **192**, 1196 (1961)

Steinbuch, M., Quentin, M., Peioudier, L.: Specific technique for the isolation of human α_2-macroglobulin. Nature (Lond.) **205**, 1225 (1965)

Tagnon, H. J., Soulier, J. P.: Anticoagulant activity of the trypsin inhibitor from soya bean flour. Proc. Soc. exp. Biol. (N.Y.) **61**, 440 (1946)

Tagnon, H. J., Soulier, J. P.: The effect of intravenous injection of trypsin inhibitor on the coagulation of blood. Blood **3**, 1161 (1948)

Telesforo, P., Semeraro, N., Verstraete, M., Collen, D.: The inhibition of plasmin by antithrombin III-heparin complex in vitro in human plasma and during streptokinase therapy in man. Thrombos. Res. **7**, 669 (1975)

Trautschold, I., Werle, E.: Spektrophotometrische Bestimmung des Kallikreins und seiner Inaktivatoren. Hoppe-Seylers Z. physiol. Chem. **325**, 48 (1961)

Trautschold, I., Werle, E., Fritz, H.: Zur Biochemie des Transylol. In: Gross, R., Kroneberg, G. (Eds.): Neue Aspekte der Trasylol-Therapie, p. 3. Stuttgart: Schattauer 1966

Trautschold, I., Werle, E., Händle, H., Sebening, H.: Neuere experimentelle Ergebnisse über Proteaseninhibitoren. Schicksal des Kallikrein-Trypsin-Inaktivators (Trasylol) nach i.v. Injektion. In: Heinkel, K., Schön, H. (Eds.): Pathogenese, Diagnostik, Klinik und Therapie der Erkrankungen des exokrinen Pankreas, p. 289. Stuttgart: Schattauer 1964

Trautschold, I., Werle, E., Zickgraf-Rüdel, G.: Über den Kallikrein-Trypsin-Inhibitor. Arzneimittel-Forsch. **16**, 1507 (1966)

Trautschold, I., Werle, E., Zickgraf-Rüdel, G.: Trasylol. Biochem. Pharmacol. **16**, 59 (1967)

Ts'ao, C. H., Kline, D. L.: Plasminogen activator by reaction of streptokinase with human plasminogen. J. appl. Physiol. **26**, 634 (1969)

Tschesche, H.: Biochemie natürlicher Proteinase-Inhibitoren. Angew. Chem. **86**, 21 (1974)

Tschesche, H., Dietl, T.: Broad-specificity protease isoinhibitors for trypsin, chymotrypsin, plasmin and kallikrein from snails (Helix pomatia). Isolation, inhibition, characteristic and amino acid composition. Europ. J. Biochem. **30**, 560 (1972)

Tschesche, H., Dietl, T., Marx, R., Fritz, H.: Neue polyvalente Proteasen-Inhibitoren für Trypsin, Chymotrypsin, Plasmin und Kallikrein aus der Weinbergschnecke (Helix pomatia). Hoppe-Seylers Z. physiol. Chem. **353**, 483 (1972)

Uszynski, M., Abildgaard, U.: Separation and characterization of two fibrinolytic inhibitors from human placenta. Thrombos. Diathes. haemorrh. (Stuttg.) **25**, 580 (1971)

Uszynski, M., Uszynski-Folejewska, R.: Plasminogen activator and urokinase inhibitor in myometrium, placenta and amniotic fluid. Amer. J. Obstet. Gynec. **105**, 1041 (1969)

Vairel, E., Choay, J.: Mise en évidence d'une activité inhibitrice de l'inhibiteur de Kunitz sur une fibrinolyse expérimentale. Sem. Hôp. Paris **36**, 675 (1960)

Vairel, E., Thely, M.: Inhibiteur de trypsine de Kunitz, inhibiteur de la fibrinolyse. Ann. Biol. clin. **18**, 363 (1960)

Vogel, R., Trautschold, I., Werle, E.: Natürliche Proteinasen-Inhibitoren. In: Weitzel, G., Zöllner, N. (Eds.): Biochemie und Klinik. Stuttgart: Thieme 1966

Vogel, R., Trautschold, I., Werle, E.: Natural Proteinase Inhibitors. New York and London: Pergamon Press, 1968

Vogel, R., Werle, E.: Kallikrein inhibitors. In: Heffter, A., Heubner, W. (Eds.): Handbuch der experimentellen Pharmakologie, Vol. XXV, p. 213. Erdös, E. G., Wilde, A. F. (Eds.): Bradykinin, Kallidin and Kallikrein. Berlin-Heidelberg-New York: Springer 1970

Walton, P. L.: The hydrolysis of α-N-acetylglycyl-L-lysine methyl ester by urokinase. Biochim. biophys. Acta (Amst.) **132**, 104 (1967)

Weinland, E.: Über Antifermente. Z. Biol. **44**, 1 (1903)

Werle, E.: Zur Biochemie des Trasylol. In: Haberland, G. L., Matis, P. (Eds.): Neue Aspekte der Trasylol-Therapie, p. 49. Stuttgart-New York: Schattauer 1969

Werle, E., Maier, L.: Zur Kenntnis des Kallikrein-Inaktivators aus Kartoffeln. Biochem. Z. **322**, 414 (1952)

Werle, E., Marx, R., Trautschold, I., Reichenbach-Klinke, K.-E.: Vergleich der Proteinasen-Inhibitoren aus Lunge und Leber vom Rind mit besonderer Berücksichtigung ihres Einflusses auf Fibrinolyse und Blutgerinnung. Blut **14**, 206 (1967)

Werle, E., Zickgraf-Rüdel, G.: Natural proteinase inhibitors. Distribution, specificity, mode of action, and physiological significance. Z. klin. Chem. **10**, 139 (1972)

Synthetic Inhibitors of Fibrinolysis

F. MARKWARDT

Until relatively recent times the control of hemorrhage was restricted to simple, often inadequate local measures. With the elucidation of the mechanisms of blood coagulation and the progress in plasma fractionation the treatment of certain hemorrhagic diatheses became possible by rational substitution of deficient clotting factors. This form of treatment, however, was ineffective in bleeding caused by enhanced fibrinolytic activity of the blood. Such hyperfibrinolytic states may lead to severe and frequently uncontrollable hemorrhage arising from complex disturbances of hemostasis.

The proteolytic activity of the fibrinolytic enzyme plasmin may reduce the levels of clotting factors V and VIII and, more importantly, fibrinogen. The cross-linking regions of the α-chains of fibrinogen are digested resulting in inhibition of normal fibrin polymerization. Fibrinogen degradation products (FDP) from plasmin digestion are of growing importance. The activities attributed to FDP include anticoagulation, an ability to form complexes with fibrinogen and fibrin monomer, and the production of platelet defects.

After the pathogenetic role of excessive fibrinolysis had been clarified, it was attempted to control fibrinolytic processes with inhibitors. Since the naturally occurring inhibitors of fibrinolysis are high molecular weight polypeptides, their therapeutic use is limited. Therefore, extensive searches were made for low molecular weight synthetic inhibitors suitable for therapy. These studies led to the development of a new class of drugs, the antifibrinolytics.

To describe the therapeutically used inhibitors of fibrinolysis, it is necessary to distinguish this class of antifibrinolytics from other inhibitors whose action is only of theoretical interest. The category of synthetic antifibrinolytics in clinical use consists of the registered preparations ε-aminocaproic acid (EACA), p-aminomethylbenzoic acid (PAMBA) and trans-4-aminomethylcyclohexanecarboxylic acid-(1) (AMCA), which are reported in detail.

A. Chemistry

I. ε-Aminocaproic Acid

As long as 20 years ago, searches for a substance with antifibrinolytic properties had been made by the OKAMOTO group. Studies on numerous compounds with different chemical structures revealed the antifibrinolytic action of certain mercapto and aminocarboxylic acids (OKAMOTO, 1959, 1960a, b). Among the latter compounds, ε-aminocaproic acid (EACA) was found to be the most effective one (OKAMOTO et al.,

Table 1. Synthetic antifibrinolytics

---

1. ε-Aminocaproic acid (EACA)
   $H_2N—CH_2—CH_2—CH_2—CH_2—CH_2—COOH$
   Empirical formula: $C_6H_{13}O_2N$ Molecular weight: 131.2
   White, odorless crystalline powder or white leaflets of slightly bitter taste. Freely soluble in water, sparingly soluble in ethanol. Practically insoluble in ether and chloroform.
   Melting point: 204–206° C

2. 4-Aminomethylbenzoic acid (PAMBA)
   Empirical formula: $C_8H_9O_2N$ Molecular weight: 151.2
   White, odorless crystalline powder of slightly bitter taste. Solubility in water at 24° C = 1.5%, at 100° C = 4%

3. trans-4-Aminomethylcyclohexanecarboxylic acid-(1) (AMCA)
   Empirical formula: $C_8H_{15}O_2N$ Molecular weight: 157.2
   White, odorless crystalline powder of slightly bitter taste, freely soluble in water and alkalies, insoluble in absolute alcohol, acetone and ether.

Table 2. Antifibrinolytic effect of derivatives of EACA

Compound		Antifibrinolytic activity (%)[a]
$H_2N—(CH_2)_5—COOH$	ε-Aminocaproic acid	100
Substitution at the amino group:		
$CH_3CONH—(CH_2)_5—COOH$	ε-N-Acetylaminocaproic acid	1
$(CH_3)_2N—(CH_2)_5 - COOH$	ε-N-Dimethylaminocaproic acid	2
$H_2N—CH_2—CONH—(CH_2)_5—COOH$	ε-N-Glycylaminocaproic acid	1
$C_6H_5CONH—(CH_2)_5—COOH$	ε-N-Benzoylaminocaproic acid	1
HN ‖ C—NH—(CH_2)_5—COOH ∕ H_2N	ε-Guanidinocaproic acid	1
Substitution at the carboxyl group:		
$H_2N—(CH_2)_5—COOCH_3$	ε-Aminocaproic acid methyl ester	13
$H_2N—(CH_2)_5—COOCH_2—CH_3$	ε-Aminocaproic acid ethyl ester	11
$H_2N—(CH_2)_5—COOCH_2—CH_2—CH_3$	ε-Aminocaproic acid propyl ester	13
$H_2N—(CH_2)_5—COOCH(CH_3)CH_3$	ε-Aminocaproic acid isopropyl ester	3
$H_2N—(CH_2)_5—CONH_2$	ε-Aminocaproic acid amide	1
$H_2N—(CH_2)_5—CONH—NH_2$	ε-Aminocaproic acid hydrazide	1

[a] To compare the antifibrinolytic activity of the inhibitors, their inhibitory action on the fibrinolytic processes measured by plasma lysis test was used. Inhibitor concentrations were determined, which prolong the normal lysis time 3-fold, and compared to that of EACA.

1959). This easily synthetizable substance of low toxicity (Table 1) was employed in Japan in the therapy of pathological fibrinolysis (SATO, 1954; ABE and SATO, 1958; MIKATA et al., 1969). In subsequent years, EACA was used therapeutically also in other parts of the world. It was the first representative of a new class of drugs, the antifibrinolytics.

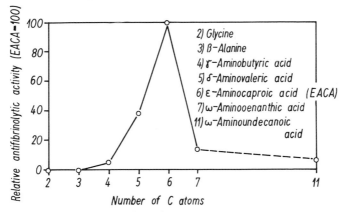

Fig. 1. Antifibrinolytic activity of ω-amino acids

The first potent synthetic fibrinolytic inhibitor was also the agent which had been studied most intensively in vitro and in vivo. The white crystalline substance is freely soluble in water. Its properties and those of the other antifibrinolytic agents are listed in Table 1.

Studies on the relationship between chemical structure and antifibrinolytic activity of EACA (LANDMANN and MARKWARDT, 1963; LOHMANN et al., 1963, 1964; MARKWARDT et al., 1963, 1964; OKAMOTO and HIJIKATA, 1975) have shown that the free amino and carboxylic groups are structural requirements for antifibrinolytic activity (Table 2). Substitution on one or the other group leads to a loss of activity. Esterification of the carboxylic group causes a significant reduction in activity (NAGAMATSU et al., 1963; MURAMATU et al., 1965a, b; IWAMOTO et al., 1968; IWAMOTO and ABIKO, 1969). Studies on homologous aminocarboxylic acids showed that the antifibrinolytic activity depends decisively on the chain length and thus on the distance between the essential amino and carboxylic groups (SJOERDSMA and NILSSON, 1960; LOHMANN et al., 1963). Compounds with longer or shorter aliphatic chains than that of EACA are less potent (Fig. 1).

II. Cyclic Aminocarboxylic Acids

The study of the antifibrinolytic activity of a series of cyclic compounds with terminal amino or carboxylic groups (Table 3) led to the identification of p-aminomethylbenzoic acid (PAMBA) a compound far more potent than EACA (LOHMANN et al., 1963, 1964; LANDMANN and MARKWARDT, 1964; MARKWARDT et al., 1964; MARKWARDT, 1965). Other compounds with an aromatic amino group or a changed distance between the amino or carboxylic groups did not attain the inhibitory activity of EACA.

The antifibrinolytic activity of 4-aminomethylcyclohexanecarboxylic acid-(1) (AMCHA) was discovered at the same time (OKAMOTO and OKAMOTO, 1962; OSHIBA and OKAMOTO, 1962). This compound, a mixture of several stereoisomers, is less potent than PAMBA. However, its antifibrinolytic activity resides in a defined stereoisomeric form which amounts to 20–25% of the isomers. By separation of stereoisomers, a potent inhibitor of fibrinolysis, trans-4-aminomethylcyclo-

Table 3. Antifibrinolytic effect of cyclic aminocarboxylic acids

Compound		Antifibrinolytic activity (%)
H_2N—$(CH_2)_5$—COOH	ε-Aminocaproic acid (EACA)	100
H_2N—⟨benzene⟩—COOH	4-Aminobenzoic acid	0
H_2N—⟨H cyclohexane⟩—COOH	4-Aminocyclohexanecarboxylic acid-(1)	10
H_2N—CH_2—⟨benzene⟩—COOH	4-Aminomethylbenzoic acid (PAMBA)	500
H_2N—CH_2—⟨H cyclohexane⟩—COOH	cis/trans-4-Aminomethyl-cyclohexanecarboxylic acid-(1) (AMCHA)	400
H_2N—CH_2—⟨cyclohexane⟩—COOH	trans-4-Aminomethyl-cyclohexanecarboxylic acid-(1) (AMCA)	1000
H_2N—CH_2—CH_2—⟨benzene⟩—COOH	4-Aminoethylbenzoic acid	15
H_2N—CH_2—CH_2—⟨H cyclohexane⟩—COOH	4-Aminoethylcyclohexane-carboxylic acid-(1)	60
H_2N—⟨benzene⟩—CH_2—COOH	4-Aminophenylacetic acid	0
H_2N—⟨H cyclohexane⟩—CH_2—COOH	4-Aminocyclohexane-acetic acid	45
H_2N—CH_2—⟨benzene⟩—CH_2—COOH	4-Aminomethylphenyl-acetic acid	10
H_2N—CH_2—⟨H cyclohexane⟩—CH_2—COOH	4-Aminomethylcyclohexane-acetic acid	70

hexanecarboxylic acid-(1) (AMCA, trans-AMCHA) was isolated (DUBBER et al., 1964, 1965; OKAMOTO et al., 1964; MARKWARDT et al., 1966; NAITO et al., 1968; SHIMIZU et al., 1968) (for chemical properties see Table 1).

Subsequently, bicyclic and polycyclic aminocarboxylic acids were synthetized and their action on the fibrinolytic process was evaluated (BAUMGARTEN et al., 1969; LOEFFLER et al., 1970). In these studies, 4-aminomethyl-bicyclo-2,2,2-octane carboxylic acid (AMBOCA) was shown to possess a strong antifibrinolytic activity. It represents the most potent synthetic inhibitor of fibrinolysis which is presently known.

Studies on the antifibrinolytic activity of several derivatives of PAMBA (Table 4) revealed that substitution on the free carboxylic and amino groups caused an inactivation of the inhibitor, as was shown in the case of EACA (MARKWARDT and RICHTER, 1964). Similar to EACA esters, a weak residual activity remained when PAMBA was esterified. Both terminal functions of the PAMBA molecule essential for its inhibitory activity cannot be completely replaced by other basic or acidic groups. Furthermore, the antifibrinolytic action depends on the position of the aminomethyl and carboxylic groups on the ring. In case of substitution on the ring or on the methyl group, an essential part of the antifibrinolytic activity of PAMBA was retained. Moreover, a number of esters of AMCA were synthetized and exam-

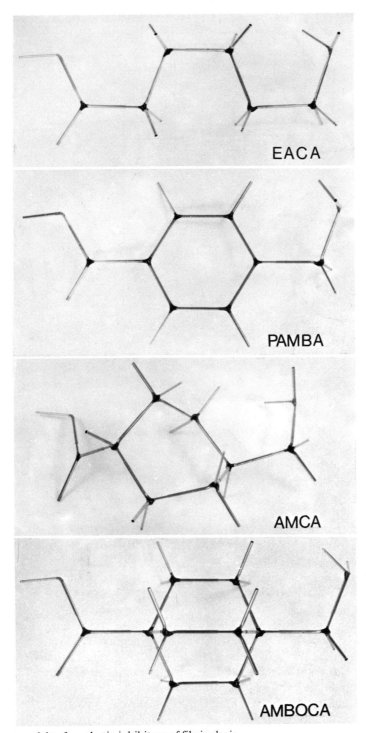

Fig. 2. Stereo models of synthetic inhibitors of fibrinolysis

Table 4. Influence of chemical changes of the PAMBA molecule on the antifibrinolytic activity

Compound	PAMBA derivative	Antifibrinolytic activity (%)[a]
$H_2N—CH_2—\langle\ \rangle—COOH$	PAMBA	100

Substitution at the carboxylic group:

$H_2N—CH_2—\langle\ \rangle—COO—CH_3$	PAMBA methyl ester	5
$H_2N—CH_2—\langle\ \rangle—COO—C_2H_5$	PAMBA ethyl ester	5
$H_2N—CH_2—\langle\ \rangle—CONH_2$	PAMBA amide	7

Substitution of the carboxylic group:

$H_2N—CH_2—\langle\ \rangle—SO_3H$	4-Aminomethylbenzene-sulphonic acid	10

Decarboxylation:

$H_2N—CH_2—\langle\ \rangle$	Benzylamine	1

Substitution at the amino group:

$H_3C—CO—HN—CH_2—\langle\ \rangle—COOH$	N-Acetyl-PAMBA	1
$(CH_3)_2N—CH_2—\langle\ \rangle—COOH$	N-Dimethyl-PAMBA	1
$H_2N—CO—HN—CH_2—\langle\ \rangle—COOH$	Carbamyl-PAMBA	1
$\begin{array}{c} H_2N \\ \diagdown \\ C—HN—CH_2—\langle\ \rangle—COOH \\ \diagup \\ HN \end{array}$	4-Guanidinomethyl-benzoic acid	1

[a] Compared to PAMBA

ined. Results obtained in vitro were very promising (Okano et al., 1972). However, these esters are quite susceptible to enzymatic esterolysis, rapidly yielding AMCA in vivo.

Studies on structure-activity relationships of synthetic antifibrinolytics allowed the assumption that the antifibrinolytic activity of these compounds is bound to their free amino and carboxylic groups which must have a defined distance between each other. As measured on stereo models (Fig. 2), in the ε-aminocaproic acid molecule the distance between the amino and carboxylic groups approximates 7 Å when the molecule is present in stretched form. Such a conformation of EACA can exist due to the flexibility of the CH_2 chain skeleton of the EACA molecule. However, in the statistical sense not every molecule of EACA takes this active conformation, which may be the reason for EACA having less inhibitory activity than PAMBA.

Table 4 (continued)

Compound	PAMBA derivative	Antifibrinolytic activity (%)[a]
Substitution of the aminomethyl group:		
H_2N–C(=NH)–⟨benzene⟩–COOH	4-Amidinobenzoic acid	18
H_2N–C(=NH)–HN–⟨benzene⟩–COOH	4-Guanidinobenzoic acid	2
Deamination:		
H_3C–⟨benzene⟩–COOH	4-Toluic acid	1
Substitution at the methylene group:		
H_2N–CH(CH_3)–⟨benzene⟩–COOH	4-(α-Amino)-ethylbenzoic acid	50
H_2N–CH(CH_2–CH_3)–⟨benzene⟩–COOH	4-(α-Amino)-propylbenzoic acid	25
Substitution on the ring:		
H_2N–CH_2–⟨benzene, OH⟩–COOH	2-Hydroxy-PAMBA	35
H_2N–CH_2–⟨benzene, O_2N⟩–COOH	3-Nitro-PAMBA	45
Changed position on the ring:		
H_2N–CH_2–⟨benzene⟩–COOH	3-Aminomethylbenzoic acid	3

The distance between both essential groups in the relatively rigid PAMBA molecule also amounts to about 7 Å. The same distance exists in 4-aminomethyl-cyclohexanecarboxylic acid-(1) when the molecule is present in chair form, and when the aminomethyl and carboxylic groups are positioned equatorially to the ring. In confirmation of earlier assumptions (LOHMANN et al., 1964; MARKWARDT et al., 1964), this form of AMCHA (trans-4-aminomethylcyclohexanecarboxylic acid-(1) = AMCA) with the specified distance between the amino and carboxylic groups was found to be the antifibrinolytically active one (ANDERSSON et al., 1965; HASSEL and GROTH, 1965). A similar distance between these groups also exists in the molecule of 4-aminomethylbicyclo-2,2,2-octane carboxylic acid.

The higher potency of the cyclic compound (in comparison with EACA) can likely be explained by the fixation of the distance of about 7 Å between the amino

Table 5. Antifibrinolytic effect of benzamidine derivatives

Compound		Antifibrinolytic activity (%)
H₂N—CH₂—⟨⟩—COOH	PAMBA	100
Benzamidine structure	Benzamidine	2
4-Aminobenzamidine structure	4-Aminobenzamidine	4
4-Amidinobenzoic acid benzyl ester structure	4-Amidinobenzoic acid benzyl ester	7
4-Amidinobenzoic acid structure	4-Amidinobenzoic acid	18
β-Naphthamidine structure	β-Naphthamidine	20
4-Amidinophenylpyruvic acid structure	4-Amidinophenylpyruvic acid	50

and carboxylic groups because of its more rigid molecular structure. The other aromatic and hydroaromatic compounds are hardly able to adjust to this distance, because they are required to turn to an energetically unfavorable conformation.

III. Derivatives of Benzamidine

Investigations of synthetic inhibitors of proteolytic enzymes revealed that derivatives of benzylamine, phenylguanidine and benzamidine are competitive inhibitors of trypsin (INAGAMI, 1964; MIX et al., 1965, 1968; GERATZ, 1966, 1967, 1969a; BAKER,

1967; BAKER and ERICKSON, 1967, 1968; LANDMANN et al., 1967). Because of the similarity in substrate specificity between trypsin and plasmin, these compounds as analogues of synthetic substrates are also effective against plasmin and other enzymes with trypsin-like specificity (MARES-GUIA and SHAW, 1965; MARKWARDT et al., 1968, 1970a, b, c, 1971a, b; MARKWARDT and WALSMANN, 1968; CHASE and SHAW, 1969; GERATZ, 1969b, 1970; WALSMANN and MARKWARDT, 1969; LANDMANN, 1970; LANDMANN and MARKWARDT, 1970; WALSMANN et al., 1972). Among these compounds, some derivatives of benzamidine possess sufficient antifibrinolytic activity. The relationships between the structure of the inhibitors and their action on plasmin were reported (MARKWARDT and LANDMANN, 1972; MARKWARDT et al., 1973, 1974; STÜRZEBECHER et al., 1974, 1976a, b; WALSMANN et al., 1974, 1975, 1976a, b, c). The antifibrinolytic activity of some benzamidine derivatives is shown in Table 5. These inhibitors do not reach the antifibrinolytic activity of PAMBA. Of special interest is 4-amidinophenylpyruvic acid (APPA) whose inhibitory effect on plasmin and thrombin was reported by MARKWARDT et al. (1970). When fibrin was used as substrate, a 50% inhibition was obtained with 0.08 mM for plasmin. In vivo, the intravenous and oral administration of APPA to rabbits blocked the effect due to streptokinase infusion (MARKWARDT, 1972). Aromatic bisamidine derivatives were reported which also cause a strong inhibition of fibrinolysis (GERATZ, 1970, 1971, 1973; WALSMANN et al., 1976b).

IV. Other Synthetic Inhibitors of Fibrinolysis

Further antifibrinolytically active compounds are known. They are derivatives of lysine and other basic amino acids (NAGAMATSU et al., 1963, 1968; MURAMATU et al., 1965a, b, 1967; MURAMATU and FUJII 1968, 1969; FUJII et al., 1972), quaternary products of EACA and other ε-aminocarboxylic acids (JOHNSON and SKOZA, 1963), primary aliphatic amines (BICKFORD and TAYLOR, 1963; BICKFORD et al., 1964), and lactams and lactones of aliphatic carboxylic acids (AUERSWALD and DOLESCHEL, 1967; DOLESCHEL and AUERSWALD, 1967). The activity of these compounds is approximately equal to that of EACA.

Substances with a much weaker antifibrinolytic activity are the low molecular weight polypeptides (ANTOPOL and CHRYSSANTHOU, 1963; BIANCHINI, 1964) and oligopeptides formed by certain bacteria (AOYAGI et al., 1969), organic dyes (GEIGER, 1952), antibiotics (NETER, 1942; WASSERMANN, 1952; v. KAULLA and HENKEL, 1953), serotonin (SANDBERG et al., 1961; TSITOURIS et al., 1962), sialic acid (RUBIN and RITZ, 1967), carbon disulphide (SAITA et al., 1963), and various other compounds (BARR et al., 1963). Furthermore, there are compounds which cause non-specific inactivation of plasmin, such as urea and methylamine (NORMAN, 1957), cysteine and mercaptoethanol (MOOTSE and CLIFFTON, 1960) as well as compounds which block the catalytic mechanism of plasmin and plasminogen activators, such as organophosphates (MOUNTER and SHIPLEY, 1958; MOUNTER and MOUNTER, 1963; SUMMARIA et al., 1968; GROSKOPF et al., 1969b), N^{α}-tosyllysine chloromethyl ketone (ABIKO et al., 1968; GROSKOPF et al., 1969a), esters of guanidinobenzoic acid (CHASE and SHAW, 1969, 1970; LANDMANN and MARKWARDT, 1970; MARKWARDT et al., 1970) and aminoalkylbenzene sulfofluorides (MARKWARDT et al., 1971b; WALSMANN et al., 1972).

B. Mode of Action

The Japanese workers believed that the antifibrinolytic effect of EACA was caused by inhibition of the fibrinolytic enzyme plasmin (OKAMOTO, 1960a, b). However, other studies on the mechanism of action allowed the assumption that the effect is more likely caused by inhibition of plasmin activation (ABE and SATO, 1958, 1959; ABLONDI et al., 1959; ALKJAERSIG et al., 1959a; IGAWA et al., 1959). Studies on the mechanism of action of cyclic aminocarboxylic acids seemed to confirm this assumption, so that the inhibition of plasminogen activation was considered to be the principal mechanism of antifibrinolytic effects. However, the finding that antifibrinolytics cause an inhibition of the specific action of plasmin on fibrin, and some work which failed to confirm the predominant antiactivator theory (GODAL and THEODOR, 1965; EGEBLAD, 1966; MAXWELL and ALLEN, 1966; LANDMANN, 1967a, b, 1970; AMBRUS, et al., 1968; LUKASIEWICZ and NIEWIAROWSKI, 1968), have led to more recent additional studies on the mechanism of action (LANDMANN, 1973; THORSEN and ASTRUP, 1974; THORSEN, 1975, 1977).

I. Influence on the Activation of Plasminogen

The interpretation that synthetic antifibrinolytics act mainly as inhibitors of plasminogen activation had its origin in the findings of ALKJAERSIG and coworkers (1959a). Their fundamental studies showed that the proteolytic (caseinolytic) activity which results from streptokinase-induced plasminogen activation will decrease when EACA is added to the system prior to activation. When the inhibitor is added after activation, it exerts only a slight influence on casein hydrolysis. This antiactivator action was confirmed by several authors. An example is given in Figure 3. In this study, plasmin activity from urokinase-induced plasminogen activation was determined by hydroly-

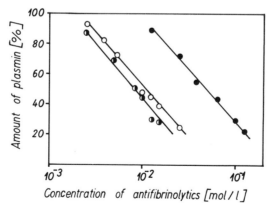

Fig. 3. Inhibition of plasminogen activation by PAMBA (◍), AMCA (○), and EACA (●). Incubation of 16.5 caseinolytic units plasminogen with inhibitor and 500 Ploug units urokinase at pH 7.5, 25° C. Interruption of activation after 5 min by addition of 8×10^{-3} M TAME (TAME esterase activity was determined by continuous titration using a pH Stat assembly)

Table 6. Influence of antifibrinolytic agents and benzamidine derivatives on ester hydrolysis by urokinase and on plasminogen activation by urokinase and streptokinase

	Urokinase AGLME[a] K_i (mM)	Urokinase Plasminogen K_i (mM)	Streptokinase Plasminogen K_i (mM)
EACA	19.0	55.0	50.0
PAMBA	1.5	3.0	4.5
AMCA	2.0	4.0	6.0
4-aminobenzamidine	0.012	0.015	0.02
4-amidinophenylpyruvic acid	0.01	0.008	0.01
β-naphthamidine	0.005	0.006	0.01

[a] AGLME = N$^\alpha$-acetylglycyl-L-lysine methyl ester

sis of the ester substrate N$^\alpha$-toluenesulfonyl-L-argininemethyl ester (TAME). In the presence of antifibrinolytic agents the plasminogen activation was inhibited, whereas the esterolytic activity of plasmin was not impaired.

When using streptokinase as activator, the inhibitory action was not due to an inhibition of the reaction between streptokinase and plasmin, which leads to the activator activity, but to a blockade of the activator formed (MARKUS, 1961; LING et al., 1965; ROBBINS et al., 1965; SUMMARIA et al., 1968).

Thus, the antifibrinolytics possess an inhibitory action on plasminogen activation induced by streptokinase, urokinase and tissue kinase. However, this antiactivator action occurs only at relatively high concentrations of antifibrinolytics. On the other hand, a strong antifibrinolytic effect of these compounds was observed at essentially lower concentrations. Inhibitor constants (K_i) were determined to compare the inhibitory action of the compounds on the hydrolysis of the ester substrate and on plasminogen activation by urokinase and streptokinase (Table 6). The antifibrinolytics are extremely weak inhibitors of the kinases tested. Other authors observed only a weak inhibitory effect of antifibrinolytics on the ester hydrolysis by urokinase (LORAND and MOZEN, 1964; SHERRY et al., 1964; LORAND and CONDIT, 1965; WALTON, 1967). The relative efficacy of the antifibrinolytics in the inhibition of plasminogen activation differs from their antifibrinolytic action. Thus, with respect to the antiactivator action PAMPA surpasses the activity of AMCA, whereas the antifibrinolytic action of AMCA exceeds that of PAMBA.

Antifibrinolytics as well as benzamidine derivatives were found to be competitive inhibitors of plasminogen activating enzymes (MARKWARDT et al., 1970a, c; LAND-MANN, 1973). Although the benzamidine derivatives proved to be highly potent inhibitors of plasminogen activation, their antifibrinolytic effect is weaker than that of the antifibrinolytics (Table 5).

Consequently, there exists no correlation between the potency of the tested compounds in the inhibition of plasminogen activation and in their antifibrinolytic activity. The demonstrated antiactivator activity does not seem to be decisive for the antifibrinolytic action of these agents. However, a participation of this effect in the action of the antifibrinolytics in the blood cannot be excluded.

II. Influence on Plasmin

The only possible explanation for the antifibrinolytic action would be the inhibition of fibrin degradation by plasmin. The antiplasmin action of the antifibrinolytics was repeatedly demonstrated. However, the extent and characteristics of this inhibitory action appeared to be contradictory. Several authors observed an inhibition of plasmin only at concentrations that were 10–100 fold higher than those required for the inhibition of plasminogen activation (SHERRY et al., 1959; ALKJAERSIG, 1961; ANDERSSON et al., 1965). Other studies showed that an inhibition of plasmin occurred also at low concentrations of antifibrinolytics (CELANDER and GUEST, 1960; FUKUTAKE et al., 1960; CELANDER et al., 1961a,b; PAPPENHAGEN et al., 1962; SCHMUTZLER and BECK, 1962; BICKFORD et al., 1964; MAKI and BELLER, 1966). The reason for these contradictions may be found in the type of substrate used. Fundamental differences were observed in the case of inhibition of plasmin action on non-specific protein or synthetic substrates as compared to inhibition of plasmin action on its physiologic substrate fibrin (SKOZA et al., 1968: AMBRUS et al., 1970; THORSEN et al., 1974).

1. Inhibition of Proteolytic and Esterolytic Activity

An inhibition of plasmin action on casein was observed only in the presence of extremely high concentrations of antifibrinolytics (0.1–1.0 M) (ABLONDI et al., 1959; ALKJAERSIG et al., 1959a, b; IGAWA et al., 1959; OKAMOTO and OKAMOTO, 1962; OSHIBA and OKAMOTO, 1962; BERGHOFF and GLATZEL, 1964; DUBBER et al., 1964, 1965; AMBRUS et al., 1968; WALSMANN and MARKWARDT, 1969). The same or higher inhibitor concentrations are necessary to inhibit the hydrolysis of p-toluenesulfonyl-L-argininemethyl ester (TAME). Lysine esters and the chromogenic amide substrate N^α-benzoyl-DL-arginine-p-nitroanilide (BAPNA) are better suited to demonstrate the antiplasmin action (OKAMOTO and OKAMOTO, 1962; OSHIBA and OKAMOTO, 1962; AMBRUS et al., 1968; MARKWARDT et al., 1968; WALSMANN and MARKWARDT, 1969; LANDMANN, 1970). Inhibitor constants were determined in the same order of magnitude as measured in the case of the inhibition of plasminogen activation (Table 7). Compared with the antifibrinolytics, benzamide derivatives possess a stronger inhibitory effect on the plasmin hydrolysis of non-specific protein and ester substrates.

Table 7. Influence of antifibrinolytic agents and benzamidine derivatives on the hydrolysis of the synthetic substrate N^α-benzoyl-DL-arginine-p-nitroanlide (A) and on fibrinogen degradation (B) by plasmin

	A K_i (mM)	B I_{50} (mM)
EACA	53.0	40.0
PAMBA	7.5	5.0
AMCA	25.0	20.0
4-aminobenzamidine	0.13	0.2
4-amidinophenylpyruvic acid	0.04	0.1
β-naphthamidine	0.06	0.15

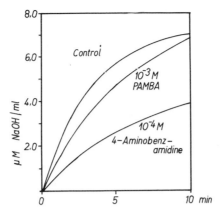

Fig. 4. Influence of PAMBA and 4-aminobenzamidine on fibrinogen degradation by plasmin (titrimetric determination)

Since plasmin hydrolyzes peptide and ester bonds of the basic amino acids arginine and lysine, it is believed that the antifibrinolytics and the benzamidine derivatives react with the substrate-binding center of the enzyme because of their structural relationship to these amino acids. In this way, a displacement of the substrate occurs and, depending on the inhibitor affinity for the binding site, the enzyme activity is more or less inhibited. Since plasminogen activators exhibit the same substrate specificity as plasmin, and activation of the pro-enzyme occurs by cleavage of an arginyl peptide bond, the inhibitor action of the antifibrinolytics and benzamidine derivatives on plasminogen activation can be explained in principle in the same way.

The plasmin-catalyzed fibrinogen degradation was inhibited to the same extent by antifibrinolytics as the hydrolysis of non-specific protein substrates (GODAL and THEODOR, 1965; LUKASIEWICZ and NIEWIAROWSKI, 1968; LUKASIEWICZ et al., 1968; LANDMANN, 1973). However, benzamidine derivatives exert a stronger inhibitory effect on fibrinogen degradation by plasmin (Fig. 4). Moreover, disc electrophoretic investigations of fibrinogen degradation products formed under the influence of plasmin revealed that the degradation sequence of fibrinogen was not impaired by antifibrinolytics. Thus, these inhibitors have no qualitative influence on fibrinogenolysis.

2. Inhibition of Fibrinolytic Activity

The action of plasmin on its physiologic substrate, i.e. the process of fibrin degradation, is strongly inhibited (CELANDER and GUEST, 1960; CELANDER et al., 1961b; EGEBLAD, 1966; MAKI and BELLER, 1966; LANDMANN, 1967b, 1973; AMBRUS et al., 1968; LUKASIEWICZ et al., 1968; WALSMANN and MARKWARDT, 1969). In this case the antifibrinolytics attain or surpass the potency of benzamidine derivatives (Table 7). The action of the antifibrinolytics on fibrinolysis is thought to be mainly the result of specific inhibition of fibrin degradation by plasmin. This effect is a strong one, and it is quantitatively correlated with the antifibrinolytic action. The efficacy of inhibition of plasmin-catalyzed fibrin degradation by synthetic antifibrinolytics (EACA<

PAMBA < AMCA) closely parallels that of plasma clot lysis. This specific action seems to be caused by a competitive mechanism (LANDMANN, 1973).

The finding that antifibrinolytics primarily inhibit the action of plasmin on fibrin, but do hardly influence the hydrolysis of other substrates, allows the conclusion that the inhibitors react with fibrin. The reaction is believed to occur at the stage of fibrinogen, and that a conformationally altered fibrin is formed which can be degraded only with difficulty by plasmin. It was observed that fibrin clots formed in the presence of EACA or AMCA are not easily dissolved by plasmin or other proteolytic enzymes (MAXWELL et al., 1967; AMBRUS et al., 1968). Nephelometric and thromb-elastographic investigations of clot structure (DONALDSON, 1964; EGEBLAD, 1966; MAXWELL, 1966; MAXWELL and ALLEN, 1966; LUKASIEWICZ and NIEWIAROWSKI, 1968; MAXWELL et al., 1968, 1970) lend further support to this assumption. Other investigators were unable to confirm a general resistance of fibrin clots formed in the presence of antifibrinolytics (LANDMANN, 1973).

Compared to other proteolytic enzymes, plasmin, which has relatively little activity against other protein substrates, obviously possesses the strongest ability to degrade insoluble fibrin into soluble degradation products (HEIMBURGER, 1962; ROKA, 1967; SCHWICK, 1967). The antifibrinolytics possibly inhibit this specific action of plasmin (LUKASIEWICZ et al., 1968; ABIKO and IWAMOTO, 1970; LANDMANN, 1973).

The results of the present investigation can be summarized in a hypothesis demonstrated schematically in Figure 5. The specific reaction of plasmin with fibrin is believed to be produced by an interaction of a specific binding center A' on the enzyme with a characteristic chemical structure A on fibrin monomers. The substrate is fixed to the enzyme by this reaction in such a way that among the peptide bonds (B), potentially hydrolyzable by plasmin, a particular bond C of strategical signifi-

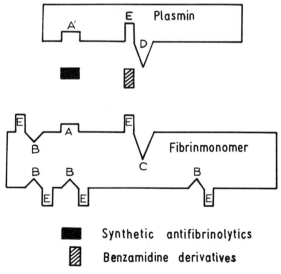

Fig. 5. Concept of the mechanism of action of antifibrinolytics and benzamidine derivatives in the process of fibrin dissolution by plasmin (according to LANDMANN, 1973)

cance for effective solubilization of fibrin, is brought into the neighborhood of the hydrolytic group of the enzyme D. Consequently, a favored hydrolysis of that bond is brought about. The antifibrinolytics, as well as bicyclic and polycyclic inhibitors described recently (BAUMGARTEN et al., 1969; LOEFFLER et al., 1970), are thought to be structurally related to group A on the surface of fibrin monomers. Thus the antifibrinolytics may also be bound to the specific center A' and so cause a displacement of fibrin and a competitive inhibition of the hydrolysis of the prominent peptide bond C. The relationship between structure and observed activity suggests that group A is possibly a lysyl residue.

This hypothesis on the mechanism of the antifibrinolytic action of ω-amino acids (LANDMANN, 1973) has been provided with experimental evidence by THORSEN et al. (1974) and IWAMOTO (1975). Accordingly, antifibrinolytics inhibit proteolysis of fibrin by competing with fibrin for sites on plasmin, which are different from the active center and most likely located in the heavy chain. This prevents a functional interaction between the active center on the plasmin-light chain and fibrin.

III. Influence on Other Enzymes

Similar to the described competitive inhibitor mechanism of antifibrinolytics against proteolytic enzymes that hydrolyze peptide and ester bonds of basic amino acids, the antifibrinolytics possess also an inhibitory effect on trypsin (ABLONDI et al., 1959; AUERSWALD and DOLESCHEL, 1962; GERATZ, 1962, 1963; MARKWARDT et al., 1964, 1965, 1968; TRETTIN, 1964; MURAMATU et al., 1965c; TRETTIN and MIX, 1965; LANDMANN, 1967a, b; LANDMANN et al., 1969). However, when compared to their antifibrinolytic activity, the antitrypsin effect of synthetic antifibrinolytics is weak. A still weaker effect is exerted on the clotting enzyme thrombin and the kinin-liberating enzyme kallikrein, which are also proteinases with trypsin-like substrate specificity. A weak inhibitory effect of the antifibrinolytics on another esteroproteolytic enzyme, the C1 esterase of the complement system, and its activation (ASGHAR et al., 1973; SOTER et al., 1975) were described (TAYLOR and FUDENBERG, 1964; BASCH, 1965; MURAMATU et al., 1972). The activity of chymotrypsin is not impaired by synthetic antifibrinolytics (LANDMANN, 1967a). An inhibition of the action of pepsin by AMCA was reported (DUBBER et al., 1964). Furthermore, it was shown that EACA inhibits carboxypeptidase B (FOLK, 1956; WINTERSBERGER et al., 1962; WOLFF et al., 1962). An inhibition of the kinin-destroying activity of human plasma, which is believed to be caused by a carboxypeptidase B-like enzyme, was also described (BISHOP and MARGOLIS, 1963; ERDÖS et al., 1963). In our investigations, the degradation of bradykinin in human plasma was not significantly inhibited by EACA, PAM-BA, and AMCA concentrations as usually employed for therapeutic use (HAUSTEIN and MARKWARDT, 1966).

IV. Physico-Chemical Effects

Based on their chemical structure, the antifibrinolytics possess a strong dipole moment that enables them to alter the dielectric constant of a solvent. Presumably, the ability of EACA to improve significantly the solubility of plasminogen and plasmin at physiological pH is due to this non-specific effect (BAUMGARTEN and COLE, 1961;

MOSESSON, 1962; BERGSTRÖM, 1963). This property of EACA is utilized in several methods of plasmin purification (WALLEN, 1962; ALKJAERSIG, 1964). The increase in the activity of plasmin in the presence of EACA and cyclic aminocarboxylic acids is also attributed to this effect (ALKJAERSIG et al., 1959a; IGAWA et al., 1959; LAND-MANN and MARKWARDT, 1963). This phenomenon is observed in purified systems. An influence in vivo can hardly be imagined, so that it is considered unimportant at the concentrations normally reached in blood during therapeutic use. Studies by ABIKO et al. (1969) revealed that EACA and AMCA form complexes with plasmino-gen which exhibit a small dissociation only. Presumably, plasminogen cannot be activated in these complexes, which is thought to be one of the reasons for the antifibrinolytic effect of the inhibitors.

EACA seems to possess a desaggregating effect on intermolecular interactions between proteins (LING et al., 1967). This action, which is possibly caused also by the above mentioned influence on the solvent, was utilized in the preparation of the streptokinase-plasmin activator complex and several coagulation factors (DAVIES et al., 1964; BARG et al., 1965; HUMMEL et al., 1966; DE RENZO et al., 1967; BUCK et al., 1968). The inhibition of antigen-antibody reactions by EACA can be explained in the same way (ATCHLEY and BHARGAVAN, 1962).

C. Assay Methods

Data on the chemical and physical properties of EACA were reported by several authors (GABRIEL and MAASS, 1899; CZEREPKO, 1958; CZEREPKO et al., 1959; STRIEGLER, 1963). The analysis of PAMBA and its hydrogenated form AMCA, and the procedures for pharmaceutical-chemical investigation of the commercial prepa-rations, were described (KLÖCKING et al., 1965; MAYER et al., 1966). In the following, mainly those procedures are presented which are used for the determination of antifibrinolytic agents in biological material.

I. Chemical Methods

Several procedures were described for the chemical detection of antifibrinolytic agents in body fluids and organs (THOMAS, 1959; MCNICOL et al., 1962; WOLOSOW-ICZ et al., 1963; MARKWARDT et al., 1964, 1966; TAKADA et al., 1964a, b; ANDERSSON et al., 1965; MELANDER et al., 1965; SHEPHERD et al., 1973). After suitable prepara-tion of the biological material the samples are deproteinized by precipitation or by ultrafiltration. The antifibrinolytics EACA, PAMBA, and AMCA are aminocarbox-ylic acids with a terminal amino group. For the chemical quantitative determination of these substances mainly the reactions of the aliphatic amino group are utilized. Therefore, other amino acids and various compounds that interfere with the determi-nation must be removed from the deproteinized samples. A quantitative separation of the antifibrinolytics from other ninhydrin-positive substances is carried out by column chromatographic pre-separation on the highly basic ion exchanger Dowex 2 or the highly acidic cation exchanger Lewatit S 100, and by subsequent chromato-graphy of the amino acids on Amberlite IT 120 or Dowex 50. One-dimensional ascending chromatography of the pre-purified biological material on paper impregnated with the highly acidic cation exchanger was used successfully. An elimination of α-amino acids by their conversion into copper complexes was proposed (JOHNSON and SKOZA, 1961)

Furthermore, a thin-layer chromatographic method on fluorescein containing cellulose (KÄSER and GUGLER, 1965), and a high-voltage electrophoretic procedure (SJOERDSMA and HANSON, 1959) were used for the isolation of EACA. One-dimensional paper chromatography of the deproteinized extracts in the solvent mixture n-butanol/acetic acid/water (4:1:5, vol/vol/vol) was found to be suited for the isolation of PAMBA (MARKWARDT et al., 1964).

For the colorimetric determination of the isolated antifibrinolytics the ninhydrin reaction was used. The solvent-free chromatograms were treated with ninhydrin reagent and, after drying, were fixed with copper reagent. The relatively stable copper complex was determined either densiometrically, or colorimetrically at 508 nm after elution with methanol or ethanol/NaCl 20% (4:1). Other authors reported the conversion of the isolated antifibrinolytic agent with ninhydrin in the eluate.

To avoid difficulties arising from the susceptibility to disturbances of the ninhydrin reaction, the aminocarboxylic acids were converted with 1-fluoro-2,4-dinitrobenzene (FDNB) into the corresponding DNP amino acids (SKOZA and JOHNSON, 1964; MARKWARDT et al., 1967a). These methods, in connection with thin-layer chromatography, were used as rather simple procedures for the determination of synthetic antifibrinolytics in biological material.

Technique: 1.0 ml blood plasma, urine or organ extract containing no more than 2.0 mg of the antifibrinolytic agent is mixed with 0.1 ml 70% perchloric acid. The precipitate is centrifuged. 0.5 ml of the deproteinized solution is mixed with 0.35 ml 5% FDNB, saturated with potassium bicarbonate, and shaken for 2 h at room temperature. All FDNB-reactive compounds present in this mixture are dinitrophenylated. Thereafter, 0.5 ml ethanol and 0.15 ml concentrated hydrochloric acid are added. An aliquot of this solution is spotted linearly on a silica gel-G plate and subjected to ascending chromatography in the solvent system chloroform/ethyl acetate/glacial acetic acid (94:4:2). In order to obtain sufficient separation of dinitrophenylated urine, additional chromatography in the solvent mixture chloroform/methanol/concentrated ammonia (95:3:2) is necessary. The self-color of the DNP amino acids allows one to observe the separation. Following separation the DNP-EACA, DNP-PAMBA or DNP-AMCA spots are scraped off and eluted with 1.0 ml 1% sodium bicarbonate. After centrifugation of the silica gel the extinction of the supernatant is measured at 360 nm. Upon separation of 150 µl of the dinitrophenylation mixture the lower detection limit is approximately 10 µg of antifibrinolytic agents per ml of deproteinized extract.

II. Biological Methods

For the quantitative assay of EACA, PAMBA or AMCA the antifibrinolytic action of these substances can be utilized. Because of the natural biological activity of the intact molecule these procedures possess a higher specificity than the chemical methods, which are only based on the detection of a functional group. Separation of the

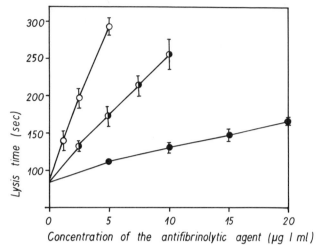

Fig. 6. Dependence of lysis time of human citrated plasma on the concentration of antifibrinolytics (measured in plasma lysis test) ○ AMCA, ◐ PAMBA, ● EACA

naturally occurring amino acids in the deproteinized plasma is not necessary because they do not display any antifibrinolytic activity (WOLOSOWICZ et al., 1963). For the biological assay of antifibrinolytics the plasma lysis test was used (MARKWARDT et al., 1967)

Technique: 0.2 ml human citrated plasma is mixed at 37° C with 0.1 ml inhibitor-containing deproteinized extract, 0.1 ml streptokinase (500 U/ml) and 0.1 ml thrombin (50 NIH U/ml). After clotting, a glass bead (4 mm diameter) is placed on the surface of the clot and the time from the addition of thrombin until the bead falls freely to the bottom of the test tube is measured. To obtain a calibration curve, increasing amounts of the respective antifibrinolytic agent are added to the plasma lysis mixture. The obtained lysis times are plotted against the inhibitor concentration (Fig. 6). The lysis time of the test sample is compared to that of the calibration curve. In biological assays the lower detection limit depends on the specific antifibrinolytic activity. For EACA it amounts to about 10 µg, for PAMBA 2 µg, and for AMCA 1 µg per ml of solution.

To estimate the concentrations in the blood, the method can be used in a simplified manner by directly measuring lysis times in plasma. Prior to the administration of the antifibrinolytic agent a blood sample (1 vol. 3.8% sodium citrate, 4 vol. blood) is taken and citrated plasma is prepared by centrifugation for 15 min at 600 g. To obtain a calibration curve, 0.2 ml aliquots of the control citrated plasma are mixed with 0.1 ml antifibrinolytic of increasing concentration, 0.1 ml streptokinase and 0.1 ml thrombin. The measured lysis times are plotted against the concentration of the antifibrinolytic. To estimate the blood level after administration of the antifibrinolytic agent, 0.5–1.0 ml citrated blood is taken at different time intervals, and 0.2 ml of the respective plasma is mixed with 0.1 ml buffer, 0.1 ml streptokinase and 0.1 ml thrombin. The antifibrinolytic agent in plasma can then be calculated by comparing the obtained lysis time of the test plasma with that of the calibration curve with control plasma.

D. Experimental Pharmacology

I. Toxicity

The results obtained in studies of the acute toxicity of therapeutically used synthetic antifibrinolytics are summarized in Table 8, indicating low toxicity. This was also demonstrated by subcutaneous injection of EACA into rabbits and dogs ($LD_{50} > 0.6$ g/kg) (ZAITSEVA, 1965). Determinations of the toxicity of AMCA in rabbits revealed LD_{50} values of 1.4 g/kg i.v., 3.4 g/kg i.p., 4.0 g/kg s.c., and > 3.0 g/kp p.o. (SIREN, 1970). The toxicity of derivatives of p-aminomethylbenzoic acid was within the range of values of the parent substance (Table 8). The esters were an exception in that they displayed a significantly greater toxic effect after intravenous injection than from oral administration.

Animal experiments showed that the synthetic antifibrinolytics are relatively well tolerated after subchronic or chronic administration. EACA doses of 0.1 g per day in rats and 0.8 g per day in dogs, which were added to the food for 30 days, had no effect on growth and development or other vital functions (LANG and BITZ, 1955; KASTRO et al., 1964). Experiments to determine the chronic toxicity revealed that oral administration of 0.5–5.0 g/kg per day in rats over 3 months did not produce any toxic effect. There were no indications of tissue damage in histological examinations of the liver, heart, lungs, and kidneys of these animals. However, with respect to fertility, differences existed between EACA-treated animals and their controls. Subchronic EACA application to female rats, however, caused disturbed fetal development in all cases (MELANDER et al., 1965). In a group of male rats treated with 5.0 g/kg per day the fertility decreased by 50%, whereas in a group of female rats it was not influenced (ENEROTH and GRANT, 1966). Physiological and pathologic-anatomical examinations revealed that animals treated with high doses of EACA (up to 2.6 g/kg per day) showed signs of dehydration and renal impairment (RITZEL and WÜTHRICH, 1964). Squamous epithelial cells, erythrocytes and leukocytes were found in the urine. The symptoms appeared most frequently during the fifth week of EACA application. The

Table 8. Acute toxicity of synthetic antifibrinolytic agents (LD_{50} in g/kg)

	Mouse			References	Rat			References
	i.v.	i.p.	p.o.		i.v.	i.p.	p.o.	
EACA	8.0	9.0	—	(1)	—	~10.0	—	(6)
	3.0	—	12.0	(2)	3.2	—	16.5	(2)
	—	8.1	—	(3)				
	4.9	—	>20.0	(4)				
PAMBA	1.6	2.7	>15.0	(1)	—	>2.5	—	(7)
AMCHA	1.6	—	>15.0	(2)	1.8	—	>15.0	(2)
AMCA	1.5	—	—	(2)	1.2	—	—	(2)
	1.4	4.2	>10.0	(4)	0.9	2.1	11.2	(5)
	1.3	2.5	12.5	(5)				

(1) MARKWARDT et al., 1972; (2) MELANDER et al., 1965; (3) KASTRO et al., 1964; (4) FOUSSARD-BLANPIN and BRETAUDEAU, 1965; (5) SIREN, 1970; (6) LANG and BITZ, 1955; (7) MARKWARDT et al., 1965.

histological examination of the kidneys showed extratubular concretions in the cortico-medullary border. Subcutaneous injection of 500 mg EACA over 10 days led to pathological alterations of liver cells and portal vein. However, these changes did not occur after application of lower doses (REZAKOVICH, et al., 1966).

The effect of subchronic PAMBA administration (250 mg/kg per day) in aqueous solution by means of a probang over 6 weeks was studied in rats. The chronic toxicity was followed after addition of PAMBA to the standard food over 9 months, with an average intake of 100 mg PAMBA per day. In both series of experiments no toxic side-effects or changes in food intake and body weight were observed. Autopsy and histological examinations of the liver, heart, lungs, and aorta did not show any pathological alterations. Teratogenic effects and disturbances of fertility were not observed in rats (MARKWARDT et al., 1964).

AMCHA was administered subchronically to rats for 12 weeks in oral doses of 0.5–5.0 g/kg per day. Toxic side-effects did not appear. The histological examination did not reveal any alterations. Disturbances of fertility, as they were observed after application of EACA, were absent (MELANDER et al., 1965).

The subacute toxicity of AMCA was studied in rats after oral application of 0.25–1.0 g/kg per day for 2 weeks. AMCA did not influence growth, the organs of the animals showed no pathological alterations, and the blood picture was normal. Subchronic tests in rats after administration of 1.0–5.0 g AMCA per day revealed that the growth of the animals, the composition of the serum protein fractions, as well as the white and red blood cell counts remained normal. Oral administration of 1 g/kg to dogs caused a reduction in growth rate and moderate diarrhea. Compared to control dogs, the weight of the ovaries of test females was significantly lower. After oral application of up to 5 g/kg per day to mice and rats teratogenic effects and disturbances of fertility were not observed (SIREN, 1970). Light and electron microscopic studies of arteries and other tissues from dogs subjected to chronic fibrinolytic inhibition with AMCA were made by STEENBLOCK and CELANDER (1968).

II. Side-Effects

To clarify whether antifibrinolytic agents display further pharmacodynamic effects in addition to their specific antifibrinolytic action, these substances were studied on several pharmacological parameters (FIDELSKI et al., 1970).

At concentrations which are normally attained in the blood during therapeutic use, EACA exerted sympathomimetic effects (RAMOS et al., 1961b; FOUSSARD-BLAN-PIN and BRETAUDEAU, 1965). Intravenous injection of more than 120 mg/kg into cats and dogs caused a rise in blood pressure, dilatation of the pupils, and contraction of the nictitating membrane. Prior application of sympatholytics and pretreatment with reserpine did not inhibit these effects. The sympathomimetic effects might have been caused by liberation of catecholamines and inhibition of amine uptake (LIPMANN et al., 1965; LIPMANN and WISHNICK, 1965; OBIANWU, 1967a, b; ANDEN et al., 1968; STITZEL et al., 1968). On isolated hearts of cats and rabbits, EACA doses of 10–40 mg exerted positive inotropic effects. High doses of EACA (3.6–4.5 g/kg) produced cardiotoxic effects, mainly arrhythmias (CUMMINGS and WELTER, 1966). In the isolated guinea-pig ileum, bath concentrations of 1 mg/ml led to relaxation. However, EACA did not possess any inhibitory action on the contractions induced by acetylcholine, histamine or serotonin (MCFADDEN, 1965). Thus, after oral doses of 500 mg/kg or i.p. administration of 250 mg/kg in rats, changes in blood pressure were not observed (CUMMINGS and WELTER, 1966), whereas the blood pressure dropped after i.v. injection of 100–500 mg into rabbits (OTTO-SERVAIS and LECOMTE, 1961). Intravenous injection of 50–200 mg EACA/kg into dogs caused diuresis which was attributed to an inhibition of Na^+ and Cl^- reabsorption in the proximal tubule (AUERSWALD and DOLESCHEL, 1967). Moreover, studies in dogs showed that EACA doses of 0.3–1.4 g/kg caused hyperkalemia (CAROL and TIZE, 1966). EACA is believed to prevent the increase in capillary permeability caused by intradermal histamine injections (LEFEBVRE et al., 1962; COPLEY and CAROL, 1964).

PAMBA proved to be a pharmacologically indifferent compound (MARKWARDT et al., 1964; MARKWARDT and KLÖCKING, 1965). On a series of isolated organs (rat ileum, uterus, diaphragm, rabbit aorta, frog heart) PAMBA did not exert any noticeable effects at bath concentrations of up to 1.0 mg/ml. The effects of PAMBA on blood pressure and respiration were studied in cats anesthetized with urethanechloralose. Intravenous doses of up to 20 mg/kg were without effect, and blood pressure responses to adrenaline injections were not influenced. The actions of EACA and AMCA on the cardiovascular systems of the cat, rabbit, guinea-pig, dog, and rat were determined by MARMO et al. (1971). In vitro evaluations were also made on intestinal, uterine, and cardiac muscle, and on coronary blood flow.

Antiallergic and antiphlogistic effects: Based on several animal experiments, EACA is believed to exert an inhibitory action on the antigen-antibody reaction (ATCHLEY and BHARGAVAN, 1962; JOHANOVSKY and ŠKAVRIL, 1962; ARNET, 1963; GILETTE et al., 1963 a, b; MUSIALOWICZ et al., 1965; AUERSWALD and DOLESCHEL, 1966; FRICK and FRICK, 1967; WOLD et al., 1967; NOFERI et al., 1969; RENOUX et al., 1973). Moreover, immunosuppressive and antiallergic (YOKOI, 1960; AUSTEN and BROCKLEHURST, 1961; SALMON, 1961; ZWEIFACH et al., 1961; NEUBAUER, 1963; WÜTHRICH et al., 1963; TOIVANEN and TOIVANEN, 1964; ROWINSKI and HAGER, 1966; GARTENMANN, 1968; RAAB, 1968) as well as antiphlogistic effects (FLANDRE et al., 1964; HÖLLER and LINDNER, 1965; YAMASAKI et al., 1967) were reported. These effects cannot yet be explained satisfactorily. They are most likely caused in part by an inhibition of proteolytic enzymes which might be of pathogenic importance in these processes. Other investigators did not observe antiallergic effects of EACA (GANS and KRIVIT, 1961; LECOMTE et al., 1964; TOIVANEN et al., 1965; TCHORZEWSKI, 1966) or of PAMBA or AMCA (HAUSTEIN, 1967; HAUSTEIN and HAUSTEIN, 1967), and other studies did not reveal antiphlogistic properties of EACA (ALLISON et al., 1963; ALLISON and LANCASTER, 1965). The antiradiation effect of EACA found in animal experiments has also remained unclear (RUDAKOVA et al., 1965; DANYSZ et al., 1966; POSPISIL et al., 1968).

Antiproteolytic effects: Based on the antiproteolytic action of antifibrinolytics, attempts have been made to prevent experimental pancreatitis by their use. Neither the course of pancreatitis nor the mortality were influenced by EACA (HUREAU et al., 1964, 1966; DIWOK et al., 1965; MARTIN et al., 1965). Pancreatic necrosis induced by trypsin injection into the pancreatic duct of rats was also not influenced by prior administration of PAMBA.

Antagonistic effect on p-aminobenzoic acid: Because of certain structural similarities between PAMBA and p-aminobenzoic acid, which is known as a growth-promoting substance for bacteria and as a constituent of folic acid, the question arises whether PAMBA may exert p-aminobenzoic acid-like or -antagonistic effects.

Studies with Gram-positive and Gram-negative microorganisms *(Staphylococcus aureus, Escherichia coli, Bacillus subtilis)* showed that PAMBA possessed neither bacteriostatic nor growth-promoting activity. In primary and permanent cell cultures (amnion and HeLa cells) PAMBA caused neither inhibition nor promotion of growth or any other morphological alterations. Sulfonamide-sensitive test germs *(Shigella flexneri)* were used to study whether PAMBA displays antagonistic effects against the action of sulfonamides. While the bacteriostatic effect of 200 µg sulfisoxazole was completely abolished by 50 µg p-aminobenzoic acid/ml, the application of up to 200 µg PAMBA/ml had no influence on sulfonamide activity. Thus, in contrast to the structurally related sulfonamides or p-aminobenzoic acid, PAMBA had no influence on cell growth (MARKWARDT et al., 1964).

III. Pharmacokinetics

The therapeutic action and effectiveness of an antifibrinolytic agent requires maintenance of sufficiently high concentrations of the substance in the blood. For this reason, the time course of absorption and elimination of the antifibrinolytics was determined in animal experiments (Table 9).

Table 9. Pharmacokinetic data on antifibrinolytics in rabbits

Substance	Dose (mg/kg)	Elimination constant k_2 (h^{-1})	Half-life $T_{1/2}$ (min)	Distribution quotient	Invasion constant k_1 (h^{-1})	Enteral absorption (%)	Excretion in 24-h urine (% of administered dose) i.v.	p.o.
EACA	100	0.70 ± 0.20	64 (46– 84)	0.28	0.83 ± 0.06	55 ± 3	40 ± 4	25 ± 3
PAMBA	100	0.89 ± 0.20	47 (37– 64)	2.93	0.49 ± 0.05	38 ± 2	42 ± 8	18 ± 4
AMCA	20	0.72 ± 0.04	59 (42–118)	1.25	0.13 ± 0.04	49 ± 5	65 ± 12	27 ± 1

1. EACA

The pharmacokinetics of EACA in rabbits are shown in Table 9. After oral administration the blood level reached a maximum in 2–3 h. A similar time course of the blood level was found in rats and dogs (WOLOSOWICZ et al., 1963; MELANDER et al., 1965). In mice, a half-life of 120 min was determined. Simultaneously with EACA excretion, the excretion of other amino acids increased in the urine of rats (LANG and BITZ, 1955). Observations on the metabolism have been published earlier (THOMAS and GOERNE, 1914; COPLEY, 1929). After feeding large amounts of EACA, γ-aminobutyric acid and adipic acid were found in the urine besides EACA in unchanged form. Furthermore, the excretion of glutamic acid was enhanced. Obviously, degradation of EACA occurs by two routes: β-Oxidation yields γ-aminobutyric acid, which is partly carboxylated to glutamic acid; and adipic acid forms by oxidative deamination. Further studies revealed that the absorption of EACA occurs via passive diffusion through the intestinal mucosa (EVERED et al., 1967).

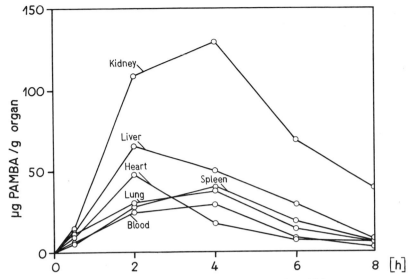

Fig. 7. Distribution of PAMBA after oral doses of 250 mg/kg in rabbits

2. PAMBA

Studies on the absorption and elimination of PAMBA showed that it is well absorbed after oral and intramuscular administration (Table 9). The blood level reached a maximum 2–3 h after oral administration, and 30–60 min after intramuscular injection. An orientation on the distribution of PAMBA in the organism was obtained by studies in rats and rabbits. Thus, PAMBA is relatively rapidly absorbed, and after 30 min it is detectable in plasma, erythrocytes and several organs (heart, lungs, liver, kidneys, spleen). Because of its renal excretion the concentration is highest in the kidneys. It requires about 8 h for plasma concentrations of PAMBA to decrease below the lower detection limit (Fig. 7). In rats, oral doses of 250 mg/kg per day over 6 weeks dit not cause a cumulation of the compound. Also in these animals, PAMBA was no longer detectable 8 h after the last dose. Its metabolic fate was investigated in man by MARKWARDT and KLÖCKING (1965a).

3. AMCA

Data on the absorption and elimination of AMCA are given in Table 9. Similar results were also obtained by others with AMCA and AMCHA (MELANDER et al., 1965). Studies in rats and mice revealed that AMCA is able to cross the placental barrier (SIREN, 1970). There is no evidence of metabolization of trans-4-amino-methylcyclohexanecarboxylic acid-(1) (ANDERSSON et al., 1971). A significant increase in the content of active compounds in the 24-h urine after acidic or after enzymatic hydrolysis by β-glucuronidase was not observed. Hydrolyzable metabolites, such as N-acetyl AMCA or AMCA glucuronide, dit not occur (KLÖCKING, 1968).

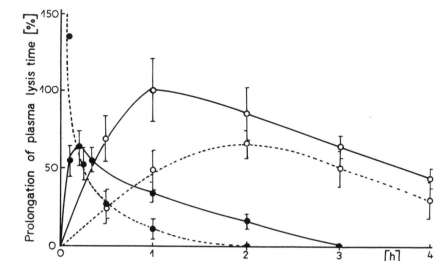

Fig. 8. Antifibrinolytic activity in rabbit plasma after oral (○) or i.v. (●) administration of 100 mg PAMBA/kg (–––) and 142 mg PAMBA-EE (——————)

4. EACA and PAMBA Derivatives

Studies on derivatives of synthetic antifibrinolytic agents (MARKWARDT and RICHTER, 1964) showed that substitution on the carboxyl or amino group will yield compounds with only a slight antifibrinolytic effect in vitro. In vivo investigations revealed that the esters of EACA, PAMBA, and AMCA are hydrolyzed in the organism, presumably in the liver, resulting in the antifibrinolytically effective free amino-carboxylic acids (Fig. 8). After oral administration, p-aminomethylbenzoic acid ethyl ester (PAMBA-EE) is more rapidly absorbed than PAMBA. Thus, the use of p-aminomethylbenzoic acid as the ethyl ester assures more rapid increase in the PAMBA level of the blood. Since the ester is rapidly hydrolyzed, its vasodilator action does not become apparent (MARKWARDT et al., 1967b).

Further investigations of homologous PAMBA esters revealed that the methyl and n-propyl esters are also hydrolyzed at about the same velocity as PAMBA-EE. Degradation of the butyl, amyl, and benzyl esters proceeds more slowly. Substitution products of the amino nitrogen of PAMBA (N-acetyl PAMBA) are not changed during body transfer and, therefore, they remain antifibrinolytically ineffective in vivo. p-(α-Amino)ethylbenzoic acid (αPAEBA), a substitution product of PAMBA, was excreted in the urine for the most part in unchanged form. Demethylation was not observed. Additional studies on the influence of chemical modifications of the PAMBA molecule on its pharmacokinetics were carried out (KLÖCKING, 1968).

IV. Antifibrinolytic Action

1. Prevention of Experimental Fibrinolysis

To demonstrate the antifibrinolytic action in vivo, the inhibitory effect of antifibrinolytic agents in hyperfibrinolytic states produced by streptokinase or urokinase

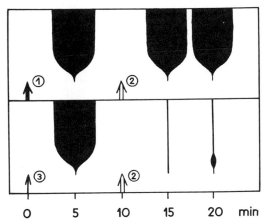

Fig. 9. Influence of EACA ① (200 mg/kg i.v.) on streptokinase-induced ② (2500 U/kg i.v.) fibrinolysis in rabbits. Injection of 0.9% NaCl ③. Thrombelastographic measurements

infusions into rabbits or dogs was utilized (MILLER et al., 1959; BELKO et al., 1963; MARKWARDT and KLÖCKING, 1965b, c, 1966a; KLÖCKING and MARKWARDT, 1969; TAKEDA et al., 1972).

To estimate the intensity of the antifibrinolytic effect in vivo, the amount of antifibrinolytic agents required to prevent fibrinolysis induced by subsequent injection of a constant amount of streptokinase was ascertained in rabbits. The antifibrinolytic agent was injected 10 min before streptokinase. Five and 10 min after streptokinase injection blood was taken by venipucture. Fibrinolysis was considered to be completely inhibited when the thrombelastogram did not show any changes compared to the control thrombelastogram, which was recorded prior to the injection. In rabbits the fibrinolysis induced by 25000 U streptokinase was prevented by 200 mg EACA/kg (for example see Fig. 9). When using the cyclic compounds, $^1/_{10}$ of the amount of EACA was sufficient.

To characterize further the antifibrinolytic action, attempts were made to interrupt streptokinase-induced and maintained fibrinolysis by injection of the antifibrinolytic agent. Experiments were carried out in rabbits anesthetized with urethane (1.2 mg/kg i.p.). Blood was withdrawn from the dissected and cannulated carotid artery. Streptokinase was infused for 60 min into the marginal ear vein. To estimate the increase in fibrinolysis and to control its course, spontaneous whole blood clot lysis, thrombin times and fibrinogen levels were determined. Moreover, thrombelastograms were recorded. As demonstrated in Figure 10, continuous i.v. infusion of 400 U streptokinase/kg/min caused extensive fibrinolysis. By i.v. injection of 25 mg PAMBA or AMCA/kg, fibrinolysis was immediately terminated and, despite continued streptokinase infusion, the tested parameters normalized. To obtain the same effects with EACA, a tenfold dose (200–300 mg/kg) was necessary.

2. Hemostatic Effect

The hemostatic effect of the antifibrinolytic agents was estimated in rabbits undergoing intensive generalized fibrinolysis in the presence of decreased prothrombin levels.

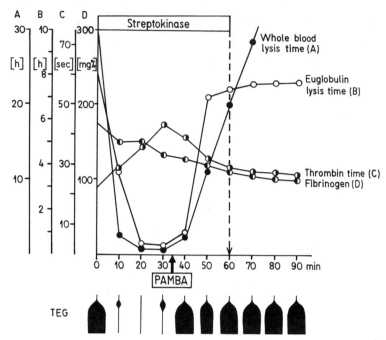

Fig. 10. Influence of PAMBA (10 mg/kg i.v.) on streptokinase-induced fibrinolysis $(4000\,U \times kg^{-1} \times min^{-1})$

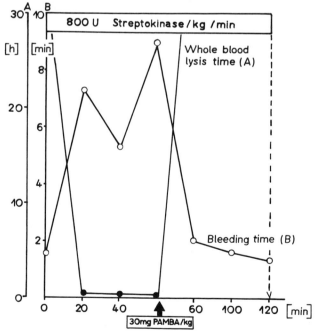

Fig. 11. Influence of PAMBA on bleeding time in rabbits pretreated with phenprocoumon after administration of streptokinase

A decrease in the prothrombin level was produced after oral pretreatment with 250 mg phenprocoumon/kg. Prothrombin was assayed by quantitative hirudin titration (MARKWARDT, 1958). On the 3rd day after anticoagulation the prothrombin level had decreased on the average to 50% of normal. At this time, a hyperfibrinolytic state was produced by infusion of 800 U streptokinase/kg/min into the marginal ear vein. Blood was withdrawn from the dissected and cannulated carotid artery. Bleeding time was determined by blotting blood every 15 s from an incision in the rabbit ear (about 3 mm long and 1 mm deep). During streptokinase infusion, bleeding time was prolonged five- to tenfold, as is demonstrated in Figure 11. Secondary bleeding from the incision occurred throughout the experiment. Upon administration of 30 mg PAMBA/kg 60 min after the beginning of streptokinase infusion, bleeding time returned to normal.

3. Other Effects Connected with the Inhibition of Fibrinolysis

When cultivating animal tissues in fibrin containing media, lysis zones may form around the explant and the fibrin medium may become liquefied (GOLDHABER et al., 1947). Due to this phenomenon, tissue cultivation is difficult, and continuous cultivation in clotted plasma or fibrin films is impossible. Therefore, it is of importance that this complication be prevented by addition of synthetic antifibrinolytics to the culture medium. To inhibit fibrinolysis in explants, a concentration of 0.005 M EACA or 0.001 M PAMBA was found to be adequate (MARKWARDT and PERLEWITZ, 1963).

Of further interest are studies on the influence of antifibrinolytics on organ transplantation in animals. By the use of EACA the survival times of skin and kidney transplants in rats and dogs were prolonged (GILETTE et al., 1963a; ZUKUOSKI et al., 1965). For this purpose, the N-acetyl derivative of EACA is thought to be more potent than EACA itself (BERTELLI et al., 1964a, b). The transplantation of animal tumors is greatly facilitated under EACA treatment (BONMASSAR et al., 1963; GILETTE et al., 1963a; CLIFFTON and AGOSTINO, 1964; DIOMEDE-FRESA and FUMAROLA, 1964; HAUSTEIN, 1967).

Because of the assumed relationship between blood coagulation and arteriosclerosis, the influence of EACA on arteriosclerotic changes in the vessel walls of experimental animals was studied. The investigations led to conflicting results (WENGER et al., 1963; KWAAN and ASTRUP, 1964; STUDER et al., 1964; KATO et al., 1970). PAMBA fed together with an atherogenic diet did not increase the rate of arteriosclerosis (MARKWARDT et al., 1964).

The inhibition of the Sanarelli-Shwartzman phenomenon or of endotoxin shock, as it was described by several authors (RAMOS et al., 1961a; SPINK and VICK, 1961; SPINK et al., 1964) could not be confirmed in studies with EACA and PAMBA (HAUSTEIN and MARKWARDT, 1965). On the contrary, EACA was found to enhance the Sanarelli-Shwartzman phenomenon (LEE, 1962; BELLER and MITCHELL, 1965). It is believed that disseminated intravascular coagulation (DIC) is provoked during endotoxin-induced Sanarelli-Shwartzman reactions. Systemic fibrinolysis secondary to DIC is a compensatory mechanism to produce lysis of intravascular clots formed by DIC, and the possibility must be accepted that the antifibrinolytics may increase microthrombosis by inhibiting the lysis of intravascular fibrin (MARGARETTEN et al., 1964; BELLER et al., 1967; BERGENTZ et al., 1972; SALDEEN et al., 1972; LOGAN et al.,

1973; BUSCH et al., 1974; MARKWARDT et al., 1975; MINN and MANDEL, 1975). Animal experiments showed that experimental thrombosis can be more frequently produced in animals treated with EACA than in controls (NORDÖY, 1963; NORD-STRÖM and ZETTERQUIST, 1969). The severity and extent of DIC and glomerular damage produced in animals by injection of thrombokinase or thrombin are increased by simultaneous administration of antifibrinolytics (VASSALI et al., 1963; MARKWARDT et al., 1975).

4. Combination with Naturally Occurring Inhibitors

The naturally occurring protease inhibitors and the synthetic antifibrinolytic agents differ in their mechanisms of action. Therefore, a mutual potentiation of effects is expected when both types of inhibitors are combined for the inhibition of fibrinolysis. Such a supra-additive effect was demonstrated by several authors using different methods (SCHMUTZLER and BECK, 1962; EGEBLAD and ASTRUP, 1963; MARKWARDT et al., 1964; SCHULTZ, 1965; ABIKO and IWAMOTO, 1970).

In vitro combination of synthetic inhibitors with protease inhibitors showed a potentiation of antifibrinolytic effects. However, the mixture of inhibitors of the same type produced only a clear additive effect, as is demonstrated by isobolograms (Fig. 12).

Moreover, supra-additive effects of a combination of antifibrinolytics were shown in animal experiments. Intravascular fibrinolysis induced by streptokinase injection was less strongly inhibited by a defined dose of either a synthetic antifibrinolytic agent or of a protease inhibitor alone, than by simultaneous administration of the half dose of each of both types of inhibitors (Fig. 13).

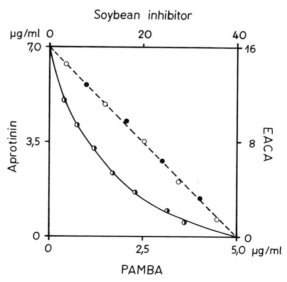

Fig. 12. Isobolograms of the inhibition of streptokinase-induced fibrinolysis (100 U/ml) in human plasma by combinations of antifibrinolytic agents ● PAMBA+EACA, ○ aprotinin+soybean inhibitor, ◑ PAMBA+aprotinin

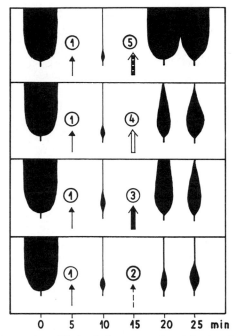

Fig. 13. Combination effects of antifibrinolytic agents after injection into rabbits. ① = 20000 U streptokinase/kg, ② = 0.9% NaCl, ③ = 3 mg PAMBA/kg, ④ = 3 mg aprotinin/kg, ⑤ = 1.5 mg PAMBA + 1.5 mg aprotinin/kg

From these experiments it is concluded that simultaneous application of antifibrinolytic agents of different modes of action causes sufficient inhibition even with greatly reduced dosage. When using inhibitor combinations therapeutically, it has to be kept in mind that, because of the different absorption, distribution and elimination characteristics of the respective antifibrinolytic agents, their blood levels may reach different values, so that the combination effect cannot be expected to be uniform at any one time and at every site of the organism.

The synthetic antifibrinolytics markedly potentiate also the inhibitory action of endogenous inhibitors (THORSEN, 1977). This may be due to the antifibrinolytic effect of the ω-amino-carboxylic acids on fibrinolysis in plasma and is probably of great importance for the clinical effectiveness of these drugs during antifibrinolytic therapy. Interestingly, COLLEN et al. (1972) reported an increased turnover of plasminogen during treatment with AMCA.

E. Clinical Pharmacology

I. Pharmacokinetics

Because blood is both the transport organ and the site of action of antifibrinolytics, their blood level and its fluctuations are of decisive importance. Therefore, to estimate their action in vivo, studies on absorption, distribution and elimination are of particular interest (Table 10).

Table 10. Pharmacokinetic data on antifibrinolytics in man

Sub-stance	Dose (mg/kg)	Elimination constant k_2 (h^{-1})	Half-life $T_{1/2}$ (min)	Distribution quotient	Invasion constant k_1 (h^{-1})	Enteral absorption (%)	Excretion in 24-h urine (% of administered dose)	
							i.v.	p.o.
EACA	37.5	0.40 ± 0.07	103 (88–127)	0.32	1.08 ± 0.08	79 ± 10	63 ± 3	55 ± 8
PAMBA	7.5	0.70 ± 0.10	60 (52– 71)	0.66	0.34 ± 0.02	69 ± 2	63 ± 17	36 ± 5
AMCA	7.5	0.65 ± 0.03	64 (61– 67)	0.33	0.74 ± 0.06	56 ± 10	80 ± 5	35 ± 18

1. EACA

Investigations of absorption and elimination of EACA in man revealed that it is rapidly and nearly completely absorbed from the gastrointestinal tract (see Table 10) (NILSSON et al., 1960; McNICOL et al., 1961a, 1962; HIEMEYER and RASCHE, 1965; NIEWIAROWSKI and WOLOSOWICZ, 1966; KALLER, 1967; KLÖCKING and MARK-WARDT, 1970). Experiments with radioactively labeled EACA confirmed these results (JOHNSON et al., 1962). From a single oral dose the EACA concentration in the blood reached its maximum after about 2 h. After intravenous injection, EACA is relatively rapidly eliminated from the blood. The half-life is about 1–2 h. Eighty to 100% of the administered dose are excreted in the urine within 12 h. Therefore, it is believed that only a small amount of the absorbed EACA is metabolized. After i.v. application of ^{14}C labeled EACA, small amounts of CO_2 were found as metabolite. From clearance tests it is concluded that EACA is eliminated by glomerular filtration and that additional tubular secretion occurs. Because of the renal elimination of EACA, its level in the urine is particularly high. After absorption, EACA is distributed also to the extracellular space and it easily crosses the erythrocyte membrane. Repeated administration for the maintenance of high plasma concentrations over a long period of time produced an increase in extravascular and intracellular concentrations of EACA. Upon termination of administration the plasma concentration decreases rapidly because of renal elimination, and EACA present in the intracellular space diffuses gradually into plasma. Consequently, after long continuous administration EACA elimination proceeds more slowly than after a single dose.

2. PAMBA

Studies on the absorption and elimination in healthy subjects revealed that the compound is well absorbed from the oral and intramuscular routes (MARKWARDT and KLÖCKING, 1965a, b; KLÖCKING, 1966b, 1967). The biological half-life is 1 h. Already 15 min after an oral dose PAMBA was detectable in the blood. The blood level reached a maximum 2–3 h after administration and had decreased below the lower detection limit after 8 h. When given intramascularly, the maximum concentration of PAMBA in the blood was reached in about 30–60 min. After intravenous injection the PAMBA level in the blood decreased sharply, and after 3–5 h the inhibitor was no longer detectable. In the 24-h urine, 50–70% of PAMBA were found in unchanged form. Up to 50% of the administered dose were excreted within the first 3 h. Two to three days after administration only traces of PAMBA (i.e. less than 2%) were found in the urine. To study the renal elimination, the clearance of PAMBA was determined after continuous i.v. infusion of 5 and 10 mg/kg body weight. Calculation of the clearance ratio revealed that the amount of PAMBA excreted in the urine was higher than that which would be eliminated by glomerular filtration alone, so that, as in the case of EACA, an additional tubular secretion must be assumed. Since PAMBA is not a lipophilic compound, its transfer from serum to the cerebrospinal fluid is difficult. After a single i.v. injection of a therapeutic dose, PAMBA was not detectable in the cerebrospinal fluid. It is, however, able to cross the placental barrier.

Since only 50–70% of PAMBA are excreted in unchanged form, the remaining portion is thought to be excreted as an inert metabolic product. Obviously, during the body passage no hydroxylation of the aromatic ring of PAMBA occurs, for no signs of the appearance of hydrobenzoic acids were found. Consequently, O-glucuronic acid conjugation of PAMBA is unlikely. N-glucuronic acid conjugation was excluded, since after incubation of the 24-h urine with β-glucuronidase the content of free PAMBA did not increase. Moreover, a conjugation of PAMBA with glycine was not observed. After hydrolysis with sulphuric acid the amount of free PAMBA in the urine samples increased on the average by 20%, so that a portion of the administered PAMBA is believed to be converted into an antifibrinolytically ineffective compound from which PAMBA can be released by hydrolysis. From collected urine of patients who had received PAMBA, the metabolic product was isolated by chromatography and electrophoresis and identified as N-acetyl PAMBA. Quantitative determinations revealed that 10–15% of the administered PAMBA are excreted in the urine as N-acetyl PAMBA. The excretion of N-acetyl PAMBA runs approximately parallel with that of PAMBA (Markwardt and Klöcking, 1965a, 1966b).

Thus, the metabolism of PAMBA proceeds in the same way as that of the sulfonamides. Usually, acetylation occurs in the organism mainly at amino groups linked directly to aromatic rings (aromatic amines), whereas acetylation as observed with PAMBA (aliphatic amino group) represents an exception. As demonstrated by pharmacologic examinations on N-acetyl PAMBA, this metabolite is a pharmacologically inert compound.

After application of PAMBA as 10% ointment (Ung. lanetti) only small amounts (<1%) were detected in the 24-h urine, whereas the same amount of PAMBA ethyl ester led to a considerably higher excretion (6%) of PAMBA in the urine (Würbach et al., 1967).

3. PAMBA Derivatives

As was shown in animal experiments with PAMBA ethyl ester, esterification of the carboxyl group in the PAMBA molecule leads to a more rapid absorption (invasion constant $k_1 = 2.82\ h^{-1}$) also in man. After oral administration a more rapid increase in the blood level is reached with PAMBA ethyl ester (Fig. 14). The higher lipid solubility of PAMBA ethyl ester decisively determines the rate of absorption. The ester reaches the blood more quickly than PAMBA and is there hydrolyzed. The

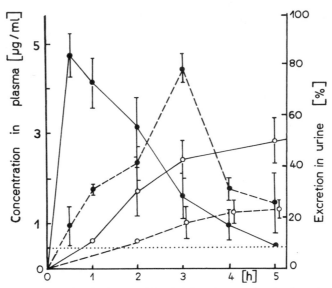

Fig. 14. PAMBA concentration in human blood (●) and excretion in the urine (○) after oral administration of 7,4 mg PAMBA/kg (– – –) or 10.7mg PAMBA-EE/kg (———)

highest rate of hydrolysis was found in the liver and kidneys. The hydrolytic activity of the blood, however, is sufficient for the rapid and complete biotransformation of the ester, whereby the blood level of PAMBA increases rapidly. Since the rate of hydrolysis of the ester is greater than that of its absorption, practically no ester is detectable in the blood. Thus, the undesired pharmacodynamic effects of the ester do not occur (MARKWARDT and RICHTER, 1964; KLÖCKING, 1967; MARKWARDT et al., 1967b; KLÖCKING et al., 1973).

Compared to PAMBA, substitution of one hydrogen of the methylene group, 4-(α-aminoethyl)-benzoic acid, results in altered pharmacokinetics in man. After oral doses (invasion constant $k_1 = 1.45\ h^{-1}$) the blood level increases more rapidly, the rate of absorption is diminished ($57 \pm 4\%$), and the half-life is 2 h (VOGEL and KLÖCKING, 1969).

4. AMCA

The pharmacokinetic data of AMCA are shown in Table 10. Accordingly, the half-life is about 1 h. Other authors reported AMCA half-lives of the same order of magnitude (ANDERSSON et al., 1965, 1971; DONNER and HOUSKOVA, 1967; KALLER, 1967). Studies on the distribution performed by measuring the AMCA content in organ samples taken after oral doses of 20 mg/kg during surgical operations revealed that AMCA is present in muscular and adipose tissues, in the kidneys and prostate and, in particularly high concentrations, in the bladder. AMCA is absorbed relatively slowly and incompletely from the gastrointestinal tract. Maximum blood levels are obtained 2–5 h after a single oral dose. Small amounts of AMCA are detectable in the blood for up to 24 h. After intravenous injection, 80–90% of the dose are found in the 24-h urine in unchanged form. Because of the incomplete absorption, only about 50% of orally given AMCA are excreted in the 24-h urine. No metabolite of AMCA is known. In the human organism, hydroxylation and conjugation with glucuronic acid do not take place. Furthermore, there is no evidence of N-acetylation of AMCA.

II. Therapeutic Uses

In general, hyperfibrinolytic bleeding cannot be stopped by conventional measures such as blood and fibrinogen transfusions. Plasminogen, which is part of the transfused blood, is activated to plasmin. Fibrinogen is degraded and yields degradation products which impair the process of hemostasis. Therefore, bleeding from pathological fibrinolysis is sustained rather than arrested by infusions of whole blood, plasma or fibrinogen. A causal treatment of fibrinolytic hemorrhage is possible only by the use of antifibrinolytics. Indications for their use arise in conditions of pathological fibrinolysis which, because of the increase in localized or generalized fibrinolysis, can result in overt hemorrhage. There are many reports on the use of antifibrinolytics in the therapy of fibrinolytic bleeding (for references see MARKWARDT et al., 1972), and several authors in various countries have demonstrated the value of antifibrinolytic therapy with synthetic antifibrinolytics (among others: NILSSON et al., 1961; MARCHAL et al., 1962, 1963, 1964; McNICOL, 1962; STEICHELE and HERSCHLEIN, 1962; BOUVIER, 1963; DETTORI and PONARI, 1963; LACOMBE, 1963; LEGER, 1963; MARX, 1963; POLUSCHKIN and BARKAGAN, 1963; LENOIR et al., 1964; McNICOL and DOUGLAS, 1964; NIEWIAROWSKI, 1964, 1965; PERLICK, 1964; SAMAMA, 1964; VAIREL et al., 1964; SWEENEY, 1965; MARKWARDT, 1966; MARKWARDT and LANDMANN, 1967; VOGEL and SUNDERMANN, 1970).

1. Mode of Action

The antifibrinolytic action of synthetic antifibrinolytic agents is attributed to an inhibition of fibrin degradation by plasmin. Consequently, after addition of an antifibrinolytic agent to blood having enhanced fibrinolytic activity, the fibrin clots formed are believed to be protected from rapid dissolution. The therapeutic effect of antifibrinolytics is a hemostatic one.

Hemostasis is the aim of antifibrinolytic therapy, and a large number of publications show that the hemostatic effect of antifibrinolytics is actually exerted in vivo (DAPUNT and SCHWARZ, 1964; HAGELSTEN and NOLTE, 1964; BONNAR and CRAWFORD, 1965; SUNDERMANN and VOGEL, 1967; HOROWITZ and SPIELVOGEL, 1971; for further references see MARKWARDT et al., 1972). The prompt arrest of fibrinolytic bleeding after administration of inhibitors can hardly be explained by a competitive inhibition of plasminogen activation, which needs to be followed by clearance of circulating plasmin. Since the hemostatic effect is displayed during generalized hyperplasminemic states, i.e. after plasminogen activation, the prevention of fibrin dissolution by the inhibition of plasmin seems to explain the observed phenomena. Even small amounts of fibrinogen, which are still present during prolonged hyperplasminemia, might suffice for effective formation of a hemostatic plug by blood platelets. Further inhibitory actions of the antifibrinolytics on the fibrinolytic system seem to be of certain importance in vivo. During therapeutic use of inhibitors both an improvement of impaired hemostasis and an inhibition of pathologically activated fibrinolysis occur. Prolongation of whole blood and plasma lysis times or normalization of the thrombelastograms can be expected, since these test systems contain antifibrinolytic agents. Prolongation of lysis times as well as shortening of thrombin times and an increase in the fibrinogen level are observed (Fig. 9). Such effects must be considered as the consequence of an inactivation of the fibrinolytic system. Presumably, the inhibitory effects of the antifibrinolytics on plasminogen activation and fibrinogenolysis by plasmin seem to play a certain role in vivo. However, it is believed that the strong hemostatic effect of the antifibrinolytics in fibrinolytic bleeding is not exclusively caused by such a depression of the activity of the fibrinolytic system. Obviously, the specific inhibition of plasmin action on fibrin represents the most important therapeutic quality of action, and it is responsible for the hemostatic effect.

2. Side-Effects

The use of EACA in man causes relatively few side-effects. In some cases, large doses of EACA produce disturbances of orthostasis. After oral administration, gastrointestinal complaints (abdominal pain, diarrhea, vomiting) were reported, which passed off when the dose was reduced or stopped (STEFANINI and MARIN, 1958; MCNICOL et al., 1961b; NILSSON et al., 1961, 1966; ANDERSSON and LINDSTEDT, 1963; ANDERSSON, 1964; LUDWIG and MEHRING, 1965; BÖHNEL and STACHER, 1966). Moreover, clot formation in the renal pelvis was observed, leading in most cases to transient anuria (JUNG and DUCKERT, 1960; HILGARTNER, 1966; LINDGARDH and ANDERSSON, 1966; GOBBI, 1967; ITTERBECK et al., 1968). Allergic reactions appeared only infrequently during EACA treatment (SACK et al., 1962). After EACA administration a fall in blood pressure was reported (STRAUB, 1966; SWARTZ et al., 1966). Since chronic administration of large doses of EACA to animals led to a decrease in fertility and to disturbances in fetal development, the question arises whether the use of EACA during pregnancy, particularly within the first trimester, may represent a risk. Until now, such effects were not observed in women. Patients who became pregnant during EACA treatment gave birth to normal children (ANDERSSON et al, 1965). Since EACA is eliminated for the most part through the kidneys, patients with reduced renal function may accumulate the drug and may reach undesirably high plasma levels.

After administration of PAMBA to healthy subjects, as well as after its therapeutic use, side-effects were not observed. Long-term treatment with PAMBA up to a total dose of 1600 g did not produce discomfort, allergic reactions were not reported, and careful clinical examination did not reveal any signs of organ damage. Thrombotic and embolic states did not develop (VOGEL, 1969; VOGEL and SUNDERMANN, 1970).

During clinical use of AMCA only vertigo was reported (ANDERSSON et al., 1964).

3. Contraindications

Starting from the assumption that fibrin formation (blood coagulation) and fibrin dissolution (fibrinolysis) are in a physiological equilibrium, occlusions of vessels might occur during antifibrinolytic therapy as a consequence of the inhibitory action on the dissolution of intravascularly formed fibrin. However, during the use of synthetic antifibrinolytics an enhanced tendency to clotting was not observed. Thrombosis during EACA treatment was reported (GRALNIK and GREIP, 1971). However, detailed studies revealed that postoperative thromboembolism occurred with about the same frequency as in the controls (McNICOL et al., 1961b; ANDERS-SON, 1964). Systematic studies of the influence of PAMBA on plasmatic coagulation factors and blood platelet functions, as well as clinical and autopsy findings, revealed that this drug exerts no thrombosis-promoting or producing effect. In patients with a disposition to thrombosis, the general use of inhibitors might involve a risk, so that in these cases care should be exercised when antifibrinolytics are used (NILSSON et al., 1961; NAEYE, 1962).

The fibrinolytic system plays a decisive role in consumption coagulopathy and disseminated intravascular coagulation (DIC). The formation of microthrombi is usually accompanied by excessive fibrinolysis as a repair mechanism for the removal of fibrin deposits (KLIMAN and McKAY, 1958; IATRIDIS, 1966; JOHNSON and MER-SKEY, 1966; ASTRUP, 1968; PHILIPS et al., 1968; WILSON et al., 1971). Therefore, microthrombosis is increased by the inhibition of fibrinolysis, as was demonstrated in many animal experiments (see D, IV, 3).

Antifibrinolytics should be used only when heparinization was not successful and excessive fibrinolysis has been demonstrated.

4. Indications

Acute and chronic localized fibrinolytic bleeding as well as primary generalized hyperfibrinolytic states are principal indications. The secondary increase in fibrinolysis as the consequence of intravascular (and in most cases diffuse) coagulation processes does not commonly represent an indication for antifibrinolytics (see E, II, 3).

a) Bleeding After Operations on Activator-Rich Organs

Fibrinolytic bleeding occurring after operation or trauma is believed to be caused by an inflow of tissue activators into the blood. The fibrinolytic activity in human organs can be determined by measuring the lysis zones formed by explants on fibrin plates. Thus, a traumatically caused liberation of activators of fibrinolysis can be estimated. The activator content of several organs varies in dependence on age, sex, and functional state. Therefore, the measured values show a relatively wide variability. However, specific organs have been identified in which fibrinolysis of a particularly high degree may occur after injury. Experience has shown that extensive operations on the lungs, brain, uterus, prostate, adrenals, and thyroid gland are often accompanied by bleeding that can hardly be stopped.

Hyperfibrinolytic states, which occur quite frequently during surgery, do not necessarily lead to clinically established hemorrhagic diatheses. In case of uncontrollable bleeding during operations in activator-rich regions, a pathological increase in fibrinolysis has to be taken into account. Bleeding caused by the inflow of tissue activators into the blood represents an indication for the use of antifibrinolytics. As demonstrated in Fig. 15, fibrinolysis was prevented or interrupted in this way and bleeding rapidly arrested.

There are numerous reports on the use of antifibrinolytics in bleeding after operations on the thorax (MARCHAL et al., 1963; BARKAGAN et al., 1965; SCHMIDT and AMRIS, 1966; VOGEL, 1966; LUKASZCZYK and ORZEL, 1968), after abdominal surgery (ROUSSELOT et al., 1962; ANDERSSON and LINDSTEDT, 1963; LEGER et al., 1963; GROSSI et al., 1964; GUIMBRETIERE and LEBEAUPIN, 1964; HELLINGER and VOGEL, 1966; MESTER et al., 1967), after neurosurgery (NORLEN and THULIN, 1967; 1969; GIBBS and CORKILL, 1971; PATTERSON and HARPEL, 1971), as well as after cardiovascular surgery (AMBRUS et al., 1971; MCCLURE and IZSAK, 1974).

b) Bleeding in the Region of the Oral, Nasal and Pharyngeal Mucosa

Bleeding occurring after surgery on the nasopharynx or after stomatological operations may be propagated by increased localized fibrinolysis. Gingival tissue (GUSTAFSSON and NILSSON, 1961) and saliva (ALBRECHTSEN and THAYSEN, 1955; SCHULTE and VORBAUER, 1965) contain activators of fibrinolysis. Furthermore, in the region of the oral or nasal mucosa there are multiple possibilities of activating the fibrinolytic system, since a part of the nasal mucosa is moistened by kinase-containing lachrymal fluid, the mucosa of the inferior concha is rich in plasminogen activator, and the salivary glands belong to the most activator-rich organs. A further possibility of activation is given by streptococci that are frequently found in the oral cavity. Besides oral or parenteral administration of antifibrinolytic agents, such bleeding can also be treated locally by rinsing with an antifibrinolytic solution and subsequent tamponade with an impregnated wad. Postoperative bleeding after dental extraction or tonsillectomy can be controlled in this way.

This use of antifibrinolytics is reported in postoperative bleeding after dental extraction (COOKSEY et al., 1966; ROTHE, 1967; EGLI and SCHRÖDER, 1968; ANDRÄ and SCHLOTTMANN, 1969) after tonsillectomy (BERGER and DINSON, 1964; DUMAY and DANCE, 1964; GHILARDI et al., 1965; IWASAWA, 1967; KHALFEN, 1967; NUERNBERGK, 1967; CONTICELLO et al., 1968; TANNER, 1968; SCHOFFKE, 1970; PELL, 1973).

c) Bleeding in the Gastrointestinal Tract

In experimental studies gastric venous blood was shown to have considerably more fibrinolytic activity than gastric arterial blood. Antifibrinolytics may become a new factor in the management of bleeding from acute gastric erosions (REDLEAF et al., 1963; NOER, 1964; THOMSON et al., 1973) and ulcerative colitis (SALTER and READ, 1970).

d) Bleeding in the Urinary Tract

Urine contains urokinase which causes a dissolution of fibrin clots in the renal pelvis, ureters, and bladder. When those organs are damaged, the healing lesion is exposed to repeated fibrinolytic attacks, since plasminogen in the wound-covering fibrin is activated by activators which are liberated from the damaged tissue, as well as by urokinase contained in the urine, whereby hemorrhages may occur. Such hemorrhages are frequently observed after operations on the bladder or prostate, where urokinase is in intimate contact with the damaged tissue. In contrast to naturally occurring proteinase inhibitors synthetic antifibrinolytics are excreted for the most part in the urine in active form. Therefore, fibrinolytic processes in the urinary tract

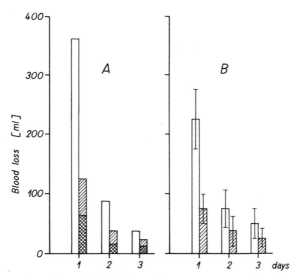

Fig. 15. Hemostatic effect of antifibrinolytics. Average postoperative blood loss following prostatectomy A) in three groups of 25 patients each under treatment with EACA (in dosages of approx. 20 and 10 g per day) *(hatched column)*. Control patients received no antifibrinolytic treatment (according to ANDERSSON, 1972); B) in two groups of 20 patients each under treatment with PAMBA (100 mg i.v. 4 times per day on the first and second day, then 250 mg p.o. 4 times per day) *(hatched column)* and placebo (according to MARKWARDT et al., 1972).

can be arrested by their use, so that EACA, PAMBA or AMCA are preferentially indicated for the treatment of fibrinolytic bleeding in that area. An example is demonstrated in Figure 15 (FETTER et al., 1961; McNICOL et al., 1961b; ANDERSSON, 1962; SACK et al., 1962; ABOULKER et al., 1963; KOLLER, 1963; LADEHOFF and OTTE, 1963; GIBBA and TETTERINO, 1964; LASSNER, 1965; ROUFFILANGE et al., 1965; AL-BEET, 1966; ANDERSSON et al., 1966; HELLINGER, 1966a, b, 1967; OSWALD et al., 1966; SCHMUTZLER and FÜRSTENBERG, 1966; KIRKMAN, 1967; LUDVIK and PECHERSTOR-FER, 1967; NEEF et al., 1967; PREUSSER et al., 1967; STORM, 1967; SZABADOS, 1967; WÖLFER et al., 1967; ZINN, 1968; HEDLUND, 1969; ROSDY et al., 1969; SAUERLAND, 1969; VESSEY et al., 1969; WARREN, 1969; SZELESTEI and KELEMEN, 1970; ANDERSSON and BOEMINGHAUS, 1972; NABER et al., 1973).

In general, antifibrinolytic treatment is started only after surgery, and it is continued until macroscopic hematuria is no longer observed. If blood reappears in the urine during the postoperative period antifibrinolytic treatment must be continued. Preoperative administration of antifibrinolytics does not reduce the blood loss during surgery, since hemorrhages are generally caused by an opened artery in the vesical cervix or in the prostatic cavity and not by fibrinolysis.

Antifibrinolytics are not only used in postoperative bleeding in the urinary tract, but also in the treatment of so-called essential hematuria, which is caused by renal lesions whose healing is significantly retarded because of the urokinase activity in the urine (ANDERSSON, 1962; ZMERLI et al., 1962; IMMERGUT and STEVENSON, 1965; SUNDERMANN and VOGEL, 1965; HELLINGER, 1966b; VOGEL and SUNDERMANN,

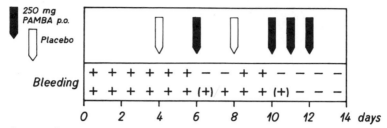

Fig. 16. Influence of PAMBA on recurrent uterine bleeding (according to FLÄHMIG et al., 1965)

1966; HOFFMANN and KLÖCKING, 1967; HOFFMANN and VOGEL, 1967; VOGEL et al., 1967; ZHILA, 1968; BILINSKY et al., 1969; RO et al., 1970; ANDERSSON, 1972; SILVER-BERG et al., 1974).

When bleeding in the urinary tract is treated with antifibrinolytics, it has to be kept in mind that inhibition of fibrinolysis may cause fibrin clots to remain in the renal pelvis and ureters, thus possibly blocking the urinary passages (COGGINS and ALLEN, 1972).

e) Uterine Bleeding

Fibrinolytic processes caused by liberation of activators from the endometrium play an important role in physiologic and pathologic uterine hemorrhages. The activator content of the endometrium varies with the menstrual cycle. During the secretory phase it is particularly high. In menstruation, the tissue activator is liberated and triggers localized fibrinolysis, resulting in a high fibrinolytic activity of the uterine blood (HUGGINS et al., 1943; ALBRECHTSEN, 1956a, b; ELLERT and NOLT, 1956; BELLER and GRAEFF, 1957).

Pathologically increased localized fibrinolytic activity might be the cause of me-norrhagia. Antifibrinolytics inhibit fibrinolytic processes in the uterus, whereby the extent of pathological bleeding is reduced. In order that physiological uterine bleeding shall not be impaired, antifibrinolytics are used only after menstruation has started. In case of primary hemorrhagic disorders (hemophilia, thrombocytopathy) uterine bleeding may be increased by localized fibrinolysis. One of the causes, i.e., localized fibrinolysis, may be eliminated with the help of antifibrinolytic therapy.

Antifibrinolytic treatment of metrorrhagia and menorrhagia was reported by several authors (SATO et al., 1959; ALBRECHTSEN and SKJØDT, 1963; BAKSHEEV et al., 1964; MALENE, 1964; NIESERT et al., 1964; FLÄHMIG et al., 1965, 1967; FRANÇOIS, 1965; LUDWIG and MEHRING, 1965; NILSSON and BJÖRKMAN, 1965; NILSSON and RYBO, 1965; KOUTSKY et al., 1967; LINZ, 1967; BOSTARD, 1969; NAGY et al., 1970; HERSCHLEIN et al., 1972) (Fig. 16).

f) Bleeding in Obstetrical Complications

Under unfavorable conditions of pathologic delivery and obstetrical complications, activators of fibrinolysis can enter the circulation. This event may occur during damage to the uterus, artificial abortion, manual removal of placenta, premature abruption of placenta, intra-uterine death of the fetus, or amniotic fluid embolism. In these cases, intensive reactions were observed which led to fatal afibrinogenemic bleedings. The use of antifibrinolytics was repeatedly reported (MARZETTI, 1964; BONNAR and CRAWFORD, 1965; DELECOUR et al., 1965; GANS, 1965; SCHILD, 1965; AZBUKINA, 1966; BONHOMME and LEMAIRE, 1966; LORIA-MENDEZ et al., 1966; CORRAL et al., 1967; SIEG and FLÄHMIG, 1967; BUDYKA, 1968; HARMS, 1968; SHILKO et al., 1968; RUZICSKA et al., 1970; SLUSKY, 1970; RYBO and WESTERBERG, 1972; ISAKSON, 1973). It is difficult to decide whether there exists a primary increase in fibrinolysis as a consequence of hyperplasminemia, or whether diffuse intravascular coagulation with secondary fibrinolysis prevails. Examination of the blood generally revealed signs of both processes, which result in defibrination with hemorrhagic diatheses. Several differential diagnostic methods were described to clarify whether the main cause of these processes was coagulation or fibrinolysis. When fibrin deficiency is caused by excessive coagulation, interruption of the coagulation process by heparin is necessary in addition to fibrinogen substitution. There exist different opinions on the usefulness of inhibitors of fibrinolysis. When intravascular coagulation is suspected, application of antifibrinolytics will carry the risk of preventing the resolution of intravascularly formed clots. Therefore, the application of antifibrinolytics in reactive fibrinolysis is only justified when the clinical picture indicates excessive lysis. Problems concerning the administration of inhibitors of fibrinolysis in obstetrical bleedings, which are caused by defibrination, were reported (ELSNER, 1962; BELLER, 1963; STAMM et al., 1963; GRAEBER et al., 1964).

g) Subarachnoidal Bleeding

Recently, considerable interest was shown in the use of antifibrinolytics in the treatment of patients with subarachnoidal hemorrhages and intracranial aneurysms. The administration of these agents to laboratory animals both maintained and strengthened experimentally produced intravascular thrombi (MULLAN et al., 1964; PATTERSON and HARPEL, 1971). In patients with recent subarachnoidal hemorrhage the antifibrinolytics seemed to have prevented premature recurrence of bleeding during the acute treatment interval (MULLAN and DAWLEY, 1968; NORLEN and THULIN, 1970; TOVI et al., 1972; SMITH and UPCHURCH, 1973; TOVI, 1973; CORKILL, 1974) (Fig. 17). Arteriopathic complications were observed during treatment of subarachnoidal hemorrhage with EACA (SONNTAG and STEIN, 1974).

h) Bleeding in Carcinoma and Leukemia

In malignant neoplasms of activator-rich organs, e.g. carcinoma of the prostate, an excessive production of plasminogen activators occurs. These are liberated into the circulating blood and trigger extensive fibrinolysis which may cause spontaneous hemorrhages. In certain cases of acute leukemia a generalized fibrinolysis of high degree develops in a similar way. In general, hemorrhages appear as extensive secondary hematomas and as hemorrhages from the primary tumor. Since these hemorrhages are mainly caused by an excessive production of activator, they can be controlled with the aid of antifibrinolytics. The use of antifibrinolytics in carcinoma of the prostate was reported (ANDERSSON and NILSSON, 1961, 1969; JOSSO et al., 1962; WINKELMANN et al., 1962; ANDERSSON, 1963; MARCHAL et al., 1963; SIGSTAD and LAMVIK, 1963; STOCKER and MAIER, 1964; SUGIURA, 1966; ANDERSSON and NILSSON, 1969). Since in some cases of acute leukemia bleeding cannot be controlled by EACA (NILSSON et al., 1961), the protease of leukocytes is believed to participate in

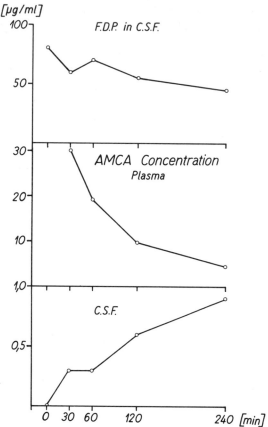

Fig. 17. Fibrinogen degradation products *(FDP)* in cerebro-spinal fluid *(CSF)* and AMCA concentration in plasma and CSF after a single i.v. dose of 1 g AMCA in man (according to TOVI et al., 1972)

the development of generalized fibrinolysis in addition to specific proteolytic processes (CAVIEZEL et al., 1964). Further problems arise when secondary fibrinolysis has developed from the liberation of tissue activators as a consequence of intravascular fibrin precipitation. Contrary to earlier assumptions, recent studies have shown that these bleedings following neoplastic disease are mainly caused by consumption coagulopathy and not by primary hyperfibrinolysis.

i) Extracorporeal Circulation

Extracorporeal circulation during surgery nearly always causes fibrin deposition in the heart-lung machine, and excessive lytic activity can often be detected in the patient's blood at the end of perfusion. There exist multiple reasons for the activation of coagulation and lysis mechanisms. The contact with foreign surfaces and with the air in the pump plays a significant role. Moreover, surgical interventions and oxygen deficit may cause tissue damage, which in turn may lead to the liberation of activators of fibrinolysis. Defibrination accompanied by increased fibrinolytic activity occasionally causes fatal bleeding immediately after perfusion. For this reason, the use of antifibrinolytics, such as naturally occurring as well as synthetic protease inhibitors, is recommended for the inhibition of fibrinolysis (MARCHAL et al., 1960; GROSSI et al., 1961; MARX and BORST, 1961; GANS and KRIVIT, 1962; MARGGRAF, 1962; WINKELMANN and HIEMEYER, 1962; MASCART, 1963; SAMAMA et al., 1963; TICE et al., 1963a b, 1964). Since heparin is generally administered as anticoagulant during operations involving extracorporeal circulation, prophylactic antifibrinolytic therapy is justified without prior establishment of diagnosis to differentiate between primary and secondary fibrinolysis.

k) Control of Therapeutic Fibrinolysis

After it had become possible to induce fibrinolysis in the organism and to perform thrombolytic therapy, antifibrinolytics have gained growing importance as antidotes. Already the first experiments with streptokinase were accompanied by incidents in the sense of hyperplasminemia. Because hyperplasminemia disappears when streptokinase application is stopped, antifibrinolytics are only infrequently used for termination of fibrinolytic therapy. The use of EACA was reported by several authors (ALKJAERSIG et al., 1959b; FLETCHER et al., 1959; FISCHBACHER, 1961; GIBELLI,

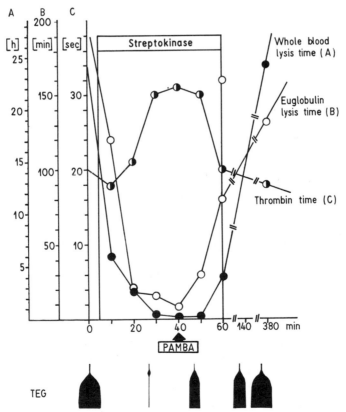

Fig. 18. Influence of PAMBA (1 mg/kg i.v.) on streptokinase-induced fibrinolysis $(2000 \, U \times kg^{-1} \times h^{-1})$ in man

1962). An example of the use of PAMBA as antidote of fibrinolytic therapy with streptokinase is shown in Figure 18. Proposals to perform fibrinolytic therapy with simultaneous administration of EACA (Nilsson and Olow, 1962; Olow, 1963; Olow and Nilsson, 1963) have been rejected because there are no advantages in this procedure (Hiemeyer and Rasche, 1965).

l) Bleeding of Unknown Etiology

The lack and inadequacy of effective hemostatic agents led to the use of antifibrinolytics in the therapy of bleedings that cannot be attributed directly to increased fibrinolysis. Because of the apparent therapeutic results it is assumed that the role of fibrinolysis as contributing factor in disturbances of hemostasis is more important than commonly believed. Therefore, the therapeutic use of antifibrinolytics in bleeding that is difficult to control seems to be justified also in those cases where no fibrinolysis has been detected. However, consumption coagulopathy must be fully excluded.

The diagnostic use in bleeding of unknown etiology has been proposed. When bleeding stops after administration of an antifibrinolytic agent, fibrinolysis is suggested; if not, other causes have to be taken into account (Roth, 1962).

m) Thrombocytopenia and Hemophilia

In the presence of thrombocytopenia the clots formed after injury are poor in platelets. Compared to normal platelet-containing fibrin clots, they are more easily attacked by the fibrinolytic enzyme (Sherry and Alkjaersig, 1957). Even a relatively slight fibrinolytic activity may lead to clot lysis and overt bleeding. Presumably, the hemostatic effect of antifibrinolytics in thrombocytopenia occurs through inhibition of lysis (Cattan et al., 1963; Fletcher, 1963; Croizat et al., 1964; Mey et al., 1967).

The fact that bleeding in hemophilia can be arrested by antifibrinolytics is of particular interest. These findings allow the assumption that fibrinolysis is an important etiological factor. Several workers believe that during the decay of platelets in the process of coagulation activators of fibrinolysis are released, leading to acute predominance of fibrinolysis over the weak and insufficient clotting activity of the hemophilic blood. A great number of publications deal with this problem (Abe et al., 1962; Poulain et al., 1964; Mainwaring and Keidan, 1965; Ritz, 1965; Tsevrenis and Mandalaki, 1965; Creveld and Vos-Bongaardt, 1966; Gugler et al., 1966; Marin et al., 1966; Poulain and Josso, 1966; Garbin and Gerofalo, 1967; Herxheimer and Capel, 1967; Hodge and Reid, 1967; Reid et al., 1967; Biggs and Hayton-Williams, 1968; Gobbi, 1968; Itterbeck et al., 1968; Corrigan, 1972; Storti et al., 1972; Rainsford, 1973).

No significant decrease in spontaneous bleeding was obtained with the prophylactic use of EACA (Gordon et al., 1965; Strauss et al., 1965). Successful arrest of bleeding by antifibrinolytics was reported after dental extraction in hemophiliacs (Fonio, 1964, 1966; Reid et al., 1964; Paddon, 1967; Cooksey, 1968; Giordano et al., 1968; Tavenner, 1968; Kontras et al., 1969; Walsh et al., 1971; Bjorlin and Nilsson, 1973). Since localized fibrinolysis in the oral cavity is maintained by activators from saliva or gingival tissue, this represents an additional complication in hemophilia. The formation of a wound cover is facilitated by inhibition of the fibrinolytic process.

n) *Wound Healing*

As was shown by ASTRUP (1959), fibrinolytic processes play a role in wound healing. Connective tissue cells enter the fibrin deposits in the wound and cause cellular organization of the clot. Studies in experimental animals showed that wound healing is impaired by increased fibrinolytic activity in the blood (BENZER et al., 1963, 1964). Correspondingly, improved wound healing occurs when the activity is decreased by protease inhibitors (FLANDRE et al., 1966). Therefore, further indications emerge for the use of synthetic inhibitors of fibrinolysis. Successful treatments of infected necrotic wounds with EACA were reported (ROLLE, 1965). Furthermore, studies on homotransplantation of human skin under EACA treatment are of interest (BOGDANOV et al., 1964).

o) *Allergic Reactions*

Several workers used EACA in the treatment of diseases that were not caused by pathological fibrinolysis. Beginning with studies in experimental animals which revealed an antiallergic effect of the antifibrinolytics, attempts were made to treat allergic diseases with antifibrinolytics. EACA was found to be particularly effective in allergic dermatoses (YOKOYAMA and HATANO, 1959; HATANO et al., 1962; ARNET et al., 1963; McFADDEN, 1965; SAKURANE and YAMAGUCHI, 1965). The tuberculin reaction was found to be decreased by the use of EACA (ITOGA and YOGO, 1959; STACHER, 1962; LOWNEY, 1964). Furthermore, successes in EACA treatment of bronchial asthma, allergic transfusion reactions and other allergic diseases were reported (STACHER, 1962; ARNET et al., 1963; BADELMANN et al., 1965). However, the conclusions drawn from these successes are not convincing. Clinical studies with PAMBA did not show antiallergic effects. Moreover, therapeutic studies in rheumatic disease and scleroderma led to different results (ROTSTEIN et al., 1963; LAUGIER, 1964; LENOIR et al., 1964; REQUE, 1965). Indications not usually associated with fibrinolysis include angioneurotic edema (LUNDH et al., 1968; CHAMPION and LACHMANN, 1969; FRANK et al., 1972; SHEFFER et al., 1972).

5. Administration and Dosage

Depending on the absorption and elimination characteristics of synthetic antifibrinolytics in man, as well as on the blood levels required for the inhibition of fibrinolytic processes, the dosages of synthetic antifibrinolytics vary between compounds.

Therapy with EACA needs relatively large doses. For prevention of fibrinolysis a plasma level of 10^{-3} M EACA (13 mg-%) is required. Because of the relatively rapid elimination a single oral or intravenous dose of EACA does not maintain this level in the blood for a sufficiently long period of time. For optimal therapeutic effects an initial dose of 4–5 g is given, and the EACA level is maintained by further doses of 1 g/h. For prophylaxis, oral administration of 5–10 g per day is adequate.

To interrupt fibrinolytic processes with the more potent cyclic amino carboxylic acids, much smaller amounts suffice. In case of PAMBA, i.v. or i.m. initial doses of 50–100 mg are adequate. Additional administration depends on the clinical course and the results of clotting tests. In the absence of a response the initial dose is followed by a continuous infusion of 100 mg per hour intravenously. In case of oral administration, 250 mg are given as a single dose. In general, the same dose is repeated in intervals of 4–8 h until bleeding is arrested.

AMCA is generally administered in doses of 250–500 mg by slow i.v. injection and, if necessary, by subsequent continuous infusion of 250 mg per hour. When given orally, 250 mg 4–6 times per day are usually satisfactory. Treatments should not exceed 7 days.

References

Abe, T., Sato, A.: Inhibitory activity of ε-aminocaproic acid upon fibrinolysis. Acta haemat. jap. **21**, 305 (1958)

Abe, T., Sato, A.: Reaction mechanism between ε-aminocaproic acid and plasmin, tissue activator and trypsin. Keio J. Med. **8**, 219 (1959)

Abe, T., Sato, A., Kazama, M., Matsumara, T.: Effect of ε-aminocaproic acid in haemophilia. Lancet **1962 II**, 405

Abiko, Y., Iwamoto, M.: Plasminogen-plasmin system. VII. Potentation of antifibrinolytic action of a synthetic inhibitor, tranexamic acid, by α_2-macroglobulin antiplasmin. Biochim. biophys. Acta (Amst.) **214**, 411 (1970)

Abiko, Y., Iwamoto, M., Shimizu, M.: Plasminogen-plasmin system. II. Purification and properties of human plasmin. J. Biochem. (Tokyo) **64**, 751 (1968)

Abiko, Y., Iwamoto, M., Tomikawa, M.: Plasminogen-plasmin system. V. A stoichiometric equilibrium of plasminogen and a synthetic inhibitor. Biochim. biophys. Acta (Amst.) **185**, 424 (1969)

Ablondi, F., Hagan, J. J., Philips, M., Renzo, E. C. de: Inhibition of plasmin, trypsin and the streptokinase-activated fibrinolytic system by ε-aminocaproic acid. Arch. Biochem. **82**, 153 (1959)

Aboulker, P., Lassner, J., Samama, M., Casubolo, M.: L'action de l'acide epsilon amino caproïque sur le saignement en chirurgie urinaire. Anesth. Analg. Réanim. **20**, 581 (1963)

Albeet, L.: Über die hämostatische Wirkung der Epsilon-Amino-Kapronsäure nach suprapubischer transvesikaler Prostatektomie. Z. Urol. **59**, 425 (1966)

Albrechtsen, O. K.: The fibrinolytic activity in the human endometrium. Acta endocr. (Kbh.) **23**, 207 (1956a)

Albrechtsen, O. K.: The fibrinolytic activity of menstrual blood. Acta endocr. (Kbh.) **23**, 219 (1956b)

Albrechtsen, O. K., Skjødt, P.: The effect of epsilonamino-caproic acid on uterine haemorrhage. Acta obstet. gynec. scand. **42**, 160 (1963)

Albrechtsen, O. K., Thaysen, J. H.: Fibrinolytic activity in human saliva. Acta physiol. scand. **35**, 138 (1955)

Alkjaersig, N.: The activation of plasminogen *in vitro* and *in vivo*. In: MacMillan, R. L., Mustard, J. F., (Eds.): Anticoagulants and Fibrinolysins, p. 365. London: Pitman Medical Publishing Co. Ltd. 1961

Alkjaersig, N.: Purification of human plasminogen by DEAE-sephadex chromatography. Fed. Proc. **21**, 64 (1962)

Alkjaersig, N.: The purification and properties of human plasminogen. Biochem. J. **93**, 171 (1964)

Alkjaersig, N., Fletcher, A. P., Sherry, S.: ε-Aminocaproic acid: an inhibitor of plasminogen activation. J. biol. Chem. **234**, 832 (1959a)

Alkjaersig, N., Fletcher, A. P., Sherry, S.: The mechanism of clot dissolution by plasmin. J. clin. Invest. **38**, 1086 (1959b).

Allison, F., Jr., Lancaster, M. G.: Pathogenesis of acute inflammation. VI. Influence of osmolarity and certain metabolic antagonists upon phagocytosis and adhesiveness by leucocytes recovered from man. Proc. Soc. exp. Biol. (N.Y.) **119**, 56 (1965)

Allison, F., Jr., Lancaster, M. G., Crostwaite, J. L.: Studies on the pathogenesis of acute inflammation. V. An assessment of factors that influence *in vitro* the phagocytic and adhesive properties of leucocytes obtained from rabbit peritoneal exudate. Amer. J. Path. **43**, 75 (1963)

Ambrus, C. M., Ambrus, J. L., Lassman, H. B., Mink, I. B.: Studies on the mechanism of action of inhibitors of the fibrinolytic system. Ann. N. Y. Acad. Sci. **146**, 430 (1968)

Ambrus, C. M., Ambrus, J. L., Lassman, H. B., Mink, I. B.: On the heterogeneity of activity by various types of plasmins and the spectra of inhibition of some plasmin inhibitors. Res. Commun. Chem. Pathol. Pharmacol. **1**, 67 (1970)

Ambrus, J. L., Schimert, G., Lajos, T. Z., Ambrus, L. M., Mink, I. B., Lassman, H. B., Moore, R. H., Melzer, J.: Effect of antifibrinolytic agents and estrogens on blood loss and blood coagulation factors during open heart surgery. J. Med. **2**, 65 (1971)

Andén, N. E., Henning, M., Obianwu, H.: Effect of epsilon-amino-caproic acid on adrenergic nerve function and tissue monoamine levels. Acta pharmacol. (Kbh.) **26**, 113 (1968)

Andersson, L.: Treatment of so-called essential haematuria with fibrinolytic inhibitor (epsilon-aminocaproic acid). Acta chir. scand. **124**, 355 (1962)

Andersson, L.: Fibrinolytic states in prostatic disease and their treatment with epsilon-amino-caproic acid. Acta chir. scand. **126**, 251 (1963)

Andersson, L.: Antifibrinolytic treatment with epsilon-aminocaproic acid in connection with prostatectomy. Acta chir. scand **127**, 559 (1964)

Andersson, L.: Antifibrinolytic drugs in the treatment of urinary tract haemorrhage. Progr. Surg. **10**, 76 (1972)

Andersson, L., Lindstedt, E.: Fibrinolysis and bleeding following appendectomy. Acta chir. scand. **126**, 362 (1963)

Andersson, L., Nilsson, I. M.: Effect of ε-amino-n-caproic acid (ε-ACA) on fibrinolysis and bleeding conditions in prostatic disease. Acta chir. scand. **121**, 291 (1961)

Andersson, L., Nilsson, I. M.: AMCA (aminomethyl cyclohexane carboxylic acid, cyklokapron) a potent haemostatic agent in urinary tract bleeding. Scand. J. Urol. Nephrol. **3**, 169 (1969)

Andersson, L., Nilsson, I. M., Björkman, E.: Anwändning av ε-aminocapron-syra vid olika blödning-stillstand. Sydsvenska Lärkarsällskapets förh. Obstet. and Gynec. **2**, 136 (1964)

Andersson, L., Nilsson, I. M., Colleen, S., Granstrand, B., Melander, B.: Role of urokinase and tissue activator in sustaining bleeding and the management thereof with EACA and AMCA (Symposion). N. Y. Acad. Sci. "Chemistry, Pharmacology and Clinical Applications of Proteinase Inhibitors". New York: 1966

Andersson, L., Nilsson, I. M., Liedberg, G., Nilsson, L., Rybo, G., Eriksson, O., Granstrand, B., Melander, B.: Antifibrinolytica. Vergleichende Untersuchungen von trans-4-(Aminomethyl)-cyclohexancarbonsäure, Aminocapronsäure und p-Aminomethylbenzoesäure. Arzneimittel-Forsch. **21**, 424 (1971)

Andersson, L., Nilsson, I. M., Niléhn, J.-E., Hedner, U., Granstrand, B., Melander, B.: Experimental and clinical studies on AMCA, the antifibrinolytically active isomer of p-aminomethyl cyclohexane carboxylic acid. Scand. J. Haemat. **2**, 230 (1965)

Andersson, L., Nilsson, I. M., Olow, B.: Fibrinolytic activity in man during surgery. Thrombos. Diathes. haemorrh. (Stuttg.) **7**, 391 (1962)

Andrä, A., Schlottmann, M.: Klinische Erfahrungen mit dem Antifibrinolytikum p-Aminomethylbenzoesäure (PAMBA) in der chirurgischen Stomatologie. Medicamentum (Berl.) **10**, 162 (1969)

Antopol, M., Chryssanthou, C.: Possible significance of bradykinin in the Shwartzman and other phenomena. Ann. N. Y. Acad. Sci. **104**, 346 (1963)

Aoyagi, T., Takeuchi, T., Matsuzaki, A., Kawamura, K., Kondo, S., Hamada, M., Maeder, K., Umezawa, H.: Leupeptins, new protease inhibitors from actinomycetes. J. Antibiot. (Tokyo) **22**, 283 (1969)

Arnet, A.: Untersuchungen über das experimentelle Kaninchenasthma. Allergie u. Asthma **9**, 272 (1963)

Arnet, A., Neubauer, H.-W., Schuppli, R.: Klinische und experimentelle Untersuchungen über die Wirkung der ε-Amino-Capron-Säure bei allergischen Zuständen. Dermatologica (Basel) **127**, 94 (1963)

Asghar, S. S., Pondman, K. W., Cormane, R. H.: Inhibition of C1r, C1s and generation of C1s by amidino compounds. Biochim. biophys. Acta (Amst.) **317**, 539 (1973)

Astrup, T.: Die Bedeutung der Fibrinolyse. Med. Grundlagenforsch. **2**, 197 (1959)

Astrup, T.: Blood coagulation and fibrinolysis in tissue culture and tissue repair. Biochem. Pharmacol. Suppl. 1968, p. 241

Atchley, W. A., Bhargavan, N. V.: Inhibition of antigen antibody reactions by aminocarboxylic acids. Science **138**, 528 (1962)

Auerswald, W., Doleschel, W.: Über den Einfluß der ε-Aminokapronsäure auf die Aktivierung von Chymotrypsinogen durch Trypsin. Wien. med. Wschr. **112**, 619 (1962)

Auerswald, W., Doleschel, W.: The influence of ε-aminocaproic acid and related compounds on antigen-antibody reaction. Brit. J. exp. Path. **47**, 525 (1966)

Auerswald, W., Doleschel, W.: Lactones as inhibitors of the fibrinolytic system. Science **156**, 1244 (1967)

Austen, K. F., Brocklehurst, W. E.: Anaphylaxis in chopped guinea pig lung. II. Enhancement of the anaphylactic release of histamine and slow reacting substance by certain dibasic aliphatic amino acids and inhibition by monobasic fatty acids. J. exp. Med. **113**, 541 (1961)

Azbukina, L. N.: Anwendung von Protaminsulfat und ε-Aminokapronsäure bei Blutungen in der Geburtshilfe (russ.). Akuš. i. Ginek. **42**, 51 (1966)

Baker, B. R.: Design of active-site-directed irreversible enzyme inhibitors. The organic chemistry of the enzymic activ-site. New York-London-Sidney: Wiley 1967

Baker, B. R., Erickson, E. H.: Irreversible enzyme inhibitors. CVI. Proteolytic enzymes. I. Trypsin-inhibitor complexes. J. med. Chem. **10**, 1123 (1967)

Baker, B. R., Erickson, E. H.: Irreversible enzyme inhibitors. CXV. Proteolytic enzymes. V. Active-site-directed irreversible inhibitors of trypsin derived from p-(phenoxyalkoxy) benzamidines with a terminal sulfonyl fluoride. J. med. Chem. **11**, 245 (1968)

Baksheev, M. S., Karavonov, A. G., Karavanov, O. A.: ε-Aminocapronsäure zur Behandlung dysfunktioneller uteriner Hämorrhagien (russ.). Akuš. i Ginek. **3**, 42 (1964)

Barg, W. F., Jr., Boggiano, E., Renzo, E. C. de: Interaction of streptokinase and human plasminogen. II. Starch gel electrophoretic demonstration of a reaction product with activator activity. J. biol. Chem. **240**, 2944 (1965)

Barkagan, Z. S., Burjanov, I. B., Kompaneets, E. J., Lapa, W. A., Eremin, G. F., Mitelman, L. S., Serčenko, W. I., Slotgayer, N. R.: Zur Charakterisierung der hämostatischen Wirkung von ε-Aminokapronsäure (russ.). Probl. Gemat. **10**, 20 (1965)

Barr, F. S., Brent, B. J., Holtman, D. F.: In vitro antifibrinolytic activity of various compounds. Amer. J. Physiol. **204**, 45 (1963)

Basch, R. S.: Inhibition of the third component of the complement system by derivatives of aromatic amino acids. J. Immunol. **94**, 629 (1965)

Baumgarten, W., Cole, R. B.: Human plasminogen-streptokinase complex: The question of the existence of a separate activator entity. Thrombos. Diathes. haemorrh. (Stuttg.) **5**, 605 (1961)

Baumgarten, W., Priester, L. I., Stiller, D. W., Duncan, A. E. W., Ciminera, J. L., Loeffler, L. J.: 4-Aminomethylbicyclo [2.2.2.]-octane-1-carboxylic acid, a new potent antifibrinolytic agent. Its evaluation by *in vitro* assay procedures. Thrombos. Diathes. haemorrh. (Stuttg.) **22**, 263 (1969)

Belko, J. S., Warren, R., Regan, E. E., Simpson, R. G.: Induced fibrinolytic activity and hypofibrinogenemia (Effect of epsilon-amino-caproic acid). Arch. Surg. **86**, 396 (1963)

Beller, F. K.: Fibrinogenopathia intra partum. Blut **9**, 65 (1963)

Beller, F. K., Graeff, H.: Gerinnungsphysiologische und Plasma-Eiweißuntersuchungen bei normalen (Menses) und pathologischen uterinen Blutungen. Arch. Gynäk. **188**, 411 (1957)

Beller, F. K., Mitchell, P.: Production of the generalized Shwartzman reaction by protease inhibitors. Fed. Proc. **24**, 155 (1965)

Beller, F. K., Mitchell, P. S., Gorstein, F.: Fibrin deposition in the rabbit kidney produced by protease inhibitors. Thrombos. Diathes. haemorrh. (Stuttg.) **17**, 427 (1967)

Benzer, H., Blümel, G., Piza, F.: Zusammenhänge zwischen fibrinolytischer Aktivität des Blutes und aseptischen Wundheilungsstörungen im Tierexperiment. Langenbecks Arch. klin. Chir. **302**, 463 (1963)

Benzer, H., Blümel, G., Piza, F.: Experimentelle Untersuchungen über die Beeinflussung der aseptischen Wundheilung durch einen Proteasen-Inhibitor. Wien. klin. Wschr. **76**, 363 (1964)

Bergentz, S.-E., Ljungqvist, U., Lewis, D. H.: The distribution of platelets, fibrin, and erythrocytes in various organs following thrombin infusion: An experimental study in dogs with and without antifibrinolytic therapy. Surgery **71**, 190 (1972)

Berger, M., Dinson, H.: Un antihémorragique de choix en otorhino-laryngologie infantile: le capromol Choay, acide epsilon aminocaproïque. Rev. Laryng. **85**, 1071 (1964)

Berghoff, A., Glatzel, H.: Untersuchungen mit einem Plasmin-Präparat unter Verwendung des Kaseinspaltungstestes: Die Aktivität von Plasmin-Novo und seine Hemmbarkeit durch Epsilon-aminocapronsäure und Trasylol. Thrombos. Diathes. haemorrh. (Stuttg.) 12, 418 (1964)

Bergström, K.: Purification and properties of plasminogen, p. 140. Abstracts 9th Congr. Europ. Soc. Haemat. Lissabon: 1963

Bertelli, A., Bisiani, M., Cerrini, L., Confalonieri, A., Libro, V., Lodi, E., Proto, M.: Prolonged survival of kidney homotransplants in dog treated by epsilon acetamide caproic acid. Nature (Lond.) 201, 209 (1964a)

Bertelli, A., Bonmassar, E., Genovese, E., Lami, V., Rossano, M. A., Trabucchi, jr. E.: Etude sur les homogreffes cutenées dans des rats traités avec le dérivé acétylé de l'acide epsilon-amino-caproïque. Arch. int. Pharmacodyn. 152, 189 (1964b)

Bianchini, P.: Attivita antifibrinolitica di alcuni polipeptidi biologicamente affivi. Farmaco, Ed. sci. 18, 763 (1964)

Bickford, A. F., Taylor, F. B.: Effect of omega-amino-carboxylic acids on fibrinogenolysis. Fed. Proc. 22, 442 (1963)

Bickford, A. F., Taylor, F. B., Sheena, R.: Inhibition of the fibrinogen-plasmin reaction by ω-aminocarboxylic acids and alkylamines. Biochim. biophys. Acta (Amst.) 92, 328 (1964)

Biggs, R., Hayton-Williams, D. S.: Epsilon-aminocaproic acid in the treatment of hemophilia. Brit. dent. J. 124, 157 (1968)

Biliński, B. T., Kandel, G. L., Rabiner, S. F.: Epsilon aminocaproic acid therapy of hematuria due to heterozygous sickle cell diseases. J. Urol. (Baltimore) 102, 95 (1969)

Bishop, E., Margolis, J.: Studies on plasma kinins. II. Some properties of the kinin-destroying enzyme. Aust. J. exp. Biol. med. Sci. 41, 307 (1963)

Björlin, G., Nilsson, I. M.: Tooth extractions in hemophiliacs after administration of a single dose of factor VIII or factor IX concentrate supplemented with AMCA. Oral Surg. 36, 482 (1973)

Böhnel, J., Stacher, A.: Die Therapie mit ε-Aminokapronsäure. Wien. med. Wschr. 116, 157 (1966)

Boeminghaus, F.: Intravesikale Applikation von Antifibrinolytika nach Eingriffen an der Prostata. Z. Urol. 65, 771 (1972)

Bogdanov, B., Stern, P., Vajs, E.: Beitrag zur Homotransplantation der Menschenhaut. Experientia (Basel) 20, 683 (1964)

Bonhomme, J., Lemaire, J.: Le traitement et la prophylaxe des hémorragies par incoagulabilité sanguine en obstétrique. Rev. franç. gynéc. obstét. 61, 749 (1966)

Bonmassar, E., Prada, A., Robotti, C. A.: The acetyl derivative of epsilon aminocaproic acid as an agent favoring the induction and development of Ehrlichs carcinom in the rat. Boll. Soc. ital. Biol. sper. 39, 1230 (1963)

Bonnar, J., Crawford, J. M.: Haemorrhagic diathesis due to abruption placentae treated by fibrinogen, epsilon-aminocaproic acid, and hysterotomy. Lancet 1965I, 241

Bostard, P.: Un traitement meniable et efficace des hémorragies utérines fonctionelles: L'acide epsilon-amonocaproïque. Sem. thér. 45, 546 (1969)

Bouvier, C. A.: Physiopathologie de l'hémostase. Le rôle du système fibrinolytique dans certaines diathéses hémorragiques. Rev. méd. Suisse rom. 83, 595 (1963)

Brockway, W. J., Castellino, F. J.: The mechanism of the inhibition of plasmin activity by epsilon-aminocaproic acid. J. biol. Chem. 246, 4641 (1971)

Buck, F. F., Hummel, B. C. W., Renzo, E. C. de: Interaction of streptokinase and human plasminogen. V. Studies on the nature and mechanism of formation of the enzymatic site of the activator complex. J. biol. Chem. 243, 3648 (1968)

Budelmann, H., Bürgi, H., Regli, J.: ε-Aminocaproic acid in asthma. Lancet 1965II, 643

Budyka, L. A.: Die Wirkung von ε-Aminokapronsäure, angewendet während der Geburt, auf das Blutgerinnungssystem des Neugeborenen (russ.). Vop. Ohrany Materin. Dets. 13, 31 (1968)

Busch, C., Lindquist, O., Saldeen, T.: Respiratory insufficiency in the dog induced by pulmonary microembolism and inhibition of fibrinolysis. Effect of defibrinogenation, leucopenia and thrombocytopenia. Acta chir. scand. 140, 255 (1974)

Carrol, H. J., Tize, D. A.: The effects of epsilon-aminocaproic acid upon potassium metabolism in the dog. Metabolism 15, 449 (1966)

Cattan, A., Schwarzenberg, L., Schneider, M., Amiel, J. L., Mathe, G.: Essai de traitement par l'acide epsilon-aminocaproïque de patients atteints de syndromes hémorragiques, en particulier de syndromes liés à une thrombocytopénie. Presse méd. 71, 2037 (1963)

Caviezel,O., Vollery,M., Vannotti,A.: Fibrinolyse leucocytaire. Schweiz. med. Wschr. **94**, 1016 (1964)

Celander,D.R., Guest,M.M.: Epsilon-aminocaproic acid (EACA) as inhibitor of various components of the fibrinolytic system. Physiologist **3**, 36 (1960)

Celander,D.R., Messer,D., Guest,M.M.: The fibrinolytic system: a review of its therapeutic significance and control, with particular emphasis on its inhibition by ε-aminocaproic acid. Tex. Rep. Biol. Med. **19**, 16 (1961a)

Celander,D.R., Naschke,M.D., Guest,M.M.: The effect of ε-aminocaproic acid on fibrinolysin and on activators of profibrinolysin. Tex. Rep. Biol. Med. **19**, 50 (1961b)

Champion,R.H., Lachmann,P.J.: Hereditary angiooedema treated with ε-aminocaproic acid. Brit. J. Derm. **81**, 763 (1969)

Charytan,C., Purtilo,D.: Glomerular capillary thrombosis and acute renal failure after ε-aminocaproic acid therapy. New Engl. J. Med. **280**, 1102 (1969)

Chase,T., Shaw,E.: Comparison of the esterase activities of trypsin, plasmin, and thrombin on guanidinobenzoate esters. Titration of the enzymes. Biochemistry **8**, 2212 (1969)

Chase,T., Jr., Shaw,E.: Titration of trypsin, plasmin, and thrombin with p-nitrophenyl p′-guanidinobenzoate HCl. In: Perlmann,G.E., Lorand,L. (Eds.): Methods in Enzymology. XIX: Proteolytic Enzymes, p. 20. New York—London: Academic Press, 1970

Cliffton,E.E., Agostino,D.: Effect of inhibitors of fibrinolytic enzymes on development of pulmonary metastase. J. nat. Cancer Inst. **33**, 753 (1964)

Coggins,J.T., Allen,T.D.: Insoluble fibrin clots within urinary tract as consequence of epsilon aminocaproic acid therapy. J. Urol. (Baltimore) **107**, 647 (1972)

Collen,D., Tytgat,G., Claeys,H., Verstraete,M., Wallén,P.: Metabolism of plasminogen in healthy subjects: effect of tranexamic acid. J. clin. Invest. **51**, 1310 (1972)

Conticello,S., Lombardo,C., Terranova,R.: Comportamento dell'attivitá fibrinolitica plasmatica in soggetti adeno-tonsillectomizzati dopo trattamento antifibrinolitico. Ann. Laring. (Torino) **67**, 610 (1968)

Cooksey,M.W.: Epsilon-aminocaproic acid in the treatment of hemophilia. Brit. dent. J. **124**, 157 (1968)

Cooksey,M.W., Perry,C.B., Raper,A.B.: Epsilon-aminocaproic acid therapy for dental extractions in hemophiliacs. Brit. med. J. **1966II**, 1633

Copley,A.L., Carol,B.: Inhibiting action of epsilon-amino caproic acid on capillary permeability in guinea pigs tested with new quantitative method based on Straus' peroxydase procedure. Variance and covariance analyses. Life Sci. **3**, 65 (1964)

Corkill,G.: Earlier operation and antifibrinolytic therapy in the management of aneurysmal subarachnoid haemorrhage: Review of recent experience in Tasmania. Med. J. Aust. **1**, 468 (1974)

Corley,R.C.: Amino acid catabolism. II. The fate of β-alanine and ε-aminocaproic acid in the phlorhizinized dog. J. biol. Chem. **81**, 545 (1929)

Corral,F.S., González,S., Inocente,J.M.: Tratamiento profiláctico u las hipocoagulabilidades obstétricas. Rev. clin. Inst. matern. (Lisboa) **18**, 225 (1967)

Corrigan,J.J.: Oral bleeding in hemophilia: treatment with epsilon aminocaproic acid and replacement therapy. J. Pediat. **80**, 124 (1972)

Creveld,S.van, Vos-Bongaardt,C.M.de: Die Anwendung von Epsilon-Aminokapronsäure bei Hämophilie. Maandschr. Kindergeneesk. **34**, 285 (1966)

Croizat,P., Revol,L., Thouverez,J.P., Belleville,J., Brunat,Y.: A propos d'un syndrome hémorragique complexe traité par l'acide epsilon-amino-caproïque. Lyon méd. **211**, 403 (1964)

Cummings,J.R., Welter,A.N.: Cardiovascular studies on aminocaproic acid. Toxicol. appl. Pharmacol. **9**, 57 (1966)

Czerepko,K.: Der papierchromatographische Nachweis von ε-Caprolactam und ε-Amino-capronsäure. Mikrochim. Acta **1958**, 638

Czerepko,K., Lüdy-Tenger,F., Barrollier,J.: Papierchromatographische Trennung von ε-Caprolactam und ε-Aminocapronsäure. Z. analyt. Chem. **170**, 455 (1959)

Danysz,A., Kocmierska-Grozdzka,D., Prokopowicz,J., Worowski,K., Rejniak,L.: Investigation on the mechanism of radioprotective action of EACA. Sborn. véd. Praci lék. Fak. (Karlovy Univ.) **9**, 725 (1966)

Dapunt, O., Schwarz, P.: Inkomplette puerperale Uterusinversion mit konsekutiver Hypofibrinogenämie. Wien. klin. Wschr. **76**, 588 (1964)

Davies, M. C., Englert, M. E., Renzo, E. C. de: Interaction of streptokinase and human plasminogen.
I. Combining of streptokinase and plasminogen observed in the ultracentrifuge under a
variety of experimental conditions. J. biol. Chem. **239**, 2651 (1964)

Delecour, M., Monnier, J. C., Vankemmel, P.: L'interêt de l'acide epsilon-amino-caproïque dans
le traitement des fibrinolyses obstétricales (A propos de 2 observations). Sem. thér. **41**, 461 (1965)

Dettori, A. G., Ponari, O.: Attuali indirizza di terapia negli stati iperfibrinolitici. Clin. ter. **27**,
97 (1963)

Diomede-Fresa, V., Fumarola, D.: Influenza dell'acido epsilon-aminocaproico sulla insorgenza e
sullo soiluppo de sarcoma da benzo [a] pirene. Tumori **50**, 25 (1964)

Diwok, K., Gülzow, M., Trettin, H.-J.: Die Wirkung der ε-Aminocapronsäure auf die
experimentelle Pankreatitis der Ratte. Z. ges. inn. Med. **20**, 111 (1965)

Doleschel, W., Auerswald, W.: Vergleichende Untersuchungen über die Hemmwirkung von
Caprolactam und analogen Verbindungen auf Kinine und Faktoren des fibrinolytischen
Systems. Wien. med. Wschr. **117**, 137 (1967)

Donaldson, V. H.: Activation of partially purified plasminogen in the presence of ε-aminocaproic
acid. J. Lab. clin. Med. **63**, 213 (1964)

Donner, L., Houskova, J.: On the action mechanism of some fibrinolysis inhibitors. Thrombos.
Diathes. haemorrh. (Stuttg.) **18**, 439 (1967)

Dubber, A. H., McNicol, G. P., Douglas, A. S.: Amino methyl cyclohexane carboxylic acid.
(AMCHA), a new synthetic fibrinolytic inhibitor. Brit. J. Haemat. **11**, 237 (1965)

Dubber, A. H., McNicol, G. P., Douglas, A. S., Melander, B.: Some properties of the antifibrinolytic
active isomer of aminomethylcyclohexane carboxylic acid. Lancet **1964 II**, 1317

Dumay, J. J., Dance, P.: Utilisation de l'acide epsilon-aminocaproïque (Hémocaprol) en
chirurgie oto-rhino-laryngologique. Sem. Hôp. Paris **18**, 1595 (1964)

Egeblad, K.: Effects of ε-aminocaproic acid on fibrin clot lysis. Thrombos. Diathes. haemorrh.
(Stuttg.) **15**, 173 (1966)

Egeblad, K., Astrup, T.: ε-Aminocaproic acid and urinary trypsin inhibitor: Potentiated
inhibition of urokinase induced fibrinolysis. Proc. Soc. exp. Biol. (N.Y.) **112**, 1020 (1963)

Egli, H., Schröder, F.: Experimentelle Untersuchungen und klinische Beobachtungen zur antifibrinolytischen und hämostyptischen Wirkung von Epsilon-Tachostyptan. Dtsch. Zahn-,
Mund- u. Kieferheilk. **50**, 386 (1968)

Ellert, R., Nold, B.: Gerinnungsphysiologische Studien am Menstrualblut. Schweiz. med.
Wschr. **86**, 999 (1956)

Elsner, P.: Pathogenese und Therapie fibrinopenischer und fibrinolytischer Blutungen in der
Gynäkologie und Geburtshilfe. Thrombos. Diathes. haemorrh. (Stuttg.) Suppl. **8**, 27 (1962)

Eneroth, G., Grant, C. A.: ε-Aminokapronsäure und Verringerung der Fertilität männlicher
Ratten. Acta pharm. suec. **3**, 115 (1966)

Erdös, E. G., Renfrew, A. G., Sloane, E. M., Wohler, J. R.: Enzymatic studies on bradykinin and
similar peptides. Ann. N. Y. Acad. Sci. **104**, 222 (1963)

Evered, D. F., Jones, M. R., Randall, H. G.: Transport of the amino acids, 1-amino cyclopentane-1-
carboxylic acid and ε-aminocaproic acid, across intestinal mucosa in vitro. Biochem.
Pharmacol. **16**, 1767 (1967)

Fetter, D. R., Tocantins, L. M., Cottone, R. N., Brosseau, C., Bowman, W. D.: Effect of epsilon
aminocaproic acid on bleeding after prostatectomy. J. Urol. (Baltimore) **85**, 970 (1961)

Fidelski, R., Konopka, P., Niedworok, J., Tchorzewski, H.: Biological properties of epsilon amino
caproic acid (EACA) Polfa in the light of experimental studies. Mater med. pol. **1**, 44 (1970)

Fischbacher, W.: Beitrag zur fibrinolytischen Therapie mit Streptokinase und Fibrinolysin.
Thrombos. Diathes. haemorrh. (Stuttg.) **6**, 547 (1961)

Flähmig, M., Sieg, U., Vogel, G.: Fibrinolytische Störungen im uterinen Blut und ihre Beeinflußbarkeit durch p-Aminomethylbenzoesäure (PAMBA). Münch. med. Wschr. **107**,
2007 (1965)

Flähmig, M., Sieg, U., Vogel, G.: Das Bild der fibrinolytischen Störung im uterinen Blut und
ihre Beeinflußbarkeit durch PAMBA. Folia haemat. (Lpz.) **87**, 41 (1967)

Flandre, M. O., Damon, M., Peillex, F., François, P.: Action de l'acide ε-aminocaproïque sur la
formation du tissu conjonctoire inflammatoire. C. R. Soc. biol. (Paris) **158**, 615 (1964)

Flandre, M. O., Damon, M., Secchi, M. J.: Action de l'acide acétyl-epsilon-aminohéxanoïque sur la cicatrisation. Thérapie **21**, 431 (1966)

Fletcher, A.: Severe hemorrhagic purpura in an 89-year-old man. Spectacular cure by intravenous injections of epsilon-aminocaproic acid. Rev. Path. gén. **63**, 773 (1963)

Fletcher, A. P., Alkjaersig, N., Sherry, S.: The maintenance of a sustained thrombolytic state in man. I. Induction and effects. J. clin. Invest. **38**, 1096 (1959)

Folk, J. E.: A new pancreatic carboxypeptidase. J. Amer. chem. Soc. **78**, 3541 (1956)

Fonio, A.: Über die kombinierte Blutstillung bei Zahnextraktionen an Hämophilen. Schweiz. med. Wschr. **94**, 1561 (1964)

Fonio, A.: Über Behandlungsversuche an Hämophilen mit Epsilon-Aminokapronsäure (Epsamon). Schweiz. med. Wschr. **96**, 1723 (1966)

Foussard-Blanpin, O., Bretaudeau, J.: Etude pharmacodynamique d'un inhibiteur de la fibrinolyse: l'acide epsilon-aminocaproïque. Anesth. Analg. Réanim. **22**, 481 (1965)

François, S.: A propos du traitement des méno-métrorragies par l'hémocaprol. Sem. thér. **41**, 39 (1965)

Frank, M. M., Sergent, J. S., Kane, M. A., Alling, D. W.: Epsilon aminocaproic acid therapy of hereditary angioneurotic edema. New Engl. J. Med. **286**, 808 (1972)

Frick, G., Frick, U.: Zur Rolle der basophilen Leukozyten und Mastzellen in Fibrinolyse und Allergie. III. Wirkung einer allergischen Sofortreaktion ohne und mit Vorbehandlung durch ε-Aminocapronsäure oder p-Aminomethylbenzoesäure auf Zahl und Degranulierung von basophilen Leukozyten. Folia haemat. (Lpz.) **88**, 1 (1967)

Fujii, A., Tanaka, K., Cook, E. S.: Antistaphylococcal and antifibrinolytic activities of N-alpha-(omega-aminoacyl-L-lysines). J. med. Chem. **15**, 378 (1972)

Fukutake, K., Shida, K., Arakawa, T., Kato, K.: Analysis of fibrinolysis by the use of epsilon-aminocaproic acid: Preliminary report. Blood **15**, 690 (1960)

Gabriel, S., Maass, T. A.: Über ε-Aminocapronsäure. Ber. dtsch. chem. Ges. *1899*, II, 1266

Gans, H.: Use of epsilon aminocaproic acid. Surg. Gynec. Obstet. **120**, 576 (1965)

Gans, H., Krivit, W.: Study of fibrinogen and plasminogen concentrations in rabbits during anaphylactic shock. J. Lab. clin. Med. **58**, 259 (1961)

Gans, H., Krivit, W.: Problems in hemostasis in open heart surgery. III. Epsilon aminocaproic acid as an inhibitor of plasminogen-activator activity. Ann. Surg. **155**, 268 (1962)

Garbin, S., Garofalo, E.: Due casi di emofilia. A trattati con acido epsilon-aminoproico (EACA). Minerva pediat. (Torino) **19**, 1979 (1967)

Gartenmann, C.: Choc anaphylactique et protéases. Absence d'activité antianaphylactique des antifibrinolytiques de synthèse chez le lapin. Rev. franç. Allerg. **8**, 15 (1968)

Geiger, W. B.: Involvement of a complement-like factor in the activation of blood protease. J. Immunol. **69**, 597 (1952)

Geratz, J. D.: The effect of aliphatic amino acids on the activation of trypsinogen and on the stability of trypsin solutions. Biochim. biophys. Acta (Amst.) **56**, 599 (1962)

Geratz, J. D.: The inhibitory effect of ω-amino acids and guanidino acids on the activation of α-chymotrypsinogen and trypsinogen. Arch. Biochem. **102**, 327 (1963)

Geratz, J. D.: p-Aminobenzamidine as inhibitor of trypsinogen activation. Experientia (Basel) **22**, 73 (1966)

Geratz, J. D.: p-Amidinophenylpyruvic acid: A new highly effective inhibitor of enterokinase and trypsin. Arch. Biochem. **118**, 90 (1967)

Geratz, J. D.: Synthetic inhibitors and ester substrates of pancreatic kallikrein. Experientia (Basel) **25**, 483 (1969a)

Geratz, J. D.: Inhibitory effect of aromatic diamidines on trypsin and enterokinase. Experientia (Basel) **25**, 1254 (1969b)

Geratz, J. D.: Inhibition of thrombin, plasmin and plasminogen activation by amidino compounds. Thrombos. Diathes. haemorrh. (Stuttg.) **23**, 486 (1970)

Geratz, J. D.: Inhibition of coagulation and fibrinolysis by aromatic amidino compounds. An in vitro and in vivo study. Thrombos. Diathes. haemorrh. (Stuttg.) **25**, 391 (1971)

Geratz, J. D.: Structure-activity relationships for the inhibition of plasmin and plasminogen activation by aromatic diamidines and a study of the effect of plasma proteins on the inhibition process. Thrombos. Diathes. haemorrh. (Stuttg.) **29**, 154 (1973)

Ghilardi,F., Voena,G., Busca,G.: Osservazioni sull'attivazione della fibrinolisi nelle emorragia da tonsillectomi e sul trattamento con l'acido epsilon-aminocaproico. Ann. Laring. (Torino) **64**, 55 (1965)

Gibba,A., Tetterino,E.: Fibrinolisi acuta dopo prostatectomia. Trattamento e risoluzione con l'acido aminocaproico. Minerva urol. (Torino) **16**, 19 (1964)

Gibbs,J.R., Corkill,A.G.L.: Use of an anti-fibrinolytic agent (tranexamic acid) in the management of ruptured intracranial aneurysms. Postgrad. med. J. **47**, 199 (1971)

Gibelli,A.: Richerche sull'azione antifibrinolitica dell'acido epsilon-amino-caproico. III. L'azione dell'acido epsilon-aminocaproico quale antidoto degli agenti trombolitici (plasmina, streptochinasi). Gazz. int. Med. Chir. **67**, 2444 (1962)

Gilette,R.W., Findley,A., Conway,H.: Prolonged survival of homograft in mice treated with EACA. Transplantation **1**, 116 (1963a)

Gilette,R.W., Findley,A., Conway,H.: Effect on tumor homografts on treating hosts with antiproteolytic enzyme compounds. Proc. Soc. exp. Biol. (N.Y.) **112**, 964 (1963b)

Giordano,M.D., Watkins,R.S., Radivoyevitch,M.: Dental extractions in hemophilic patients on aminocaproic prophylaxis. Further experience with two additional cases. Oral Surg. **26**, 160 (1968)

Gobbi,F.: Use and misuse of aminocaproic acid. Lancet **1967 II**, 472

Gobbi,F.: L'acido epsilon-aminocaproico nella terapia dell'emofilia. Clin. ter. **46**, 55 (1968)

Godal,H.C., Theodor,I.: In vitro inhibition of streptokinase-induced proteolysis by trasylol and epsilon aminocaproic acid. Scand. J. clin. Lab. Invest. **17**, Suppl. 84, 199 (1965)

Goldhaber,P., Corman,I., Ormsbee,R.A.: Experimental alteration of the ability of tumor cells to lyse plasma clots in vitro. Proc. Soc. exp. Biol. (N.Y.) **66**, 590 (1947)

Gordon,A.M., McNicol,G.P., Dubber,A.H.C., McDonald,G.A., Douglas,A.S.: Clinical trial of epsilon-aminocaproic acid in severe hemophilia. Brit. med. J. **1965**, 1632

Graeber,W., Bach,H.G., Lau,H., Sackreuther,W.: Defibrinierungsblutung bei der vorzeitigen Placentalösung. Gynaecologia (Basel) **158**, 89 (1964)

Gralnick,H.R., Greipp,P.: Thrombosis with epsilon aminocaproic acid therapy. Amer. J. clin. Path. **56**, 151 (1971)

Groskopf,W.R., Hsieh,B., Summaria,L., Robbins,K.C.: Studies on the active center of human plasmin. The serine and histidine residue. J. biol. Chem. **244**, 359 (1969a)

Groskopf,W.R., Summaria,L., Robbins,K.C.: Studies on the active center of human plasmin. Partial amino acid sequence of a peptide containing the active center serine residue. J. biol. Chem. **244**, 395 (1969b)

Grossi,C.E., Moreno,A.H., Rousselot,L.M.: Studies on spontaneous fibrinolytic activity in patients with cirrhosis of the liver and its inhibition by epsilon amino caproic acid. Ann. Surg. **153**, 383 (1961)

Grossi,C.E., Rousselot,L.M., Panke,W.F.: Control of fibrinolysis during portocaval shunts. J. Amer. med. Ass. **187**, 115 (1964)

Gugler,E., Käser,H., Bütler,R.: Die Anwendung von Epsilon-Aminokapronsäure in der Behandlung der Hämophilie. Schweiz. med. Wschr. **96**, 386 (1966)

Guimbretière,J., Lebeaupin,P.R.: Acide epsilon-aminocaproïque. Premiers résultats thérapeutiques dans certains syndromes hémorragiques. Anesth. Analg. Réanim. **21**, 339 (1964)

Gustafsson,G.T., Nilsson,I.M.: Fibrinolytic activity in fluid from gingival crevice. Proc. Soc. exp. Biol. (N.Y.) **106**, 277 (1961)

Hagelsten,J., Nolte,H.: Operative und postoperative Blutungen mit besonderer Berücksichtigung der Fibrinolyse. Anaesthesist **13**, 263 (1964)

Harms,W.: Über die Behandlung geburtshilflicher und gynäkologischer Blutungen mit einem neuen Antifibrinolytikum. Med. Welt (Stuttg.) **1968**, I, 643

Hassel,O., Groth,P.: Cis-trans relationship between the two amino acids obtained by hydrogenation of p-aminomethylbenzoic acid. Acta chem. scand. **19**, 1709 (1965)

Hatano,H., Yamamoto,K., Kono,N., Usui,K.: Clinical use of AMCHA on certain dermatoses. Keio J. Med. **11**, 127 (1962)

Haustein,K.-O., Markwardt,F.: Über den Einfluß von Hemmstoffen der Blutgerinnung und Fibrinolyse auf das Sanarelli-Shwartzman-Phänomen. Thrombos. Diathes. haemorrh. (Stuttg.) **13**, 60 (1965)

Haustein, K.-O., Markwardt, F.: Über den Einfluß von Antifibrinolytika auf die Aktivierung des Kininsystems durch Fibrinolysevorgänge. Acta biol. med. germ. **16**, 658 (1966)

Haustein, U.-F.: Zur Wirkung des Antifibrinolytikums p-Aminomethylbenzoesäure (PAMBA) auf die Transplantationsimmunität von Mäusen. Allergie u. Asthma **13**, 229 (1967)

Haustein, U.-F., Haustein, K.-O.: Zur Wirkung synthetischer Antifibrinolytika auf allergische Reaktionen. Derm. Wschr. **153**, 1274 (1967)

Hedlund, P. O.: Antifibrinolytic therapy with cyclokapron in connection with prostatectomy. Scand. J. Urol. Nephrol. **3**, 177 (1969)

Heimburger, N.: Neuere Erkenntnisse über den Mechanismus der Fibrinolyse unter besonderer Berücksichtigung der Fibrinagar-Elektrophorese. Behringwerk-Mitt. Heft **41**, 84 (1962)

Hellinger, J.: Die Behandlung schwerer Fibrinolyseblutungen nach Prostatektomie mit p-Aminomethylbenzoesäure. Urol. int. (Basel) **21**, 61 (1966a)

Hellinger, J.: Die Bedeutung lokaler Fibrinolysesteigerungen bei der symptomatischen Hämaturie und ihre Hemmung durch p-Aminomethylbenzoesäure. Z. Urol. **59**, 633 (1966b)

Hellinger, J.: Die Anwendung von PAMBA in der Urologie. Folia haemat. (Lpz.) **88**, 187 (1967)

Hellinger, J., Vogel, G.: Zur Klinik und Therapie fibrinolytischer Blutungen in der Chirurgie unter besonderer Berücksichtigung des neuen Antifibrinolytikums p-Aminomethylbenzoesäure (PAMBA). Bruns' Beitr. klin. Chir. **213**, 478 (1966)

Herschlein, H. J., Steichele, D. F., Briel, R.: Untersuchungen über die antifibrinolytische Wirkung der p-Aminomethylbenzoesäure PAMBA auf die lokale Aktivierung der Fibrinolyse im menschlichen Scheidengewebe und Myometrium. Med. Welt (Stuttg.) **23**, 1540 (1972)

Herxheimer, A., Capel, L. H.: Aminocaproic acid in hemophilia and menorrhagia. Drug. Ther. Bull. **5**, 63 (1967)

Hiemeyer, V., Rasche, H.: Der Einfluß von Epsilon-Aminokapronsäure auf die Streptokinase-induzierte Thrombolyse. Klin. Wschr. **43**, 930 (1965)

Hilgartner, M. W.: Intrarenal obstruction in haemophilia. Lancet **1966**, II, 486

Hodge, S. M., Reid, W. O.: The use of EACA in preventing or reducting hemorrhages in the hemophiliac. Thrombos. Diathes. haemorrh. (Stuttg.) **18**, 179 (1967)

Höller, H., Lindner, A.: Zur Pharmakologie der ε-Aminocapronsäure. Wien. klin. Wschr. **77**, 693 (1965)

Hoffmann, W., Klöcking, H.-P.: Klinische Erfahrungen mit dem neuen Antifibrinolytikum p-Aminomethylbenzoesäure (PAMBA). Pädiat. Pädol. **3**, 59 (1967)

Hoffmann, W., Vogel, G.: Die Behandlung essentieller und symptomatischer Hämaturien im Kindesalter mit Antifibrinolytika. Folia haemat. (Lpz.) **88**, 263 (1967)

Horowitz, H. I., Spielvogel, A. R.: Hemostasis. In: Bang, N. U., Beller, F. K., Deutsch, E., Mammen, E. F. (Eds.): Thrombosis and Bleeding Disorders. Theory and Methods, p. 412. Stuttgart: Thieme, New York—London: Academic Press, 1971

Huggins, C., Vail, V. C., Davis, M.: Fluidity of menstrual blood; proteolytic effect. Amer. J. Obstet. Gynec. **46**, 78 (1943)

Hummel, B. C. W., Buck, F. F., Renzo, E. C. de: Interaction of streptokinase and human plasminogen. III. Plasmin and activator activities in reaction mixtures of streptokinase and human plasminogen or human plasmin of various molar ratios. J. biol. Chem. **241**, 347 (1966)

Hureau, J., Audhoui, H., Vayre, P., Vairel, E.: Place de l'acide ε-amino-caproïque parmi les inhibiteurs de protéases. C. R. Soc. Biol. (Paris) **158**, 17 (1964)

Hureau, J., Vairel, E., Martin, E., Vayre, P.: Comparative study of some properties of sodium salt of N-acetylamino-6-hexanoic and ε-amino-caproic acids. C. R. Soc. Biol. (Paris) **160**, 746 (1966)

Iatridis, S. G.: Fibrinolysis and intravascular coagulation. Separate or associated mechanisms. Thrombos. Diathes. haemorrh. (Stuttg.) Suppl. **20**, 53 (1966)

Igawa, T., Watanabe, H., Amano, M., Okamoto, S.: Viscosimetric study of the action of ε-amino-caproic acid on human plasmin. Keio J. Med. **8**, 225 (1959)

Immergut, M. A., Stevenson, T.: Use of epsilon amino caproic acid in control of hematuria associated with hemoglobinopathias. J. Urol. (Baltimore) **93**, 110 (1965)

Inagami, T.: The mechanism of the specificity of trypsin catalysis. I. Inhibition by alkyl ammonium ions. J. biol. Chem. **239**, 787 (1964)

Isaksson, G.: Treatment of obstetric bleeding with antifibrinolytics. Cent. Afr. J. Med. **19**, 98 (1973)

Itoga,G., Yogo,T.: The inhibitory effect of epsilon-aminocaproic acid on the tuberculin reaction. Keio J. Med. **8**, 289 (1959)

Itterbeck,H.van, Vermylen,J., Verstraete,M.: High obstruction of urine flow as a complication of the treatment with fibrinolysis inhibitors of haematuria in haemophiliacs. Acta haemat. (Basel) **39**, 237 (1968)

Iwamoto,M.: Plasminogen-plasmin system. IX. Specific binding of tranexamic acid to plasmin. Thrombos. Diathes. haemorrh. (Stuttg.) **33**, 573 (1975)

Iwamoto,M., Abiko,Y.: Further kinetic studies on the inhibition of fibrinolysis by synthetic inhibitors. J. Biochem. (Tokyo) **65**, 821 (1969)

Iwamoto,M., Abiko,Y., Shimizu,M.: Plasminogen-plasmin system. III. Kinetics of plasminogen activation and inhibition of plasminogen-plasmin system by some synthetic inhibitors. J. Biochem. (Tokyo) **64**, 759 (1968)

Iwasawa,T.: Klinische Wirkung von Transamin, einem Antiplasmin, in der Oto-rhinolaryngologie (jap.) Otolaryngology **39**, 195 (1967)

Johanovský,I., Škavril,F.: Inhibition of the formation of hypersensitivity pyrogen from delayed hypersensitive cell extract by protease inhibitors in vitro. Immunology **5**, 469 (1962)

Johnson,A.J., Merskey,C.: Diagnosis of diffuse intravascular clotting. Its relation to secondary fibrinolysis and treatment with heparin. Thrombos. Diathes. haemorrh. (Stuttg.) Suppl. **20**, 161 (1966)

Johnson,A.J., Skoza,L.: Chemical determination of ε-aminocaproic acid, an inhibitor of plasminogen activation. Fed. Proc. **20**, 59 (1961)

Johnson,A.J., Skoza,L.: Amino acids and their derivates, as inhibitors of fibrinolysis. Fed. Proc. **22**, 442 (1963)

Johnson,A.J., Skoza,L., Claus,E.: Observations on epsilon aminocaproic acid. Thrombos. Diathes. haemorrh. (Stuttg.) **7**, 203 (1962)

Josso,F., Castets,J.B., Zmerli,S., Chaperon,C., Auvert,J.: Guérison spectaculaire d'un accident fibrinolytique aïgu, déclenché par une résection endoscopique d'un cancer de la prostate et obtenue grace à l'emploi d'un produit nouveau: l'acide epsilon amino-caproïque. J. Urol. néphrol. **68**, 898 (1962)

Jung,E.G., Duckert,F.: Wirkung von Plasmin (Fibrinolysin) auf die Gerinnungsfaktoren. Schweiz. med. Wschr. **90**, 1239 (1960)

Käser,H., Gugler,E.: Die dünnschichtchromatographische Bestimmung der ε-Aminocapronsäure (EACS) in Serum und Urin. Z. klin. Chem. **3**, 33 (1965)

Kaller,H.: Enterale Resorption, Verteilung und Elimination von 4-Aminomethylcyclohexancarbonsäure (AMCHA) und ε-Aminocapronsäure (ACS) beim Menschen. Naunyn-Schmiedebergs Arch. Pharmak. exp. Path. **256**, 160 (1967)

Kastro,B., Prokopowicz,J., Serwatko,A.: Untersuchung der akuten und chronischen Toxizität der ε-Aminocapronsäure (pol.). Acta physiol. pol. **15**, 439 (1964)

Kato,N., Morimatsu,M., Tanaka,K., Hori,A.: Effects of trans-4-aminomethylcyclohexane carboxylic acid as an antifibrinolytic agent on arterial wall and experimental atherosclerotic lesions in rabbit. Thrombos. Diathes. haemorrh. (Stuttg.) **24**, 85 (1970)

Kaulla,K.N.von, Henkel,W.: Beeinflussen Antibiotika fibrinolytische Vorgänge in vitro? Klin. Wschr. **31**, 40 (1953)

Khalfen,L.N.: Über die Pathogenese der Blutung bei Tonsillektomien und die Anwendung der ε-Aminokapronsäure zu ihrer Prophylaxe (russ.). Vestn. Oto-rino-laring. **29**, 76 (1967)

Kirkman,N.F.: Post-prostatectomy haematuria. Treatment with epsilon-aminocaproic acid. Brit. J. Surg. **54**, 1026 (1967)

Kliman,A., McKay,D.G.: The prevention of the generalized Shwartzman reaction by fibrinolytic activity. Arch. Path. **66**, 715 (1958)

Klöcking,H.-P.: p-Aminomethylbenzoesäureäthylester — ein oral wirksames Antifibrinolytikum. Z. ärztl. Fortbild **61**, 880 (1967)

Klöcking,H.-P.: Pharmakologische Untersuchungen über 4-Aminomethylbenzoesäure und ihre Derivate. Habil.-Schrift, Med. Akademie Erfurt, 1968

Klöcking,H.-P., Knauer,H., Markwardt,F.: Über die antifibrinolytische Wirkung von araliphatischen Estern und Amiden der p-Aminomethylbenzoesäure. Acta biol. med. germ. **30**, K9 (1973)

Klöcking,H.-P., Markwardt,F.: Tierexperimentelle Verfahren zur Testung von Fibrinolytika und Antifibrinolytika. Folia haemat. (Lpz.) **92**, 84 (1969)

Klöcking,H.-P., Markwardt,F.: Über die Pharmakologie des Antifibrinolytikums p-Aminomethylbenzoesäure. Haematologia, Suppl. 1, 175 (1970)

Klöcking,H.-P., Markwardt,F., Richter,M.: Zur Analytik von p-Aminomethylbenzoesäure,
einem neuen Antifibrinolytikum. Pharmazie 20, 554 (1965)

Koller,F.: Über die Therapie der postoperativen Blutung und Thrombose bei Prostatektomie
unter besonderer Berücksichtigung der ε-Aminocapronsäure. Helv. chir. Acta 30, 514 (1963)

Kontras,S.B., Steiner,D., Kramer,N.: Use of epsilon-aminocaproic acid in hemophiliacs for
dental extractions. Ohio St. med. J. 65, 391 (1969)

Koutsky,J., Padovec,J., Jirasek,J.E., Rybak,M., Hladovec,J., Mansfeld,V.: Die antifibrinolytische Therapie der gynäkologischen Blutungen. Folia haemat. (Lpz.) 88, 151 (1967)

Kwaan,H.C., Astrup,T.: Aortic arteriosclerosis in rabbits, fed inhibitors of fibrinolysis. Arch.
Path. 78, 474 (1964)

Lacombe,M.: Antifibrinolytic agents. Un. méd. Can. 92, 683 (1963)

Ladehoff,A.A., Otte,E.: Inhibitory effect of epsilon aminocaproic acid on fibrinolytic activity
and bleeding in transvesical prostatectomy. Scand. J. clin. Lab. Invest. 15, 239 (1963)

Landmann,H.: Vergleichende Untersuchungen über Antifibrinolytika. Folia haemat. (Lpz.) 87,
106 (1967a)

Landmann,H.: Der Einfluß von p-Aminomethylbenzoesäure (PAMBA) auf die Aktivität
proteolytischer Fermente. Verh. dtsch. Ges. exp. Med. 12, 233 (1967b)

Landmann,H.: Synthetische Hemmstoffe des Plasmins. Haematologia Suppl. 1, 169 (1970)

Landmann,H.: Studies on the mechanism of action of synthetic antifibrinolytics. A comparison
with the action of derivatives of benzamidine on the fibrinolytic process. Thrombos. Diathes.
haemorrh. (Stuttg.) 29, 253 (1973)

Landmann,H., Markwardt,F.: Über die Hemmstoffe der Fibrinolyse. Verh. Ges. exper. Med.
DDR, Bd. 4, 32. Dresden-Leipzig: Theodor Steinkopff 1963

Landmann,H., Markwardt,F.: The action of the new antifibrinolytic agent p-aminomethylbenzoic acid (PAMBA). Xth Congr. Int. Soc. Haematol. Abstr. G: 67, Stockholm: 1964

Landmann,H., Markwardt,F.: Irreversible synthetische Inhibitoren der Urokinase. Experientia
(Basel) 26, 145 (1970)

Landmann,H., Markwardt,F., Kazmirowski,H.-G., Neuland,P.: Zusammenhänge zwischen
chemischer Konstitution und Antitrypsinwirkung bei Derivaten der 4-Aminomethyl-benzoe-
säure und anderen strukturverwandten zyklischen Verbindungen. Hoppe-Seylers Z. physiol.
Chem. 348, 745 (1967)

Landmann,H., Markwardt,F., Perlewitz,J.: Die Beeinflussung der Wirkung des Trypsins auf
die Blutgerinnung durch natürliche und synthetische Trypsin- und Thrombininhibitoren.
Thrombos. Diathes. haemorrh. (Stuttg.) 22, 552 (1969)

Lang,K., Bitz,H.: Über den Stoffwechsel der ε-Aminocapronsäure. Biochem. Z. 324, 495 (1955)

Lassner,J.: L'emploi de l'acide epsilon aminocaproïque en chirurgie prostatique. Anesth. Analg.
Réanim. 22, 475 (1965)

Laugier,P.: Attempt of treatment of three cases of scleroderma with epsilon-aminocaproic acid.
Bull. Soc. franç. Derm. Syph, 71, 645 (1964)

Lecomte,J., Salmon,J., Lambert,P.H.: Absence d'activité antianaphylactique de l'acide ε-aminocaproïque chez le rat. C.R. Soc. Biol. (Paris) 158, 1759 (1964)

Lee,L.: Reticuloendothelial clearence of circulating fibrin in the pathogenesis of the generalized
Shwartzman reaction. J. exp. Med. 115, 1065 (1962)

Lefèbvre,P., Salmon,J., Lecomte,J., Cauverberge,H. van: Influence de l'acide ε-aminocaproïque
sur l'augmentation de la perméabilité vasculaire provoquée, chez le rat, par l'histamine. Son
action sur le purpura engendré, chez la souris par l'huile de croton. C. R. Soc. Biol. (Paris) 156,
183 (1962).

Léger,L.: Current status of our ideas on fibrinolysis. Prevention and treatment with enzyme
inhibitors. Acta chir. belg. 62, 655 (1963)

Léger,L., Lande,M., Fournet,R.: Prévention et traitement par l'acide epsilon-aminocaproïque
des syndromes fibrinolytiques en chirurgie. Presse méd. 71, 969 (1963)

Lenoir,P., Turpin,J., Pawlotsky,Y., Noury,S., Gouffault,J., Bourel,M.: Résultats cliniques
obtenus par l'usage d'un antifibrinolytique. Thérapie 19, 1651 (1964)

Lindgardh,G., Andersson,L.: Clot retraction in the kidneys as a probable cause of anuria during
treatment of haematuria with ε-aminocaproic acid. Acta med. scand. 180, 469 (1966)

Ling,C.M., Summaria,L., Robbins,K.C.: Mechanism of formation of bovine plasminogen activator from human plasmin. J. biol. Chem. **240**, 4213 (1965)

Ling,C.-M., Summaria,L., Robbins,K.C.: Isolation and characterization of bovine plasminogen activator from a human plasminogen-streptokinase mixture. J. biol. Chem. **242**, 1419 (1967)

Linz,O.: Über die Behandlung funktioneller uteriner Blutungsstörungen mit Epsilon-Aminokapronsäure („EACA", Berlin-Chemie). Dtsch. Gesundh.-Wes. **22**, 1652 (1967)

Lipmann,W., Wishnick,M.: Effects of the administration of epsilon-aminocaproic acid on catecholamine and serotonin levels in the rat and dog. J. Pharmacol. exp. Ther. **150**, 196 (1965)

Lipmann,W., Wishnick,M., Buyske,D.A.: The depletion of norepinephrine from the heart by epsilon-amino-caproic acid. Life Sci. **4**, 281 (1965)

Loeffler,L.J., Britcher,S.F., Baumgarten,W.: Bridged bicyclic and polycyclic amino acids. Potent new inhibitors of the fibrinolytic process. J. med. Chem. **13**, 926 (1970)

Logan,L.J., Rapaport,S.I., Kuefler,P.: Failure of heparin, epsilon aminocaproic acid, or both agents to prevent increased fibrinogen levels after endotoxin in rabbits. Proc. Soc. exp. Biol. (N.Y.) **142**, 321 (1973)

Lohmann,K., Markwardt,F., Landmann,H.: Über neue Hemmstoffe der Fibrinolyse. Naturwissenschaften **50**, 502 (1963)

Lohmann,K., Markwardt,F., Landmann,H.: Zusammenhänge zwischen Konstitution und Wirkung bei Hemmstoffen der Fibrinolyse. Thrombos. Diathes. haemorrh. (Stuttg.) **10**, 424 (1964)

Lorand,L., Condit,E.V.: Ester hydrolysis by urokinase. Biochemistry **4**, 265 (1965)

Lorand,L., Mozen,M.M.: Ester hydrolyzing activity of urokinase preparations. Nature (Lond.) **201**, 392 (1964)

Loria Mendez,M., Karchmer,S., Dominguez,J.L.: Uso del acido epsilon caproico en el tratemiento de la hipofibrinogenemia obstetrica. Ginec. Obstet. Méx. **21**, 997 (1966)

Lowney,E.D.: Effects of epsilon-aminocaproic acid on the tuberculin reaction in man. J. invest. Derm. **42**, 243 (1964)

Ludvik,W., Pecherstorfer,M.: Beeinflussung der Blutung nach suprapubischer Prostatektomie durch die Epsilon-Aminokapronsäure. Wien. klin. Wschr. **79**, 384 (1967)

Ludwig,H., Mehring,W.: Zur Behandlung uteriner Blutungen mit ε-Aminocapronsäure. Fortschr. Med. **83**, 585 (1965)

Lukasiewicz,H., Niewiarowski,S.: In vitro studies on the mechanism of the antifibrinolytic action of E-aminocaproic acid. Thrombos. Diathes. haemorrh. (Stuttg.) **19**, 584 (1968)

Lukasiewicz,H., Niewiarowski,S., Worowski,K.: The plasmin inhibition by synthetic antifibrinolytic agents in relation to the type of substrate. Biochim. biophys. Acta **159**, 503 (1968)

Lukaszczyk,E., Orzel,S.: Opanowanie preparatem PAMBA wzmożonej aktywnosci fibrynolitycznej po resekcji tkanki plucnej. Pol. Tyg. lek. **23**, 1526 (1968)

Lundh,B., Laurell,A.B., Wetterquist,H., White,T.: A case of hereditary angioneurotic oedema successfully treated with ε-aminocaproic acid. Studies on C'1 esterase inhibitor, C'1 activation, plasminogen level and histamine metabolism. Clin. exp. Immunol. **3**, 733 (1968)

Mainwaring,D., Keidan,S.E.: Fibrinolysis in haemophilia: The effect of epsilon-aminocaproic acid. Brit. J. Haemat. **11**, 209 (1965)

Maki,M., Beller,F.K.: Comparative studies of fibrinolytic inhibitors in vitro. Thrombos. Diathes. haemorrh. (Stuttg.) **16**, 668 (1966)

Malene,Y.: Traitements des méno-métrorragies par l'hémocaprol (acide epsilon aminocaproïque). Sem. thér. **40**, 505 (1964)

Marchal,G., Bilski-Pasquir,G., Samama,M., Casubolo,L.: Lugar del acide epsilon-aminocaproico en los estados fibrinoliticos. Rev. clin. esp. **95**, 17 (1964)

Marchal,G., Duhamel,G., Samama,M., Flandrin,G.: Fibrinolyse aigue révélatrice d'un cancer de la prostate avec métastases osseuses. Efficacité de l'acide ε-aminocaproïque. Bull. Soc. Méd. Hôp. Paris **114**, 143 (1963)

Marchal,G., Samama,M., Leroux,M.E.: Les agents actuels de la thérapeutique antifibrinolytique. Sem. Hôp. Paris **38**, 1985 (1962)

Marchal,G., Samama,M., Mirabel,J., Vaysse,J.: Fibrinolyse cataclysmique au cours d'un traitement chirurgical d'une tétralogie de Fallot en circulation extracorporelle. Résultats encourageants in vitro d'un agent antifibrinolytique. Sem. Hôp. Paris **36**, 1994 (1960)

Marchal,G., Weiss,M., Dubost,C., Samama,M., Yver,J.: Acquisitions récentes de la fibrinolyse hémorragique en chirurgie et son traitement. Proc. 9th Congr. Europ. Soc. Haemat. Lisbon 1963, 1397

Mares-Guia,M., Shaw,E.: Studies on the active center of trypsin. The binding of amidines and guanidines as models of substrate side chain. J. biol. Chem. **240**, 1579 (1965)

Margaretten,W., Zunker,H.O., McKay,D.G.: Production of the generalized Shwartzman reaction in pregnant rats by intravenous infusion of thrombin. Lab. Invest. **13**, 552 (1964)

Marggraf,W.: Beobachtungen über Fibrinolysen in der Chirurgie, ihre Prophylaxe und gezielte Behandlung mit Inhibitoren. Bruns' Beitr. klin. Chir. **205**, 121 (1962)

Marini,M.P., Arturi,F., Crolle,G.: Terapia delle emorragie postestrattine negli emofilici con acido epsilon-aminocaproico (EACA). Haematologica **51**, 553 (1966)

Markus,G.: On the heterogenity of streptokinase-induced plasmin. In: Anticoagulants and Fibrinolysins (MacMillan,R.C., Mustard,J.F. Eds.), p. 376. London: Pitman Medical Publishing Co. Ltd. 1961

Markwardt,F.: Die quantitative Bestimmung des Prothrombins durch Titration mit Hirudin. Naunyn Schmiedeberg's Arch. exp. Path. Pharmak. **232**, 487 (1958)

Markwardt, F.: Die Entwicklung von Fibrinolysehemmstoffen. Mitteilung der Deutschen Akademie der Naturforscher Leopoldina. Reihe 3, 11, p. 149 (1965)

Markwardt,F.: Antifibrinolytika, eine neue Arzneistoffklasse. Internist (Berl.) **7**, 400 (1966)

Markwardt,F.: Gerinnungsphysiologische Analyse der Wirkung synthetischer Thrombininhibitoren. Thrombos. Diathes. haemorrh. (Stuttg.) **27**, 99 (1972)

Markwardt,F., Drawert,J., Walsmann,P.: Einfluß von Benzamidinderivaten auf die Aktivität von Serum- und Pankreaskallikrein. Acta biol. med. germ. **26**, 123 (1971a)

Markwardt,F., Haustein,K.-O., Klöcking,H.-P.: Die pharmakologische Charakterisierung des neuen Antifibrinolytikums p-Aminomethylbenzoesäure (PAMBA). Arch. int. Pharmacodyn. **152**, 223 (1964)

Markwardt,F., Haustein,K.-O., Landmann,H.: Zusammenhänge zwischen Konstitution und antifibrinolytischer Wirkung der ε-Aminocapronsäure. Second International Pharmacological Meeting, Prague, August 1963, Biochemical Pharmacology, Conference Issue, p. 242, 1963

Markwardt,F., Klöcking,H.-P.: Über das Stoffwechselschicksal der p-Aminomethylbenzoesäure (PAMBA) beim Menschen. Acta biol. med. germ. **14**, 519 (1965a)

Markwardt,F., Klöcking,H.-P.: Zur Pharmakologie des Antifibrinolytikums p-Aminomethylbenzoesäure (PAMBA). Medicamentum (Berl.) **6**, 297 (1965b)

Markwardt,F., Klöcking,H.-P.: p-Aminomethylbenzoesäure (PAMBA), ein neues Antifibrinolytikum. Tierexperimentelle Untersuchungen. Münch. med. Wschr. **107**, 2000 (1965c)

Markwardt,F., Klöcking,H.-P.: Tierexperimentelle Untersuchungen der Wirkung synthetischer Antifibrinolytika. Acta biol. med. germ. **17**, 746 (1966a)

Markwardt,F., Klöcking,H.-P.: Über Anwendung und Stoffwechselschicksal des neuen Antifibrinolytikums p-Aminomethylbenzoesäure. Z. ges. inn. Med. **21**, 18 (1966b)

Markwardt, F., Klöcking,H.-P.,Landmann,H.: Vergleichende Untersuchungen über Antifibrinolytika. Thrombos. Diathes. haemorrh. (Stuttg.) **15**, 561 (1966)

Markwardt,F., Klöcking,H.-P., Nowak,G.: Antithrombin- und Antiplasminwirkung von 4-Amidinophenylbrenztraubensäure (APPA) in vivo. Thrombos. Diathes. haemorrh. (Stuttg.) **24**, 240 (1970a)

Markwardt,F., Klöcking,H.-P., Richter,M.: Die Kombinationswirkung von Fibrinolysehemmstoffen. Acta biol. med. germ. **12**, 522 (1964)

Markwardt,F., Klöcking,H.-P., Richter,M.: Die Bestimmung synthetischer Antifibrinolytica in Körperflüssigkeiten und Organen. Pharmazie **22**, 83 (1967a)

Markwardt,F., Klöcking,H.-P.,Vogel,G.: Untersuchungen zur Anwendung von p-Aminomethylbenzoesäureäthylester als Antifibrinolytikum. Z. ges. inn. Med. **22**, 569 (1967b)

Markwardt,F., Landmann,H.: Antifibrinolytika. Jena: Fischer 1967

Markwardt,F., Landmann,H.: Struktur-Wirkungs-Beziehungen bei Proteaseninhibitoren. Verh. dtsch. Ges. exp. Med. **9**, 125 (1972)

Markwardt,F., Landmann,H., Hoffmann,A.: Die Hemmung der Trypsinogen- und Chymotrypsinogenaktivierung durch p-Aminomethylbenzoesäure (PAMBA) und andere Aminocarbonsäuren. Naturwissenschaften **51**, 635 (1964)

Markwardt, F., Landmann, H., Hoffmann, A.: Über den Einfluß der p-Aminomethylbenzoesäure auf die Aktivierung proteolytischer Fermente. Hoppe-Seylers Z. physiol. Chem. **340**, 174 (1965)

Markwardt, F., Landmann, H., Klöcking, H.-P.: Fibrinolytika und Antifibrinolytika. Jena: Fischer 1972

Markwardt, F., Landmann, H., Vogel, G.: Die Entwicklung des neuen Antifibrinolytikums p-Aminomethylbenzoesäure (PAMBA). Dtsch. Gesundh.-Wes. **19**, 2320 (1964)

Markwardt, F., Landmann, H., Walsmann, P.: Comparative studies on the inhibition of trypsin, plasmin, and thrombin by derivatives of benzylamine and benzamidine. Europ. J. Biochem. **6**, 502 (1968)

Markwardt, F., Nowak, G., Meerbach, W., Rüdiger, K.-D.: Studies in experimental animals on disseminated intravascular coagulation (DIC). Thrombos. Diathes. haemorrh. (Stuttg.) **34**, 513 (1975)

Markwardt, F., Perlewitz, J.: Die Hemmung der fibrinolytischen Wirkung von Gewebekulturen durch Antifibrinolytika. Naturwissenschaften **50**, 502 (1963)

Markwardt, F., Richter, M.: Über die antifibrinolytische Wirkung von Derivaten der p-Aminomethylbenzoesäure (PAMBA). Acta biol. med. germ. **13**, 719 (1964)

Markwardt, F., Richter, P., Stürzebecher, J., Wagner, G., Walsmann, P.: Synthetische Inhibitoren der Serinproteinasen. 6. Mitteilung: Über die Hemmung von Trypsin, Plasmin und Thrombin durch Phenylbrenztraubensäuren mit verschiedenen basischen Substituenten. Acta biol. med. germ. **33**, K 1 (1974)

Markwardt, F., Richter, M., Walsmann, P., Landmann, H.: The inhibition of trypsin, plasmin, and thrombin by benzyl 4-guanidinobenzoate and 4'-nitrobenzyl 4-guanidinobenzoate. FEBS Letters **8**, 170 (1970b)

Markwardt, F., Walsmann, P.: Über die Hemmung des Gerinnungsfermentes Thrombin durch Benzamidinderivate. Experientia (Basel) **24**, 25 (1968)

Markwardt, F., Walsmann, P., Drawert, J.: Über den Einfluß synthetischer Trypsininhibitoren auf die kininliberierende Wirkung von Trypsin und Pankreaskallikrein. Acta biol. med. germ. **24**, 401 (1970c)

Markwardt, F., Walsmann, P., Landmann, H.: Hemmung der Thrombin-, Plasmin- und Trypsinwirkung durch Alkyl- und Alkoxybenzamidine. Pharmazie **25**, 551 (1970d)

Markwardt, F., Walsmann, P., Richter, M., Klöcking, H.-P., Drawert, J., Landmann, H.: Aminoalkylbenzolsulfofluoride als Fermentinhibitoren. Pharmazie **26**, 401 (1971b)

Markwardt, F., Walsmann, P., Stürzebecher, J., Landmann, H., Wagner, G.: Synthetische Inhibitoren von Serinproteinasen. 1. Mitteilung: Über die Hemmung von Trypsin, Plasmin und Thrombin durch Ester der Amidino- und Guanidinobenzoesäure. Pharmazie **28**, 327 (1973)

Marmo, E., Ungaro, B., Giordano, L.: Sugli effetti cardio-vascolari di alcuni anti-fibrinolitici (Trasylol, ac. epsilon-amino-caproico, ac. tranexamico). Minerva cardioangiol. **19**, 86 (1971)

Martin, E., Hureau, J., Vayre, P., Audhony, H.: Etude anatome-pathologique de la pancréatic aigue hémorrhagique et nécrosante expérimentale. Arch. Mal. Appar. dig. **54**, 195 (1965)

Marx, R.: Wirkungsweise der Fibrinolytika und Antifibrinolytika. Thrombos. Diathes. haemorrh. (Stuttg.) Suppl. **3**, 27 (1963)

Marx, R., Borst, H.: Störungen der Blutgerinnung und Blutstillung nach extrakorporaler Zirkulation. Thoraxchirurgie **9**, 75 (1961)

Marzetti, L.: Treatment of hemorrhagic diseases with epsilon-aminocaproic acid in obstetrics and gynecology. Clin. obstet. ginec. **66**, 311 (1964)

Mascart, P.: A propos du contrôle de la fibrinolyse au cours des circulations extracorporelles. Acta chir. belg. **62**, 677 (1963)

Maxwell, R. W.: Enhancement of inhibition of fibrinolysis by reversible plasmin inhibitors. Fed. Proc. **25**, 498 (1966)

Maxwell, R. E., Allen, D.: Interactions of ε-aminocaproic acid with the thrombin clotting and fibrinolytic system. Nature (Lond.) **209**, 211 (1966)

Maxwell, R. E., Lewandowski, V., Nickel, V. S., Nawrocki, J. W.: Substrate modification and the mechanism of potentiation of plasmin inhibition by ω-amino acid. Thrombos. Diathes. haemorrh. (Stuttg.) **18**, 99 (1967)

Maxwell, R. E., Nawrocki, J. W., Nickel, V. S.: Some complexities of multiple inhibitor interactions in fibrinolytic systems. Thromb. Diathes. haemorrh. (Stuttg.) **19**, 117 (1968)

Maxwell,R.E., Nawrocki,J.W., Nickel,V.S.: Multiple inhibitor interactions in the control of fibrinolysis. In: Schor,J.M. (Ed.). Chemical Control of Fibrinolysis-Thrombolysis. Theory and Clinical Applications, p. 287. New York-London-Sidney-Toronto: Wiley 1970

Mayer,W., Erbe,S., Horn,W.: Vorschlag zum DAB 5 Aminomethylbenzoesäure. Pharmazie **21**, 543 (1966)

McClure,P.D., Izsak,J.: The use of epsilon-aminocaproic acid to reduce bleeding during cardiac bypass in children with congenital heart disease. Anesthesiology **40**, 604 (1974)

McFadden,S.W.: Über die Wirkung der Epsilon-Amino-Capronsäure auf einige allergische und immunologische Phänomene. Dermatologica (Basel) **130**, 107 (1965)

McNicol,G.P.: Disordered fibrinolytic activity and its control. Scot. med. J. **7**, 266 (1962)

McNicol,G.P., Douglas,A.: ε-Aminocaproic acid and other inhibitors of fibrinolysis. Brit. med. Bull. **20**, 233 (1964)

McNicol,G.P., Fletcher,A.P., Alkjaersig,N., Sherry,S.: Absorption, distribution and excretion of epsilon aminocaproic acid (EACA). Fed. Proc. **20**, 58 (1961a)

McNicol,G.P., Fletcher,A.P., Alkjaersig,N., Sherry,S.: The use of epsilon aminocaproic acid. A potent inhibitor of fibrinolytic activity, in the management of postoperative hematuria. J. Urol. (Baltimore) **86**, 829 (1961b)

McNicol,G.P., Fletcher,A.P., Alkjaersig,N., Sherry,S.: Impairment of hemostasis in the urinary tract: the role of urokinase. J. Lab. clin. Med. **58**, 34 (1961c)

McNicol,G.P., Fletcher,A.P., Alkjaersig,N., Sherry,S.: Plasma amino acid chromatography with ion exchange resin loaded paper: assay of ε-aminocaproic acid. J. Lab. clin. Med. **59**, 7 (1962)

Melander,B., Gliniecki,G., Granstrand,B., Hanshoff,G.: Biochemistry and toxicology of Amikapron; the antifibrinolytically active isomer of AMCHA (a comparative study with ε-aminocaproic acid). Acta pharmacol. (Kbh.) **22**, 340 (1965)

Mester,E., Detky,B., Füsy,J.: Durch Fibrinolyse verursachte postoperative Blutungen in der chirurgischen Praxis. Zbl. Chir. **92**, 1429 (1967)

Mey,U., Sundermann,A., Vogel,G.: Begleitfibrinolyse bei hämatologischen Erkrankungen und ihre Beeinflussung durch PAMBA. Folia haemat. (Lpz.) **87**, 80 (1967)

Mikata,I., Hasegawa,M., Igarashi,T., Shirakura,N., Hoshida,M., Toyama,K.: Clinical use of ipsilon for the prevention of the allergic reaction from blood transfusion. Keio J. Med. **8**, 319 (1969)

Miller,J.M., Robinson,D.R., Jackson,D.A., Collier,C.S.: Reversal by ipsilon of lytic system in blood stream produced in rabbits by streptokinase. Arch. Surg. **78**, 33 (1959)

Minn,S.K., Mandel,E.E.: Experimental disseminated intravascular coagulation. Effect of heparin and e-aminocaproic acid on tests of hemostatic function. Thrombos. Res. **6**, 235 (1975)

Mix,H., Trettin,H.-J., Gülzow,M.: Zusammenhänge zwischen Konstitution und Wirkung primärer Amine und Aminosäuren bei der Inhibierung von Trypsin. Hoppe-Seylers Z. physiol. Chem. **343**, 52 (1965)

Mix,H., Trettin,H.-J., Gülzow,M.: 4-Guanidino-benzoesäurebenzylester und 4-Guanidino-benzoesäure-4'-nitrobenzylester: Neue hochwirksame Trypsininhibitoren. Hoppe-Seylers Z. physiol. Chem. **349**, 1237 (1968)

Mootse,G., Cliffton,E.E.: The effect of cycsteine and mercaptoethanol on plasmin. Amer. J. Cardiol. **6**, 399 (1960)

Mosesson,W.M.: The preparation of human fibrinogen free of plasminogen. Biochim. biophys. Acta (Amst.) **57**, 204 (1962)

Mounter,L.A., Mounter,M.E.: The inhibition of hydrolytic enzymes by organophosphorus compounds. J. biol. Chem. **238**, 1079 (1963)

Mounter,L.A., Shipley,B.A.: The inhibition of plasmin by toxic phosphorus compounds. J. biol. Chem. **231**, 855 (1958)

Mullan,S., Beckman,F., Vailati,G., Karasick,J., Dabben,G.: An experimental approach to the problem of cerebral aneurysm. J. Neurosurg. **21**, 838 (1964)

Mullan,S., Dawley,J.: Antifibrinolytic therapy for intracranial aneurysms. J. Neurosurg. **28**, 21 (1968)

Muramatu,M., Fujii,S.: Inhibitory effects of ω-guanidino acid esters on trypsin, plasmin, thrombin and plasma kallikrein. J. Biochem. (Tokyo) **64**, 807 (1968)

Muramatu,M., Fujii,S.: Inhibitory effects of ω-amino acid esters on the activities of trypsin, plasmin and thrombin. J. Biochem. (Tokyo) **65**, 17 (1969)

Muramatu, M., Hayakumo, Y., Fujii, S.: Synthetic inhibitors of trypsin, plasmin and chymotrypsin. J. Biochem. (Tokyo) **62**, 408 (1967)

Muramatu, M., Onishi, T., Makino, S., Fujii, S., Yamamura, Y.: Inhibition of caseinolytic activity of plasmin by various synthetic inhibitors. J. Biochem. (Tokyo) **57**, 402 (1965a)

Muramatu, M., Onishi, T., Makino, S., Fujii, S., Yamamura, Y.: Inhibition of fibrinolytic activity of plasmin by various synthetic inhibitors. J. Biochem. (Tokyo) **57**, 450 (1965b)

Muramatu, M., Onishi, T., Makino, S., Hayakumo, Y., Fujii, S.: Inhibition of tryptic activity by various synthetic inhibitors. J. Biochem. (Tokyo) **58**, 214 (1965c)

Muramatu, M., Shiraishi, S., Fujii, S.: Inhibitory effects of omega amino and omega guanidino acid esters on the first component of human complement. Biochim. biophys. Acta (Amst.) **285**, 224 (1972)

Musialowicz, J., Jezuita, J., Bielecki, M.: The effect of epsilon-aminocaproic acid on the antigen-antibody reaction. Brit. J. exp. Path. **46**, 274 (1965)

Naber, K., Bichler, K. H., Mueller, K. H., Sommerkamp, H., Jöhrens, H., Porzsolt, F.: Veränderungen der Blutgerinnung beim chirurgischen Eingriff an der Prostata, Konsequenzen für die prophylaktische Therapie mit Antifibrinolytika. Helv. chir. Acta **40**, 519 (1973)

Naeye, R. L.: Thrombolytic state after a hemorrhagic diathesis, a possible complication of therapy with ε-aminocaproic acid. Blood **19**, 694 (1962)

Nagamatsu, A., Okuma, T., Hayashida, T., Yamamura, Y.: Studies on antiplasminic agents. Chem. pharm. Bull. **16**, 211 (1968)

Nagamatsu, A., Okuma, T., Watanabe, M., Yamamura, Y.: The inhibition of plasmin by some amino acid derivatives. J. Biochem. (Tokyo) **54**, 491 (1963)

Nagy, J., Gáti, J., Losonczy, H., Than, E.: Dauerbehandlung mit Antifibrinolytika bei Hypermenorrhoe. Haematologia, Suppl. **1**, 221 (1970)

Naito, T., Okano, A., Kadoya, S., Miki, T., Inaoka, M., Moroi, R., Shimizu, M.: Medicinal-chemical studies on antiplasmin drugs. II. Separation of stereoisomers of 4-aminomethyl-cyclohexanecarboxylic acid and assignment of their configuration. Chem. pharm. Bull. **16**, 728 (1968)

Neef, H., Preusser, K. P., Anger, G.: PAMBA-Prophylaxe bei Prostatektomien. Folia haemat. (Lpz.) **88**, 197 (1967)

Neter, E.: Effect of tyrothricin and actinomycin A upon bacterial fibrinolysis and plasma coagulation. Proc. Soc. exp. Biol. (N. Y.) **49**, 163 (1942)

Neubauer, H. W.: Neuere Medikamente zur Behandlung des anaphylaktischen Schocks bei Versuchstieren. Dermatologica (Basel) **126**, 124 (1963)

Niesert, W., Schneider, J., Stegmann, H., Winckelmann, G.: Uterus myomatosus mit Hypofibrinogenämie, passagerer Fibrinolyse und Thrombopenie. Geburtsh. u. Frauenheilk. **24**, 594 (1964)

Niewiarowski, S.: Inhibitoren der Fibrinolyse zur Behandlung von Hämorrhagien, hämorrhagischen Diathesen und anderen pathologischen Erscheinungen. I. Spezifische Inhibitoren der Fibrinolyse (pol.) Pol. Arch. Med. wewnęt. **34**, 211 (1964)

Niewiarowski, S.: Untersuchungen über die hämostatische Wirkung von ε-Aminocapronsäure (EACA). Z. ges. inn. Med. **20**, 323 (1965)

Niewiarowski, S., Wolosowicz, N.: The in vivo-effect of ε-aminocaproic acid (EACA) on human plasma fibrinolytic system. Thrombos. Diathes. haemorrh. (Stuttg.) **15**, 491 (1966)

Nilsson, I. M., Andersson, L., Björkman, S. E.: Epsilon aminocaproic acid (EACA) as a therapeutic agent based on 5 year's clinical experience. Acta med. scand. Suppl. 448 (1966)

Nilsson, I. M., Björkman, S. E.: Experiences with ε-aminocaproic acid (ε-ACA) in the treatment of profuse menstruation. Acta med. scand. **177**, 445 (1965)

Nilsson, I. M., Björkman, S. E., Andersson, L.: Clinical experiences with ε-aminocaproic acid (ε-ACA) as an antifibrinolytic agent. Acta med. scand. **170**, 487 (1961)

Nilsson, I. M., Olow, B.: Fibrinolysis induced by streptokinase in man. Acta chir. scand. **123**, 247 (1962)

Nilsson, I. M., Sjoerdsma, A., Waldenström, J.: Antifibrinolytic activity and metabolism of ε-aminocaproic acid in man. Lancet **1960**, I, 1322

Nilsson, L., Rybo, G.: Treatment of menorrhagia with epsilon aminocaproic acid. A double blind investigation. Acta obstet. gynec. scand. **44**, 467 (1965)

Noer, G. H.: Behandling av gastrointestinal blödning med epsilon-aminokapronsyre. Norske Laegeforen. **84**, 676 (1964)

Noferi, A., Volpari, A. L., Mancuso, A.: Efetto dell'acido epsilon-amino-caproico (EAC) sulla reazione cutanea specifica di tipo immediato e sul transporto passivo locale della sensibilita all Praussnitz-Küster. Folia allerg. (Roma) **16**, 169 (1969)

Nordöy, A.: Experimental venous thrombosis in rats. Increased formation during inhibition of the fibrinolytic system with epsilon amino caproic acid. Thrombos. Diathes. haemorrh. (Stuttg.) **9**, 427 (1963)

Nordström, S., Zetterqvist, E.: Effects of epsilon-aminocaproic acid (EACA) and trasylol on thromboplastin-induced intravascular coagulation, studied in dogs with iodine-labelled fibrinogen. Acta physiol. scand. **76**, 93 (1969)

Norlén, G., Thulin, C. A.: Experiences with epsilon-aminocaproic acid in neurosurgery (a preliminary report). Neurochirurgia (Stuttg.) **10**, 81 (1967)

Norlén, G., Thulin, C. A.: The use of antifibrinolytic substances in ruptured intracranial aneurysms. Neurochirurgia (Stuttg.) **12**, 100 (1969)

Norlén, G., Thulin, C. A.: Preliminära erfarenheter av antifibrinolytisk behandling vid intrakraniella blödningar. In: Antifibrinolytisk terapi, p. 73. Stockholm: AB Kabi 1970

Norman, P. S.: Effect of urea and methylamine on plasmin. Proc. Soc. exp. Biol. (N. Y.) **96**, 709 (1957)

Nuernbergk, W.: Hyperfibrinolytische Blutungen in der HNO-Heilkunde und ihre Behandlung mit PAMBA. Folia haemat. (Lpz.) **87**, 72 (1967)

Obianwu, H. O.: Inhibition of the dual amine uptake concentration mechanisms of the adrenergic neurone by ε-aminocaproic acid. J. Pharm. (Lond.) **19**, 54 (1967a)

Obianwu, H. O.: Disposition of ^{3}H-epsilon aminocaproic acid and its interaction with adrenergic neurones. Brit. J. Pharmacol. **31**, 244 (1967b)

Okamoto, S.: Plasmin and antiplasmin. Their pathologic physiology. Keio J. Med. **8**, 211 (1959)

Okamoto, S.: Refer to British Patent Nr. 770693 (Mitsubishi Kasei Kogyo, Co., Ltd.) filed 1954, patented 1957, Refer to USA Patent Nr. 2939817, filed 1953, patented 1960a

Okamoto, S.: Epsilon amino caproic acid and its suppressing effects on some biological phenomena associated with activated plasmin in the circulatory blood. Proc. 8th Congr. Int. Soc. Hematol. Tokyo 1960b, III, 1606

Okamoto, S., Hijikata, A.: Rational approach to proteinase inhibitors. Drug Design **6**, 143 (1975)

Okamoto, S., Nakajima, T., Okamoto, U., Watanabe, H., Iguchi, Y., Igawa, T., Chien, C.-C., Hayashi, T.: A suppressing effect of ε-amino-n-caproic acid on the bleeding of dogs, produced with the activation of plasmin in the circulatory blood. Keio J. Med. **8**, 247 (1959)

Okamoto, S., Okamoto, U.: Amino-methyl-cyclohexanecarboxylic acid: AMCHA. A new potent inhibitor of the fibrinolysis. Keio J. Med. **11**, 105 (1962)

Okamoto, S., Sato, S., Takada, Y., Okamoto, U.: An active isomer (trans form) of AMCHA and its antifibrinolytic (antiplasminic) action *in vitro* and *in vivo*. Keio J. Med. **13**, 177 (1964)

Okano, A., Inaoka, M., Funabashi, S., Iwamoto, M., Isoda, S., Moroi, R., Abiko, Y., Hirata, M.: Medicinal-chemical studies on antiplasmin drugs: 4. Chemical modification of trans-4-aminomethyl-cyclohexanecarboxylic acid and its effect on antiplasmin activity. J. med. Chem. **15**, 247 (1972)

Olow, B.: Studies on the effect of streptokinase infusions in thrombembolic disease. Acta chir. scand. **126**, 7 (1963)

Olow, B., Nilsson, I. M.: Fibrinolysis induced by streptokinase in man. II. Further studies with large doses of streptokinase alone and streptokinase combined with epsilon-aminocaproic acid. Acta chir. scand. **125**, 593 (1963)

Oshiba, S., Okamoto, S.: Influence of AMCHA on the activity of fibrinolysin (plasmin). Keio J. Med. **11**, 117 (1962)

Oswald, K., Mörl, F. K., Matis, P.: Postoperative Blutstillung durch Epsilon-Aminocapronsäure unter vorsorglicher Gerinnungshemmung. Med. Welt (Stuttg.) **1966**, I, 817

Otto-Servais, M., Lecomte, J.: Inhibition par l'acide ε-aminocaproïque des réactions anaphylactiques générales du lapin. C. R. Soc. Biol. (Paris) **155**, 2050 (1961)

Paddon, A. J.: The use of aminocaproic acid as supplementary treatment of the haemophiliac undergoing surgery. J. dent. Ass. S. Afr. **22**, 64 (1967)

Pappenhagen, A. R., Koppel, J. L., Olwin, J. H.: Use of fluorescein-labeled fibrin for the determination of fibrinolytic activity. J. Lab. clin. Med. **59**, 1039 (1962)

Patterson, R. H., Jr., Harpel, P.: The effect of epsilon aminocaproic acid and tranexamic acid on thrombus size and strength in a simulated arterial aneurysm. J. Neurosurg. **34**, 365 (1971)

Pell, G.: Tranexamic acid — its use in controlling dental-postoperative bleeding in patients with defective clotting mechanisms. Brit. J. oral. Surg. **11**, 155 (1973)

Perlick, E.: Zur therapeutischen Anwendung von ε-Aminocapronsäure und anderen Antifibrinolytika. Dtsch. Gesundh.-Wes. **19**, 900 (1964)

Philips, L. L., Margaretten, W., McKay, D. G.: Changes in the fibrinolytic enzyme system following intravascular coagulation induced by thrombin and endotoxin. Obstet. and Gynec. **100**, 319 (1968)

Poluschkin, B. V., Barkagan, Z. S.: ε-Aminocapronsäure als ein Hemmstoff der Fibrinolyse, Eigenschaften und klinische Anwendung (russ.). Klin. Med. (Mosk.) **41**, 3/25 (1963)

Pospisil, J., Skala, E., Beran, M.: Use of epsilon-amino-caproic acid in experimental animals in the course of acute radiation sickness. Strahlentherapie **135**, 346 (1968)

Poulain, M., Josso, F.: Traitment des hématuries chez les hémophiles, études de 62 cas chez 40 hémophiles. Bibl. haemat. (Basel) **26**, 115 (1966)

Poulain, M., Renard, M. J., Josso, F.: Essai d'appréciation statistique de l'action préventive de l'acide epsilon-aminocaproïque sur les complications hémorragiques de l'hémophilie. Hémostase **4**, 307 (1964)

Preusser, K. P., Neef, H., Anger, G.: Die Beeinflussung der Hämaturie nach Prostatektomie durch die p-Aminomethylbenzoesäure (PAMBA). Langenbecks Arch. klin. Chir. **317**, 117 (1967)

Raab, W.: Influence of antifibrinolytic substances on allergic reactions. Experiments with ε-aminocaproic acid and amino-methylcyclohexane-carbonic acid. Experientia (Basel) **24**, 250 (1968)

Rainsford, S. G., Jouhar, A. J., Hall, A.: Tranexamic acid in the control of spontaneous bleeding in severe haemophilia. Thrombos. Diathes. haermorrh. (Stuttg.) **30**, 272 (1973)

Ramos, A. O., Chapman, L. F., Corrado, A. F.: Inhibition of the local Shwartzman-phenomenon by the administration of epsilon-aminocaproic acid. Arch. int. Pharmacodyn. **132**, 270 (1961 a)

Ramos, A. O., Chapman, L. F., Corrado, A. F., Fortes, V. A.: Sympathomimetic action of the epsilon-aminocaproic acid. Arch. int. Pharmacodyn. **132**, 274 (1961 b)

Redleaf, P. D., Davis, R. B., Kucinski, C., Hoilund, L., Gans, H.: Amyloidosis with an unusual bleeding diathesis. Observations on the use of epsilon amino caproic acid. Ann. intern. Med. **58**, 347 (1963)

Reid, W. O., Hodge, S. M., Cerutti, E. R.: The use of EACA in preventing or reducing hemorrhages in the hemophiliac. Thrombos. Diathes. haemorrh. (Stuttg.) **18**, 179 (1967)

Reid, W. O., Lukas, O. N., Francisco, J., Geisler, P. H., Erslev, A. J.: The use of epsilon-aminocaproic acid in the management of dental extractions in the hemophiliac. Amer. J. med. Sci. **248**, 184 (1964)

Renoux, M., Lerolle-Mollaret, P. E., Gonin, J., Chahinian, P.: Inhibition de l'anaphylaxie cutanée passive du rat par l'acide epsilon amino caproïque. Path. et Biol. (Paris) **21**, 171 (1973)

Renzo, E. C. de, Boggiano, E., Barg, W. F., Jr., Buck, F. F.: Interaction of streptokinase and human plasminogen. IV. Further gel electrophoretic studies on the combination of streptokinase with human plasminogen or human plasmin. J. biol. Chem. **242**, 2428 (1967)

Reque, P. G.: The treatment of systemic sclerosis: with special reference to epsilon aminocaproic acid. Sth. med. J. (Bgham, Ala.) **58**, 319 (1965)

Rezakovic, D., Nikulin, A., Stern, P.: Beitrag zur Kenntnis der Wirkungsweise und der Toxikologie der ε-Aminokapronsäure, Blut **12**, 262 (1966)

Ritz, N. D.: Fibrinolytic activity in hemophilia and the use of epsilon aminocaproic acid. J. Med. **65**, 2914 (1965)

Ritzel, G., Wüthrich, R.: Zur Wirkungsweise der ε-Aminocapronsäure. Schweiz. med. Wschr. **94**, 267 (1964)

Ro, J. S., Knutrud, O., Stormorken, H.: Antifibrinolytic treatment with tranexamic acid (AMCHA) in pediatric urinary tract surgery. J. pediat. Surg. **5**, 315 (1970)

Robbins, K. C., Ling, C., Summaria, L.: Mechanism of formation of bovine plasminogen activator from human plasmin. Fed. Proc. **24**, 452 (1965)

Roka, L.: Diskussions-Résumé. Thrombos. Diathes. haemorrh. (Stuttg.) Suppl. **22**, 67 (1967)

Rolle, J.: Epsilon-Aminocapronsäure. Übersicht und Diskussion der therapeutischen Wirkungs-breite. Chir. Praxis **9**, 209 (1965)

Rosdy, E., Biro, J., Szendroi, Z.: Die Anwendung von Antifibrinolytika in der Urologie. Acta chir. Acad. Sci. hung. **10**, 25 (1969)

Roth, F.: Die Beeinflussung gesteigerter proteolytischer Vorgänge mit einem neuen Ferment-hemmer. Geburtsh. u. Frauenheilk. **22**, 975 (1962)

Rothe, G.: Anwendung von PAMBA in der Zahn- und Kieferheilkunde. Folia haemat. (Lpz.) **87**, 67 (1967)

Rotstein, J., Gilbert, M., Estrin, I.: Antifibrinolytic drug in treatment of progressive systemic scle-rosis. J. Amer. med. Ass. **184**, 517 (1963)

Rouffilange, F., Picard, P., Radiguet de la Bastaie, P.: A propos de l'emploi de l'acide epsilon-amino-caproïque en urologie. Hémostase **5**, 405 (1965)

Rousselot, L. M., Grossi, C. E., Panke, W. F.: Altérations des facteurs de coagulation et fibrinolyse chez les cirrhotiques au cours des anastomoses porto-caves. Presse méd. **70**, 1975 (1962)

Rowinski, W. A., Hager, E. B.: Immunosuppressive effect of epsilon-amino caproic acid (EACA). J. surg. Res. **6**, 58 (1966)

Rubin, H., Ritz, N. D.: The inhibitory effect of sialic acid on fibrinolysis. Thrombes. Diathes. haemorrh. (Stuttg.) **17**, 23 (1967)

Rudakova, S. F., Zhukova, N. A., Khnychev, S. S., Susanyan, T. A., Kozlova, J. J.: Einige neue Aspekte über die durch ε-Aminokapronsäure auf den Organismus ausgeübte Wirkung (russ.) Vestn. Akad. med. Nauk **20**, 74 (1965)

Ruzieska, G., Dzvonyár, J., Gulyás, P., Baros, S.: Anwendung von Acepramin bei der Behandlung geburtshilflicher Koagulopathien. Haematologia, Suppl. **1**, 245 (1970)

Rybo, G., Westerberg, H.: The effect of tranexamic acid (AMCA) on postoperative bleeding after conization. Acta obstet. gynec. scand. **51**, 347 (1972)

Sack, E., Spaet, T. H., Gentile, R. L., Hudson, P. B.: Reduction of postprostatectomy bleeding by epsilon-aminocaproic acid. New Engl. J. Med. **266**, 541 (1962)

Saita, G., Sbertoli, C., Farina, G., Galli, T.: Azione del sulfuo dicarbonio sulla fibrinolisi. Med. Lavoro **54**, 45 (1963)

Sakurane, K., Yamaguchi, M.: Die klinische Wirkung von ε-Aminocapronsäure auf Ekzem, Der-matitis und andere Hautkrankheiten, vermutlich allergischen Ursprungs (jap.). Hifu to Hinyo **18**, 434 (1965)

Saldeen, T., Bagge, L., Busch, C., Rammer, L.: Delayed fibrin elimination from the lungs and pulmonary damage after intravenous injection of thrombin in rats with endogenous inhibition of the fibrinolytic system. Forensic Sci. **1**, 115 (1972)

Salmon, J.: Inhibition du purpura thrombopénique immunologique par l'acide ε-aminocaproïque. Thrombos. Diathes. haemorrh. (Stuttg.) **6**, 172 (1961)

Salter, R. H., Read, A. E.: Epsilon-aminocaproic acid therapy in ulcerative colitis. Gut **11**, 585 (1970)

Samama, M.: Fibrinolysis and epsilon-aminocaproic acid. Sangre (Barcelona) **9**, 367 (1964)

Samama, M., Weiss, M., Yver, J., Dubost, C., Marchal, G.: L'hyperactivité fibrinolytique au cours de la chirurgie cardiaque avec circulation extracorporelle. Etude portant sur 280 interventions. Acta chir. belg. **62**, 664 (1963)

Sandberg, H., Tsitouris, G., Bellet, S., Schraeder, J., Feinberg, L.: The antifibrinolytic properties of serotonin. Fed. Proc. **20**, 59 (1961)

Sato, S.: Clinical and laboratory studies on the effect of the administration of ε-aminocaproic acid. Med. Dig. **17**, 14 (1954)

Sato, S., Ishibashi, Y., Endo, T., Watanabe, T., Nakajima, K.: Clinical use of ε-amino-n-caproic acid on metropathia hemorrhagica. Keio J. Med. **8**, 267 (1959)

Sauerland, D.: Fibrinolytische Spätblutungen nach Prostatektomie. Erfolgreiche Behandlung mit Cohnscher Fraktion in Verbindung mit Epsilon-Aminocapron-Säure. Zbl. Chir. **93**, 546 (1969)

Schild, W.: Antifibrinolytische Therapie in der Geburtshilfe und Gynäkologie. Gynaecologia (Basel) **160**, 39 (1965)

Schmidt, A., Amris, C. J.: Blodtabet ved thoraxoperationer under behandling med epsilon-amino-kapronsyre. Ugeskr. Laeg. **128**, 817 (1966).

Schmutzler, R., Beck, E.: Die Wirkung von ε-Aminocapronsäure und Trasylol auf die Fibrinolyse. Schweiz. med. Wschr. **92**, 1368 (1962)

Schmutzler, R., Fürstenberg, H.: Fibrinolyse und Blutverlust nach Prostata-Operationen und deren Beeinflußbarkeit durch Antifibrinolytika. ε-Aminicapronsäure und Kallikrein-Inhibitor Trasylol. Dtsch. med. Wschr. **91**, 297 (1966)

Schoffke, S.: Zur haemostatischen Prophylaxe der Tonsillektomie-Nachblutung. Medicamentum (Berl.) **11**, 211 (1970)

Schulte, W., Vorbauer, J.: Fibrinolytische Effekte beim Kontakt von Speichel und Blut. Dtsch. Zahn-, Mund- u. Kieferheilk. **44**, 23 (1965)

Schulz, K.: Antifibrinolyse durch einen neuen Proteaseninhibitor. Z. ges. inn. Med. **20**, 325 (1965)

Schwick, H. G.: Biochemie der Fibrinolyse. Thrombos. Diathes. haemorrh. (Stuttg.) Suppl. **22**, 27 (1967)

Sheffer, A. L., Austen, K. F., Rosen, F. S.: Treatment of hereditary angioedema with trans-AMCHA. J. Allergy **49**, 133 (1972)

Shepherd, J. A., Nibbelink, D. W., Stegink, L. D.: Rapid chromatographic technique for the determination of epsilon-aminocaproic acid in physiological fluids. J. Chromatogr. **86**, 173 (1973)

Sherry, S., Alkjaersig, N.: Studies on the fibrinolytic enzyme of human plasma. Thrombos. Diathes. haemorrh. (Stuttg.) **1**, 264 (1957)

Sherry, S., Fletcher, A. P., Alkjaersig, N., Sawyer, W. D.: ε-Aminocaproic acid "a potent antifibrinolytic agent". Transact. Ass. Amer. Phycns **75**, 62 (1959)

Shilko, N. A., Borsuk, G. T., Gurova, I. F.: Prophylaxe und Behandlung von uterinen Blutungen während der Geburt mit ε-Aminokapronsäure (russ.). Vop. Ohrany Materin. Dets. **13**, 63 (1968)

Shimizu, M., Aoyagi, T., Iwamoto, M., Abiko, Y., Naito, T., Okana, A.: Medicinal chemical studies on antiplasmin drugs. I. Establishment of the screening assay method for antiplasmin drugs and the superiority of trans-4-aminomethylcyclohexane-carbolitic acid (tranexamic acid to cis-form. Chem. pharm. Bull. **16**, 357 (1968)

Sieg, U., Flähmig, M.: Die Bedeutung der Fibrinolysesteigerung bei Nachgeburtsblutungen und ihre Behandlung mit PAMBA. Folia haemat. (Lpz.) **87**, 51 (1967)

Sigstad, H., Lamvik, J.: Haemorrhagic diathesis, fibrinolysis and fibrinogenopenia in prostatic cancer. Report of a case. Acta med. scand. **173**, 215 (1963)

Silverberg, D. S., Dossetor, J. B., Eid, T. C., Mant, M. J., Miller, J. D. R.: Arteriovenous fistula and prolonged hematuria after renal biopsy: treatment with epsilon aminocaproic acid. Canad. med. Ass. J. **16**, 671 (1974)

Sirén, M.: Toxikologi och farmakologi. In: Antifibrinolytisk terapi, p. 9. Stockholm: AB Kabi, 1970

Sjoerdsma, A., Hanson, A.: Determination of ε-aminocaproic acid by means of high-voltage paper electrophoresis. Acta chem. scand. **13**, 2150 (1959)

Sjoerdsma, A., Nilsson, I. M.: Aliphatic amino compounds as inhibitors of plasminogen activation. Proc. Soc. exp. Biol. (N. Y.) **103**, 533 (1960)

Skoza, L., Johnson, A. J.: Chemical determination of epsilon aminocaproic acid (EACA) in purified systems or biological fluids. In: Blood Coagulation, Hemorrhage and Thrombosis, p. 482 Tocantins, L. M., Kazal, L. A. (Eds.). New York, London: Grune & Stratton 1964.

Skoza, L., Tse, A. O., Semar, M., Johnson, A. J.: Comparative activities of amino acid and polypeptide inhibitors on natural and synthetic substrates. Ann. N. Y. Acad. Sci. **146**, 659 (1968)

Slunsky, R.: Unsere Erfahrungen mit dem Antifibrinolytikum PAMBA in der Geburtshilfe und Gynäkologie. Zbl. Gynäk. **92**, 364 (1970)

Smith, R. R., Upchurch, J. J.: Monitoring antifibrinolytic therapy in subarachnoid hemorrhage. J. Neurosurg. **38**, 339 (1973)

Sonntag, V. K. H., Stein, B. M.: Arteriopathic complications during treatment of subarachnoid hemorrhage with epsilon-aminocaproic acid. J. Neurosurg. **40**, 480 (1974)

Soter, N. A., Austen, K., Gigli, I.: Inhibition by epsilon-aminocaproic acid of the activation of the complement system. J. Immunol. **114**, 928 (1975)

Spink, W. W., Davis, R. B., Potter, R., Chartrand, S.: The initial stage of canine endotoxin shocks as an expression of anaphylactic shock: studies on complement titers and plasma histamine concentrations. J. clin. Invest. **43**, 696 (1964)

Spink, W. W., Vick, J. A.: Endotoxin shock and the coagulation mechanism: Modification of shock with epsilon-aminocaproic acid. Proc. Soc. exp. Biol. (N.Y.) **106**, 242 (1961)

Stacher, A.: Zur Wirkung der ε-Aminocapronsäure. Wien. klin. Wschr. **74**, 771 (1962)

Stamm, H., Caflisch, A., Mall, M.: Diagnose und Therapie der Afibrinogenämie post partum. Gynaecologia (Basel) **156**, 12 (1963)

Steenblock, D. A., Celander, D. R.: A light and electron microscopic study of arteries and other tissues from dogs subjected to chronic fibrinolytic inhibition with AMCHA. Vasc. Surg. **2**, 149 (1968)

Stefanini, M., Marin, H. M.: Fibrinolysis. I. Fibrinolytic activity of extracts from nonpathogenic fungi. Proc. Soc. exp. Biol. (N.Y.) **99**, 504 (1958)

Steichele, D. F., Herschlein, H. J.: Klinik und Therapie der durch Fibrinolyse und Fibrinogenolyse hervorgerufenen Blutungen. Med. Welt (Stuttg.) **1962**, I, 141

Stitzel, R., Lundborg, P., Obianwu, H.: Subcellular distribution of (3H)-epsilon amino caproic acid and its effect on amine storage mechanisms. J. Pharm. (Lond.) **20**, 41 (1968)

Stocker, H., Maier, C.: Chronische Fibrinolyse bei Prostatakarzinom. Schweiz. med. Wschr. **94**, 1373 (1964)

Storm, C.: Suprapubic prostatectomy with preoperative dicumarol and epsilon-aminocaproic acid prophylaxis. Scand. J. Urol. Nephrol. **1**, 1 (1967)

Storti, E., Ascari, E., Turpini, R., Molinari, E., Gamba, G., Pettene, A.: Epsilon-aminocaproic acid for synovectomy in haemophilic patients. Acta haemat. (Basel) **47**, 146 (1972)

Staub, W.: ε-Aminocapronsäure. Schweiz. med. Wschr. **96**, 1080 (1966)

Strauss, H. S., Kevy, S. V., Diamond, L. K.: Ineffectiveness of prophylactic epsilon-aminocaproic acid in severe hemophilia. New Engl. J. med. **273**, 301 (1965)

Striegler, G.: Neue Arzneifertigwaren. 3. Mitteilung: Das Antifibrinolytikum ε-Aminocapronsäure. Pharm. Praxis **1963**, 256.

Studer, A., Reber, K., Lorenz, H.: Experimentelle Untersuchungen zur Frage der Bedeutung intravasaler Fibrinabscheidungen für die Entstehung arteriosklerotischer Wandveränderungen. Path. Microbiol. (Basel) **27**, 287 (1964)

Stürzebecher, J., Markwardt, F., Richter, P., Voigt, B., Wagner, G., Walsmann, P.: Synthetische Inhibitoren von Serinproteinasen. 8. Mitteilung: Über die Hemmung von Trypsin, Plasmin und Thrombin durch Amidinophenylverbindungen mit Ketostruktur. Pharmazie **31**, 450 (1976)

Stürzebecher, J., Markwardt, F., Richter, P., Wagner, G., Walsmann, P., Landmann, H.: Synthetische Inhibitoren von Serinproteinasen. 3. Mitteilung: Über die Hemmwirkung basisch substituierter Phenylcarbonsäureester gegenüber Trypsin, Plasmin und Thrombin. Pharmazie **29**, 337 (1974)

Stürzebecher, J., Markwardt, F., Voigt, B., Walsmann, P., Wagner, G.: Synthetische Inhibitoren der Serinproteinasen. 10. Mitteilung: Untersuchungen zur Hemmung von Trypsin, Plasmin und Thrombin durch 4-Amidinophenylaralkanone. Pharmazie **31**, 886 (1976)

Sugiura, H.: Some clinical experiences of "DV-79 (trans-AMCHA)" in urological diseases. Acta urol. Jap. **12**, 82 (1966)

Summaria, L., Ling, C.-M., Groskopf, W. R., Robbins, K. C.: The active site of bovine plasminogen activator. Interaction of streptokinase with human plasminogen and plasmin. J. biol. Chem. **243**, 144 (1968)

Sundermann, A., Vogel, G.: Hämaturie infolge lokaler Urokinasewirkung und ihre erfolgreiche Behandlung durch p-Aminomethylbenzoesäure (PAMBA). Münch. med. Wschr. **107**, 2003 (1965)

Sundermann, A., Vogel, G.: Klinische Erfahrungen mit p-Aminomethylbenzoesäure (PAMBA) bei schweren akuten Fibrinolyseblutungen in der Inneren Medizin. Folia haemat. (Lpz.) **87**, 22 (1967)

Swartz, C., Onesti, G., Ramirez, O., Shah, N., Brest, A. N.: Cardiac and renal hemodynamic effects of the antifibrinolytic agent, epsilon-aminocaproic acid. Curr. ther. Res. **8**, 336 (1966).

Sweeney, W. M.: Aminocaproic acid, an inhibitor of fibrinolysis. Amer. J. med. Sci. **249**, 756 (1965)

Szabados, J. C.: De toepassing van epsilonaminocapronzuur in de prostaatchirurgie. Nederl. T. Geneesk. **111**, 816 (1967)

Szelestei, T., Kelemen, Z.: Erfahrungen mit Acepramin in der Urologie unter besonderer Berücksichtigung der lokalen Anwendung. Haematologia Suppl. **1**, 193 (1970)

Takada, Y., Takada, A., Okamoto, U.: A new method of the determination of epsilon aminocaproic acid and aminomethyl cyclohexane carboxylic acid. Keio J. med. **13**, 115 (1964a)

Takada, Y., Takada, A., Okamoto, U.: A new method of the analysis of ε-aminocaproic acid (EACA) and aminomethylcyclohexane carboxylic acid (AMCHA), the potent antifibrinolytic agents. J. physiol. Soc. jap. **26**, 281 (1964b)

Takeda, Y., Parkhill, T. R., Nakabayashi, M.: Effect of heparin and epsilon-aminocaproic acid in dogs on plasmin-125-I generation in response to urokinase injections and venous injury. J. clin. Invest. **51**, 2678 (1972)

Tanner, K.: Über die Fibrinogenbehandlung von Tonsillektomie-Nachblutungen. Bibl. oto-rhino-laryng. (Basel) **1968**, 227

Tavenner, R. W.: Epsilon aminocaproic acid in the treatment of hemophilia and Christmas disease with special reference to the extraction of teeth. Brit. dent. J. **124**, 19 (1968)

Taylor, F. B., Jr., Fudenberg, H.: Inhibition of C'_1-component of complement by amino acids. Immunology **7**, 319 (1964)

Tchorzewski, A.: Effect of aminocaproic acid on anaphylactic shock in guinea pigs. Acta physiol. pol. **17**, 89 (1966)

Thomas, K., Goerne, M. H. G.: Über die Herkunft des Kreatins im tierischen Organismus. II. Mitt.: Das Verhalten der ε-Guanidino-, ε-Ureido- und ε-Amino-n-capronsäure im Organismus des Kaninchens. Hoppe-Seylers Z. physiol. Chem. **92**, 163 (1914)

Thomas, K., Stalder, K.-H., Stegemann, H.: Stoffwechselversuche mit ε-Aminokapronsäure. Hoppe-Seylers Z. physiol. Chem. **317**, 276 (1959)

Thomson, J. M., Turner, L., Poller, L.: Inhibition of gastric plasmin activity by epsilon amino-caproic acid (EACA). Ann. Surg. **53**, 340 (1973)

Thorsen, S.: Differences in the binding to fibrin of native plasminogen and plasminogen modified by proteolytic degradation. Influence of ω-aminocarboxylic acids. Biochim. biophys. Acta (Amst.) **393**, 55 (1975)

Thorsen, S.: Influence of fibrin on the effect of 6-aminohexanoic acid on fibrinolysis caused by tissue plasminogen activator or urokinase. In: Davidson, J. F., Samama, M., Desnoyers, P. (Eds.) Progress in Chemical Fibrinolysis and Thrombolysis, Vol. 3. New York: Raven Press 1977

Thorsen, S., Astrup, T.: Substrate composition and the effect of ε-aminocaproid acid on tissue plasminogen activator and urokinase-induced fibrinolysis. Thrombos. Diathes. haemorrh. (Stuttgart) **32**, 306 (1974)

Thorsen, S., Kok, P., Astrup, T.: Reversible and irreversible alterations of human plasminogen indicated by changes in susceptibility to plasminogen activators and in response to ε-aminocaproic acid. Thrombos. Diathes. haemorrh. (Stuttg.) **32**, 325 (1974)

Tice, D. A., Reed, G. E., Clauss, R. H., Worth, M. H.: Hemorrhage due to fibrinolysis occurring with open-heart operations. J. thorac. Surg. **46**, 673 (1963a)

Tice, D. A., Worth, M. H., Clauss, R. H., Reed, G. E.: The inhibition of fibrinolytic activity associated with cardio-vascular operations by Trasylol. J. Amer. med. Ass. **184**, 213 (1963b)

Tice, D. A., Worth, M. H., Clauss, R. H., Reed, G. E.: The inhibition of trasylol of fibrinolytic activity associated with cardiovascular operations. Surg. Gynec. Obstet. **119**, 71 (1964)

Toivanen, P., Mäntyjärvi, R., Toivanen, A.: Complement-fixing antibodies to adenovirus in rabbits and guinea pigs treated with 6-mercaptopurine or ε-aminocaproic acid. Acta path. microbiol. scand. **63**, 221 (1965)

Toivanen, P., Toivanen, A.: The effect of ε-aminocaproic acid on adjuvant arthritis in rats. Experientia (Basel) **20**, 579 (1964)

Tovi, D.: The use of antifibrinolytic drugs to prevent early recurrrent aneurysmal subarachnoid haemorrhage. Acta neurol. scand. **49**, 163 (1973)

Tovi, D., Nilsson, I., Thulin, C.-A.: Fibrinolysis and subarachnoid haemorrhage. Inhibitory effect of tranexamic acid. Acta neurol. scand. **48**, 393 (1972)

Trettin, H. J.: Zur Hemmung der Aktivierung proteolytischer Enzyme im Rattenpankreashomo-genat und des α-Chymotrypsinogen durch ε-Aminocapronsäure und p-Aminomethylbenzoe-säure. Z. ges. inn. Med. **19**, 729 (1964)

Trettin, H. J., Mix, H.: Hemmung der Pankreas-Zymogenaktivierung durch Guanidinverbin-dungen. Hoppe-Seylers Z. physiol. Chem. **340**, 24 (1965)

Tsevrenis, H., Mandalaki, T.: Haematuria in a haemophiliac treated with E-aminocaproic acid. Lancet **1965**, I, 610

Tsitouris, G., Sandberg, H., Bellet, S., Feinberg, L. J., Schraeder, J.: The effects of serotonin on inhibition of the plasmin-plasminogen fibrinolytic system in vitro. J. Lab. clin. Med. **59**, 25 (1962)

Vairel, E., Lande, M., Leger, L.: Acide epsilon-amino-caproïque et fibrinolyse. Presse méd. **72**, 945 (1964)

Vassali, P., Simon, G., Rouiller, C.: Electron microscopic study of glomerular lesions resulting from intravascular fibrin formation. Amer. J. Path. **43**, 579 (1963)

Vecsey, D., Czuczor, H., Bankuti, P.: Blutungs- und Thromboseprophylaxe bei Prostatektomie. Med. Welt (Stuttg.) **1969**, II, 1666

Vogel, G.: Klinische Erfahrungen nir dem neuen Antifibrinolytikum p-Aminomethylbenzoesäure (PAMBA). Z. ges. inn. Med. **21**, 57 (1966)

Vogel, G.: Klinische und gerinnungsphysiologische Untersuchungen mit 4-Aminomethylbenzoesäure, 4-Aminomethylbenzoesäure-Äthylester und 4-(α-Aminoäthyl)-benzoesäure bei Hämostasestörungen. Habil. Schrift Erfurt (1969)

Vogel, G., Klöcking, H.-P.: Klinische Untersuchungen mit Derivaten von p-Aminomethylbenzoesäure. Folia haemat. (Lpz.) **92**, 93 (1969)

Vogel, G., Sundermann, A.: Nierenblutungen auf dem Boden einer vermutlichen Steigerung der Urokinaseaktivität. Folia haemat. (Lpz.) **85**, 70 (1966)

Vogel, G., Sundermann, A.: Beobachtungen bei der Langzeitbehandlung mit synthetischen Fibrinolysehemmstoffen. Haematologia Suppl. **1**, 217 (1970)

Vogel, G., Sundermann, A., Kresch, K.: Die fibrinolytische Aktivität des Urins und ihre Beeinflußbarkeit durch natürliche und synthetische Fibrinolysehemmstoffe. Folia haemat. (Lpz.) **88**, 182 (1967)

Wallén, P.: Studies on the purification of human plasminogen. I. The preparation of a partially purified human plasminogen with a low spontaneous proteolytic activity. Ark. Kemi **19**, 451 (1962)

Walsh, P. N., Rizza, C. R., Matthews, J. M., Eipe, J., Kernoff, P. B. A., Coles, M. D., Bloom, A. L., Kaufman, B. M., Beck, P., Hanan, C. M., Biggs, R.: Epsilon-aminocaproic acid therapy for dental extractions in hemophilia and Christmas disease: a double blind controlled trial. Brit. J. Haemat. **20**, 463 (1971)

Walsmann, P., Horn, H., Landmann, H., Markwardt, F., Stürzebecher, J., Wagner, G.: Synthetische Inhibitoren der Serinproteinasen. 5. Mitteilung: Über die Hemmung von Trypsin, Plasmin und Thrombin durch araliphatische Amidinoverbindungen mit Ätherstruktur sowie Ester der 3- und 4-Amidinophenoxyessigsäure. Pharmazie **30**, 386 (1975)

Walsmann, P., Horn, H., Markwardt, F., Richter, P., Stürzebecher, J., Vieweg, H., Wagner, G.: Synthetische Inhibitoren der Serinproteinasen. 11. Mitteilung: Über die Hemmung von Trypsin, Plasmin und Thrombin durch neue Bisamidinoverbindungen. Acta biol. med. germ. **35**, K1 (1976a)

Walsmann, P., Markwardt, F.: Über die Entwicklung von synthetischen Thrombinhemmstoffen. Verh. dtsch. Ges. exp. Med. **22**, 214 (1969)

Walsmann, P., Markwardt, F., Richter, P., Stürzebecher, J., Wagner, G., Landmann, H.: Synthetische Inhibitoren von Serinproteinasen. 2. Mitteilung: Über die Hemmwirkung von Homologen der Amidinobenzoesäure und ihrer Ester gegenüber Trypsin, Plasmin und Thrombin. Pharmazie **29**, 333 (1974)

Walsmann, P., Markwardt, F., Stürzebecher, J., Vieweg, H., Wagner, G.: Synthetische Inhibitoren von Serinproteinasen. 7. Mitteilung: Über die Hemmung von Trypsin, Plasmin und Thrombin durch Amidinobenzylsulfide und -sulfone sowie N-(Amidinobenzyl)-N-(aryl)- und N-(Amidinobenzyl)-N-(aralkyl)-amine. Pharmazie **31**, 170 (1976b)

Walsmann, P., Markwardt, F., Stürzebecher, J., Voigt, B., Wagner, G.: Synthetische Inhibitoren von Serinproteinasen. 9. Mitteilung: Über die Hemmung von Trypsin, Plasmin und Thrombin durch Amidinophenyl-, Amidinobenzyl- und β-(Amidinophenyl)äthyl-aryl-Ketone. Pharmazie **31**, 733 (1976)

Walsmann, P., Richter, M., Markwardt, F.: Inaktivierung von Trypsin und Thrombin durch 4-Amidinobenzolsulfofluorid und 4-(2-Aminoäthyl)-benzolsulfofluorid. Acta biol. med. germ. **28**, 577 (1972)

Walton, P. L.: The hydrolysis of α-N-acetylglycyl-L-lysine methyl ester by urokinase. Biochim. biophys. Acta (Amst.) **132**, 104 (1967)

Warren, J. W.: New anti-hemorrhagic agent, epsilon aminocaproic acid for control of hemorrhage after transurethral prostatic resection: a control study. J. Kans. med. Soc. **70**, 173 (1969)

Wasserman, A. E.: Effect of tyrothricin upon fibrinolysis mediated by streptokinase. Proc. Soc. exp. Biol. (N.Y.) **80**, 582 (1952)

Wenger, R., Kriehuber, E., Holzner, H., Kaufmann, F.: Weitere tierexperimentelle Untersuchungen über die Arteriosklerose-Entstehung. Z. Kreisl.-Forsch. **52**, 577 (1963)

Wilson, III., J. E., Frenkel, E. P., Pierce, A. K., Johnson, R. L. jr., Winga, E. R., Curry, G. C., Mierzwiak, D. S.: Spontaneous fibrinolysis in pulmonary embolism. J. clin. Invest. **50**, 474 (1971)

Winckelmann, G., Hiemeyer, V.: Fibrinolyse beim extrakorporalen Kreislauf. Thoraxchirurgie **10**, 580 (1962)

Winckelmann, G., Schirmeister, J., Helms, M.: Fibrinolyse als Blutungsursache beim metastasierenden Magencarcinom. Klin. Wschr. **40**, 748 (1962)

Wintersberger, E., Cox, D. J., Neurath, H.: Bovine pancreatic procarboxypeptidase B. I. Isolation, properties, and activation. Biochemistry **1**, 1069 (1962)

Wold, R. T., Reid, R. T., Farr, R. S.: The effect of epsilon-aminocaproic acid on antigen-antibody reactions. J. Immunol. **99**, 797 (1967)

Wölfer, E., Mihalecz, K., Karatson, A., Nagy, J.: Durch Fibrinolyse bedingte Operationskomplikation und ihre Behandlung im Anschluß an Prostataoperationen. Z. Urol. **60**, 853 (1967)

Wolff, E. C., Schirmer, E. W., Folk, J. E.: The kinetics of carboxypeptidase B activity. I. Kinetic parameters. J. biol. Chem. **237**, 3094 (1962)

Wolosowicz, N., Niewiarowski, S., Czerepko, K.: Method for determining ε-aminocaproic acid (EACA) in blood plasma, based on the properties of this compound. Thrombos. Diathes. haemorrh. (Stuttg.) **10**, 308 (1963)

Würbach, G., Klöcking, H.-P., Kahlert, G.: Zur perkutanen Resorption von synthetischen Antifibrinolytika. Arch. klin. exp. Derm. **230**, 245 (1967)

Wüthrich, R., Rieder, H.-P., Ritzel, G.: Beeinflussung der experimentellen allergischen Encephalomyelitis durch ε-Aminocapronsäure. Experientia (Basel) **19**, 421 (1963)

Yamasaki, H., Tsuji, H., Kitamura, M.: Antiinflammatorische Wirkung des Antiplasmins, der ε-Aminocapronsäure (EACA) und der Trans-4-aminomethylcyclohexancarbonsäure (AMCHA) bei Ratten (jap.). Folia pharmacol. jap. **63**, 560 (1967)

Yokoi, M.: Untersuchungen über spezifische Inhibitoren des Plasminsystems und ihre physiologische Wirkung. III. Einige biologische Wirkungen der ε-Aminocapronsäure auf Tiere (jap.). J. physiol. Soc. jap. **22**, 1109 (1960)

Yokoyama, K., Hatano, H.: Clinical use of ε-amino-n-caproic acid on eczema or other kinds of skin diseases suspected to be allergic. Keio J. Med. **8**, 303 (1959)

Zaitseva, R. I.: Antifibrinolytische und toxische Eigenschaften der ε-Aminocapronsäure unter experimentellen Bedingungen (russ.) Farmakol. Toksikol. **28**, 196 (1965)

Zhila, V. V.: Essentielle Hämaturie und ihre Behandlung mit Fibrinolysehemmstoffen (russ.). Vrach. delo **2**, 82 (1968)

Zinn, D.: Untersuchungen des neuen Antifibrinolytikums "Styptosolut" bei der suprapubischen transvesikalen Prostatektomie. Med. Welt (Stuttg.) **1968**, II, 1644

Zmerli, S., Josso, F., Moulonguet, A., Auvert, J.: De la cure des hématuries rénales par un inhibiteur de l'urokinase fibrinolytique. J. Urol. Néphrol. **68**, 901 (1962)

Zukuoski, C. F., Sachatello, C. R., Tinsley, E. A.: Prolongation of canine renal allograft survival by epsilon-aminocaproic acid, an in vitro inhibitor of complement. Surgery **58**, 167 (1965)

Zweifach, B. W., Nagler, A. L., Troll, W.: Some effects of proteolytic inhibitors on tissue injury and systemic anaphylaxis. J. exp. Med. **113**, 437 (1961)

Author Index

Subject Index

Acetylcholine   90, 108, 279
Acetylsalicylic acid   384
Acrosin   9
Activator: see Plasminogen activator
Adenylcyclase   284
Adrenalectomy   275, 277
Adrenaline   90, 108, 122, 209, 274, 275, 280, 284, 432
Afibrinogenemia   74
Agkistrodon rhodostoma venom enzyme: see Ancrod, arvin, arwin, thromboserpentin, venacil
Agmatine   216
Aldosterone   284
Alloxan   289
Alprenolol   277, 278
AMBOCA   514, 515, 517
AMCA   111, 115, 512, 517, 524, 525
   antifibrinolytic activity   513, 514, 523, 524, 527, 528, 535, 538
   assay   526—528
   dosage   554
   hemostatic effect   536, 537, 547, 550
   inhibition of plasmin   522, 523
   inhibition of plasminogen activation   9, 520, 521
   inhibition of urokinase   220, 221, 521
   pharmacokinetics   532, 533, 542
   physicochemical effects   525, 526
   side-effects   530—532, 544
   toxicity   529, 530
AMCHA   533
   antifibrinolytic activity   513, 514
   toxicity   529
p-Aminomethylbenzoic acid: see PAMBA
4-Aminomethyl-bicyclo-2,2,2-octane carboxylic acid: see AMBOCA
cis/trans-4-Aminomethylcyclohexanecarboxylic acid-(1): see AMCHA
trans-4-Aminomethylcyclohexanecarboxylic acid-(1): see AMCA
Aminophylline   298
Aminopyrine   242
AM protease   338
   fibrinolytic activity   442

preparation   441
properties   441, 442
Ancrod: see also Arvin, arwin, thromboserpentin, venacil
Ancrod   453
   assay   459, 460
   clinical trials   471—475
   dosage   471, 472
   effect on bleeding   466
   effect on blood viscosity   468, 469
   effect on fibrinogen   85, 454—456, 460, 463—465
   effect on plasminogen   465, 466
   effect on platelets   455, 467
   effect on thrombus formation   469, 470
   effect on wound healing   468
   indications   473
   inhibitors   458
   pharmacokinetics   462, 463
   properties   454, 459
      immunologic   459, 475
   side-effects   476
   substrates   457—459
   toxicity   460—462
   in transplantation   471
Angina pectoris gravis   195
Angiotensin   90, 283
Angiotensinogen   283
Anthranilic acid derivatives   247, 257—260, 264
Antifibrinolytic agents, synthetic: see also AMCA, AMCHA, EACA, PAMBA
Antifibrinolytic agents, synthetic
   assay   129, 526—528
   contraindications   544, 545
   dosage   553, 554
   hemostatic effect   535, 536, 543, 545—552
   indications   545—553
   mode of action   520—525, 543
   pharmacokinetics   532, 533, 540, 541
   side-effects   530—532, 544
   structure-activity relationships   512—519
   therapy   537, 543, 545, 551
   in tissue culture   537
   toxicity   529, 530
   in transplantation   537

Handbook of Experimental Pharmacology

Continuation of "Handbuch der experimentellen Pharmakologie"

Heffter-Heubner, New Series

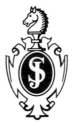

Springer-Verlag
Berlin
Heidelberg
New York

Handbook of Experimental Pharmacology

Continuation of "Handbuch der experimentellen Pharmakologie"

Heffter-Heubner, New Series

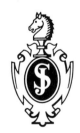

Springer-Verlag
Berlin
Heidelberg
New York